Clinical Reasoning in the Health Professions

Clinical Reasoning in the Health Professions

Fifth Edition

Edited by

JOY HIGGS, AM, PhD, MHPEd, BSc, PFHEA

Emeritus Professor in Higher Education
Charles Sturt University
Sydney, New South Wales, Australia

GAIL M. JENSEN, PhD, PT, FAPTA

Professor, Dept of Physical Therapy and Dept of Medical Humanities; Vice Provost for Learning and
*   Assessment, Dean Emerita*
School of Pharmacy and Health Professions
Creighton University
Omaha, Nebraska, United States

STEPHEN LOFTUS, PhD, MSc, BDS

Adjunct Associate Professor of Medical Education
William Beaumont School of Medicine
Oakland University
Rochester, Michigan, United States

FRANZISKA V. TREDE, PhD, MHPEd, Diploma of Physiotherapy
Professor in Higher Education and Professional Practice
Education Portfolio
University of Technology Sydney
Sydney, New South Wales, Australia

SANDRA GRACE, PhD, MSc, DipEd, BA

Professor of Integrative Medicine
Faculty of Health
Southern Cross University
Lismore, New South Wales, Australia

ELSEVIER

Publisher's note: *Elsevier* takes a neutral position with respect to territorial disputes or jurisdictional claims in its published content, including in maps and institutional affiliations.

First edition 1995
Second edition 2000
Third edition 2008
Fourth edition 2019

Notices

Practitioners and researchers must always rely on their own experience and knowledge in evaluating and using any information, methods, compounds or experiments described herein. Because of rapid advances in the medical sciences, in particular, independent verification of diagnoses and drug dosages should be made. To the fullest extent of the law, no responsibility is assumed by Elsevier, authors, editors or contributors for any injury and/or damage to persons or property as a matter of products liability, negligence or otherwise, or from any use or operation of any methods, products, instructions, or ideas contained in the material herein.

ISBN: 978-0-443-11097-9

Content Strategist: Andrae Akeh
Content Project Manager: Tapajyoti Chaudhuri
Design: Mark Rogers
Marketing Manager: Deborah J. Watkins

Printed in India.

Last digit is the print number: 9 8 7 6 5 4 3 2 1

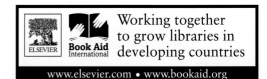

CONTENTS

PART 4
Clinical Reasoning and the Professions

PART 5
Pedagogy

PREFACE

In this fifth edition of *Clinical Reasoning in the Health Professions*, we put forward special insights that emphasise the current challenges and future needs faced by health care professionals and the many workers, educational experts and government regulators today. The first part, 'The Future of Health Care', grounds messages that the COVID-19 pandemic brought to the surface for healthcare. They centre around the well-being of populations and highlight social justice, make global megatrends apparent, appreciate foresight and emphasise 'wicked problems' that epitomise well-being.

The book connects clinical reasoning in individual clinician-patient encounters at the micro level with public health and global perspectives at the meta level. One message of the book is that healthcare disciplines can no longer afford to educate and practise in silos. The future of clinical reasoning integrates biophysical with social, economic and environmental well-being and requires inter-, multi- and transdisciplinary perspectives. We have delved into how we educate our healthcare workers and communities about public health: firstly with ethical decision making, next sustainable development goals, then social determinants of health and finally, blending scientific and cultural knowledges with a particular emphasis on First Nation peoples' ontologies.

The core of the book builds upon these two comprehensive introductions that are new to this fifth edition: our central message of clinical reasoning as the core competency of professional practice, which epitomises professional judgement, epistemic fluency, duty of care, the solution around problem spaces and embodying metacognition.

This fifth edition offers a fresh focus across the health professions. There is a lot of talk about interprofessional education and collaborative practice but we are slow in putting this into practice. The reality is we remain in our own educational lanes. Not so with this book that takes a cross-professions look. By bringing authors together across health professions, networks and relationships emerge that lead to various outcomes from collaborative scholarship in education and practice. Collaboration is critical to the continual act of working and learning together and pushing the boundaries of knowledge and practice in clinical reasoning. While we are making progress, there is still so much more work to be done with collective efforts that inspire and lead in learning together for advancing collaborative practice and education.

And finally, we have spelled out and given many different visions of education to bring clinical reasoning to life: work-integrated learning, using communities of practice, combining professional and shared knowledges and combining capability and competency to achieve expertise.

In this book we move from an emphasis solely on competency and expertise, which in the past has conjured up ideas of mastering and knowing a lot about very specific things. Now we want to emphasise capability, collaboration and collective agency.

Joy Higgs
Gail M. Jensen
Stephen Loftus
Franziska V. Trede
Sandra Grace

ACKNOWLEDGEMENTS

The editors would like to acknowledge and extend their thanks for the input of contributors to all previous editions, which laid an important foundation for the ideas that have been extended in this volume.

We are deeply indebted to our world-wide authors, and especially to Steven Cork and Geoff Scott, contributors to the first two chapters of this book, for their many insights into our expanding concept of clinical reasoning.

CONTRIBUTORS

ROLA AJJAWI, BAPPSC(PHYSIO)HONS, PHD
Professor Education Research
Centre for Research in Assessment and Digital Learning
Deakin University
Melbourne, Victoria, Australia

JOSE F. AROCHA, MA, PHD
Associate Professor
School of Public Health and Health Systems
University of Waterloo
Waterloo, Ontario, Canada

RACHEL BACON, BAPPSC, MSC, PHD
Associate Professor
Faculty of Health
University of Canberra
Bruce, Australian Capital Territory, Australia

RYAN BATENHORST, MED, NRP
Director of the Department of Paramedicine
Creighton University
Omaha, Nebraska, United States

INGRID BERG, DO, MA
Palliative Medicine Physician; Assistant Professor of
    Medicine
Departments of Medicine and Medical Humanities
Creighton University
Omaha, Nebraska, United States

**NICOLE BLAKEY, BN, GRAD DIP CRITICAL CARE,
MN**
Deputy Head of School (Melbourne)
Senior Lecturer
School of Nursing, Midwifery & Paramedicine
Australian Catholic University
Melbourne, Victoria, Australia

HENNY P.A. BOSHUIZEN, PHD
Professor Emeritus
Faculty of Educational Sciences
Open Universiteit
Heerlen, The Netherlands

ROSEMARY BRANDER, BSC (PT), MSC, PHD
Assistant Professor (Adjunct)
School of Rehabilitation Therapy and
    Department of Biomedical and Molecular Sciences
Queen's University
Kingston, Ontario, Canada

**ABRAM L. BRUMMETT, MA (HISTORY), MA
(PHILOSOPHY), PHD**
Assistant Professor
Department of Foundational Medical
    Studies
Oakland University William Beaumont
    School of Medicine and Corewell Health
    William Beaumont University Hospital
Rochester, Minnesota, United States

CHRIS CHAPPARO, MA, PHD
Associate Professor
Discipline of Occupational Therapy
Sydney School of Health Sciences;
Faculty of Medicine and Health
The University of Sydney
Australia

NICOLE CHRISTENSEN, PT, MAPPSC, PHD
Professor
Department of Physical Therapy
Samuel Merritt University
Oakland, California, United States

DENISE M. CONNOR, MD
Professor of Clinical Medicine
University of California
San Francisco;
Gold-Headed Cane Endowed Teaching Chair in
  Internal Medicine;
Director
Anti-Oppression Curriculum Initiative
School of Medicine
San Francisco, California, United States

CINDY COSTANZO, RN, CNL, PHD
Senior Associate Dean
Graduate School
Department Chair for Interdisciplinary Studies
Creighton University
Omaha, Nebraska, United States

JENNIFER COX, BSC, BMEDSC(HONS), PHD
Course Director | Oral Health
Dentistry & Dental Implantology
Charles Sturt University
Orange, New South Wales, Australia

RACHEL DAVENPORT, BSC(HONS), PHD,
MSPA, CPSP
Senior Lecturer
Department of Clinical and Community Health
La Trobe University
Bundoora, Victoria, Australia

GURPREET DHALIWAL, MD
Professor of Medicine
University of California at San Francisco;
Site Director
Internal Medicine Clerkships
San Francisco VA Medical Center
San Francisco, California, United States

JANINE MARGARITA DIZON, BSPT, MSPT, PHD
Research Fellow
International Centre for Allied Health Evidence
  (ICAHE)
University of South Australia
Adelaide, South Australia, Australia

JOY DOLL, OTD, OTR/L
Associate Professor
School of Pharmacy and Health
  Professions
Creighton University
Omaha, Nebraska, United States

STEVEN J. DURNING, MD, PHD, FACP
Professor and Vice Chair
Department of Medicine;
Director
Center for Health Professions Education
  (CHPE)
Uniformed Services University
Bethesda, Maryland, United States

CAROLINE FAUCHER, OD, PHD, FAAO
Associate Professor and Associate Director
Undergraduate Studies
École d'optométrie
Université de Montréal
Montréal, Quebec, Canada

RICK FLOWERS, BAHONS, MA(GEOG/ANTHR),
GRDIPADULTED, PHD
Senior Lecturer, Teaching and Learning
  Director
School of International Studies and
  Education
University of Technology Sydney
Sydney, New South Wales, Australia

SANDRA GRACE, PHD, MSC, DIPED, BA
Professor of Integrative Medicine
Faculty of Health
Southern Cross University
Lismore, New South Wales, Australia

EMILY GREENBERGER, MD
Assistant Professor
Department of Medicine
The Robert Larner
MD College of Medicine at the University of
  Vermont
Burlington, Vermont, United States

AMY M. HADDAD, PhD, MFA, FAAN
Professor Emerita
School of Pharmacy and Health Professions
Creighton University
Omaha, Nebraska, United States

JOY HIGGS, AM, PhD, MHPEd, BSc, PFHEA
Emeritus Professor in Higher Education
Charles Sturt University
Sydney, New South Wales, Australia

GAIL M. JENSEN, PhD, PT, FAPTA
Professor, Dept of Physical Therapy and Dept of
 Medical Humanities; Vice Provost for Learning and
 Assessment, Dean Emerita
School of Pharmacy and Health Professions
Creighton University
Omaha, Nebraska, United States

**ROBYN B. JOHNSON, BAppSc(SPEECH
PATHOLOGY), CPSP, PhD**
Health Professions Education Lead (Speech
 Pathology)
Sydney School of Health Sciences
Faculty of Medicine and Health
University of Sydney
Sydney, New South Wales, Australia

**MARK JONES, CertPT, BS(PSYCH),
GRAD DIP ADVAN MANIP THER, MAppSc
(MANIP PHYSIO)**
Adjunct Senior Lecturer – Physiotherapy
Allied Health & Human Performance Academic Unit
University of South Australia
Adelaide, South Australia, Australia

**DAVID R. KAUFMAN, BA (PSYCHOLOGY),
MA (EDUCATIONAL PSYCHOLOGY), PhD
(EDUCATIONAL PSYCHOLOGY)**
Associate Professor
Department of Biomedical Informatics
Arizona State University;
Research Affiliate
Mayo Clinic
Scottsdale, Arizona, United States

BELINDA KENNY, PhD
Director of Academic Program (Speech
 Pathology)
School of Health Sciences
Western Sydney University
Sydney, New South Wales, Australia

**SHIVA KHATAMI, DDS, PhD,
DIPLOMA OF THE AMERICAN BOARD OF
ORTHODONTICS**
ART Orthodontics
Davie, Florida;
Associate Professor
Department of Orthodontics
Nova Southeastern University
Fort Lauderdale, Florida, United States

OLGA KOSTOPOULOU, MSc, PhD
Reader in Medical Decision Making
Imperial College
London, United Kingdom

KATHRYN N. HUGGETT, PhD
Robert Larner
MD Professor in Medical Education;
Director
The Teaching Academy;
Assistant Dean for Medical Education
The Larner College of Medicine at the University of
 Vermont
Burlington, Vermont, United States

**TRACY LEVETT-JONES, RN, BN,
DipAppSc(NURSING), MEd & WORK, PhD**
Distinguished Professor
School of Nursing and Midwifery
University of Technology
Sydney, New South Wales, Australia

STEPHEN LOFTUS, PhD, MSc, BDS
Adjunct Associate Professor of Medical
 Education
William Beaumont School of Medicine
Oakland University
Rochester, Michigan, United States

MICHAEL MACENTEE, LDSI, PHD(TCD), FRCDC, FCAHS, FFDRCSI
Professor Emeritus
Faculty of Dentistry
University of British Columbia
Vancouver, British Columbia, Canada

ANNA MAIO, MD
General Internal Medicine
Adjunct Associate Professor of Medicine
Creighton University
Omaha, Nebraska, United States

CATHERINE MAITLAND, BA (HONS), DIP HEALTH, GRAD DIP ADULT ED, MED, PHD
Research Lead
Australian Network on Disability
Sydney, New South Wales, Australia

MARIA A. MARTIMIANAKIS, MA, MED, PHD
Associate Professor and Director of Medical
   Education Scholarship
Department of Paediatrics;
Scientist and Strategic Lead International
Wilson Centre
Faculty of Medicine
University of Toronto
Toronto, Ontario, Canada

W. CARY MOBLEY, BS(BIOLOGY), BS(PHARMACY), PHD
Clinical Associate Professor
University of Florida College of Pharmacy
Gainesville, Florida, United States

ROBIN MOORMAN-LI, PHARMD, BCACP, NBC-HWC
Clinical Associate Professor;
Assistant Director
Jacksonville Campus
University of Florida College of Pharmacy
Gainesville, Florida, United States

GINA MARIA MUSOLINO, PT, DPT, MSED, EDD
College of Public Health and Health Professions
University of Florida
Gainesville, Florida, United States

MARIA MYLOPOULOS, PHD
Associate Professor
Department of Paediatrics;
Scientist
The Wilson Centre
University of Toronto
Toronto, Ontario, Canada

SIRISHA NARAYANA, MD
Associate Professor of Clinical Medicine;
Academy Chair for Excellence in Foundational Teaching
Division of Hospital Medicine
Department of Medicine
University of California
San Francisco, California, United States

MARK C. NAVIN, PHD
Professor and Chair of Philosophy
Oakland University
Rochester, Michigan;
Clinical Ethicist
Corewell Health
Southfield, Michigan, United States

PATRICK NEWMAN, MD, MPH
Department of Pediatrics
University of California San Francisco School of
   Medicine
San Francisco, California, United States

GEOFFREY R. NORMAN, PHD
Professor Emeritus
Department of Health Research Methods, Evidence
   and Impact
McMaster University
Hamilton, Ontario, Canada

RAINE OSBORNE, PT, DPT, EDD, FAAOMPT
Assistant Professor
Department of Physical Therapy
University of North Florida
Jacksonville, Florida, United States

ROBIN PAP, NDIPEMC, BTECHEMC, HDIPHED, MSCMED(EMERGMED), PHD
School of Health Sciences
Western Sydney University
Sydney, New South Wales, Australia

VIMLA L. PATEL, DSc, PhD, FACMI
Cognitive Studies in Medicine and Public Health
The New York Academy of Medicine and Biomedical
　Informatics
Columbia University
New York, New York, United States

**NARELLE PATTON, SFHEA, B.APP.SC. (PHYS),
MHLTHSC (OMT), PHD, GRAD CERT RESEARCH
MANAGEMENT**
Associate Dean (Partnerships and Workplace
　Learning)
Faculty of Science
Charles Sturt University
Albury, New South Wales, Australia

JACQUELINE PICH, PHD, BNURS HONS (I), BSC
Associate Professor
Deputy Head of School Teaching and Learning
University of Technology
Sydney, New South Wales, Australia

NICOLE PIEMONTE, PHD
Associate Professor of Medical Humanities
Assistant Dean for Student Affairs
Peekie Nash Carpenter Endowed Chair in Medicine
Creighton University, School of Medicine, Phoenix
　Regional Campus
Phoenix, Arizona, United States

JUDY RANKA, BSC(OT), MA, HLTHSCD
Director and Principal Occupational Therapist
Occupational Performance Network
The University of Sydney
Sydney, New South Wales, Australia

JOSEPH J. RENCIC, MD
Professor of Medicine
Boston University Chobanian and Avedisian School
　of Medicine
Boston, Massachusetts, United States

BARBARA J. RITTER, EDD, FNP-BC, CNS
Adjunct Professor
Family Nurse Practitioner Program
Sonoma State University
Rohnert Park, California, United States

ERICA K. SALTER, BA, PHD, HEC-C
Associate Professor of Health Care Ethics and
　Pediatrics
Department of Pediatrics
Gnaegi Center for Health Care Ethics
Saint Louis University
St. Louis, Missouri, United States

HENK G. SCHMIDT, PHD
Professor of Psychology
Institute of Psychology
Erasmus University
Rotterdam, South Holland, The Netherlands

**ALAN SCHWARTZ, BA(COGNITIVE SCIENCE AND
WOMEN'S STUDIES), MS(ORGANIZATIONAL
BEHAVIOUR AND INDUSTRIAL RELATIONS),
PHD(COGNITIVE PSYCHOLOGY)**
The Michael Reese Endowed Professor of Medical
　Education
Departments of Medical Education and
　Pediatrics
University of Illinois
Chicago, Illinois, United States

GEOFF SCOTT, PHD
Chair and Clinical Professor
Environmental Health Sciences
Arnold School of Public Health
University of South Carolina
Columbia, South Carolina, United States

**MAREE SIMPSON, BPHARM,
BSC (HONS), GRADCERT UNIV TEACH &
LEARN, PHD**
Adjunct Associate Professor
Charles Sturt University
Orange, New South Wales, Australia

**PAUL SIMPSON, BED(PREHOSP), BHSC,
GCCLINED, MSCM(CLINEPI), PHD, ICP**
Associate Professor
School of Health Sciences
Western Sydney University
Sydney, New South Wales, Australia

MEGAN SMITH, BAppSc (PHYSIO), GCUT&L, MAppSc (CARDIOPULMPHYSIO), PhD
Executive Dean
Faculty of Science and Health
Charles Sturt University
Wagga Wagga, New South Wales, Australia

REBECCA SUTHERLAND, PhD
Lecturer and Speech Pathologist
Faculty of Medicine and Health
Sydney School of Health Sciences
University of Sydney
Sydney, New South Wales, Australia

CATHERINE SUTTLE, BSc(OPTOMETRY), GradCert(UNIVERSITY LEARNING AND TEACHING), PhD
Lecturer Optometry and Visual Science
School of Health and Psychological Sciences
City, University of London
London, United Kingdom

JILL E. THISTLETHWAITE, MBBS, MMED, PhD, FRCGP, FRACGP
Health Professions Education Consultant;
Adjunct Professor
University of Technology Sydney;
Clinical Chair
Hospital Non-specialist Program
Health Education and Training Institute (HETI)
NSW Health
Sydney, New South Wales, Australia

ALIKI THOMAS, BSc(OT), MEd, PhD
Assistant Professor
School of Physical and Occupational Therapy;
Research Scientist
Center for Medical Education
McGill University Centre for Interdisciplinary
   Research in Rehabilitation of Greater Montreal
Montreal, Quebec, Canada

FRANZISKA V. TREDE, PhD, MHPED, DIPLOMA OF PHYSIOTHERAPY
Professor in Higher Education and Professional Practice
Education Portfolio
University of Technology Sydney
Sydney, New South Wales, Australia

ROBERT L. TROWBRIDGE, MD
Professor of Medicine
Tufts University School of Medicine
Maine Medical Center
Boston, Massachusetts, United States

RUTH VO, BNutrDiet(HONS), MHSc(EDU), PhD
Professional Identity Coach, Dietitian & Author
Praxcess
Sydney, New South Wales, Australia

HsingChi von BERGMANN, MSc, PhD
Professor;
Director
Health Science Professionals - Education Research;
Faculty of Dentistry
University of British Columbia
Vancouver, British Columbia, Canada

JASON A. WASSERMAN, BA(PHILOSOPHY), MA(MEDICAL SOCIOLOGY), PhD
Professor
Department of Foundational Medical Studies;
Founding Director
Center for Moral Values in Health and Medicine
Oakland University William Beaumont School of
   Medicine
Rochester, Michigan, United States

THILAN P. WIJESEKERA, MD, MHS
Assistant Professor
Director of Clinical Reasoning
Department of Internal Medicine
Yale School of Medicine
New Haven, Connecticut, United States

MICHAEL J. WITTE, MD, FAAFP
Consultant and Healthcare Leader Coach and Mentor
Western Clinicians Network
Petaluma, California, United States

MEREDITH YOUNG, PhD
Assistant Professor
Department of Medicine;
Research Scientist
Centre for Medical Education
McGill University
Montreal, Quebec, Canada

NICOLE A. YOSKOWITZ, PhD
Licensed Psychologist
Metro NY DBT Centre
Florham Park, New Jersey, United States

MOHAMMAD S.Y. ZUBAIRI, MD, MED, FRCPC
Developmental Paediatrician
Holland Bloorview Kids Rehabilitation Hospital
Clinical Team Investigator
Bloorview Research Institute;
Assistant Professor
Department of Paediatrics
University of Toronto
Toronto, Ontario, Canada

PART 1

The Future of Healthcare
The Big Picture of Clinical Decision Making

The aim of Part 1 is to expand on our previous publications on clinical reasoning. While the present book continues to deal with clinical reasoning as a core notion of the health professions, this first part introduces *futures thinking* as it relates to planning of public health. The book as a whole has many messages which relate to how differently health professionals currently learn how to practise the specific roles and nuances of what it takes to develop the expertise of their particular profession. It also spells out what it means to be a health professional in general, and particularly one who has to cope with planning a future that sets forth the best interest of the whole population.

The intent of futures thinking that is considered here is to plan for a preferred way of thinking that imagines a future and works towards it. In terms of health, futures thinking sets out the parameters, ethics and challenges of public health and helps populations work to meet these goals. With a challenge as large and pervasive as the COVID-19 pandemic, health professions have switched their focus from not only being the best their profession can be but also being part of the best healthcare system they can be. Health professionals now need to take into account such issues as planning education that can deal with contingency management, disaster management, emergency medicine, climate control, national preventative medicine, indigenous and underprivileged issues, national public health tragedies, refugees and war. Dealing with these issues requires the technology and science that underpin our guidance for governments and populations to make sense of public health.

Such a health system requires engagement of governments, world leaders (e.g. the UN, WHO), climate experts, scientists and ethical experts, along with local communities to set guidelines for global healthcare, and it requires standards to govern all aspects of practice. For instance, the Australian Commission on Safety and Quality in Health Care 'works in partnership with patients, consumers, clinicians, managers, policy makers and healthcare organisations to achieve a sustainable, safe and high-quality health system' (https://www.safetyandquality.gov.au/standards/nsqhs-standards). In another example, in the US, the National Standards for Culturally and Linguistically Appropriate Services recommend standards to be applied to healthcare. These standards affect the cultural sensitivity of healthcare by taking account of religion, ethnicity, race, national origin, language and gender in the care provided. Adopting such standards for public health places social justice, ethical decision making and the combination of clinical reasoning and the socialization of healthcare practices at the forefront of health planning.

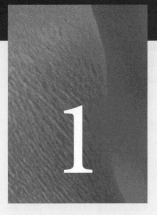

1

THE FUTURE OF HEALTHCARE

JOY HIGGS ■ SANDRA GRACE

CHAPTER OUTLINE

CHAPTER AIMS

The aims of this chapter are:

- to examine our reasons for expanding the focus of this book from clinical reasoning in the health professions to include a focus on future health, in particular the future of decision making for the health of the whole population, the future of healthcare, including how nations and regions develop the foresight and strategies to deal with the future of population health, and how the practice of healthcare and clinical decision making is making a difference to the future of healthcare
- to elucidate how standards are making a difference to healthcare for the common good, social justice and quality of life for all
- to describe the megatrends that could shape healthcare futures
- and to describe how changes arising from these events effect changes in professional education.

INTRODUCTION

Understanding Change

Change is a certainty and the fast pace of change in the 21st century is universal with no part of our lives remaining unaffected. This includes changes in technology, work, political systems, how goods and services are provided, how we are cared for and care for others, how our children grow up, the nature of our relationships and how we communicate with each other, what we eat and how food is produced, changes in the natural world, our notions of social justice and fairness, how we cool and heat our houses, public buildings and shared public spaces, even changes to the very air that we breathe. Reactions to this fast pace of change include excitement, curiosity, greed, exploitation, hope, anxiety, alienation, blame, avoidance and bewilderment. We hope that our responses include a sense of the possibility that the world could be a better place for future generations. What is certain is that it will be a vastly different place that our children and grandchildren inhabit, in terms of what, where and

3

how they will work. While the rate of change may very possibly be overwhelming, we do not want to be passive or immobilized bystanders. We need to be able to recognize and anticipate change that is not in the greater good versus change that is needed to adapt healthcare to the changing world. Resisting the former change while encouraging the latter makes sense when considering the common good but the opposite might be true for some private interests. Uncritical followers of, or colluders in, changes that are not for the greater good (e.g. conservatives resisting change globally) will simply be joining bandwagons without interrogating their potential benefit and implications.

The Future of Decision Making for the Health of the Whole Population

This book (the fifth edition) sees Clinical Reasoning in the Health Professions in a wider context. We have introduced a section relating to the COVID-19 pandemic that looks at the way clinical reasoning is moderated by the rules and regulations of public health and the management of decision making by governments in the light of the financial and public health restrictions we faced in the pandemic. We are also currently facing climate influences on the health of the whole population and a heightened awareness of the role of science, technologies, government restrictions and information systems in decision making, politics and management in public health. The way we treat decision making is changing, not only because of the substantial changes in our education, but also because of the substantial impact on the way we manage our healthcare systems. Our preferred public healthcare future is healthcare for the common good, which affords social justice for all concerned, that is, healthcare which provides for resilience of populations and equity of management by governments in the broad context of healthcare.

The fourth edition of this book expanded our views of clinical reasoning in the health professions; it challenged each profession to interrogate patient care thoroughly. It focused on decision making as central to health policy and the conjectural nature of medical practice: 'Because health outcomes are probabilistic, most decisions are made under conditions of uncertainty' (Kaplan and Frosch, 2005, p. 525). The fourth edition introduced an encultured view of clinical

reasoning that set out the *knowing, being* and *identity* in practice and examined the challenges faced by health professionals seeking to perform excellence in practice and who do so with regard to cultural understanding and duty of care. This can be described as a narrower (clinical) view of decision making.

This first chapter talks about the broader view of health (well-being). This is important in determining 'whether societies flourish or languish, including how they cope with adverse events and conditions' (Eckersley, 2010, p. 108). Eckersley refers to this as the forgotten dimension of social resilience; it is often forgotten in healthcare. 'Not only does population health affect the ability of societies to withstand adversity, it can shape how they respond to it–whether in ways that make things better or worse' (Eckersley, 2010, p. 105). How societies have faced the challenge of the pandemic in setting a broader framework for contemplating and envisioning the future of health (in its broad sense of well-being) and how well we have coped with these challenges are discussed in Chapters 1 and 2 of this edition. The remainder of the book considers the impact of this in the narrower sense of clinical health.

FUTURES THINKING

In this chapter we draw attention to futures thinking, which means thinking about the future in a structured and systematic way. 'Two important assumptions of futures thinking are that the future is unknowable in detail; and preparing for the future … is very risky over medium to long-term horizons' (Schwartz, 2003, p. 30). We are not dealing with pre-set futures, but rather with *desirable* futures that address our *preferred* future for social justice and the greater good. So here we have the contributions that we think futures thinking can make to anticipating and preparing for future challenges and opportunities of clinical reasoning and the management of public health, taking a particular (normative) view of futures thinking in support of social justice (Börjeson et al., 2006; Cork et al., 2023).

The Future of Healthcare: Creating Preferred Futures

Foresight as it relates to preferred healthcare is about imagining, sharing visions of preference and having the will (and resilience) and the power to make it happen. Foresight in relation to the health of the whole population has been described as:

the systematic process of developing a range of views of possible ways in which the future could develop, and understanding these sufficiently well to be able to decide what decision may be taken today to create the best possible tomorrow. More specifically, technology foresight can be a combination of systemic efforts used to assist planning in technology and science towards innovation and improvements in the quality of life (James, 2001, p. 6).

Moore and Milkoreit (2020) make the point that in much futures thinking there are three failures: failure to comprehend the real situation, failure to appreciate the social dimensions of the issues and failure to imagine alternative futures. One of the reasons for the third of these failures is the way the brain is organized, which causes us to form visions of the future based on past experiences. Creating preferred futures involves thinking that goes beyond past experiences.

First, we need to ask who is involved in healthcare, thinking about the future of healthcare and/or currently creating preferred futures:

- The people who need healthcare: (everyone) all ages, all socioeconomic categories, all cultures, all population categories (including indigenous and refugee populations), all communities
- The people who provide healthcare: all professionals and carers
- The institutions and people who educate and train the providers
- The organizations and administrative systems that provide the healthcare and organize the regulation of the system
- The governments that operate and provide funding for healthcare
- The legal system that regulates healthcare and provides law enforcement
- The providers and systems of emergency management
- Who else could be involved?

Second, we need to consider who provides and funds healthcare:

- Governments, the public sector
- Aid agencies
- Voluntary bodies
- Employer purchasers of health benefits, the private sector
- Who else can provide and fund healthcare?

Third, we need to consider who plans and controls this healthcare currently and who are the recipients of the preferred futures:

- A range of people with imagination, intelligence, good will, ethics, social justice, wisdom and ethical justice, and good guidelines
- Leaders of the healthcare industry, for example, the United Nations, the World Health Organization (WHO), leaders of professional organizations, research leaders, regional leaders and national bodies, disaster management bodies, refugee agencies.
- People with negative attributes such as greed and self-interested power could also control healthcare. These people are likely to provide inequitable healthcare or may be the source of injustices and life-threatening and endangerment situations.

Finally, we need to consider all the precipitants of healthcare problems in relation to:

- Chronic illnesses
- Pandemics
- Emergency healthcare
- Acute care
- Mental health
- Refugee health and conditions of war
- Underprivileged and minority groups

Futures thinking at both an individual and a societal level requires the psychological capacities for such imagining (Cork et al., 2023). However, building futures thinking at societal level faces numerous challenges, including having institutional arrangements in place so that futures thinking can influence decision making. Ultimately what matters is that futures thinking can anticipate the challenges and opportunities and therefore allow policy for sustainable and just healthcare to be strategic and timely. Futures thinking, when done well, brings diverse people and ideas together to improve imagination about possible futures. This process is also important for helping people agree on preferred futures. People do not agree on every aspect of preferred futures and the challenge is therefore to identify the core things that people do agree on and that allow different people to meet different needs (Cork et al., 2023).

PLANNING A SOLUTION THAT DEMONSTRATES FORESIGHT ABOUT THE FUTURE OF HEALTHCARE

It is critical that we plan our preferred health future with care – care that is based on foresight, using imagining to explore multiple possible futures, identifying visions of preferred futures and considering what might be required to achieve such futures when faced with possible challenges as well as opportunities. The solutions we arrive at will demand funding, embedded ethical approaches, efficient information systems and appropriate standards and regulations of healthcare.

Funding

Securing funding is one strategy for facing the future of healthcare, providing optimal healthcare and preventative healthcare options; perhaps the answer is to have as much healthcare as we can afford (and share it fairly). To decide what we can afford we need to anticipate what the challenges and opportunities might be and what the costs and benefits of different actions might be. Foresight can help by anticipating what mix of challenges and opportunities might need to be addressed in different futures and, therefore, what levels of healthcare might be required.

For years there have been calls for more investment in preventive health, but it is still not popular among those who profit from responding to illness and disaster. Foresight can support preventive health by anticipating what challenges and opportunities might arise and exploring the costs and benefits of preventive versus reactive measures. In relation to challenges and opportunities, foresight can also explore the futures in which there might be more or less political and public support for prevention versus reaction.

We can elect governments that prioritize equity and social justice (Sutherland and Till, 1993). We can call for climate control and a healthy planet for all species. We can develop new views of the professions to look at sharing knowledge between patients and professionals. Healthcare professionals need to use foresight to anticipate the sorts of challenges and opportunities they might face in different futures, the funding that might be required to meet the challenges and/or take the opportunities, and consider what early warning signs might alert them to when it might be appropriate to prepare and implement different strategies.

Ethics

A number of ethical matters arose during the COVID-19 pandemic. These included how to allocate scarce resources such as vaccines and therapeutics within and between countries, when to mandate vaccines and masks, when to issue vaccine passports, whether and how to conduct health surveillance and how to monitor international and intranational inequities. Ethical values such as fairness, equity, solidarity and trust have been prominent in discussions at a global level. Many recent futures-thinking projects have explored alternative directions of change in attitudes across societies as key uncertainties. For example, extremes of individualism versus communitarianism have major implications for how fairness and ethics are defined, recognized and addressed (Cork et al., 2023). COVID-19 and the recent resurgence of tensions between progressive and conservative schools of thought have suggested that there will be uncertainty about how ethical issues are interpreted and acted on in alternative futures (S. Cork, personal communication, 15 February 2023). We need to consider carefully how we integrate ethics into our decision making. This requires ethics to be at the starting point of decision making and our stated values to be an essential part of decision making in the future, and for ethicists to be included in the policy-making process. Moreover, agreement across societies will be true in relation to some ethical issues but not necessarily all. Healthcare professionals will need to engage with people across society to understand different stances on ethics and identify strategies that work with different stances. 'The COVID-19 pandemic has been marked by moral failures. We cannot expect to correct these moral failures without improving the ways in which ethical values and commitments are incorporated into the policy-making process' (World Health Organization, 2022, p. vi).

Information Systems

An important aspect of optimizing future health management is planning technologies that provide for optimal health information systems. Information systems must not only be suitable for the users (providers, recipients), timely, appropriate for the education levels of participants and security conscious, but they must also keep in touch with expert wisdom and with the ethics of use. In short, they need to be suitable for the complexity of the magnitude and ethnicity of the systems of healthcare to be provided (Wager et al., 2022).

However, control of information and disinformation have become major issues and are likely to be major drivers of alternative futures. In particular, the collection of, and access to, health data are likely to be contentious issues that drive the types of healthcare systems we see in alternative futures. For example, we are likely to see increasing ability to collect and to analyse data on people's health via technologies that can be deployed at the level of individuals in their homes and that offer many opportunities for real-time diagnoses and treatment of health issues. However,

these possibilities also run up against concerns about privacy and misuse of data. In alternative futures we could see integrated, efficient and effective healthcare systems at one extreme or fragmented systems that perpetuate inequalities of access to healthcare across societies at the other, depending on socioeconomic circumstances and attitudes towards new technologies (S. Cork, personal communication, 15 February 2023).

Standards and Regulations of Healthcare

Standards are essential to healthcare. The National Safety and Quality Health Service Standards were developed by the Australian Commission on Safety and Quality in Health Care in collaboration with the Australian Government, states and territories, the private sector, clinical experts, patients and carers. The standards provide a nationally consistent statement of the level of care consumers can expect from health service organizations. The Australian Commission on Safety and Quality in Health Care works in partnership with patients, consumers, clinicians, managers, policy makers and healthcare organizations to achieve a sustainable, safe and high-quality health system (Australian Commission on Safety and Quality in Health Care, 2022) (Box 1.1).

BOX 1.1
THE NATIONAL SAFETY AND QUALITY HEALTH SERVICE STANDARDS

Clinical Governance, which describes the clinical governance and safety and quality systems that are required to maintain and improve the reliability, safety and quality of healthcare and improve health outcomes for patients.

Partnering with Consumers, which describes the systems and strategies to create a person-centred health system by including patients in shared decision making, to ensure that patients are partners in their own care and that consumers are involved in the development and design of quality healthcare.

Preventing and Controlling Healthcare-Associated Infection, which describes the systems and strategies to prevent infection, to manage infections effectively when they occur and to limit the development of antimicrobial resistance through prudent use of antimicrobials, as part of effective antimicrobial stewardship.

Medication Safety, which describes the systems and strategies to ensure that clinicians safely prescribe, dispense and administer appropriate medicines to informed patients, and monitor use of the medicines.

Comprehensive Care, which describes the integrated screening, assessment and risk identification processes for developing an individualized care plan, to prevent and minimize the risks of harm in identified areas.

Communicating for Safety, which describes the systems and strategies for effective communication between patients, carers and families, multidisciplinary teams and clinicians, and across the health service organization.

Blood Management, which describes the systems and strategies for the safe, appropriate, efficient and effective care of patients' own blood, as well as other supplies of blood and blood products.

Recognizing and Responding to Acute Deterioration, which describes the systems and processes to respond effectively to patients when their physical, mental or cognitive condition deteriorates.

Australian Commission on Safety and Quality in Health Care, 2022. The National Safety and Quality Health Service Standards. Commonwealth of Australia. https://www.safetyandquality.gov.au/standards/nsqhs-standards.

These standards are designed to ensure quality of care at the clinical level. In the United States, the Culturally and Linguistically Appropriate Services (CLAS) system was set up by the US Department of Health and Human Services, Office of Minority Health (2000). It recommends the National Standards for CLAS that are applied to healthcare. These affect the cultural sensitivity of healthcare by taking account of religion, ethnicity, race, national origin, language and gender in the care provided (Box 1.2).

In future, all standards will need to be developed with the kind of shared vision for equitable healthcare that is demonstrated in the National Standards for CLAS. In particular, foresight will be an essential tool to enable our preferred healthcare to be equitably delivered throughout the world. Future healthcare

---

BOX 1.2
NATIONAL STANDARDS FOR CULTURALLY AND LINGUISTICALLY APPROPRIATE SERVICES IN HEALTHCARE

The National CLAS Standards are intended to advance health equity, improve quality and help eliminate healthcare disparities by establishing a blueprint for health and healthcare organizations to:

Principal Standard:

1. Provide effective, equitable, understandable and respectful quality care and services that are responsive to diverse cultural health beliefs and practices, preferred languages, health literacy and other communication needs.

Governance, Leadership and Workforce:

2. Advance and sustain organizational governance and leadership that promotes CLAS and health equity through policy, practices and allocated resources.
3. Recruit, promote and support a culturally and linguistically diverse governance, leadership and workforce that are responsive to the population in the service area.
4. Educate and train governance, leadership and workforce in culturally and linguistically appropriate policies and practices on an ongoing basis.

Communication and Language Assistance:

5. Offer language assistance to individuals who have limited English proficiency and/or other communication needs, at no cost to them, to facilitate timely access to all healthcare and services.
6. Inform all individuals of the availability of language assistance services clearly and in their preferred language, verbally and in writing.
7. Ensure the competence of individuals providing language assistance, recognizing that the use of untrained individuals and/or minors as interpreters should be avoided.

8. Provide easy-to-understand print and multimedia materials and signage in the languages commonly used by the populations in the service area.

Engagement, Continuous Improvement and Accountability:

9. Establish culturally and linguistically appropriate goals, policies and management accountability and infuse them throughout the organization's planning and operations.
10. Conduct ongoing assessments of the organization's CLAS-related activities and integrate CLAS-related measures into measurement and continuous quality improvement activities.
11. Collect and maintain accurate and reliable demographic data to monitor and evaluate the impact of CLAS on health equity and outcomes and to inform service delivery.
12. Conduct regular assessments of community health assets and needs and use the results to plan and implement services that respond to the cultural and linguistic diversity of populations in the service area.
13. Partner with the community to design, implement and evaluate policies, practices and services to ensure cultural and linguistic appropriateness.
14. Create conflict and grievance resolution processes that are culturally and linguistically appropriate to identify, prevent and resolve conflicts or complaints.
15. Communicate the organization's progress in implementing and sustaining CLAS to all stakeholders, constituents and the general public.

CLAS, Culturally and linguistically appropriate services. US Department of Health and Human Sciences Office of Minority Health, 2000. National standards for culturally and linguistically appropriate services (CLAS) in health and health care. https://thinkculturalhealth.hhs.gov/clas/standards.

standards may also need to address the emerging issues of managing false information and theft of information.

Foresight in the Time of COVID-19

Foresight methodologies allow individuals and organizations to envision different future scenarios and promote greater future resilience in relation to health promotion. These include scenarios for possible, likely and desirable futures that can be used to guide decision making (Armstrong et al., 2023). Analyses of scenarios and trends engage increasingly diverse 'disciplinary and other knowledges' (Cork et al., 2023, p. 4). Several challenges have been identified by Cork et al. (2023), including cultural biases (most future-thinking studies reflecting Western interpretations), constraints on human imagining associated with cognitive processing and the need for futures thinking at societal scale. The authors also noted the emergence of models for achieving transformations in the way people relate to the planet.

Models for improving healthcare have also been developed. For example, the WHO Western Pacific Regional Office brought experts from government departments and policy areas together with external experts in innovative forums or think tanks. These think tanks identified themes that were synthesized into 12 dimensions of the new future. Fig. 1.1 illustrates the breadth and complexity of changes that could emerge (Gariboldi et al., 2021). The 12 dimensions relate to society, health, politics and governments and technology.

Healthcare Practice and Clinical Decision Making

We argue that clinical decision making must now be considered in the broader context of sustainable and equitable future healthcare, thereby extending our understanding of decision making beyond the narrower clinical environment. This was the case during the COVID-19 pandemic when external factors such as government mandates and access to healthcare services changed the clinical decision-making process. Two key focuses emerge when clinical decision making is conceptualized in this broader context: (1) the importance of team-based decision making and (2) prioritizing the integration of ethics into all clinical decisions.

Team-Based Decision Making

There is an increasing focus on team-based decision making to provide the collaborative care that is often required for optimal health outcomes for patients. However, more needs to be done. In Australia, for example, the number of general medical practitioners per head of population is currently the highest it has ever been, albeit unevenly distributed throughout the country (Breadon et al., 2022). However, doctors are overwhelmed by increasingly complex disease presentations that often require more time than the standard 15-minute consultation. Access to healthcare could be greatly improved if allied health practitioners were able to conduct some of the noncritical tasks that currently fall to doctors: for example, screening of musculoskeletal injuries by radiographers without medical referral (Nancarrow et al., 2013). Team-based care can not only serve greater numbers of patients without reducing the safety and quality of care (Korner et al., 2016; O'Leary et al., 2012), but also reduce the load on general practitioners.

It is important to note here that the increasing focus on team-based decision making could always be overtaken by radically different possibilities that could emerge in the future. For example, it is possible that individuals could, wisely or unwisely, demand greater input to their own health management than is currently possible or imaginable.

Ethical Decision Making in Clinical Practice

Another important change that will become increasingly necessary is the deliberate integration of ethical considerations into clinical decision making, including considering the ethical implications not only for individual patients and health professionals but also for societies, healthcare systems and global environments. This is particularly important in an era of generative artificial technologies, inequitably distributed resources and pressures on public funding.

KEY MEGATRENDS THAT SHAPE HEALTHCARE FUTURES

Megatrends refer to 'the great forces in human and technology development that affect the future in all areas of human activity, in a horizon of 10 to 15 years' (Naisbitt and Aubrdene, 1991). Megatrends will

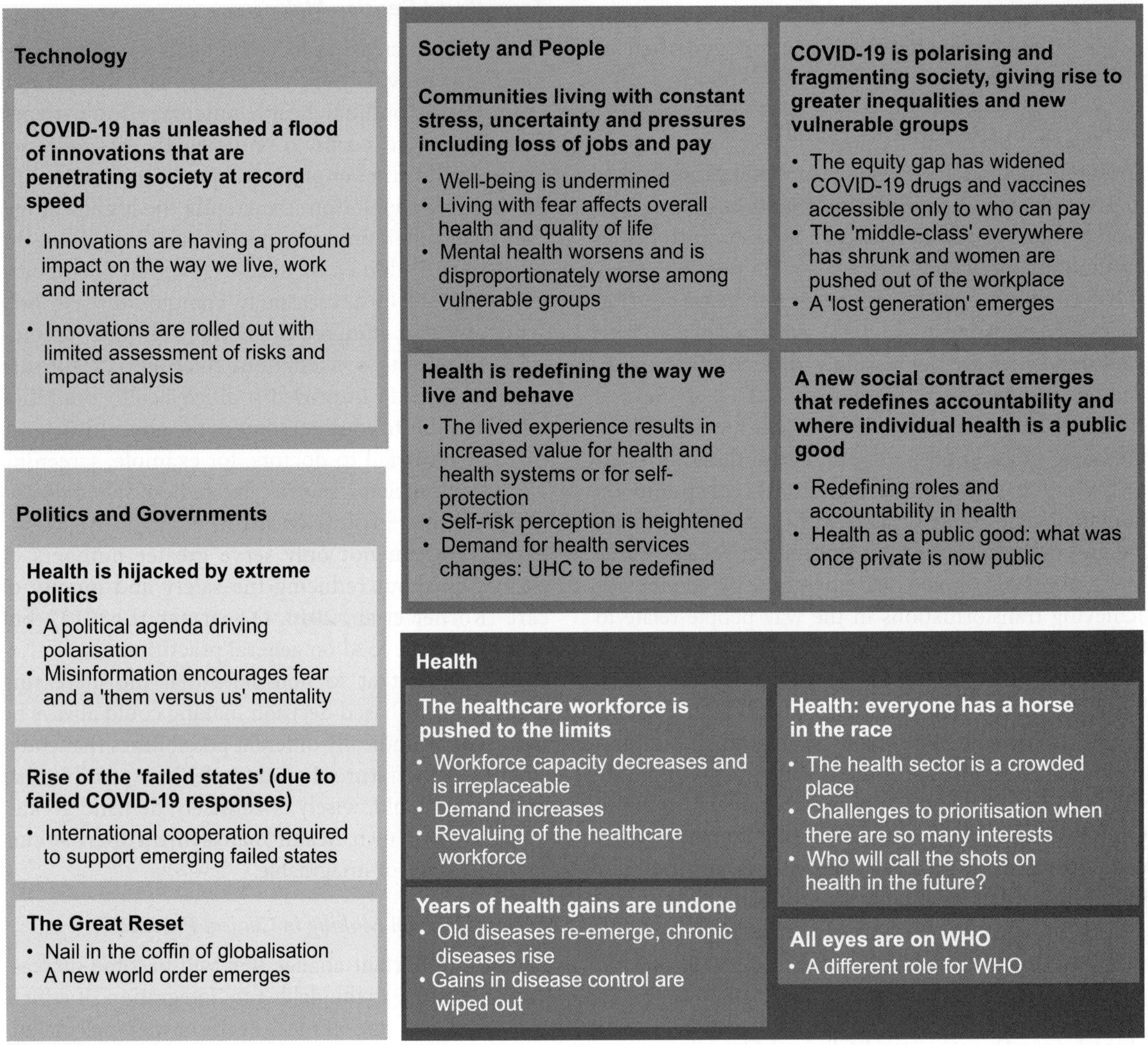

Technology

COVID-19 has unleashed a flood of innovations that are penetrating society at record speed

- Innovations are having a profound impact on the way we live, work and interact
- Innovations are rolled out with limited assessment of risks and impact analysis

Politics and Governments

Health is hijacked by extreme politics

- A political agenda driving polarisation
- Misinformation encourages fear and a 'them versus us' mentality

Rise of the 'failed states' (due to failed COVID-19 responses)

- International cooperation required to support emerging failed states

The Great Reset

- Nail in the coffin of globalisation
- A new world order emerges

Society and People

Communities living with constant stress, uncertainty and pressures including loss of jobs and pay

- Well-being is undermined
- Living with fear affects overall health and quality of life
- Mental health worsens and is disproportionately worse among vulnerable groups

Health is redefining the way we live and behave

- The lived experience results in increased value for health and health systems or for self-protection
- Self-risk perception is heightened
- Demand for health services changes: UHC to be redefined

COVID-19 is polarising and fragmenting society, giving rise to greater inequalities and new vulnerable groups

- The equity gap has widened
- COVID-19 drugs and vaccines accessible only to who can pay
- The 'middle-class' everywhere has shrunk and women are pushed out of the workplace
- A 'lost generation' emerges

A new social contract emerges that redefines accountability and where individual health is a public good

- Redefining roles and accountability in health
- Health as a public good: what was once private is now public

Health

The healthcare workforce is pushed to the limits

- Workforce capacity decreases and is irreplaceable
- Demand increases
- Revaluing of the healthcare workforce

Years of health gains are undone

- Old diseases re-emerge, chronic diseases rise
- Gains in disease control are wiped out

Health: everyone has a horse in the race

- The health sector is a crowded place
- Challenges to prioritisation when there are so many interests
- Who will call the shots on health in the future?

All eyes are on WHO

- A different role for WHO

Fig. 1.1 ■ The 12 dimensions of the new future. (With permission from Gariboldi, M.I., Lin, V., Bland, J., Auplish, M., Cawthorne, A., 2021. Foresight in the time of COVID-19. Lancet Reg. Health. West Pac. 6, 100049.)

resonate with health professionals currently in practice and will shape the possibilities for healthcare futures. The following key megatrends were identified by Deloitte (2016):

1. **Discontinuity**
   Predictions are typically based on continuity from the past, where possibilities can be imagined. With ongoing disruptions, the patterns of the past become difficult to discern and possible futures become harder to imagine. Financial austerity also stifles innovation. Discontinuity will be the new normal, making patterns of the past difficult to discern and obstructing the emergence of reimagined health and well-being policy.

2. **Demographic shifts**
   Climate change, urbanization, human mobility, increased chronic care, changing substance use and global pandemics such as viral illness

and mental health decline are key shifts in today's world. Population demands, and hence demographic changes, have enormous influence on health futures. Alternatives, such as collaborative, community-based management of chronic disease, will need to be developed and strengthened. Genome technology is also likely to strongly influence population-based approaches to care delivery.

3. **Digitalized futures: technology and healthcare innovation**

   Soft changes such as the move towards inner technologies (embedded in the human body) are increasing. Expanding global co-creation of value, innovation and new technologies are increasingly shared across borders. 'Open health' (health information that is readily accessible), peer-to-peer health and community-based health that enable sharing of knowledge and innovation are critical shifts.

4. **Globalized industries and commodification**

   Over the past 50 years, we have witnessed the emergence of highly influential conglomerates (e.g. large pharmaceutical, technological, private healthcare and insurance industries). Their impacts have been proprietary and based on the commodification of healthcare. A new era has emerged in which democratization of health, education, science and arts is disrupting dominant models of private enterprise and government. Disruptions have come mainly from macro changes such as the shift to healthcare wellness, the emergence of large economic communities such as the Association of Southeast Asian Nations (ASEAN) and the shift of power among healthcare stakeholders.

5. **Universal or nonuniversal provision of healthcare**

   Universal healthcare as a system is controversial because many claim it is financially unsustainable. There is a trend to move into more privatized systems, a commodification of healthcare. However, moving away from universal healthcare is likely to cause spiralling health costs and inequity. The association between economic inequity and health is well established. In the long run, the interests of the wealthy are best served by supporting and subsidizing global health equity.

6. **Politics**

   Traditional policy and regulation making will no longer work as we move into value-based care. Policy makers must drive accountability of all parties and providers, whether public or private. Policy development suffers from lack of bottom-up systematic redesign, including areas that are typically outside the system. Four levels of change are required:

   - Measuring illness prevention and wellness
   - Shifting from hospital to home care
   - Changing the culture of the worldview of the health system
   - Moving from 'the doctor knows best' to 'I am the expert of my body'

   It is likely that change will be driven by innovation disrupting the current system.

Deprofessionalization

Another trend that is directly affecting health professionals and the future of healthcare is deprofessionalization. Deprofessionalization, or the loss of autonomy of the professions, has reportedly been occurring for several decades, driven by the open health trends previously described where health information is sought from Internet sources and others with similar conditions rather than directly from health professionals during consultations (Cork and Alford, 2019). One of the key themes explored here was declining trust in professions. Trust in authority in general has been a major uncertainty in futures thinking for many decades and is likely to continue to be a major uncertainty that influences political support and funding for healthcare systems, the nature of those systems and how effectively they are implemented (Read et al., 2021). Three main factors – the market, technology and human ingenuity – support these trends (Table 1.1), which ultimately shift control of knowledge and expertise from the professions to the whole of society (Susskind and Susskind, 2015). It is likely that different generations and cohorts will experience different challenges, but two key issues have been identified: (1) future skills are likely to be

TABLE 1.1
Possible Evolution of Professional Work

Stage	When?	Characteristics
Professions as crafts	Past	Expert, bespoke services; knowledge and its application controlled
Standardization	Emerging now	Sharing of knowledge; agreement on approaches; standardization checklists
Systematization	Early signs now	Systems, technology and tools assist, or replace, human experts in carrying out professional tasks
Externalization	Medium- to long-term future	Online services, charged for; online services for no charge; free access to information commons

multidisciplinary and related to problem-solving; and (2) a smaller proportion of the population might be employed in the professions (Cork and Alford, 2019).

The implications for health professionals are significant: multidisciplinary skills, including collaborative clinical reasoning and teamwork, are needed for currently practising health professionals and students and should be a priority in continuing professional development and undergraduate education. New healthcare roles will continue to emerge (e.g. health assistant roles, roles where professionals from one health profession take on some of the tasks of another). Roles to assist health professionals understand and use AI and other digital technologies in the delivery of healthcare will also need to be created.

REFLECTION POINT

- On thinking about this chapter, how can you incorporate the broader perspective of public health in your clinical reasoning?

SUMMARY

This chapter has focused on futures thinking and an expanded understanding of clinical reasoning that encompasses social justice and the health and well-being of the whole population. This expanded understanding was prompted by the COVID-19 pandemic, which has irrevocably changed the world in many ways. We have considered future health and healthcare for the whole population and highlighted the importance of collaborative clinical decision making and ethical practice. Planning to mediate our preferred future involves considerations of funding, ethics, information systems, science and technology, standards and megatrends. Health practitioner roles are already changing in line with megatrends and are likely to continue to do so and with foresight and planning, equitable and socially just healthcare may be secured for everyone.

Acknowledgement

We wish to acknowledge Dr Steven Cork for his valuable assistance in this chapter.

REFERENCES

Armstrong, F., Wyns, A., Colagiuri, P., Anderson, R., Hunter, A., Arabena, K., et al., 2023. Healthy, regenerative and just: Guiding the development of a national strategy on climate, health and well-being for Australia. The Journal of Climate Change and Health, 10, 100205. https://doi.org/10.1016/j.joclim.2023.100205

Australian Commission on Safety and Quality in Health Care, 2022. The National Safety and Quality Health Service Standards. Commonwealth of Australia. Retrieved December 18 from https://www.safetyandquality.gov.au/standards/nsqhs-standards

Börjeson, L., Höjer, M., Dreborg, K.-H., Ekvall, T., Finnveden, G., 2006. Scenario types and techniques: Towards a user's guide. Futures 38, 723–739.

Breadon, P., Romanes, D., Fox, L., 2022. How do you fix general practice? More GPs won't be enough. Here's what to do. The Conversation. https://theconversation.com/how-do-you-fix-general-practice-more-gps-wont-be-enough-heres-what-to-do-195447

Cork, S., Alexandra, C., Alvarez-Romero, J.G., Bennett, E.M., Berbés-Blázquez, M., Bohensky, E., et al., 2023. Exploring alternative futures in the anthropocene. Annual Review of Environmental and Resources. 48, 25–54. https://doi.org/10.1146/annurev-environ-112321-095011

Cork, S., Alford, K., 2019. Plausible practice futures. In: Higgs, J., Cork, S., Horsfall, D. (Eds.), Challenging future practice possibilities. Brill Sense, pp. 29–40.

Deloitte. 2016. Health care foresight: Identifying megatrends. Retrieved November 15 from https://www2.deloitte.com/content/dam/Deloitte/sg/Documents/life-sciences-health-care/sg-lshc-healthcare-foresight-megatrends.pdf

Eckersley, R., 2010. Population health: A forgotten dimension of social resilience. In: Cork, S. (Ed.), Resilience and transformation: Preparing Australia for uncertain futures. CSIRO Publishing, pp. 105–120.

Gariboldi, M.I., Lin, V., Bland, J., Auplish, M., Cawthorne, A., 2021. Foresight in the time of COVID-19. The Lancet Regional Health - Western Pacific 6, 100049. https://doi.org/10.1016/j.lanwpc.2020.100049

James, M., 2001. Australia 2020: Foresight for our future. https://parlinfo.aph.gov.au/parlInfo/download/library/prspub/61G36/upload_binary/61g366.pdf;fileType=application%2Fpdf#search=%22Australia%20%20Foresight%20for%20our%20future%22

Kaplan, R.M., Frosch, D.L., 2005. Decision making in medicine and health care. Annual Review of Clinical Psychology 1 (1), 525–556. https://doi.org/10.1146/annurev.clinpsy.1.102803.144118

Korner, M., Butof, S., Muller, C., Zimmermann, L., Becker, S., Bengel, J., 2016. Interprofessional teamwork and team interventions in care: A systematic review. Journal of Interprofessional Care 30 (1), 15–18. https://doi.org/10.3109/13561820.2015.1051616

Moore, M-L., Milkoreit, M., 2020. Imagination and transformations to sustainable and just futures. Elementa Science of the Anthropocene 8 (1). https://doi.org/10.1525/elementa.2020.081

Naisbitt, J., Aubrdene, P., 1991. Megatrends 2000: Ten directions for the 1990s. William Morrow & Co.

Nancarrow, S., Roots, A., Grace, S., Moran, A., Vanniekerk-Lyons, K., 2013. Implementing large-scale workforce change: Learning from 55 pilot sites of allied health workforce redesign in Queensland, Australia. Human Resources for Health 11, 66. https://doi.org/10.1186/1478-4491-11-66

O'Leary, K.J., Sehgal, N.L., Terrell, G., Williams, M.V., 2012, Jan. Interdisciplinary teamwork in hospitals: A review and practical recommendations for improvement. Journal of Hospital Medicine (Online) 7 (1), 48–54. https://doi.org/10.1002/jhm.970

Read, L., Korenda, L., Nelson, H., 2021. Rebuilding trust in health care. Deloitte. Retrieved May 25 from https://www2.deloitte.com/us/en/insights/industry/health-care/trust-in-health-care-system.html

Schwartz, P., 2003. Inevitable surprises: Thinking ahead in a time of turbulence. Gotham.

Susskind, R., Susskind, D., 2015. The future of the professions: How technologies will transform the work of human experts. Oxford University Press.

Sutherland, H.J., Till, J.E., 1993. Quality of life assessments and levels of decision making: Differentiating objectives. Quality of Life Research 2, 297–303. https://doi.org/10.1007/BF00434801

US Department of Health and Human Sciences Office of Minority Health. 2000. National standards for culturally and linguistically appropriate services (CLAS) in health and health care. https://thinkculturalhealth.hhs.gov/clas/standards

Wager, K.A., Lee, F.W., Glaser, J.P., 2022. Health care information systems: A practical approach for health care management, 5th Ed. Wiley.

World Health Organization. 2022. Bridging the gap between ethics and decision-making in pandemics: Report of the WHO Pandemic Ethics and Policy Summit.

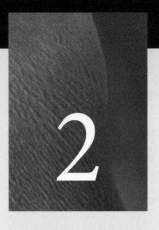

2

CONTEXTS OF CLINICAL REASONING
Navigating a World of Increasing Complexity

FRANZISKA V. TREDE ■ GEOFF SCOTT

CHAPTER AIMS

The aims of this chapter are:

■ to articulate the key sources that inform the development of a comprehensive world view of clinical decision making
■ to position decision making within the social, cultural and political determinants of positive health outcomes
■ to identify the key principles of effective clinical decision making and change leadership for this area.

OVERVIEW

This chapter provides a summary of the key sources of information that can be used to sharpen the world view of clinical decision making and the policy and educational initiatives that support it. What is explored is of relevance not just to clinicians but also to policy makers, clinical educators and their students.

It is argued that sound clinical decisions need to be underpinned not only by scientific evidence but also by a high level of cultural competence and personal ethics and an understanding of the impact that broader global influences have on health outcomes. This is especially important when routines break down, when faced with a key practice dilemma, a time when things go awry, or when confronted with a perplexing diagnostic moment. It is then that professional capability is most tested and it is then that being clear on where one stands in relation to the broader set of perspectives, outlined in this chapter, and the values that underpin them come into play. A central message of the chapter is that clinical decisions are not value free. Of particular importance is the role played by the United Nations 17 Sustainable Development Goals (SDGs) and the other key sources reviewed in the chapter in appropriately reading the unique and complex combination of broader influences of each practice situation and matching a uniquely suited decision (Hunt, 1976). The chapter concludes by drawing out some of the key implications from the issues raised for action at the macro, meso and micro levels. In doing this it highlights the importance of clinicians giving focus not just to treating individual symptoms but also to advocating collectively for, and supporting, actions that address the broader social, cultural, economic, political and environmental causes of poor health outcomes that are embedded in the SDGs.

OUR CONTEMPORARY CONTEXT

We are living in times of relentless disruption. The world is increasingly connected, global and complex. Zygmunt Bauman (2012) labelled our contemporary context 'liquid times'. He asserted that practices such as decision making have no time to solidify before the next decision needs to be made. The consequences of one decision lead to the next decision having to be made. Linear thinking that follows one-dimensional decision-making processes and is based on trust in one disciplinary knowledge source alone is no longer enough to solve wicked global problems. Horst Rittel and Melvin Webber (1973) used the term 'wicked problems' to identify problems that are ill-defined, unique, have no stopping rule or perfect solution and are nested within a range of other problems in which action relies on judgement. The challenges faced over the last few years during the COVID-19 pandemic have highlighted the importance of futures thinking and sound, transdisciplinary clinical decision making in addressing the multidimensional, 'wicked' health problems that are characteristic of the age of acceleration (Friedman, 2016; Lockwood, 2019) and uncertainty (Galbraith, 1977).

The COVID-19 pandemic, the rapidly accelerating impacts of climate change on human and ecological well-being and exponential developments in technology, along with increasing injustices and inequality leading to wars, invasions and a plethora of refugee crises, characterize our contemporary context. We can no longer pretend to live in an orderly world that is predictable and certain (Bauman, 2012). Instead of best practices and narrow conceptions of evidence, we need to accept that we are living in an imperfect world that requires multilateral and integrated decision making. The future world view of clinical decision making cannot afford to ignore the wider social, ecological, political context within which it is enacted. The world view or knowledge systems that focus on controlling variables out of context are no longer adequate. The future is transdisciplinary, relational and connected and requires an inclusive approach to decision making. We want to emphasize here that inclusive clinical decision making is not a neutral or objective act. Clinicians require courage and a considered moral stance to advance social justice in healthcare accompanied by a capacity to act because good ideas are not enough, they need to be operationalized.

- Can you list some disruptions that have changed the way you practise and make decisions?
- How do you introduce your students or clients into the wider global, complex and connected context of healthcare practices?
- What knowledge do you engage your students or clients with in their clinical decision-making processes?

Key Sources of Information for Clinical Decision Making

As professionals working in the healthcare sector, it is no longer sufficient to look only for inspiration and guidance from within the profession. In this chapter we propose engagement with wider social and economic well-being ecosystems and global alliances in order to integrate complex issues into more local decision-making practices. To navigate the contemporary context, we discuss key sources that can guide future practices for clinical decision making and the prevention of negative population health outcomes.

The United Nations' Sustainable Developmental Goals (SDGs)

The UN SDGs identify the complex, interlaced mix of changes to be addressed for a sustainable healthcare future and highlight the way in which the many social determinants of health need to be addressed concurrently if we are to achieve equitable health and well-being outcomes over the coming decades. They highlight the important role of values centred on equity, equality of access, environmental care, clean water and sanitation, human rights, decent work and harmonious societies in clinical decision making.

The 17 SDGs (Box 2.1) have been identified by a wide range of peak healthcare bodies and practitioners as a key framework in the age of acceleration and uncertainty for informing and shaping the futures thinking and foresight necessary to achieve the positive public health and well-being outcomes we desire over the coming decades. They include the work now underway to address not just SDG 3 (Good health and well-being) but the many social and ecological determinants of health embedded in the other SDGs.

SDG 3 (Good health and well-being) is being highlighted as a key dependent variable and as a core quality test for the impact of the other SDGs, which are being seen as an interlaced set of factors constituting the social and ecological determinants of positive health outcomes.

SDG 17 (Partnerships for the goals) brings into play the need to apply the key lessons of effective change leadership and implementation and highlights the need to work collaboratively in order to make progress towards achieving all of the other SDGs.

As Nunes et al. (2016) observe:

Measures of health and well-being (SDG3) can be used to assess progress in the implementation of the SDGs … The WHO argues that health and well-being are central measures of progress in achieving the SDGs as an overall strategy of the post-2015 agenda.

In this perspective, a first-order quality test in a just, equitable and sustainable world is that all people, irrespective of background, have access to high-quality healthcare and the healthy living factors embedded in the other SDGs. The COVID-19 pandemic demonstrated how, as the crisis unfolded across the world, all of these SDGs had to be addressed concurrently as they all fed into and off each other and

played a role in affecting COVID-19 health outcomes (Scott, 2022, p. 28)

The complex way in which all of the SDGs play a role in shaping health outcomes can be seen in the way in which poverty, crowded living, hunger and unclean water allow not just COVID-19 but malaria and other diseases such as TB and cholera to spread. Land clearing can increase the likelihood of more zoonotic diseases. The pollution that results from a failure to care for the environment kills. Seas rise, floods and wildfires hit and people are displaced. Poverty in developing countries drives people to take dangerous voyages and can lead to prostitution, which spreads sexually transmitted diseases and deadly variants such as HIV and AIDS. War results in not only physical but long-term mental health issues, along with ill health and early death from starvation when supply lines are broken. We saw how the gap between rich and poor countries affected the movement of key medications during the COVID-19 pandemic and how vaccine inequity differentially influenced health outcomes.

Carey and O'Mara (2022) cite Australian Bureau of Statistics data, which show that poverty dramatically increases the likelihood of sickness (the impact of the so-called social gradient where less money and lower education make access to healthcare much harder and the spread of disease and rates of illness higher). It is argued that, during the pandemic, people faced with poverty had little choice but to take jobs that exposed them more directly to COVID-19 and tended to live in the more crowded conditions that increased spread.

As the International Council of Nurses (2017, pp. 7–8) observes:

Poor health can be attributed to inequity in the conditions in which people are born, grow, live, work and age … Furthermore, the (sustainable development) goals inextricably link the social determinants of health to the full spectrum of government sectors (e.g. agriculture, water, housing, education, energy, transport, infrastructure, social development, environmental protection, governance) and not just the health sector.

On 28 July 2022, the UN General Assembly declared that everyone on the planet has a right to a healthy environment. Inger Andersen, Executive Director of the UN Environment Programme (UNEP) said ... 'It will help people stand up for their right to breathe clean air, to access safe and sufficient water, healthy food, healthy ecosystems, and non-toxic environments to live, work, study, and play' (UNEP, 2022; see also: Khosla et al., 2022).

As Sara Bennett (2015, p. 2), Professor at John Hopkins University, observed:

> In the next 15 years many of the major challenges to human health will originate outside of the health sector.

Bennett's foresight is becoming a lived reality. The following discussion draws on sources outside of the healthcare sector that have implications for the health of populations and individuals. For example, researchers such as Piracha and Chaudhary (2022) highlight the impact of poor urban design and the creation of the Urban Heat Island (UHI) effect on poor health outcomes and the technological solutions that can ameliorate its impact.

To summarize, SDG 3 is a key goal and all of the other social/ecological SDGs are the independent variables. Health professionals also need to be explicitly aware of their role and impact on their practice and to take steps to highlight their significance to policymakers in order to decrease the causes of poor health outcomes rather than only treating their symptoms.

This means highlighting how COVID-19, as noted earlier, has been a typical example of a 'wicked' multidimensional, uncertain problem, the handling of which requires not just sound clinical decision makers who are futures thinkers but also practitioners who become advocates for key preventative health measures that cover all of the SDGs.

Scott (2022) argues that the values which underpin the SDGs identify a moral purpose for the conduct of society, including the operation, focus and future's thinking for areas like health. As Hutchinson (2020, p. 3) has observed:

> In these times of unprecedented change and challenge, these goals are a clear framework to review the work we do, how we live our lives and how we individually and collectively can come together to find new ways of working, new opportunities and new ways to solve joint problems.

As cited by Scott (2022, p. 28), Roger Crisp, Professor of Moral Philosophy at the University of Oxford, links these observations to the Aristotelian virtues and 'everyday morality: courage, generosity, even temper, moderation, being a good friend (to all), justice, prudence, honesty ... virtues such as patience, tolerance and resilience, ... a life of autonomy and authenticity ... and the virtue of collaborativeness'.

REFLECTION POINT

- How are you already or how might you address the 17 UN SDGs in your teaching or clinical practice?

The World Health Organization and the Social Determinants of Health

The Social Determinants of Health (SDH) (Wilkinson and Marmot, 2003) provide another global framework for comprehensive decision making. The SDH framework identifies economic, cultural and political policies and systems as key factors influencing health outcomes for individuals. This framework is not new but its messages about the broader contextual factors influencing health and well-being remain contemporary and continue to attract attention as inequalities widen. Professionals working in the health profession need, therefore, to know about and engage with them. It is now well established that the social determinants of health have a greater impact on individuals' health than healthcare provision and lifestyle choices alone (Wilkinson and Marmot, 2003). The 10 social factors that determine health outcomes are social gradient, stress, early life, social exclusion, work, unemployment, social support, addiction, food and transport. This list aligns with the earlier discussion about the broader set of SDGs that influence SDG 3 and speaks to the need for social policies that can create conditions for healthy societies. They are also a reminder that social and economic justice are important interdependent pillars for understanding the intersections of the social, cultural, economic, environmental and medical contributions to health and well-being.

These social determinants can inform more effective decision making at all levels of the health profession from national policy to workplace cultures and clinical encounters with patients. The SDH factors raise awareness of how complex and 'wicked' decision making can get. At an individual patient level, it is effective to know, understand and take into account the 10 social determinants of health. They point to the importance of critical, contingent, responsive, holistic and diagnostic thinking about the unique situation of the patient in the broader context of the systems, structures and policies that affect them in order for the most relevant, desirable and feasible clinical decision to be made. These determinants address awareness, responsibility and capacity to act within a social health ecosystem.

REFLECTION POINT

- The workplace is one social determinant of health. Think about your workplace and scrutinize the workplace conditions. What are the decision-making protocols and norms at your workplace?
- Who makes the big decisions?
- What decision-making processes are you part of?
- What aspects of work can you influence?
- To what extent do you take into account the social determinants of health when patients consult you?

Indigenous Perspectives on Health and Well-Being

Although the social determinants of health have advanced Western understanding of health, they have not adequately explored the cultural, historical and structural determinants faced by First Nations' Peoples (Jackson Pulver et al., 2019). Western biomedical models of health continue to perpetuate deficit-based approaches implying that patients have deficits or insufficiencies, lack something or are a failure (Kennedy et al., 2022). The social determinants of health have another social layer in the context of Indigenous peoples due to structural racism, marginalization and oppression. It has been suggested that indigenous models of health involve a social ecology underpinned by values of community, reflexivity and relatedness (Jackson Pulver et al., 2019). Reflexivity by clinicians is important here because it enables them to become aware of unreflected assumptions, their own social position and professional authority. Reflexivity is key for cultural humility and cultural safety (Redfern and Bennett, 2022). Cultural safety places Indigenous peoples' experiences at the centre of healthcare. It has

been recognized as a human right that can strengthen clinical safety and patient well-being.

Improving the cultural safety and cultural responsiveness of the health system can improve access to and the quality of healthcare for Indigenous Australians. A culturally safe health system is one that respects indigenous cultural values, strengths and differences, and addresses racism and inequity. It also requires health professionals and health services to be culturally responsive, to take action to overcome racism and power imbalances and to have active engagement with Indigenous clients/patients to ensure that the system meets their needs.

(Australian Institute of Health and Welfare, 2022a, Section 3)

This text speaks not only to the social and cultural determinants in the Australian context but also to the political determinants of positive health outcomes. These insights apply to other countries where Indigenous people have been marginalized. A key component of clinical decision making in the coming years will, therefore, involve clinicians developing a more detailed understanding of their own culture and what constitutes cultural safety for First Nations peoples and greater respect for their self-determination, including an understanding of their unique connection to land, water, air, the stars, community and culture. As Wiradjuri scholar of public health Professor Lisa Jackson Pulver and colleagues (2019) emphasize, Aboriginal health has always been about health for all. In this perspective, health and well-being are intimately connected, with health entailing both cultural and relational well-being. The underpinning principles for clinical decision making in this context must, therefore, include participation, empowerment and self-determination (Mazel, 2016). Jackson Pulver et al. (2019) argue that providing equality of opportunity, better enabling processes for participation and supportive social networks are all necessary to foster a collective healing process. Kelaher et al. (2014) emphasize how, historically, the trauma of colonization and interpersonal racism experienced through the loss of language, dispossession and erasure of culture has led to internalized and institutionalized racism and, through this, negative health impacts. In this context, Fitzpatrick (2003, 2011) asserts the importance of a broader peace-building process for productive coexistence underpinned by self-awareness through critical reflection.

The SDH framework (Wilkinson and Marmot, 2003) is a good starting point for clinical decision making in this context but the earlier discussion implies that it needs to be complemented by more holistic, relational and expansive perspectives cognisant that 'Australia's First Nation Peoples are leading world citizens in the struggle for health equity and justice' (Jackson Pulver et al., 2019, p. 176). According to a widely cited definition from Aboriginal and Torres Strait Islander peoples, health and well-being is: 'Not just the physical well-being of the individual but the social, emotional and cultural well-being of the whole community. This is a whole-of-life view and it also includes the cyclical concept of life-death-life' (National Aboriginal Health Strategy Working Party, 1989, p. x). Indigenous cultures 'are based on the recognition of the central importance of land to Indigenous peoples' identity, spirituality, community and culture' (Ganesharajah, 2009, p. 26). Indigenous perspectives on health are based on participatory and collective decision making. Jackson Pulver et al. (2019, p. 187) ask us to consider 'What is the link between racism and First Peoples not achieving their self-determined strategies to improve social determinants of health?' They contend that a paradigm shift is needed, with a more nuanced perspective that includes a human rights framework, cultural understandings of health and a strength-based approach that enables self-determination and is grounded on reflexivity.

This valuing of collectivism does not align well with a medical decision-making approach that is authoritative and hierarchical. Successful decision making within indigenous contexts is underpinned by partnerships, co-creation of solutions, respectful relationships and working together using strengths-based approaches. Kennedy et al. (2022) who have Cree, Blackfoot, Métis and Settler ancestries in Canada explored indigenous perspectives of strengths-based approaches to healthcare drawing on locations from Australia, Canada, New Zealand, UK and the United States. Kennedy et al. (2022, p. 340) crystallized the following eight interconnected actions:

(1) respecting indigenous human rights,
(2) respecting indigenous knowledges and healing practices,
(3) re-centring power relationships,
(4) revitalizing culture and collective identity,
(5) cultivating individual and collective resilience,
(6) advancing equity,
(7) advancing self-determination, and
(8) capacity building with individuals and communities.

These strengths-based actions enable collective self-determination. Self-determination is about identifying choices and making decisions based on them. Key principles for indigenous well-being can be summarized to include self-determination, autonomy and community and are underpinned by the UN Declaration on the Rights of Indigenous Peoples (United Nations, 2007). The declaration which was co-written with Indigenous peoples and endured many years of rejections and requests for revisions, consists of 46 items and sets guidelines and standards for the survival, health and well-being of Indigenous peoples around the world. It recognizes self-determination and collective rights and speaks against assimilation. The four countries who initially rejected the declaration (Australia, Canada, New Zealand and the United States) have since changed their position and are now supporting it.

The importance of understanding the role of kinship, along with indigenous traditions of knowing, being and doing and cultural health practices and medicines when delivering healthcare for and with First Nation peoples, is highlighted by Griffith University (2022, p. 1) in their *Future Learn* programme.

The kinship system is fundamental to First Peoples' culture and may influence decision making in health, so it's important for you to know more about it… Traditional health practices and medicine is deeply rooted in Aboriginal and Torres Strait Islander cultural knowledge. For example, the use of bush medicines is based on local, cultural knowledge. As opposed to western, science-based medicines, it draws on Indigenous traditions of knowing, being and doing.

The Australian Institute of Health and Welfare (2022b) provides a range of resources for addressing a broad spectrum of indigenous health and social-emotional well-being issues. It notes how many of the key factors embedded in the SDGs can act as factors in this area and provides a range of guidelines on how they might be addressed. As Professor Elizabeth Elliot observed:

> To move forward non-Indigenous doctors must acknowledge that Western medicine is not the only way. (2016)

A widening perspective is called for that is attentive to the everchanging configuration of Australian society. This is a perspective that disrupts our conventional understandings, attitudes and unconscious biases; a perspective that questions who makes up the 'social' in social determinants; and a perspective that is rights-based and promotes multilevel empowerment (Jackson Pulver et al., 2019, p. 10). This is because:

- The social is dominated by the majority of the population who determine just who should and could move to embrace First Peoples' cultures, including holistic approaches to health.
- The social is made up of multiple cultures and values to be embraced with respect for all.
- Racism is a grave legal, health and well-being concern.
- Solutions involve partnerships, with strategies for multilevel empowerment and self-determination to occur.
- Accountability is paramount and must include community.
- Critical reflection will enable progress in providing social support.

REFLECTION POINT

- How might you take into account indigenous perspectives of health in your decision-making practices in order to facilitate cultural safety and positive health outcomes for First Nations peoples?
- How might non-Indigenous health professionals benefit from an indigenous perspective on health and decision making?

Engaging in Strategic Foresight

Foresight is not about predicting a single future but contemplating multiple possible futures and how to navigate them if they eventuate. It includes, therefore, thinking about what is likely to happen, what is not going to happen and what else is possible. Engaging in strategic foresight enables a more purposeful and informed decision-making practice. This form of forward and contingent thinking helps the practitioner to successfully negotiate an uncertain future by anticipating what response is likely to be most relevant, desirable and feasible (implementable) if each of the different scenarios envisaged eventuate. The Commonwealth Scientific and Industrial Research Organisation of Australia (Naughtin et al., 2022) identifies a list of future megatrends every decade and this is a potentially relevant source to consult to gain a world view of future clinical challenges and decision-making options.

The report by Naughtin et al. (2022) on 'the Seven trends that will shape the next 20 years' gives a data-driven outline of emerging trends that are likely to unfold over the coming decades. The report is another useful source for guiding future-focussed and strategic clinical decision making and once again also aligns with the collective focus of the UN SDGs. The seven megatrends in the report are:

1. Adapting to a Changing Climate (protecting livelihoods, infrastructure and quality of life)
2. Leaner, Cleaner and Greener (global push to net zero, protecting biodiversity)
3. Escalating Health Imperative (health promotion despite rising demand, demographic changes, emerging diseases and unhealthy lifestyles)
4. Geopolitical Shifts (efforts to ensure global stability, trade and economic growth)
5. Diving into Digital (rapidly growing digital and data economy)
6. Increasingly Autonomous (rise of artificial intelligence and autonomous systems)
7. Unlocking the Human Dimension (importance of diversity, equity and transparency in society)

We can take guidance from all these global and future trends for decision making in the healthcare context but for the purpose of this chapter, we want to focus especially on two trends: the escalating health imperative and unlocking the human dimension. Through the COVID-19 pandemic, escalating health imperatives in decades to come and the need for anticipatory thinking have been amplified (Naughtin et al., 2022). Population groups that have been hardest hit by the pandemic are people with mental health conditions, the ageing population, the poor and people living with chronic diseases. For these groups especially, decision making cannot be viewed in isolation from the wider context within which they live. This trend also highlights the close connection to the social determinants of health.

The second trend we highlight is 'unlocking the human dimension'. The voice of consumers, clients and citizens is becoming louder; we need to remind ourselves that patients are also consumers and citizens. They are demanding governments and professionals to be more accountable, responsible and transparent. There is an expectation to strengthen trust, fairness, ethical conduct, and environmental and social governance. Due to the Internet and rapidly advancing technologies, consumers and patients are better informed and more outspoken about their expectations of their healthcare providers (Naughtin et al., 2022). To align with this consumer trend we would argue that decision making needs to be transparent, collaborative and underpinned by respect.

REFLECTION POINT

Check the equivalent of your national research council for future trends that impact healthcare policy.
- What do these trends imply for your decision-making practices?

Implications For Action in Support of This Agenda

What, then, are the general implications for action as clinical decision-makers that emerge from the various sources of information and areas for change highlighted in this chapter?

First, we argue that the focus should be on purposeful participation of all who are affected by each initiative and that the actions taken should be comprehensively informed. Participation starts with ensuring that patients and others involved in each desired change have optimum access to resources and information. But beyond access, reasoning

through various meanings and options for action is an important collective process which underpins sound clinical decision making. It enables expert knowledge to work in combination with the lived experience of the client and others affected by each change. It requires everybody to be prepared to be challenged to rethink their values and their considered position on issues such as growth being equally good for everyone, consumption being happiness, information technology always being the answer and globalization being great. Where one stands on such assumptions can directly impact the clinical decisions made, especially when one is faced with an unexpected situation or a professional dilemma and as a result will affect the quality of the health outcomes of patients. Furthermore, action at such times requires everybody to contribute in their own distinctive way to addressing the situation and ensuring it is dealt with wisely, promptly and effectively: policy writers at the macro level, managers at the meso level and clinicians working with patients at the micro level. It also requires ensuring that the decisions made are effectively implemented and that their consequences and impact are continuously monitored and enhanced.

A second area for follow-up action is to recognize that decision making is not a neutral, scientific or rational process alone. No technical breakthrough, clinical decision or social initiative is ever value free. Decisions require a clear understanding of both the values and cultural considerations at play in each unique decision situation. Complex situations with uncertain outcomes call for practice capabilities that are uniquely human so that decisions can be made based on what is most relevant, desirable and feasible. When assessing the desirability of a particular course of action there is a profound difference between change (something becoming or being made different) and progress (a personal value judgement that the change is beneficial and worth pursuing). It is in this way that values and ethics become the engine house of change. This implies that situated professional judgement needs to be given more explicit attention in professional education and clinical decision making.

A third implication is that we need to move from talking about what needs to change to becoming more adept at actually putting desired changes into practice.

This directly addresses the issue noted at the start of this chapter that good ideas with no ideas on how to implement them are wasted ideas (Fullan and Scott, 2009). As Biermann (2022) observed:

> With 61 colleagues from around the world, we analysed more than 3,000 academic studies that scrutinised aspects of the SDGs … Unfortunately, our findings are disheartening. The SDGs have infiltrated the things people say, think and write about global sustainability challenges … But nothing has changed where it matters … Those in power now refer to the SDGs often. Yet the way they govern has not changed.

What is needed now, therefore, is to question current practices, to identify injustices and to act on them. There needs to be more focus on taking actions that are grounded in moral judgement, are implementation-focussed and address increasing injustices and widening gaps (Kreber, 2016). For internationally validated guidelines on how to take good ideas in this area and ensure they are successfully implemented see Scott (2016, pp. 28–33). Stetsenko (2019) describes this as a shift from a relational to a transformative world view for decision making. Her proposal states that:

> … it is time to move past ecological and relational approaches in their emphasis on reactive/responsive modes of agency—while preserving their important insights—and toward more explicitly political and activist accounts of agency that challenge the status quo and that are urgently needed today in our world in the state of a profound crisis and turmoil.

The sources and their key messages discussed in this chapter imply a need for a social transformation in which rational, economic decision making needs to be infused with political, cultural and global longer-term visions aimed at fostering a more positive social and planetary future. And it is here that education can play a more central role in ensuring that graduates at every level are sustainability literate, change implementation savvy, inventive (socially not just commercially) and are clear on where they stand

on the tacit assumptions driving much of society in the 21st century.

REFLECTION POINT

- How is capacity for collaborative decision making focussed on sustainability focussed healthcare enabled in your workplace?

SUMMARY

In this chapter, key sources of information and insight that healthcare decision-makers and leaders need to take into account in their daily practice and advocacy for a more sustainable healthcare future and planet have been identified. The complex ways in which the social, cultural and ecological determinants of health interact and the need for transformational agency have been highlighted.

It has been argued that high levels of health and well-being are key measures of a successful society. However, good ideas on how to achieve this do not just make their way automatically into practice. They must be deftly led, underpinned by values of social justice and sustainability and this requires the development of healthcare professionals who are not just work ready for today's world (competent) but who are, in the context of an increasingly complex, intertwined and uncertain world, prepared to make professional judgements and take a stance which helps their profession, communities and countries achieve a healthy, sustainable future for all.

At the macro level, practitioners can choose to advocate more directly for policies and action to address the social determinants of health we have outlined. At the micro level practitioners need to ensure that they are clear on where they stand on the tacit assumptions and the values embedded in the SDGs, in the SDH framework, in indigenous perspectives, the megatrends predicted by Nunes et al. (2016) and the other sources reviewed. It will be their values that will come into play whenever they are faced with a wicked clinical case or professional dilemma.

The chapter reminds us that, like life, no clinical decision or policy initiative is ever value free and that decision making is a complex practice that needs to engage with the interface of biophysical, social, cultural and political determinants of health. All of the sources identified in this chapter advocate for diversity, human rights, critical reflection and action. Without these elements the clinical decision making of the future will not make an impact to advance health for all.

Acknowledgement

We are grateful for cultural mentoring and advice from Professor Megan Williams (Wiradjuri, Palawa) and Dr Sally Fitzpatrick.

REFERENCES

Australian Institute of Health and Welfare. 2022a. Indigenous Australians and the health system. https://www.aihw.gov.au/reports/australias-health/indigenous-australians-use-of-health-services

Australian Institute of Health and Welfare, 2022b. Indigenous health and well. Australian Government, Canberra. https://www.aihw.gov.au/reports/australias-health/indigenous-health-and-well-being

Bauman, Z., 2012. Liquid modernity. Polity Books.

Bennett, S., 2015. How the SDGS can help address global health challenges. World Economic Forum. https://www.weforum.org/agenda/2015/10/how-the-sdgs-can-help-address-global-health-challenges/

Biermann, F., 2022. UN sustainable development goals failing to have meaningful impact. The Conversation. https://theconversation.com/un-sustainable-development-goals-failing-to-have-meaningful-impact-our-research-warns-185269

Carey, G., O'Mara, B., 2022. Australia is failing marginalised people, and it shows in COVID death rates. The Conversation. https://theconversation.com/australia-is-failing-marginalised-people-and-it-shows-in-covid-death-rates-177224

Elliot, E., 2016. How traditional Aboriginal medicine can help close the health gap. Poche Key Thinkers Forum, University of Sydney.

Fitzpatrick, S., 2011. What's stopping us now? Envisioning a transformed Australia through critical reflection. Journal of Australian Indigenous Issues 14 (2–3), 199–218.

Fitzpatrick, S., 2003. Imagining a truth commissioned for Australia. In: Schraner, C. (Ed.), Peace Year Book. People for Nuclear Disarmament, pp. 52–59.

Friedman, T., 2016. Thank you for being late: Thriving in the age of accelerations. Farrar, Straus and Giroux.

Fullan, M., Scott, G., 2009. Turnaround leadership for higher education. Jossey Bass.

Galbraith, J.K., 1977. The age of uncertainty. BBC.

Ganesharajah, C., 2009. Indigenous health and wellbeing: The importance of country. Native Title Research Report No1/2009, Australian Institute of Aboriginal and Torres Strait Islander Studies, Canberra, Australia.

Griffith University, 2022. Safer health care for Australia's First Peoples. Future Learn. https://www.futurelearn.com/info/courses/first-peoples-safer-healthcare/0/steps/50670

Hunt, D., 1976. Teachers' adaptation: 'Reading' and 'Flexing' to students. Journal of Teacher Education 27 (3), 268–275.

Hutchinson, B., 2020. Connect for a better future Sydney Ideas Podcast. The University of Sydney. https://www.sydney.edu.au/content/dam/corporate/documents/engage/events-sponsorships/sydney-ideas/transcript-connectfor-launch-event.pdf

International Council of Nurses, 2017. Nurses' role in achieving the Sustainable Development Goals. International Council of Nurses, Geneva.

Jackson Pulver, L., Williams, M., Fitzpatrick, S., 2019. Social determinants of Australia's First Peoples: A multi-level empowerment perspective. In: Liamputtong, P. (Ed.), Social Determinants of Health. Oxford University Press, pp. 175–214.

Kelaher, M.A., Ferdinand, A.S., Paradies, Y., 2014. Experiencing racism in health care: The mental health impacts for Victorian Aboriginal communities. Medical Journal of Australia 201 (1), 44–47.

Kennedy, A., Sehgal, A., Szabo, J., McGowan, K., Lindstrom, G., Roach, P., et al., 2022. Indigenous strengths-based approaches to healthcare and health professions education – Recognising the value of elders' teachings. Health Education Journal 81 (4), 423–438.

Khosla, R., Allotey, P., Gruskin, S., 2022. 'Reimagining human rights in global health: what will it take?' BMJ Global Health 7, e010373.

Kreber, C., 2016. Educating for civic-mindedness: Nurturing authentic professional identities through transformative higher education. Routledge: London.

Lockwood, C.J., 2019. Coping in the age of acceleration. Contemporary OB/GYN 64 (98). https://www.contemporaryobgyn.net/view/coping-age-acceleration

Mazel, O., 2016. Self-determination and the right to health: Australian Aboriginal community controlled health services. Human Rights Law Review 16, 323–355.

National Aboriginal Health Strategy Working Party. 1989. A National Aboriginal Health Strategy. National Aboriginal Health Strategy Working Party. https://catalogue.nla.gov.au/catalog/668993

Naughtin, C., Hajkowicz, S., Schleiger, E., Bratanova, A., Cameron, A., Zamin, T., et al., 2022. Our future world: Global megatrends impacting the way we live over coming decades. CSIRO, Brisbane, Australia.

Nunes, A.R., Lee, K., O'Riordan, T., 2016. The importance of an integrating framework for achieving the Sustainable Development Goals: The example of health and well-being. BMJ Global Health 1 (3), 1–12.

Piracha, A., Chaudhary, M., 2022. Urban air pollution, urban heat island and human health: A review of the literature. Sustainability 14, 1–19.

Redfern, H., Bennett, B., 2022. An intercultural critical reflection model. Journal of Social Work Practice 36 (2), 135–147.

Rittel, H.W., Webber, M.M., 1973. Dilemmas in a general theory of planning. Policy Sciences 4 (2), 155–169. https://urbanpolicy.net/wp-content/uploads/2012/11/Rittel+Webber_1973_PolicySciences4-2.pdf

Scott, G., 2016. Transforming graduate capabilities and achievement standards for a sustainable future. Office for Learning and Teaching,

National Senior Teaching Fellowship, Australian Government, Canberra. http://flipcurric.edu.au/sites/flipcurric/media/107.pdf

Scott, G., 2022. Building a wise and sustainable future: Moral purpose and challenged assumptions. In: Higgs, J., Orrell, J., Tasker, D., Patton, N. (Eds.), Shaping wise futures: A shared responsibility. Brill, Leiden and Boston, pp. 21–43.

Stetsenko, A., 2019. Radical-transformative agency: Continuities and contrasts with relational agency and implications for education. Frontiers Education 4.

United Nations Environment Program (UNEP), 2022. UN declares healthy environment a human right. UNEP. https://www.unep.org/news-and-stories/story/historic-move-un-declares-healthy-environment-human-right?mc_cid=8df3b460d6&mc_eid=98bed2ce5c

United Nations, 2007. United Nations Declaration on the Rights of Indigenous Peoples. https://www.un.org/development/desa/indigenouspeoples/declaration-on-the-rights-of-indigenous-peoples.html

Wilkinson, R., Marmot, M. (Eds.), 2003. Social determinants of health: The solid facts. WHO, Europe. https://www.euro.who.int/__data/assets/pdf_file/0005/98438/e81384.pdf

PART 2 | Understanding Clinical Reasoning

PART OUTLINE

Part 2 builds on the aim of expanding clinical reasoning in the health professions to include the future of decision making for the health of the whole population. In discussing foresight and strategies to promote social justice and quality of life for all, we focus on clinical health, rather than population health (our focus in Part 1). In this way we can expand our vision of clinical reasoning to key sources of information that underpin this expanded view of clinical reasoning. Clinical decision making is positioned within the social, cultural and political determinants of healthcare.

Clinical reasoning is the core of professional practice. Without good clinical decisions, health practitioners cannot serve the best interests of their patients. Part 2 helps readers gain a deep understanding of the nature of clinical reasoning. Key aspects of clinical reasoning are presented through an exploration of professional judgement, epistemic fluency (flexibility and skill with different ways of knowing about the world), metacognition and problem spaces. Clinical reasoning is understood as a complex process in which critical analysis and reflection take place in the context of the action and interaction with the patient.

The *complex nature* of clinical reasoning is discussed from a number of perspectives, including the cognitive and noncognitive components of clinical reasoning, the complexity associated with incorporating the biopsychosocial model, the need for a range of clinical reasoning strategies to understand patients and patients' health problems, and multiple and multidimensional problem spaces. We discuss hypothetico-deductive approaches to clinical reasoning and approaches that focus on patient narratives and understanding patients' illness experiences and recognize the increasing focus on collaborations with patients, their families and other health practitioners when making clinical decisions.

Part 2 also highlights the *reflexive nature* of clinical reasoning. Health practitioners need to be open to reflect on their practice. To do so requires the metacognitive reasoning skills to recognize situations when routine approaches to problems are likely to work or not work, the critical thinking skills to challenge assumptions, the capacity to reconstruct the problem space and the creativity to find potential solutions to 'wicked problems'. Moreover, health practitioners need to understand that clinical reasoning expertise is dynamic and fluctuates along a spectrum with novice at one end and expert at the other according to the situation, and to take that into account when making clinical decisions. They also need to recognize the potential impact of unchallenged assumptions and beliefs on their decisions.

In Part 2 we also emphasize the *encultured nature* of clinical reasoning. Clinical reasoning is a sophisticated set of capabilities that are deeply contextualized in the health practitioner's discipline, their ways of knowing, their practice model and work setting, and their communities of practice. Finally, and in keeping with the social justice focus of this edition, we present a model of *social justice-oriented* clinical reasoning that challenges readers to reflect on empowerment in clinical practice and its enactment in the clinical reasoning process.

3

CLINICAL REASONING
Challenges of Interpretation and Practice in the Current Era

JOY HIGGS ■ GAIL M. JENSEN

CHAPTER OUTLINE

CHAPTER AIMS

The aim of this chapter is to introduce key themes explored in this book in relation to:

- current understandings of the term and practice of clinical reasoning
- challenges faced by people engaged in decision making
- challenges faced by people engaged in learning and teaching clinical reasoning.

THE PRACTICE OF THE PROFESSIONS

The practice of health professionals is the way they 'walk', 'talk' and 'think' their practice: each of these is linked with clinical reasoning.

Practices are bundles of sayings and doings that have existence beyond the particular individuals engaged in them. The ways practitioners speak about what they do and the actions in which they engage are not matters of individual choice but are an intrinsic feature of the practice itself. Practices connect material conditions with people and with work. They cannot be thought of separately from the conditions in which they exist—abstracting of practice from its context is to no longer have a practice.

(Boud, 2016, p. 160)

'A richer understanding of how capable people do what they do—in workplaces and elsewhere—is necessary if we are to make more sensible use of learning cognitive spaces' (Goodyear, 2019, p. 83). Researchers who are interested in educating people for professional capabilities and professional practice including professional vision are interested in linking closer coupling of the mind, body and world.

UNDERSTANDING CLINICAL REASONING

Clinical reasoning is the core of clinical practice; it enables practitioners to make informed and responsible clinical decisions and address problems faced by their patients or clients. It involves *wise action*, meaning taking the best judged action in a specific context (Higgs, 2016), *professional action* encompassing ethical, accountable and self-regulatory decisions and conduct, and *person-centred action* that demonstrates respect for and collaboration with clients, carers and colleagues.

Simply, clinical reasoning is the thinking and decision-making processes associated with clinical practice; it is a critical capability in the health professions, central to the practice of professional autonomy that permeates clinical practice. However, there are challenges with defining and assessing it (Young et al., 2018; Daniel et al., 2019). At a complex level, clinical reasoning is a multilayered and multicomponent capability that allows practitioners to make difficult decisions in the conditions of complexity and uncertainty that often occur in healthcare. Such decisions require a high level of tolerance of ambiguity, reflexive understanding, practice artistry and collaboration.

There is no single model of clinical reasoning that best, or comprehensively, represents what clinical reasoning is in the contexts of different professions and different workplaces. The reason for this lies in several factors:

- the complex nature of the phenomenon of clinical reasoning and the consequential challenges of understanding, researching, assessing and measuring it
- the context-dependent nature of clinical decision making in action
- the inherent individuality of expertise
- the changing conceptions of quality and error in clinical reasoning
- the challenge to novices in developing clinical reasoning capabilities and to educators in facilitating this development
- the changing volume and nature of the demands of factors influencing healthcare, its costs, its consequences and its modes of operation.

Ratcliffe and Durning (2015, p. 13) provided this overview of clinical reasoning: 'although definitions and descriptions of clinical reasoning entail the cognitive operations allowing clinicians to observe, collect and analyse information, resulting in actions that take into account a patient's specific circumstances and preferences'. They added that 'many scholars now view clinical reasoning as having both cognitive and non-cognitive domains as well as being a social as opposed to an individual construct' (p. 14). These considerations are reflected in the following two definitions.

> *We define clinical reasoning as the cognitive and noncognitive process by which a health care professional consciously and unconsciously interacts with the patient and environment to collect and interpret patient data, weigh the benefits and risks of actions, and understand patient preferences to determine a working diagnostic and therapeutic management plan whose purpose is to improve a patient's well-being.*
> **(Trowbridge et al., 2015, p. xvii).**

Clinical reasoning (or practice decision making) is a context-dependent way of thinking and decision making in professional practice to guide practice actions. It involves the construction of narratives to make sense of the multiple factors and interests pertaining to the current reasoning task. It occurs within a set of problem spaces informed by the practitioner's unique frames of reference, workplace context and practice models, as well as by the patient's or client's contexts. It utilizes core dimensions of practice knowledge, reasoning and metacognition and draws on these capacities in others. Decision making within clinical reasoning occurs at micro, macro and meta levels and may be individually or collaboratively conducted. It involves meta skills of critical conversations, knowledge generation, practice model authenticity and reflexivity (Higgs, 2006).

CHALLENGES FACED BY PEOPLE ENGAGED IN CLINICAL DECISION MAKING

In this section we will explore four key challenges faced by people engaged in clinical decision making:

- dealing with a complex world
- dealing with wicked problems in a world that looks for accountability and evidence clarity
- addressing complex real-world problems, human tasks with consequences for life and quality of life
- dealing with issues associated with sharing decision-making processes and outcomes.

Challenges of Dealing With a Complex World

Bauman's (2000, 2005) 'liquid modernity' metaphor captures the values and desires that characterize the prosperous West today. Casting aside the attitudes that predominated in the second half of the 20th century (such as the vision that puts others first, the sense of mystery of things beyond us and recognition of the fallibility of human knowledge), liquid modernity challenges the ideals of service and moral responsibility of professions in meeting societal needs. Bauman's ideas highlight current trends, such as taking shortcuts to increase perceived efficiencies, outsourcing work and resources provision, being preoccupied with short-term goals and desires instead of long-term pursuits. This is seen in changing consumerist ideas such as replacing long-lasting products with shorter, fixed-term products and changing lifetime employment with casual jobs.

The liquid-modern age pursues instant gratification and constant movement (which goes beyond fluency and flexibility to volatility, fragmentation and short life spans of knowledge, tasks, work groups, etc.). This contrasts with the ongoing commitments of health professionals to patients, to best possible care, to persistence, to resilience, to carefulness and to obligations arising from and through multiprofessional teamwork. Another problem is the changing attitude towards knowledge in the liquid-modern world, where established knowledge and know-how have an increasingly shorter shelf life. Tradition and experience seem to be no longer valued.

A key issue in clinical reasoning is the demand for practitioners to be able to explain professional matters articulately and clearly to all parties and to take proper account of their own values as well as the needs and values of all those involved or influential in patient/client care. Fish and Higgs (2008) contended that responsible members of a profession need to argue their moral position, implement their roles with proper transparency and integrity, and utilize their clinical thinking, professional judgement and practice wisdom in order to serve the needs of differing individuals as well as understanding and working towards the common good.

A second key element of the complexity of the worlds of practice and healthcare today is the digital revolution, which poses both opportunities and challenges to healthcare, clinical reasoning and the making and communication of clinical decisions. Sennett (2005), reviewing culture and society for several decades in Britain and the United States, reflected on the challenges facing us all today due to the unstable, fragmentary conditions in society and work. He contended that not everyone will thrive in the face of 'hot-desking' workplaces and in 'dot.com' modelled hospital and university workplaces. O'Neill (2002) critiqued today's systems of accountability that are driven by the human resources industry and are designed to provide transparent checks on the implementation of change. The critique is that constant checking on people's work progress and outcomes in support of transparency actually damages trust and does not allow change to consolidate. Thibault (2020) identified trends for the future of health professions education including the need for better preparation in collaborative practice; stronger focus on patient, community, chronic disease and social determinants of health; greater emphasis on life-long learning across a career; and integration of information technologies into practice. All of these trends demonstrate the complexity of the world of practice.

Of particular interest, in relation to clinical reasoning, are the strategies and tools that have been developed with the goal of assisting decision making and communication. Studies in this area include the work of Chaudhry et al. (2006) who demonstrated improved quality and efficiency of health information technologies across four benchmark institutions. Buntin et al. (2011) provided support for the adoption of electronic health records and information technology. They found that such tools and strategies had largely positive benefits but that the 'human element' was critical to health information technology implementation. Chau and Hu (2002) examined different theories and strategies for implementing telemedicine; they reported variation in the acceptability of different telemedicine approaches, linked to differences in the essential characteristics of user, technology and context.

Osheroff et al. (2007, p. 141) examined the value of clinical decision support, which provides practitioners, patients and others with 'knowledge and person-specific information, intelligently filtered or presented at appropriate times, to enhance health and healthcare. It encompasses a variety of tools and inter-ventions such as computerized alerts and reminders, clinical guidelines, order sets, patient data reports and dashboards, documentation templates, diagnostic support, and clinical workflow tools'. They concluded that some healthcare institutions achieved positive benefits for knowledge users while others faced prob-lems. The demand for reliable health information to support decisions is being driven by consumerism and moves to shift the cost of care to patients and increase client input to decision making. Koch (2006) raised the concern of the potential negative impact of home telehealth on the patient–provider relation-ship particularly in relation to special user groups, such as people who are elderly or have a disability. She called for further exploration of the use of such strategies.

REFLECTION POINT

- How do you think we should go about linking the headspace of personal reasoning with the ether space of technology-enabled reasoning?
- What experience have you had in this area?
- How would you advise novices about this area?

Challenges in Addressing Wicked Problems and Accountability

Clinical reasoning and decision making is essentially professional problem solving: solving the problem or challenge of making decisions about diagnosis, prog-nosis, treatment options and preferences etc. as a way of informing healthcare actions by practitioners and clients. In Schön (1987) reminded us that the pro-cess of problem setting, i.e. the ability to identify the problem in the swampy lowland of practice, requires seeing the situation or context from multiple frames of reference. Roberts (2000) identifies three types of problems (Box 3.1) with different levels of complexity and solution/management solution.

Wicked problems (Roberts, 2000) have the follow-ing characteristics:

1. There is no definitive statement of the problem; indeed, there is typically broad disagreement on what 'the problem' is.
2. Without a definitive statement of the problem, the search for solutions is open-ended. People

---

BOX 3.1
TYPES OF PROBLEMS

Type 1 problems are 'simple problems' that enjoy a consensus on a problem definition and solution.

Type 2 problems are 'complex problems' that intro-duce conflict to the problem-solving process. Although problem solvers agree on what the prob-lem is, there is no consensus on how to solve it.

Type 3 problems are 'wicked problems' that engender a high level of conflict among the stakeholders. The problem-solving process is not bound; it is experi-enced as ambiguous, fluid, complex, political and frustrating.

Based on Roberts, N., 2000. Wicked problems and network approaches to resolution. Int. Pub. Manag. Rev., 1, pp. 1–19.

---

who have a stake in the problem and its solution, the stakeholders, play various competing and changing roles from their perspectives including framing the problem and supporting and shap-ing different solutions.

3. The problem-solving process is complex because constraints, such as resources and political rami-fications, are constantly changing.
4. Constraints also change because they are gener-ated by numerous interested parties who may bring variable levels of participation to the prob-lem solving and whose input can vary because they change their minds, fail to communicate well and change their frame of reference in addressing the problem.

The very idea of wicked problems runs contrary to the search for 'correct' answers and the unequivocal justification of clinical decisions. Consider diagnos-tic and treatment decisions, for instance. Although in some cases a clear diagnosis is straightforward and necessary, particularly in life-threatening situations, it is often the case that comorbidities exist, the clini-cal condition is rare, unfamiliar or hard to diagnose. Treatment decisions are multifactorial, facing variables such as skill levels of practitioners, available funding, resourcing and client wishes. For instance, a client/patient may aspire to a health and well-being narra-tive that runs contrary to the 'restitution narrative' (i.e. return to normality). The latter is particularly the case for people with chronic health problems (Alder and Horsfall, 2008). Further, decision paradigms and cultures vary across different professions. Again, we see clinical reasoning and decision making as complex phenomena (Young et al., 2018; Koufidis et al., 2022).

REFLECTION POINT

- Where does evidence in support of our decisions fit with these decisions and actions?

Consider the arguments put forward on expertise, on collaborative and transdisciplinary decision making and on clinical reasoning across the professions.

Challenges of Making Complex and Consequential Decisions

Orasanu and Connolly (1993), examining the real world of clinical decision making, described the characteristics of decision making in dynamic settings as follows:

- problems are ill-structured and made ambiguous by the presence of incomplete dynamic information and multiple interacting goals
- the decision-making environment is uncertain and may change while decisions are being made
- goals may be shifting, ill-defined or competing
- decision making occurs in the form of action–feedback loops, where actions result in effects and generate further information that decision makers have to react to, and use, in order to make further decisions
- decisions contain elements of time pressure, personal stress and highly significant outcomes for the participants
- multiple players act together, with different roles
- organizational goals and norms influence decision making.

To work within such a practice world requires an approach to clinical reasoning that accommodates these complexities. Higgs and colleagues (2006) described a number of key characteristics of clinical reasoning needed to address these challenges:

- clinical reasoning as a solo process is a complex, mostly invisible, process that is often largely automatic and therefore not readily accessible to others in practice or research
- clinical reasoning is linked with more visible behaviours such as recording diagnoses and treatment plans in patient histories and communicating treatment rationales in team meetings, case conferences and teaching novices
- clinical reasoning and practice knowledge are mutually developmental; each relies on the other, each gives meaning to the other in the achievement of practice and each is the source of generation and development of the other
- clinical reasoning can be implemented as a sole practitioner process or a group process
- clinical reasoning may be understood as both cognitive and collaborative processes; however, in either case there is a growing imperative, linked to increasing demands for evidence-based practice and public accountability, to make reasoning more explicit
- the idea of evidence means different things in different contexts and paradigms (Turpin and Higgs, 2017); understanding evidence is important when planning to use or require evidence-based practice
- core reasoning abilities, language and interactive behaviours are required for understanding and developing practice knowledge and clinical reasoning
- it is important to understand clinical reasoning behaviours and effectiveness (including the communication of reasoning) in relation to contextual influences, including the practice model that has been chosen or imposed
- clinical reasoning requires a range of capabilities including cognitive, metacognitive, emotional, reflexive and social capabilities
- clinical reasoning is, and for the purposes of quality assurance, should be, a reflexive process which involves practitioner(s) in critical self-reflection and ongoing development of their reasoning abilities, knowledge and communication (of reasoning) abilities.

So, what has the current era brought to this practice space that further challenges clinical reasoning practice? Some of the most critical factors, we believe, include:

- the technological and digital revolutions which have increased the use of high-level technology in healthcare (for those who can afford it) and high-tech communication and decision-making aids in the practice of clinical decision making and its communication. Examples of these trends include robotics, telehealth, use of big data and self-doctoring
- the further erosion of professionalism often linked to a decline in altruism and an increase in self-interest and expectations privilege by practitioners
- an escalation in the demand by patients/clients and carers for respectful and informed participation in clinical decision making. This has been greatly impacted by readily accessible information on the Internet
- globalization (the global spread of capitalism as an economic system) and neoliberalism (the support of a deregulated global market society) have brought increasing emphasis in healthcare (and therefore clinical decision making) on commodification of healthcare, fiscal accountability often in advance of ethical accountability, replacement of service-oriented professionals with business-oriented entrepreneurs, corporatization of professional practices, increasing litigation by consumers and more widespread adoption of systems and practices that shift the economic cost/burden of healthcare to the individual rather than the state
- the immense confusion and conflict arising from the COVID-19 pandemic (Riedel et al., 2022)
- continued growth of team-based care, shared decision making and collaborative practice.

Professionals are under increasing pressure on a number of fronts from higher demands for standards of professional competence and fiscal demands for increased productivity to external regulations that require sound evidence, efficiency and accountability. These challenges also impact professional autonomy and control. Sullivan and Benner (2005, p. 79) described this well: 'the question of how healthcare professionals can function as prudent

CASE STUDY 3.1

Misalignment of Professional Autonomy, Accountability and Evidence

Dan, a newly licensed physical therapist, was working in a clinic where the organization had a clinical standard— to achieve at least 52 minutes and four billable units with each patient. He was told that this was the expectation for maintaining productivity, and that as a skilled clinician he should be able to work with any patient for 52 minutes. If he couldn't, then he should not consider himself a skilled clinician. It did not take long for him to experience moral distress as he was trying to balance his ability to make clinical decisions about patient discharge and accountability for being a good steward of healthcare resources in balance with evidence-based practice guidelines and now organizational expectations. His patient, Joan, had adhesive capsulitis of her shoulder and had reached all of her goals. Joan was well aware of everything she needed to do after therapy, was experiencing no pain, had achieved functional goals and was ready for discharge. Dan ended up keeping the patient for only 30 minutes and was confronted by the clinic manager for not maintaining productivity for that hour with that patient. Dan was following best practice clinical guidelines and believed that as a practising physical therapist, he had professional responsibility for patient-centered quality care along with being a steward of scarce healthcare resources.

managers in the public interest, as well as engaged autonomous professionals, takes on salience in this new environment'. Now more than ever, healthcare professionals need not only strong cognitive and analytical skills but also integrity, individual self-awareness and the ability to engage in clinical reasoning that leads to wise judgement. Consider how you would respond to the situation presented in Case Study 3.1.

Challenges in Sharing Decision-Making Processes and Outcomes

Interprofessional collaboration is being promoted by healthcare organizations, governments and regulatory groups as an important means to addressing many of the complex and wicked problems in caring for patients, improving health organization performance measures, managing escalating costs and improving health outcomes (Frenk et al., 2010; Royeen et al., 2009; Thibault, 2020). (Refer to Chapters 38, 41, 43 and 45 in this book for further work on collaborative decision making.) Professional education accreditation requirements are moving rapidly in response to this need for interprofessional collaboration and setting standards for institutions to demonstrate that graduates are 'collaboration ready' (Prystajecky et al., 2017).

The successful care of patients and communities depends not only on the knowledge and expertise of the individual practitioner but the collective knowledge and distributed intelligence of the interprofessional team (Cooke et al., 2010; Jensen, 2011). This distributed intelligence of the team often requires a process of shared decision making as patients and the interprofessional team members work together in the decision-making process. The development of the specific health profession's clinical reasoning abilities is a central focus in professional education and often leaves little time for an intentional focus on shared decision making. Therefore, it is essential that the development of clinical reasoning from novice to expert has an intentional focus on key concepts. These key concepts include the critical relationship between knowledge restructuring and clinical reasoning and level of expertise, the importance of adaptive expertise and the concept of progressive problem solving, outlined in clinical reasoning expertise.

CHALLENGES FACED BY PEOPLE ENGAGED IN LEARNING AND TEACHING CLINICAL REASONING

In this section we will explore three key challenges faced by people engaged in clinical reasoning and decision making:

- intentionally building clinical reasoning teaching and learning into pressured curricula
- teaching and learning the often more tacit elements in clinical reasoning along with the ambiguous, complex realities and 'wickedness' of clinical reasoning
- learning about how professionals often have to make judgements in uncertain conditions.

REFLECTION POINT

- Which teaching and learning strategies could be used to engage learners in shared decision-making processes?
- How would you apply key ideas for the ongoing development of expertise in clinical reasoning and the concept of adaptive expertise in your clinical teaching?

Building Clinical Reasoning Into Curricula

Health sciences curricula tend to follow a number of patterns: discipline-content driven preclinical and clinical courses, problem-based courses and practice-based curricula. These vary in the attention given to clinical problem solving, clinical reasoning and clinical decision making as part of the curricula. A key goal of this book is to emphasize the importance of overtly and experientially teaching clinical reasoning as part of any curriculum. The last section of the book provides multiple examples of curriculum, learning and teaching approaches adopted across the professions including:

- application of a clinical thinking pathway for surgeons that uses a formulaic approach along with humane and individualistic approaches
- creative strategies such as deconstructing critical events, reflecting on cognitive biases as part of teaching clinical reasoning in nursing
- understanding the centrality of context in the teaching and learning of clinical reasoning in academic and workplace environments as essential.

Teaching and Learning Clinical Reasoning Complexities

We have argued that clinical reasoning – when approached deeply and in many complex circumstances – is a challenging thing to do. Fig. 3.1 illustrates the definition of clinical reasoning by Higgs (2006). This figure shows different types of decisions, multiple decision spaces (Higgs and Jones, 2008), the foundational dimensions of clinical reasoning, the players in the clinical decision-making process and meta processes framing the practices of clinical reasoning and decision making. This, or any other interpretation of clinical reasoning as a complex process, highlights the challenges that even experienced practitioners, let alone novices, face when engaging in this critical component of clinical practice.

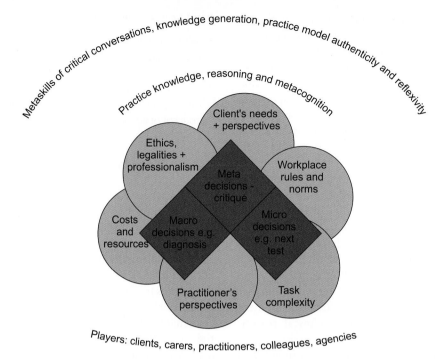

Fig. 3.1 ■ Clinical reasoning: a challenging practice (Higgs, J., 2006. The complexity of clinical reasoning: Exploring the dimensions of clinical reasoning expertise as a situated, lived phenomenon. Seminar Series, Faculty of Health Sciences, The University of Sydney, Australia.)

We also move towards the task of addressing learning clinical reasoning in the final section, from the perspective of providing learning opportunities and activities for learners, ranging from direct clinical experience, to online learning activities and self-directed learning. In each case it is the learner who needs to come to an understanding of what their job requires of them in relation to making clinical decisions, what is expected of them and what the consequences of their reasoning are for their clients, colleagues and themselves, and also which strategies they can adopt as part of their lifelong learning commitment to continue to develop their reasoning abilities. Students and novice professionals often experience insecurities when they become responsible for people's lives and well-being in clinical situations. It takes time to build up the capacity to reason well in situations that are complex and to become confident in performing this core practice.

REFLECTION POINT

As a novice or experienced practitioner reflect on these questions:

- What do I know about clinical reasoning? What does it mean in my practice?
- How well do I reason, not just in terms of avoiding errors and making sound decisions, but also in terms of working across different communities of practice (e.g. within my profession, across work teams, with my clients) as active decision-making participants?
- How can I improve my clinical decision making? What strategies work well for me? Who can I ask for help to further develop my clinical reasoning capability?

SUMMARY

In this chapter we have explored a number of arguments:

- There is no universal model of clinical reasoning that fits all settings, professions and individuals, but we recognize this as a complex phenomenon that includes cognitive and noncognitive processes.
- Dealing with a complex world presents healthcare professionals with wicked problems that

require approaches to clinical reasoning that can accommodate and address these complexities.

- Increasing demands for interprofessional collaboration and client engagement bring the need for greater understanding of shared decision making.
- The challenges in teaching and learning clinical reasoning provide great opportunities for innovation, exploration and assessment of learning.

REFERENCES

Alder, S., Horsfall, D., 2008. Beyond the restitution narrative: Lived bodies and expert patients. In: Higgs, J., Jones, M.A., Loftus, S., Christensen, N. (Eds.), Clinical reasoning in the health professions, 3rd ed. Elsevier, pp. 349–356.

Boud, D., 2016. Taking professional practice seriously: Implications for deliberate course design. In: Trede, F., McEwen, C. (Eds.), Educating the deliberate professional: Preparing for future practice. Springer, pp. 157–173.

Bauman, Z., 2000. Liquid modernity. Polity Press.

Bauman, Z., 2005. The liquid modern challenges to education. In: Robinson, S., Katulushi, C. (Eds.), Values in higher education. Aureus and the University of Leeds, pp. 36–50.

Buntin, M.B., Burke, M.F., Hoaglin, M.C., Blumenthal, D., 2011. The benefits of health information technology: A review of the recent literature shows predominantly positive results. Health Information Technology 30 (3), 464–471. https://doi.org/10.1377/hlthaff.2011.0178

Chau, P.Y.K., Hu, P.J., 2002. Investigating healthcare professionals' decisions to accept telemedicine technology: An empirical test of competing theories. Information & Management 39, 297–311.

Chaudhry, B., Wang, J., Wu, S., Maglione, M., Mojica, W., Roth, E., et al., 2006. Systematic review: Impact of health information technology on quality, efficiency, and costs of medical care. Annals of Internal Medicine 144 (10), 742–752. https://doi.org/10.7326/0003-4819-144-10-200605160-00125

Cooke, M., Irby, D., O'Brien, B., 2010. Educating physicians: A call for reform of medical school and residency. Jossey-Bass.

Daniel, D., Rencic, J., Durning, S.J., Holmboe, E., Santen, S.A., Lang, V., et al., 2019. Clinical reasoning assessment methods: A scoping review and practical guidance. Acad Med. 94 (6), 902–912. https://doi.org/10.1097/ACM.0000000000002618

Fish, D., Higgs, J., 2008. The context for clinical decision making in the 21st century. In: Higgs, J., Jones, M.A., Loftus, S., Christensen, N. (Eds.), Clinical reasoning in the health professions, 3rd ed. Elsevier, pp. 19–30.

Frenk, J., Bhutta, Z., Cohen, J., Crisp, N., Evans, T., Fineberg, H., et al., 2010. Health professionals for a new century: Transforming education to strengthen health systems in an interdependent world. Lancet 376 (9756), 1923–1958. https://doi.org/10.1016/S0140-6736(10)61854-5

Goodyear, P., 2019. Creating productive spaces for developing employability. In: Higgs, J. Crisp, Letts, W. (Eds.), Education for employability, Volume 1. Brill Sense, pp. 83–96.

Higgs, J., 2006, May 5. The complexity of clinical reasoning: Exploring the dimensions of clinical reasoning expertise as a situated, lived phenomenon. Seminar Series, Faculty of Health Sciences, The University of Sydney, Australia.

Higgs, J., 2016. Practice wisdom and wise practice: Dancing between the core and the margins of practice discourse and lived practice. In: Higgs, J., Trede, F. (Eds.), Professional practice discourse marginalia. Sense, pp. 65–72.

Higgs, J., Jones, M.A., 2008. Clinical decision making and multiple problem spaces. In: Higgs, J., Jones, M.A., Loftus, S., Christensen, N. (Eds.), Clinical reasoning in the health professions, 3rd ed. Elsevier, pp. 3–17.

Higgs, J., Trede, F., Loftus, S., Ajjawi, R., Smith, M., Paterson, M., et al., 2006. Advancing clinical reasoning: Interpretive research perspectives grounded in professional practice. CPEA, Occasional Paper 4, Collaborations in Practice and Education Advancement, The University of Sydney, Australia.

Jensen, G.M., 2011. The Forty-Second Mary McMillan Lecture: Learning: What matters most. Physical Therapy 91, 1674–1689. https://doi.org/10.2522/ptj.2011.mcmillan.lecture

Koch, S., 2006. Home telehealth: Current state and future trends. International Journal of Medical Informatics 75 (8), 565–576. https://doi.org/10.1016/j.ijmedinf.2005.09.002

Koufidis, C., Manninen, K., Nieminen, N., Wohlin, M., Silen, C., 2022. Representation, interaction, and interpretation. Making sense of the context in clinical reasoning. Medical Education 56, 98–1009. https://doi.org/10.1111/medu.14545

O'Neill, O., 2002. A question of trust. Polity Press.

Orasanu, J., Connolly, T., 1993. The reinvention of decision making. In: Klein, G.A., Orasanu, J., Calderwood, R., Zsambok, C.E. (Eds.), Decision making in action: Models and methods. Ablex, pp. 3–20.

Osheroff, J.A., Teich, J.M., Middleton, B., Steen, E.B., Wright, A., Detmer, D.E., 2007. A roadmap for national action on clinical decision support. Journal of the American Medical Informatics Association 14 (2), 141–145. https://doi.org/10.1197/jamia.M2334

Prystajecky, M., Lee, T., Abonyi, S., Perry, R., Ward, H., 2017. A case study of healthcare providers' goals during interprofessional rounds. Journal of Interprofessional Care 31 (4), 463–469. https://doi.org/10.1080/13561820.2017.1306497

Ratcliffe, T.A., Durning, S.J., 2015. Theoretical concepts to consider in providing clinical reasoning instruction. In: Trowbridge, R.L., Rencic, J.J., Durning, S.J. (Eds.), Teaching clinical reasoning. American College of Physicians, pp. 13–30.

Riedel, P., Kreh, A., Kular, V., Lieber, A., Juen, B., 2022. A scoping review of moral stressors, moral distress and moral injury in healthcare workers during COVID-19. International Journal of Environmental Research and Public Health 19, 1666. https://doi.org/10.3390/ijerph19031666

Roberts, N., 2000. Wicked problems and network approaches to resolution. International Public Management Review 1, 1–19.

Royeen, C., Jensen, G.M., Harvan, R., 2009. Leadership in interprofessional health education and practice. Jones and Bartlett Learning.

Schön, D., 1987. Educating the reflective practitioner. Jossey-Bass.

Sennett, R., 2005. The culture of the new capitalism. Yale University Press.

Sullivan, W., Benner, P., 2005. Challenges to professionalism: Work integrity and the call to renew and strengthen the social contract of the professions. American Journal of Critical Care 14, 78–84. PMID: 15608113.

Thibault, G., 2020. The future of health professions education: Emerging trends in the United States. FASEB BioAdvances 2 (12), 685–694. https://doi.org/10.1096/fba.2020-00061

Trowbridge, R.L., Rencic, J.J., Durning, S.J., 2015. Introduction/ Preface. In: Trowbridge, R.L., Rencic, J.J., Durning, S.J. (Eds.), Teaching clinical reasoning. American College of Physicians, pp. xvii–xxii.

Turpin, M., Higgs, J., 2017. Clinical reasoning and evidence-based practice. In: Hoffmann, T., Bennett, S., Del Mar, C. (Eds.), Evidence-based practice: Across the health professions. Elsevier, pp. 364–384.

Young, M., Thomas, A., Lubarsky, S., Ballard, T., Gordon, D., Gruppen, L., et al., 2018. Drawing boundaries: The difficulty in defining clinical reasoning. Academic Medicine 93, 990–995. https://doi.org/10.1097/ACM.0000000000002142

4

RE-INTERPRETING CLINICAL REASONING
A Model of Encultured Decision-Making Practice Capabilities

JOY HIGGS

CHAPTER AIMS

The aims of the chapter are:

- to re-interpret clinical reasoning as a complex practice through the lens of enculturation
- to recognize the place of social, practice and epistemic cultures in framing clinical reasoning and decision making
- to explore the connection between clinical reasoning, learning and knowing in practice
- to present a model of clinical reasoning as encultured decision-making practice capabilities.

INTRODUCTION

The complexity of clinical reasoning is inherent in the very nature of the task or challenge, faced by novice and expert alike. This challenge is to process multiple variables, contemplate the various priorities of competing healthcare needs, negotiate the interests of different participants in the decision-making process, inform all decisions and actions with advanced practice knowledge, and make decisions and take actions in the accountable context of professional ethics and community expectations. By encompassing much of what it means to be a professional (autonomy, responsibility, accountability and decision making in complex situations), clinical reasoning is imbued with an inherent mystique. This mystique is most evident in the way expert practitioners make difficult decisions with seemingly effortless simplicity and justification, and in the professional artistry and practice wisdom of experienced practitioners who produce, with humanity and finesse, individually tailored health management plans that address complicated health needs. To address and achieve these professional attributes, clinical reasoning is much more a lived phenomenon, an experience, a way of being and a chosen model of practising than simply a process. It is enacted through a set of capabilities that demonstrate current knowledge and practice expertise as well as the capacity to work in unknown and unpredictable situations.

RE-INTERPRETING CLINICAL REASONING

Many chapters in this book hint at or openly declare the need for re-interpretation of clinical reasoning for multiple reasons including:

- the escalation of research and scholarship on clinical reasoning, which is exploring the complexities and demands of clinical reasoning in a range of human, professional and institutional healthcare spaces
- the far greater current emphasis on shared decision making (among multidisciplinary teams and with clients and carers)
- the quantum shift in the use of technology and digital communication systems to aid the reasoning, communication and collaboration involved in clinical decision making
- the changing local and global contexts of healthcare and decision making including influences and challenges posed by and to evidence-based practice, changing expectations and capacities of healthcare consumers and healthcare economic factors (including escalating healthcare costs, the difficulty and even the impossibility of public funding of healthcare for all citizens, and the large proportion of populations who cannot self-fund their healthcare)
- the multiple levels of complexity inherent currently operating in the COVID-19 pandemic
- the need to see clinical reasoning as knowledge use and development in practice, not the application of prior knowledge to clinical decision making
- the need to view clinical reasoning and decision making as collaborative, holistic practices

actioned by practitioners and clients, assisted by technology as appropriate.

The re-interpretation presented in this chapter builds on the following key arguments:

- **Encultured practice**: Clinical reasoning is a way of thinking and decision making that is developed within the framework of various cultural arenas: the world of healthcare practice and the societal and organizational cultures that shape healthcare practices and systems, the multiple worlds and cultures of healthcare clients and professional practice cultures.
- **Understanding professional practice paradigms**: Clinical reasoning and decision making operate within communities of practice. To operate within these practice communities and their cultures requires a deep understanding of the practice paradigms underpinning them.
- **Knowing, being and identity in practice**: Deliberate choices and ownership by practitioners of their practice models and their approaches to reasoning and collaboration are essential for advanced practice. Informed and owned practice comprises doing, knowing, being and becoming and chosen stances on practice epistemology and practice ontology.
- **Practice-in-action**: Practice actions, knowledge, reasoning and discourse operate symbiotically; they are essential organic aspects of practice-in-action.
- **Pursuing clinical reasoning capability:** Viewed as a capability, clinical reasoning is a journey of development in self-realization, interaction and critical appraisal.

This chapter will extend this discussion and produce a revised definition of clinical reasoning and a model of modes of encultured and contextualized reasoning.

REFLECTION POINT

What do you understand as clinical reasoning? How do you go about incorporating it in your professional practice?

CLINICAL REASONING AS AN ENCULTURED PRACTICE

Clinical reasoning operates within practice settings and multiple cultures including sociopolitical and instructional cultures, client health and well-being contexts and cultures, professional practice cultures and communities of practice. These cultures are created and entered through rich social construction and interaction processes in particular, professionalization of occupations and the professional socialization of individuals entering the profession.

Culture

Culture is the characteristics, social behaviour and customs of a particular group of people (a society, community, ethnic group). It encompasses the beliefs, language, customs and the acquired knowledge of societies, so-named due to their ongoing interaction and patterns of expected social behaviour and organization. Culture is expressed through material forms (technologies, artefacts, tool usage, art and architecture) and non-material forms (politics, mythology and science). It is created and transmitted through social learning in human social groups both as a means of individual enculturation and as a way of maintaining that culture through succeeding generations. Culture can also refer to the set of shared attitudes, values, conventions, goals and social practices that characterize a particular field, discipline, institution or organization.

Sociopolitical and Institutional Cultures Impacting the World of Healthcare Practice

Healthcare practice and decisions occur within complex social, economic, global and political contexts. These contexts reflect a range of influences and trends (Fish and Higgs, 2008) including:

- *Political trends*
  - political and strategic environments that are imbued with a general failure to trust and an aversion to risk
  - a world that is fragmented, complex and uncertain.
- *Global work context trends*
  - an increased emphasis on strategies and operations that are loosely connected and short-term

  - changes in work, communication and service mechanisms linked to the digital revolution, creating unstable, fragmentary conditions (Sennett, 2005) where constant checking of progress creates instability and difficulty to flourish (O'Neill, 2002)
  - the rising demands for accountability for practice that is fiscally, evidentially and ethically defensible and more available with the Internet.
- *Communication and information trends*
  - global mass communication strategies that bring to our urgent attention the latest information and knowledge of practice, technologies, world events and dilemmas
  - escalating client access to Internet information.
- *Knowledge trends*
  - exponential knowledge and technological advances
  - transitory knowledge and the devaluing of history, tradition and practice cultures.
- *Population trends*
  - demographic changes, particularly ageing populations and an increasing number of displaced persons in many areas
  - changing patterns of disease and disability, changing locations for health services provision, an increased focus on chronic diseases and an increase in the need for complex disease management strategies.
- *Individual/lifestyle trends and expectations*
  - limited time for individuality, creativity and practice wisdom
  - increased pressures on health professionals in relation to work and life balance contexts and changing roles and expectations
  - increased client expectations of quality care and participation in clinical decision making.
- *21st Century trend in economic and factors to consider in healthcare costs*
  - the notion of doughnut economics and the influence it has on received costs (Raworth, 2019)
  - the escalating cost of healthcare
  - the poverty of many populations (especially refugees) in addressing healthcare cost.

Practice cultures are shaped by their organization's target groups, goals, structures, operational factors such as hierarchies and power, economic factors, codes of conduct, legal imperatives and the size of the organization. Organizations may be local, national or international, government-operated, public or private funded, and they can focus on primary, secondary or tertiary healthcare. The ongoing debate and pressures from economic versus professionalism imperatives is a key part of institutional healthcare cultures. This debate influences expectations held by clients and colleagues of healthcare professionals, but also expectations of the organization as a whole to provide competent and ethical services to clients.

Client Health and Well-Being Narratives and Horizons

Today we are faced with the changing behaviour and expectations of clients who have much more medical information available to them, the way society is changing (particularly in the West) in relation to the pursuit of health and well-being as a more widespread norm in the face of epidemics such as obesity and diabetes, plus changes in professional practice towards greater recognition of the role clients can play in clinical decision making, as informed experts about their own life and health situations. In addition to bringing these horizons to the decision-making table, patients, particularly those who are suffering from the COVID-19 pandemic and/or who have chronic conditions, are bringing other perspectives and narratives to their healthcare that go beyond the biomedical, cure, illness or restitution narrative. People want to replace 'normal' with 'their normal', 'the professional as expert and the patient as recipient' with 'we both have knowledge to share and perspectives to consider'. Many healthcare clients want to replace 'my role is a passive, compliant patient' with 'since much of my healthcare is in my own time, I need to be informed so that I can take sound and chosen actions' (particularly when discharged early and learning to live with chronic disability or illness).

Professional Practice

Professional practice and healthcare deals with many different challenges, including wicked problems (Roberts, 2000), in a context that looks for accountability and evidence clarity, addresses complex real-world problems, human tasks with consequences for life and quality of life, and deals with issues associated with sharing decision-making processes and outcomes. Within this arena, professions share a number of common characteristics (the expectation of ethical conduct, operation within professional codes of conduct and societal expectations of competence and professionalism) and are increasingly challenged by the complexities of the human world as well as the changing physical and technological worlds.

Yet each profession has its own culture including the norms and realizations of practice, standards, language and modes of communication, tools and artefacts of practice implementation and typical locations and situations of operation. Healthcare comprises a collective of disciplinary and professional cultures and could be thought of as a meta-culture in which key norms and ways of being and doing are manifest. For instance, across healthcare (professions and systems) we recognize the importance of duty of care for individuals and groups participating in healthcare or living in communities where health promotion seeks to impact individual and population health. The potential of healthcare interventions or restrictions to impact on people's lives and well-being is a core dimension of healthcare practice and decision making at broad community and individual levels. Such potential impact demands decisions and decision-making capabilities that are commensurate with quality of life and actions of doing good.

Communities of Practice

Professions, such as the health professions, are communities of practice that occur locally, nationally and globally. Practice communities may operate on a profession-specific or interprofessional basis within organizations. In both cases such communities demonstrate the ability to work collaboratively due to shared discourse, language, goals and practices. These shared artefacts and actions constitute dimensions of culture.

The term *communities of practice* was developed by Lave and Wenger (1991) to describe a theory of social learning that places learning 'in the context of our lived experience of participation in the world' (Wenger, 1998, p. 3). Communities of practice are dynamic and flexible as people arrive and leave and as they become more or less central to the practice of the group. Some communities of practice are formally established and managed, others are more organic and evolve, developing shared purposes based on interests or passions. Underpinning this theory are four premises: (1) people are social beings, (2) knowledge occurs in relation to valued enterprises, (3) knowing results from participating and pursuing ability in these enterprises and (4) learning produces meaningful knowledge.

Two key concepts related to communities of practice (Lave and Wenger, 1991) are:

- *situated learning*, which views learning as part of an activity in the world, in that agent, activity, and the world mutually constitute each other
- *legitimate peripheral participation*, which relates to the contention that for newcomers to a practice community, learning through activity happens legitimately from the periphery towards the core of the community of practice as they progressively become full practitioners and members of the practice community, who are integral to the maturing of the field of practice.

Professionalization and Professional Socialization

Two core processes lead to the emergence of the practice of professionals within practice cultures. First, there is the sociohistorical process of professionalization that transitioned their occupations into professions. These occupations defined and shaped themselves into autoregulated, standard-setting, occupational groups with requirements of educational entry and continued membership. Second, there is the process of professional socialization. This is an acculturation process involving entry education, reflection, professional development and engagement in professional work interactions; it enables the individual's development of the expected capabilities of the profession and a sense of professional identity and responsibility (Higgs et al., 2009). Novices become members of a particular profession, a unique social group, and

learn to be part of the culture of that group with all its privileges, requirements and responsibilities. They learn about, and make commitments to, meeting professional and discipline-specific codes of conduct and practice. Professional socialization also refers to the way in which a profession, through its educators, practitioners and leaders, socializes or inducts new members (Higgs, 2013).

Professional socialization involves both learning through practice communities and learning to be part of communities of practice. In her research on collaboration in healthcare, Croker (2011) found that most health professionals engage with multiple practice communities in their work (e.g. their discipline team, their local work area group such as in a specific workplace, and their broader professional association). Newcomers need to learn how to relate across each of these groups and communities. A key aspect of professional socialization is the way that students develop working relationships with other practitioners and team members from a range of professions.

UNDERSTANDING PROFESSIONAL PRACTICE PARADIGMS

We can relate communities of practice and practice cultures to the notion of paradigms wherein a group of practitioners (who could be researchers in a shared research paradigm or professional/clinical practitioners in a shared practice paradigm) come together to pursue common interests and goals. By sharing cultural norms, knowledge and practices members of the paradigm community function coherently as members of a group who walk, talk and think (reason) in shared, encultured ways. Over time, paradigms evolve their pursuits and methodologies and their goals often become more refined and effective in relation to the interests they serve. Paradigms proliferate and new ones emerge as interests change or evolve. This means that science (including study of the human and the physical worlds) is not static or confined to a single strategy but responds to changing interests.

A key element of learning and working in practice paradigms is recognizing and respecting the profession's practice world view (or practice ontology) and

---

BOX 4.1
ONTOLOGY AND EPISTEMOLOGY: DEFINITIONS

Ontology: What is? What exists? What types of entities really exist? What is reality (like)?

'The theory of existence, or, more narrowly, of what really exists' (Bullock and Trombley, 1999, pp. 608–609).

A branch of metaphysics, ontology 'is the science of *being* in general, embracing such issues as the nature of existence and the categorical structure of reality' (Honderich, 1995, p. 634).

'Derived from the Greek word for *being*, but a 17th century coinage for the branch of metaphysics that concerns itself with what exists' (Blackburn, 1994, p. 269).

'Ontology comes from the Greek "ontos" meaning being and "logos" meaning logic or rationale and means literally the study of being or the study of existence' (Everitt and Fisher, 1995, p. 9).

Epistemology: What is knowledge? What can we know? How do we know what we know? What counts as true knowledge?

The philosophical theory of 'knowledge, which seeks to define it, distinguish its principal varieties, identify its sources, and establish its limits' (Bullock and Trombley, 1999, p. 279).

The branch of philosophy, epistemology 'is concerned with the theory of knowledge. Traditionally, central issues in epistemology are the nature and derivation of knowledge, the scope of knowledge, and the reliability of claims to knowledge' (Flew, 1984, p. 109).

'The term derives from the two Greek words "episteme" meaning knowledge and "logos" meaning logic or rationale. In modern English, epistemology means the theory of knowledge' (Everitt and Fisher, 1995, p. 1).

---

our inquiries and action. Our interests are expressed in our knowledge (which is an activity rather than a static phenomenon) and are evident in the types of questions we ask and the strategies that we apply to search for responses to these questions. Habermas differentiated three interests: technical, practical and emancipatory (Table 4.1). Habermas (1968/1972, p. 308) contended that:

The approach of the empirical-analytic sciences incorporates a technical cognitive interest, that of the historical-hermeneutic sciences incorporates a practical one (and emanates from a concern for understanding); and the approach of critically oriented sciences incorporates emancipatory cognitive interest.

In this table, the three paradigms are interpreted according to: the practice field, interests, ontology, epistemology, methodological tools, knowledge produce, evidence and expertise, and the mode of practice they epitomize. Across the health sciences, practitioners may work in areas that are typically based on the biosciences (e.g. pathology, practices that support the cure and restitution narrative), areas with a wellness orientation (e.g. occupational therapy, narratives based on client-led ability rather than disability narratives) and areas that are collaborative, focussed on rejection of taken-for-granted rules and practices.

Practitioners who want to work deliberately in these paradigms need to pursue practice ontologies and practice epistemologies that match their paradigms. They need to understand these practice philosophy underpinnings and make them part of their being (practice ontology), knowing (practice epistemology), doing (practice embodiment), thinking (practice reasoning) and becoming (practice development). In this way practitioners develop and own their personal ontologies and epistemologies:

- ***Personal ontologies*** refers to *being* in practice, and owning and embodying an ontological world view. The ontological turn involves a shift away from technical rationality and intellectual (cognitive) capacity towards being and becoming in practice.

---

how that is linked to the way knowledge is determined and created within that practice world (or practice epistemology) (Higgs et al., 2004b) (Box 4.1). Being grounded in their own profession's practice, members of the profession typically work across multiple communities of practice with a range of frames of reference (profession-specific, interdisciplinary, organizational and workplace oriented).

Table 4.1 presents a categorization of three practice paradigms (the empirico-analytical, interpretive and critical paradigms) informed by Habermas' concept of interests. According to Habermas (1968/1972), our interests, while often hidden, reflect our specific viewpoints and values and are the motivational aspect of

	PRACTICE PARADIGM		
	Empirico-Analytical Paradigm	Historical-Hermeneutic/Interpretive Paradigm	Critical Paradigm (Critical Science)
Practice field	Natural Sciences Biomedicine	Social Sciences Wellness-oriented healthcare	Critical Science Collaborative healthcare
Interests	Technical cognitive: prediction, objective evidence	Practical cognitive: finding understanding, mediation, consensus	Emancipatory-cognitive: ▪ transformation ▪ emancipation
Ontology approach to defining reality	Positivist/empiricist ontology: the world is objective and lawful; it exists independently of the knowers	Social constructivist ontology: reality is socially constructed Hermeneutic ontology: people are being in the world of social practices and historical contexts	Historical realism: history, social practice and culture shape practice
Epistemology (nature and construction of knowledge)	To positivists knowledge arises from the rigorous application of the scientific method	In the interpretive paradigm, knowledge comprises constructions arising from the minds and bodies of knowing, conscious and feeling beings and is generated through a search for meaning	In the critical paradigm, knowledge: is emancipatory and personally developmental, requires becoming aware of how our thinking is socially and historically constructed
Methodological tools	Controlled observation	Understanding meaning, interpretations of texts	Self-reflection, group critical reflection
Knowledge product	Facts Truths	Intersubjectively negotiated meaning	Critique of natural and social influences Negotiated understanding
Evidence and expertise	Best available external evidence	Individual practice expertise	Respect for expertise of all parties
Practice	Practice is characterized as objective, pure, accountable	Practice is characterized as subjective, emotional, risky	Practice is characterized as collaborative, respectful, self-challenging and transformative

TABLE 4.1
Practice Paradigm

From Higgs, J., Trede, F., Rothwell, R., 2007. Qualitative research interests and paradigms. In: Higgs, J., Titchen, A., Horsfall, D., Armstrong, H. (Eds.), Being critical and creative in qualitative research (pp. 32–42). Hampden Press; Higgs, J., Trede, F., 2010. Philosophical frameworks and research communities. In: Higgs, J., Cherry, N., Macklin, R., Ajjawi, R. (Eds.), Researching practice: A discourse on qualitative methodologies (pp. 31–36). Sense.

This turn is primarily based on the assumption that the knowledge and skills that will be needed in future workplaces cannot be known, in advance, in detail or with any great certainty; thus, attention to 'knowing the world' and 'skills for doing' appears to be an unproductive focus for educating future professionals in higher education. Rather, 'being in the world' – pulling disparate elements of practice together into one 'assemblage of self' – needs to be at the centre of university teaching.
(Markauskaite and Goodyear, 2017, p. 54).

▪ **Personal epistemologies:** Epistemology as a broad concept (Barton and Billett, 2017) refers to the nature and origins of knowledge and encompasses how knowledge is derived, tested and validated. Personal epistemology is about people's way of knowing and how they build their knowledge base from prior experiences, and through their capacities and ongoing negotiations. Such knowledge bases evoke readiness for practice, learning and reasoning, but they can also inhibit these activities if they are narrow or unchanging.

Loftus (2009) identified the substantial influences of sociocultural factors and the personal history and socialization experiences of individual practitioners and students on the way they understood what knowledge is and how they use and name it in practice.

Further depth of information on ontological and epistemological underpinnings of different practice approaches are provided in Box 4.2.

CLINICAL REASONING AND KNOWING IN PRACTICE

Practice and knowledge are reciprocal elements; each forms part of the composite culture of professional practice. One of the responsibilities of professionals is to understand and critique the knowledge they use in practice. Professional knowledge is embedded in and arises from the context of professional practice, particularly the history of ideas and the knowledge

---

BOX 4.2
ONTOLOGIES AND EPISTEMOLOGIES

Ontological or world view perspectives differ across the practice paradigms.

■ In the positivist/empiricist ontological tradition the world is objective, since it is said to exist independently of the knowers, and it consists of phenomena or events which are orderly and lawful.

■ In the constructivist view, knowers are seen as conscious subjects separate from a world of objects; subjects who use knowledge who have theories about their practice and who behave according to tacit rules and procedures. Multiple constructed realities are recognized to occur (i.e. different people have different perceptions of reality through their attribution of meaning to events, meaning being part of the event not separate from it) (Lincoln and Guba, 1985).

■ The social constructivist view contends that reality and knowledge are socially constructed. Reality exists because we give meaning to it (Berger and Luckmann, 1985). Different cultures have different social constructions of reality. Within the interpretive tradition, the world and reality are interpreted by people in the context of historical and social practices.

■ The hermeneutic view arises from the ideas of Heidegger (1962), Merleau-Ponty (1956) and Gadamer (1975). In this hermeneutic view, there is no subject/object split; people are seen as part of the world, being in it and coping with it. They are also seen as beings for whom things have significance and value, having a world of social practices and historical contexts and as being a person in time (Leonard, 1989). This view of people and the world is a relational one (Benner and Wrubel, 1989). Unlike the constructivist view of knowledge, this knowing has no mental representation and may be embodied, that is, known by the body without cognition.

■ The (historical) realist is concerned with social structures and how macro- and micro-political, historical and socioeconomic factors influence our lives.

Epistemological perspectives or stances within research paradigms are portrayed as follows:

■ To positivists or empiricists, knowledge arises from the rigorous application of the scientific method and is measured against the criteria of objectivity, reliability and validity. In the empirico-analytical paradigm, knowledge is discovered (i.e. universal and external truths are grasped and justified), arises from empirical processes that are reductionist, value neutral, quantifiable, objective and operationalizable; statements are valid only if publicly verifiable by sense data.

■ The idealist approaches of Wilhelm Dilthey (1833–1911) and Max Weber (1864–1920) focussed on interpretive understanding (Verstehen), accessing the ideas and experiences of actors, as opposed to the explanatory and predictive approach of the physical sciences (Smith, 1983). This perspective results in a focus on human behaviour as occurring within a context and the understanding or knowledge of human behaviour as requiring an understanding of this context.

■ Constructivists view knowledge as 'an internal construction or an attempt to impose meaning and significance on events and ideas. In this perspective each person constructs a more-or-less idiosyncratic explanatory system of reality' (Candy, 1991, p. 251).

■ The social constructionist approach (McCarthy, 1996) construes knowledge as a changing and relative phenomenon and examines the social and historical constructs of knowledge in terms of what knowledge is socially produced and what counts as knowledge.

■ The (historical) realist is concerned with how we understand our lives in the context of sociocultural, historical influences. Knowledge is always influenced by social interest. In the critical paradigm, knowledge is emancipatory and personally developmental, requires becoming aware of how our thinking is socially and historically constructed and how this limits our actions, enables people to challenge learned restrictions, compulsions or dictates of habit, is not grasped or discovered but is acquired through critical debate, promotes understanding about how to transform current structures, relationships and conditions that constrain development and reform (Higgs and Titchen, 1995).

of society (Higgs et al., 2004a). The development of practice knowledge occurs within a variety of contexts including: the historical era and the cultural, social and individual perspectives of practitioners, scholars and researchers engaged in the exploration of practice and practice knowledge.

Professions evolve in sociocultural, political and historical frames of reference. Traditionally, Western thought has been dominated by the Cartesian notions that reasoning and knowing are essentially activities of individuals operating in isolation. Vygotsky (1978, 1986) and Bakhtin (1986) have challenged this idea. They argued that reasoning and knowing begin as activities embedded in social interaction and they are primarily intersubjective processes arising within cultures. We become acculturated into societies that provide us with a cognitive toolkit of knowledge and ways of using such knowledge. Professional education and training are primarily about socializing students into particular ways of knowing and thinking about the world of practice. In Vygotskian terms, professional ways of thinking and knowing are higher mental functions. Vygotsky (1978) claimed that higher mental functions, which would include clinical reasoning, are qualitatively different from lower mental functions and cannot be reduced to them. Higher mental functions need a different conceptual framework, one that takes into account their cultural and historical nature.

Professional Practice Knowledge

Professional practice knowledge evolves as a consequence of the critical use and reflection on the profession's knowledge and practice by individual professionals and the profession collectively. The exploration of the *history of ideas* (Berlin, 1979) within a practice can assist practitioners to contextualize their understanding of contemporary practice and enhance their ability to develop their knowledge and practice effectively. The discipline of the history of ideas was popularized by the American philosopher Arthur Lovejoy (1873–1962) in the 1920s (Kelley, 1990). The term *history of ideas* encompasses approaches to study that centre on how the meaning and associations of ideas change according to history (Burke, 1988). Lovejoy (1936) argued that we understand ourselves better by understanding the ways in

which we have evolved or the manner in which we have come, over time, to hold the ideas that we do. History needs to be concerned with ideas that attain a wide diffusion and to cross barriers between different disciplines and thinking, recognizing the fact that ideas that emerge at any one time usually manifest themselves in more than one direction (Lovejoy, 1936). A history of ideas approach allows us to understand the origins of ideas and place our own ideas in perspective (Adams, 1987).

Learning, both formal and self-directed, involves understanding how knowledge of the discipline is created and used in practice. Epistemology and disciplinarity are related; both are concerned with knowledge and the adaptation of knowledge in particular situations of practice (Barton and Billett, 2017). Building disciplinary knowledge, similarly, requires this understanding, as well as a recognition of how knowledge in the discipline and practice community is created, tested and validated.

Table 4.2 provides an overview of different ways of categorizing knowledge. This work illustrates how important knowledge is in practice and how much work over time has been spent by many scholars in recognizing different ways knowledge is created and used in practice. We need multiple forms of knowledge including the scientific knowledge of human behaviour and body responses in health and illness, the aesthetic perception of significant human experiences, understanding of the uniqueness of the self and others and their interactions, and an appreciation of morality and ethics. According to Kemmis and Smith (2008, p. 4) praxis 'is action that *is morally-committed and oriented and informed by traditions in a field.* It is the kind of action people are engaged in when they think about what their action will mean *in the world.* Praxis is what people do when they take into account all the circumstances and exigencies that confront them at a particular moment and then, taking the broadest view they can of what it is best to do, they act.' Clinical reasoning is embedded in praxis. In the following text, praxis is seen as a core aspect of advanced practice, both due to the expertise required to engage deeply in praxis and because it epitomizes practice that embodies ethics and morality as well as professional capabilities.

TABLE 4.2
Knowledge Categorizations

Plato (400 BC) (P) Aristotle (300 bc) (A) (in Gustavsson, 2004)*	Vico (in Berlin, 1979)	Kolb (1984)	Carper (1978) Sarter (1988)	Reason and Heron (1986)	Higgs and Titchen (1995)	Bereiter (2002) Eraut (1994, 2010)
Epistémé (P) (A) Objective knowledge, represents scientific knowledge, theoretical knowledge	Deductive knowledge: things that are true either by definition or by deduction from propositions or assumptions that are themselves true purely by definition		Interpretive knowledge (philosophical analysis)	Propositional knowledge: knowledge of things, gained through conversation, reading, etc.	Propositional knowledge: knowledge derived through research and/or scholarship; it is formal, explicit and exists in the public domain. It may be expressed in propositional statements that describe relationships between concepts or cause–effect relationships, thus permitting claims about generalizability. Or it may be presented in descriptive terms that allow for transferability of use.	Public knowledge (Bereiter, 2002) Theoretical/propositional knowledge (Schön, 1995)
	Scientific knowledge requires objectively valid, reliable and reproducible evidence. Only evidence gained by the senses, through observation, description and measurement, may be counted. Knowledge remains 'true' only for as long as it is not objectively refuted; when it fails the crucial test, it becomes obsolete, to be replaced by a superior formula/findings.		Empirical knowledge			

Continued

TABLE 4.2
Knowledge Categorizations—cont'd

Plato (400 BC) (P) Aristotle (300 bc) (A) (in Gustavsson, 2004)*	Vico (in Berlin, 1979)	Kolb (1984)	Carper (1978) Sarter (1988)	Reason and Heron (1986)	Higgs and Titchen (1995)	Bereiter (2002) Eraut (1994, 2010)
Téchnē (A) Knowledge used in the process of producing, manufacturing and creating products	Experiential knowledge is gained by personal experience. Some crucially important human knowledge exists that is distinct from and not reducible to either scientific or deductive knowledge	Experiential knowledge: concrete experience, reflective observation, abstract conceptualization, active experimentation	Aesthetic knowledge (artistic) pattern of knowing, derived from experience Personal pattern of knowing self Ethical (moral) pattern of knowing	Nonpropositional (a) Experiential knowledge from direct encounters with persons, places/things (b) Practical knowledge gained through activity and related to skills or competencies	Nonpropositional/ experience-based (a) Professional craft knowledge can be tacit and is embedded in practice; it comprises general professional knowledge gained from health professionals' practice experience and also specific knowledge about a particular client in a particular situation. (b) Personal (individual) knowledge includes the collective knowledge held by the community and culture in which the individual lives and the unique knowledge gained from the individual's life experience.	Collaborative knowledge building and knowledgeability: (stable, episodic, implicit, impressionistic, regulative) (Bereiter) Professional personal knowledge and capability: codified knowledge, accumulated memories, personal understandings, self-knowledge, metaprocesses and know-how (Eraut) Knowing in action (Schön, 1995) Actionable knowledge (Argyris, 1999) Working knowledge (Yinger and Hendricks-Lee, 1993)
Phrónēsis (A) Practical knowledge or wisdom used in the process of social interaction; incorporates ethical understanding of the values and norms that help people frame their ideas of a good life						

From Higgs, J., Jones, M., Titchen, A., 2008. Knowledge, reasoning and evidence for practice. In: Higgs, J., Jones, M., Loftus, S., Christensen, N. (Eds.), Clinical reasoning in the health professions (Third ed., pp. 151–161). Elsevier.

Developing Intellectual Virtues

Another way of revealing advanced and deliberately known practice is via Aristotle's (transl. 1999) three intellectual virtues or excellences of mind:

- *Epistêmê* is an intellectual virtue characterized as scientific, universal, invariable, context-independent knowledge. The concept is reflected in the terms *epistemology* and *epistemic*.
- *Téchnê* refers to craft or applied practice; it is an intellectual virtue characterized as context-dependent, pragmatic, variable, craft knowledge; it is governed by a conscious goal and it is oriented towards practical instrumental rationality. The concept is reflected in terms such as *technique*, *technical* and *technology*.
- *Phrónêsis* refers to practical wisdom; it is an intellectual virtue characterized by values and ethics. It involves value-based deliberation and practical judgement. It is reflective, pragmatic, variable, context-dependent and action-oriented.

These ways of knowing provide a useful point of reflection on reasoning in practice – what it is and what it can be, when knowingly practised. These virtues ask learners and practitioners to think deeply about what knowledge is, how it links to professionalism and how knowledge, reasoning and action combine in practice and to engage with these ways of knowing, doing, being and becoming in practice (Higgs, 1999; Higgs and Titchen, 2001).

Epistemic Cultures

According to Nerland and Jensen (2014; Nerland, 2016, p. 137) 'professions can be regarded as distinct knowledge cultures, constituted by a set of knowledge processes and practices that define expertise in the given area and serve to distinguish professional practitioners from other actors'. Nerland (2016) argued that to contend with the challenges related to knowledge and practice conventions faced by professional communities today, we need a perspective that accounts for multiple and dynamic dimensions of knowledge. This would involve adopting a critically reflexive approach to the use and development of knowledge processes and development practices.

Knorr Cetina (2007) contends that different expert cultures produce knowledge in distinctly different ways and she introduced the concept of epistemic cultures to represent the way that such expert and professional cultures generate and use their knowledge. She uses the term *machinery of knowledge construction* to encompass:

sets of practices, arrangements and mechanisms bound together by necessity, affinity and historical coincidence which, in a given area of professional expertise, make up how we know what we know (Knorr Cetina, 2007, p. 363).

The notion of *epistemic culture* is a rich and deep way of understanding the worlds of practice and how the discourse of practice knowledge and knowledge-grounded practice cohabit these worlds symbiotically. Epistemic cultures comprise both knowledge as practised and the disciplinary, expert-framed and social cultural settings in which knowledge and practices interact for the benefit of the participants in these cultures. Professional cultures are thus enacted and embodied through the group or profession as well as by individual practitioners. This enactment involves a critical living dialogue that occurs between practice knowledge, practice actions and practice reasoning, with each of these three existing as evolving dimensions of living practice in changing social practice arenas.

Epistemic Fluency

Beyond and within epistemic cultures we come to the idea of *epistemic fluency* (Goodyear and Zenios, 2007). Goodyear and Ellis (2007) build on the work of Morrison and Collins (1996, p. 109) who provide Collins' key terms: *epistemic forms* to refer to 'target structures that guide inquiry' and *epistemic games* to refer to 'sets of moves, constraints, and strategies that guide the construction of knowledge around a particular epistemic form'. Epistemic forms include taxonomies, models and lists. Engaging in epistemic games in one's own disciplinary field (and others) helps to build capacity to perform strategies linked to the inquiry structures of that field and others; the latter helping the learner to gain an appreciation of how others develop and use knowledge.

The concept and practice of epistemic fluency is described by Markauskaite and Goodyear (2017, p. 1) as follows: 'people who are flexible and adept with respect to different ways of knowing about the world can be said to possess epistemic fluency'. The idea of fluency, typically applied to language, the spoken word and interactive communication, is particularly useful when thinking about knowledge and clinical reasoning. First, it refers to having a command of the language and experienced practitioners with advanced clinical reasoning capabilities need to have this ability. Technical language provides the means and tools for communicating with colleagues using the rich knowledge and shared understanding embedded in discipline-specific and generic healthcare language. It is used to record notes in patient histories, write reports to referring practitioners, record information for legal or historical records and present new ideas such as research findings for the critical appraisal of the professional and scientific communities. Interpersonal (professional) language is a means for performing the actions of practice such as taking a patient's history and seeking feedback about changes in symptoms during treatments, a way of sharing viewpoints and discussing treatment options, and a tool for communicating findings, decisions, diagnoses and so on.

Linking this fluency to knowledge construction and co-construction and the derivation of knowledge from practice, we can recognize how clinical reasoning and decision making rely on epistemic fluency. Both reasoning and decision making involve understanding knowledge, appreciating different ways of knowing, using different sources and forms of knowledge in reasoning and placing different knowledge (including client's knowledge) as the influences and benchmarks that drive and determine decisions. We can think of epistemic fluency within clinical reasoning as a capability that is most clearly demonstrated by experienced and expert practitioners. Overall practice capability requires clinical reasoning fluency.

Developing Epistemic Fluency and Reasoning Conversation Capability

If we acknowledge that living cultures exist in healthcare, we recognize that culture requires communication and decision making requires conversations. At the very least these practice conversations involve the ascertainment of patients'/clients' needs/goals/expectations and practitioners'/professionals' expert input to decision making and treatment advice. Frequently,

professional practice also involves conversations and collaborative decision making among practitioners who share case management responsibilities. Ideally, practice involves conversations that incorporate and respect the multiple cultures, expert and self-knowledge perspectives of the decision-making participants (including the patients/clients and carers) and the perspectives and prerogatives of each player. In this way, rich collaborative clinical decision making is both encultured and conversational.

PURSUING CLINICAL REASONING CAPABILITY

Too often clinical reasoning is simply thought of as a process of thinking or a set of decisions that need to be made. Instead, clinical reasoning needs to be recognized as capability or a set of capabilities.

Capability refers to practice-grounded ability that is demonstrable and justifiable (Stephenson, 1998); it goes beyond technical competence and encompasses agency, ingenuity and confidence in actions including decision making, problem identification and problem solving. Capability places emphasis on being able to perform well in both known and unknown contexts and the capacity to solve complex as well as more straightforward clinical problems. Capability is required in both task and relationship aspects of practice, in working effectively with others, and confidence in the ability to navigate unfamiliar circumstances and learn from these experiences.

'Capability is a holistic concept which encompasses both current competence and future development through the application of potential. The concept is applicable across both individuals and organisation' (Cairns and Stephenson, 2009, p. 16). The three key elements of capability are: ability (current competence and perceived potential), self-efficacy (confidence in capacity to perform tasks) and values (particularly the way actions in uncertain conditions are guided by values and the capacity to articulate values).

Capability (encompasses):

- the capacity to operate in both familiar and unfamiliar circumstances
- the utilisation of creativity and imagination/innovation

- being mindful about change and open to opportunities/uncertainties
- being confident about one's abilities
- being able to engage with the social values relevant to actions
- engaging with learning as a self-directed process
- operating to formulate and solve problems.

(Cairns and Stephenson, 2009)

In the re-interpretation of clinical reasoning presented in this chapter, clinical reasoning is viewed as a set of capabilities that are cognitive, embodied, owned, collaborative and critical. Each of these words reminds us of the contexts, cultures, communities and challenges that have been presented above and they epitomize the essential responsibilities of professionals to draw all of their knowledge, reasoning and technical capabilities together in practice that is of high quality in conditions of uncertainty as well as conditions of greater simplicity, whether these situational dimensions are due to the inherent nature of the practice-reasoning task, setting, decision-making practice or the setting.

The idea of capability is strongly supported in education and other forms of practice. Eraut (2000, p. 128), for example, identifies capability as a core element in choosing an appropriate cognitive approach in given situations. He raises the question: 'What factors are likely to affect the mode of cognition employed by a particular practitioner in a particular context?' The answer, he argues, includes:

- task factors: evidence, complexity,
- practitioner factors: capability and disposition,
- contextual factors: time available and the crowdedness of the situation (the number of clients, activities, pieces of information, etc., that are competing for the practitioner's attention).

Eraut (2000) contends:

- an analytic approach is appropriate where there is 'sufficient research evidence available in which the practitioner has confidence, the problem being capable of being represented in a form which enables it to be "solved" mainly on the basis of that evidence, and the practitioner being

willing and able to do the analysis and implement the results'
- an intuitive approach is appropriate when 'the practitioner has considerable experience of similar situations'
- a deliberative approach is appropriate when the practitioner 'has both some evidence and some relevant experience, a willingness to reflect and consult and a sense of what is possible under the circumstances'.

Fig. 4.1 draws together the arguments presented earlier, in an interpretation of clinical reasoning capability, built around an encultured view of clinical reasoning that is embodied and enacted in health professional practice.

The evolution of clinical reasoning capability requires practitioners to pursue a deep understanding of reasoning as a complex arena of practice, to recognize the inherent contextualization of clinical reasoning, to value different approaches to reasoning suited to the reasoner's learning readiness, to develop advanced ability and fluency in the language and articulation of reasoning with diverse clinical decision-making partners, and to use learning strategies that draw each of these abilities and understandings into practice.

REFLECTION POINT

- How do you interpret each of the dimensions and considerations of capability presented in Fig. 4.1?
- Do they feature in your reasoning practices?

REDEFINING CLINICAL REASONING AS A RANGE OF ENCULTURED DECISION-MAKING CAPABILITIES

In this section I present my model and definition of clinical reasoning and decision making reconceptualized as a set of encultured decision-making capabilities. This definition and model build on my 25 years of extensive research and scholarship on clinical reasoning. Of particular interest in my research and education have been: the nature of practice knowledge; multiple ways of knowing; communities of practice; the symbiosis of practice knowledge and research; philosophical views of knowledge and practice; and the power of the

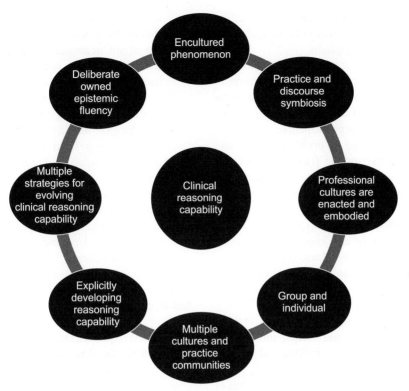

Fig. 4.1 ▓ Clinical reasoning capability.

lenses of capability and enculturation. International leaders in clinical reasoning research, scholarship and education have debated with me about the nature of clinical reasoning and how it operates in and emerges from practice. These rich debates have enriched my journey of understanding of this fascinating and vital component of professional practice.

A Revised Interpretation of Clinical Reasoning and Decision Making

Clinical reasoning is a multilayered, context-dependent way of thinking and decision making in professional practice that is embedded and enacted in health professional practice through epistemic-ontological cultures.

The **purpose** of clinical reasoning is to make sound, client-centred decisions (preferably *with* clients), guide practice stances, actions and trajectories, and optimize client health and well-being choices, pathways and outcomes.

Its key **dimensions** are the generation and use of practice knowledge, reasoning capabilities and metacognition.

It involves **metaskills** of reflexivity, knowledge generation through practice, ongoing learning and reasoning refinement, practice model authenticity constructed narratives and critical, creative conversations. The construction of **narratives** helps to make sense of the multiple factors and interests pertaining to the current reasoning task. The pursuit of **conversations** among colleagues, clients and carers helps to construct client-optimal decisions and particularized healthcare pathways. Such conversations occur when clinical reasoning is viewed as a contextualized interactive phenomenon rather than a specific process. Practitioners interact both with the task/informational elements of decision making and with the human/collaborative elements and the interests of the various decision-making participants. These conversations involve interactions based on critical appraisal of circumstances and, where possible, critical interests in promoting emancipatory practice, and the creation and implementation of particularized, person-centred healthcare programs.

It is **framed** by, and embodied in, the epistemic (knowledge) and ontological (world view) cultures of practice communities, professionalism, ethical codes of practice, community and client expectations and the needs and perspectives of its participants.

It occurs within a range of **problem spaces** and contexts framed by the unique frames of reference (interests, knowledge, abilities, values, experience) of the practitioners, patients/clients, carers and organizations involved.

It draws on **evidence** to support decision making that takes a range of forms and importance including clinical data, experience-based illness scripts (qualitative and quantitative), research findings, theoretical arguments and professional experience theorizations (Higgs, 2017; 2018).

It incorporates **judgement** and decision making at micro (e.g. deciding on next steps, interpreting observed symptoms), macro (e.g. making and producing diagnoses, treatment plans) and meta (e.g. metacognitive critique of decisions in action, evaluation of proposed actions and outcome suitability and quality) levels. Judgement is both a verb (practise, process) and a noun (product and responsibility).

It may be **individually or collaboratively** conducted. Teams are often interdisciplinary and ideally involve the client (and carers). Shared reasoning and decision making values the different inputs (knowledge, interests, perspectives) that each player bring to decision making, particularly the client.

Advanced clinical reasoning involves moving beyond the acts of clinical decision making through the pursuit of epistemic and ontological **fluency** and the informed use of the language of clinical reasoning across cultures, to enhance clinical reasoning in action as an embodied, reflexive and interactive capability that is realized through clinical decision-making conversations.

A Model of Clinical Reasoning as Encultured Decision Making (Fig. 4.2)

This model is framed by four factors:

- the task facing the decision maker(s) (left-hand side) ranging from highly complex, challenging tasks to straightforward tasks. In the centre of this continuum lie fluctuating tasks
- the 'scene' or context (right-hand side) ranging from highly fluid settings where multiple factors influence the decision-making challenge to stable, predictable situations. In the centre of this continuum lie changeable situations
- the decision-making approach (upper continuum) ranging from discipline-based, autonomous approaches to life-based, interdependent approaches
- the decision makers (lower continuum) ranging from individual and teams of professionals who lead the clinical decision making to community-based decision-making groups (including practitioners and clients).

There are five decision-making approaches identified by colours to reflect the approach:

- WHITE (Novice) Decision Making: this approach matches the demands of (more) straightforward reasoning tasks in relatively stable and predictable settings. It is typical of novices who adopt a deliberate, explicit, and studied approach to reasoning (e.g. hypothetico-deductive reasoning), and work individually or in professional teams; it relies on emerging disciplinary knowledge. This approach draws on *téchnê* and *epistêmê* intelligences.
- PURPLE (Expert) Decision Making: this approach matches the demands of (more) complex and challenging reasoning tasks in relatively fluid settings influenced by multiple factors. It is typical of acknowledged, expert clinical reasoners who adopt a complex reasoning approach to reasoning (e.g. pattern recognition) and the use of instantiated scripts (Boshuizen and Schmidt, 1992) and deep rich knowledge bases. They work individually or in professional teams. This approach draws on *epistêmê* and the embedded ethicality and depth of embodied practice or *praxis*. It demands high-level fluency and rich technical, professional, critical, epistemic, ontologic and interpersonal capability.
- ORANGE (Coconstructed) Decision Making: this approach emphasizes the demands of recent times where clients are better informed and

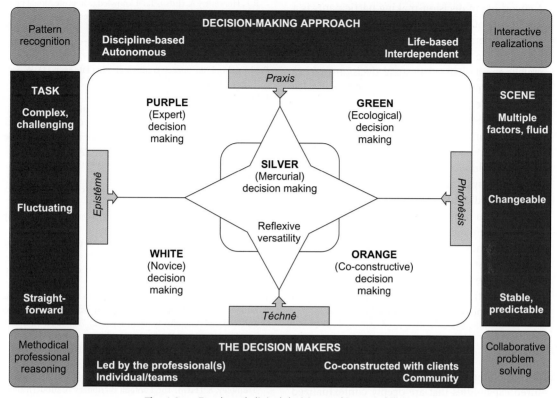

Fig. 4.2 ▨ Encultured clinical decision-making capabilities.

agentic than ever before. It can work well within the demands of (more) straightforward reasoning tasks in relatively stable and predictable settings. It may involve decision making with individual clients, groups or communities. The key element that influences this approach is co-constructed and interdependent decision making, aiming to pursue life-based rather than clinically-oriented decisions. This approach draws on *téchnê* and *phrónêsis*. It requires a willingness to share expert knowledge and capabilities with clients and a commitment to valuing the perspectives and input of others.

- GREEN (Ecological) Decision Making: this approach matches the demands of (more) complex and challenging reasoning tasks in relatively fluid settings, influenced by multiple factors. It is typical of highly experienced but nontraditional practitioners who focus on the complexity of

practice and community settings where individuals or groups of clients are looking for different narratives and solutions. The term ecological has been attached to this approach to highlight the interdependence of the decision-making parties and the need for mutual respect between them for their different perspectives and contributions. The processes of 'green' decision making are inherently dynamic and emergent. This approach draws on a strong ability in *phrónêsis* and the embedded ethicality and depth of embodied practice or *praxis*. It demands high-level (individual and collective) epistemic and ontological fluency and rich critical, technical, professional, epistemic, ontologic and interpersonal capability on the part of practitioners, as well as a willingness to share expert knowledge and capabilities with clients and a commitment to valuing the perspectives and input of others in order to realize optimal solutions to the challenges posed. Networking of decision-making participants is a key feature of this approach to decision making.

- SILVER (Mercurial) Decision Making: this is placed at the centre of the four continua, deliberately emphasizing that some decision-making approaches need to be highly versatile, reflexive and dynamic. This approach draws on *epistêmê*, *phrónêsis*, *téchnê* and *praxis* in varying ways, depending on the task, setting, practice and players. The approach is included in this model to recognize that clinical decision-making situations and players are not static and the approaches adopted need to be knowingly responsive to these changes or at times driving context changes. This approach demands a high level of reflexivity, versatility, fluency and rich technical, professional, critical, epistemic, ontologic and interpersonal capability, a willingness to share expert knowledge and capabilities with clients and a commitment to valuing the perspectives and input of others.

SUMMARY

Clinical reasoning is a sophisticated set of reflexive, encultured capabilities that are deeply contextualized in the reasoner's discipline, their ways of knowing, their owned practice model and in their work setting across multiple communities of practice. Somewhere on the journey from learning clinical reasoning as a systematic, conscious, risk-managed, novice-oriented process to the highly attuned wise practice of professional experts, practitioners should come to appreciate clinical reasoning as the most critical, integrative dimension and capability of professional practice.

REFLECTION POINT

- At the end of this chapter reflect back on what you have learned and understood more deeply about the capabilities you need for clinical reasoning.
- How might these insights influence your reasoning and practice?

REFERENCES

Adams, J., 1987. Historical review and appraisal of research on learning, retention, and transfer of human motor skills. Psychological Bulletin 10 (1), 41–74.

Argyris, C., 1999. Tacit knowledge in management. In: Sternberg, R.J., Horvath, J.A. (Eds.), Tacit knowledge in professional practice: Researcher and practitioner perspectives. Lawrence Erlbaum Associates, pp. 123–140.

Aristotle, 1999. Nicomachean ethics (T. Irwin, Transl.). Hackett Publishing.

Bakhtin, M., 1986. Speech genres and other late essays (V.W. McGee, Transl.). University of Texas Press.

Barton, G., Billett, S., 2017. Personal epistemologies and disciplinarity in the workplace: Implications for international students in higher education. In: Barton, G., Hartwig, K. (Eds.), Professional learning in the workplace for international students: Exploring theory and practice. Springer, pp. 98–111.

Bereiter, C., 2002. Education and mind in the knowledge age. Lawrence Erlbaum Associates.

Berger, P., Luckmann, T., 1985. The social construction of reality. Penguin.

Benner, P., Wrubel, J., 1989. The primacy of caring: Stress and coping in health and illness. Addison-Wesley.

Berlin, I., 1979. Against the current: Essays in the history of ideas. The Hogarth Press. ISBN: 9780701204396

Blackburn, S., 1994. The Oxford dictionary of philosophy. Oxford University Press.

Boshuizen, H.P.A., Schmidt, H.G., 1992. On the role of biomedical knowledge in clinical reasoning by experts, intermediates and novices. Cognitive Science 16 (2), 153–184. https://doi.org/10.1016/0364-0213(92)90022-M

Bullock, A., Trombley, S., 1999. The new Fontana dictionary of modern thought, 3rd ed. Harper Collins.

Burke, P., 1988. History of ideas. In: Bullock, A., Stallybrass, O., Trombley, S. (Eds.), The Fontana dictionary of modern thought, 2nd ed. Fontana, p. 388.

Cairns, L., Stephenson, J., 2009. Capable workplace learning. Sense.

Candy, P.C., 1991. Self-direction for lifelong learning. Jossey-Bass.

Carper, B.A., 1978. Fundamental patterns of knowing. Advances in Nursing Science 1, 13–23. https://doi.org/10.1097/00012272-197810000-00004

Croker, A., 2011. Collaboration in rehabilitation teams (Doctoral dissertation, Charles Sturt University, Australia).

Eraut, M., 1994. Developing professional knowledge and competence. Falmer Press.

Eraut, M., 2000. Non-formal learning and tacit knowledge in professional work. British Journal of Educational Psychology 70, 113–136. https://doi.org/10.1348/000709900158001

Eraut, M., 2010. Knowledge, working practices and learning. In: Billett, S. (Ed.), Learning through practice: Models, traditions, orientations and approaches. Springer, pp. 37–58.

Everitt, N., Fisher, A., 1995. Modern epistemology: A new introduction. McGraw Hill.

Fish, D., Higgs, J., 2008. The context for clinical decision making in the twenty-first century. In: Higgs, J., Jones, M., Loftus, S., Christensen, N. (eds.), Clinical reasoning in the health professions, 3rd ed. Elsevier, pp. 19–30.

Flew, A. (Ed.), 1984. A dictionary of philosophy, 2nd ed. Pan.

Gadamer, H.-G., 1975. Hermeneutics and social science. Cultural Hermeneutics 2, 307–316. https://doi.org/10.1177/019145377500200402

Goodyear, P., Ellis, R., 2007. The development of epistemic fluency: Learning to think for a living. Sydney University Press.

Goodyear, P., Zenios, M., 2007. Discussion, collaborative knowledge work and epistemic fluency. British Journal of Educational Studies 55 (4), 351–368. http://www.jstor.org/stable/4620577

Gustavsson, B., 2004. Revisiting the philosophical roots of practical knowledge. In: Higgs, J., Richardson, B., Abrandt Dahlgren, M. (Eds.), Developing practice knowledge for health professionals. Butterworth-Heinemann, pp. 35–50.

Habermas, J., 1968/1972. Knowledge and human interest (J.J. Shapiro, Transl.). Heinemann.

Heidegger, M., 1962. Being and time. Harper & Row.

Higgs, J., 1999, September. Doing, knowing, being and becoming in professional practice. Proceedings of the Master of Teaching Post Internship Conference. The University of Sydney.

Higgs, J., 2013. Professional socialisation including COP. In: Loftus, S., Gerzina, T., Higgs, J., Smith, M., Duffy, E. (Eds.), Educating health professionals: Becoming a university teacher. Sense, pp. 83–92.

Higgs, J., 2017. Clinical reasoning: Conversations in epistemic cultures. Pédagogie Médicale 18 (2), 51–53. https://doi.org/10.1051/pmed/2018004

Higgs, J., 2018. Judgment and reasoning in professional contexts. In: Lanzer, P. (Ed.), Textbook of catheter-based cardiovascular interventions, 2nd ed. Springer, pp. 15–25. https://link.springer.com/chapter/10.1007/978-3-319-55994-0_2

Higgs, J., Andresen, L., Fish, D., 2004a. Practice knowledge—its nature, sources and contexts. In: Higgs, J., Richardson, B., Abrandt Dahlgren, M. (Eds.), Developing practice knowledge for health professionals. Butterworth-Heinemann, pp. 51–69.

Higgs, J., Titchen, A., 1995. The nature, generation and verification of knowledge. Physiotherapy 81, 521–530. https://doi.org/10.1016/S0031-9406(05)66683-7

Higgs, J., Titchen, A. (Eds.), 2001. Professional practice in health, education and the creative arts. Blackwell Science.

Higgs, J., McAllister, L., Whiteford, G., 2009. The practice and praxis of professional decision making. In: Green, B. (Ed.), Understanding and researching professional practice. Sense, pp. 101–120.

Higgs, J., Richardson, B., Abrandt Dahlgren, M. (Eds.), 2004b. Developing practice knowledge for health professionals. Butterworth-Heinemann.

Honderich, T. (Ed.), 1995. The Oxford companion to philosophy. Oxford University Press.

Kelley, D.R., 1990. What is happening to the history of ideas? Journal of the History of Ideas 51 (1), 3–25. https://doi.org/10.2307/2709744

Kemmis, S., Smith, T.J., 2008. Enabling praxis: Challenges for Education. Sense.

Knorr Cetina, K., 2007. Culture in global knowledge societies: Knowledge cultures and epistemic cultures. Interdisciplinary Science Reviews 32 (4), 361–375. https://doi.org/10.1179/030801807X163571

Kolb, D.A., 1984. Experiential learning: Experience as the source of learning and development (vol. 1). Prentice-Hall.

Lave, J., Wenger, E., 1991. Situated learning: Legitimate peripheral participation. Cambridge University Press.

Leonard, V.A., 1989. A Heideggerian phenomenologic perspective on the concept of the person. Advances in Nursing Science 11, 40–55. https://doi.org/10.1097/00012272-198907000-00008

Lincoln, Y.S., Guba, E., 1985. Naturalistic inquiry. Sage.

Loftus, S., 2009. Language in clinical reasoning: Towards a new understanding. VDM Verlag Dr. Müller.

Lovejoy, A.D., 1936. The great chain of being: A study of the history of an idea. Harvard Press.

Markauskaite, L., Goodyear, P., 2017. Epistemic fluency and professional education: Innovation, knowledgeable action and actionable knowledge. Springer.

McCarthy, E.D., 1996. Knowledge as culture: The new sociology of knowledge. Routledge & Kegan Paul.

Merleau-Ponty, M., 1956. What is phenomenology? Cross Currents 16, 59–70.

Morrison, D., Collins, A., 1996. Epistemic fluency and constructivist learning environments. In: Wilson, B. (Ed.), Constructivist learning environments: Case studies in instructional design. Educational Technology Publications, pp. 107–119.

Nerland, M., 2016. Learning to master profession-specific knowledge practices: A prerequisite for the deliberate professional. In: Trede, F., McEwen, C. (Eds.), Educating the deliberate professional: Preparing practitioners for emergent futures. Springer, pp. 127–139.

Nerland, M., Jensen, K., 2014. Changing cultures of knowledge and professional learning. In: Billett, S., Harteis, C., Gruber, H. (Eds.), International handbook of research in professional and practice-based learning. Springer, pp. 611–640.

O'Neill, O., 2002. A question of trust. Polity Press.

Reason, P., Heron, J., 1986. Research with people: The paradigm of cooperative experiential enquiry. Person-Centred Review 1, 457–476.

Raworth, K., 2019. Doughnut Economics, Seven ways to think like a 21st century economist. Chelsea Green Publishing.

Roberts, N., 2000. Wicked problems and network approaches to resolution. International Public Management Review 1, 1–19.

Sarter, B., 1988. Paths to knowledge: Innovative research methods for nursing. National League for Nursing.

Schön, D.A., 1995. The reflective practitioner: How professionals think in action. Ashgate, Aldershot Hants.

Sennett, R., 2005. The culture of the new capitalism. Yale University Press.

Smith, J.K., 1983. Quantitative versus qualitative research: An attempt to clarify the issue. Educational Researcher 12, 6–13.

Stephenson, J., 1998. The concept of capability and its importance in higher education. In: Stephenson, J., Yorke, M. (Eds.), Capability and quality in higher education. Kogan Page, pp. 1–13.

Vygotsky, L.S., 1978. Mind in society: The development of higher psychological processes. Harvard University Press.

Vygotsky, L.S., 1986. Thought and language (A. Kozulin, Transl.). MIT Press.

Wenger, E., 1998. Communities of practice: Learning, meaning, and identity. Cambridge University.

Yinger, R., Hendricks-Lee, M., 1993. Working knowledge in teaching. In: Day, C., Calderhead, J., Denicolo, P. (Eds.), Research on teacher thinking: Understanding professional development. Falmer Press, pp. 100–123.

5

MULTIPLE SPACES OF ENGAGEMENT AND INFLUENCE IN CLINICAL DECISION MAKING

JOY HIGGS ■ MARK JONES

CHAPTER OUTLINE

CHAPTER AIMS

The aims of this chapter are:

- to examine reasoning strategy choices
- to reflect on professional development implications for the practitioner-as-reasoner.

INTRODUCTION

Clinical decision making involves people, information, evidence, goals and connections. Each of these elements of decision making operate in situations which could be thought of as spaces where engagement and influences interact. Clinical reasoning could be interpreted as operating in spaces in which different clinical situations are considered, healthcare problems, needs or issues are addressed, particular influences are experienced and unique sets of people are engaged in providing client care. Kassirer and colleagues (2010, p. 311) define the problem space as 'the subject's representation of the task environment that permits the consideration of different problem solutions and sets limitations on possible operations that can be applied to the problem; a sort of maze of mental activity through which individuals wander when searching for a solution to a problem'.

In Fig. 5.1 the core players – the client and the clinician – can be seen at the centre addressing the client's clinical needs/problems. Moving outwards, this core team is joined by other people who play a role in the client's care: the healthcare team, carers and other support people such as community services agencies. Many factors influence all of these core and surrounding interactions.

Client Spaces

The role for the client as a consumer of healthcare is rather different from the dependent patient role of traditional medicine, where 'autonomy' of health professionals is underpinned by bias towards clinical-centred decision making. Consumers of healthcare are becoming increasingly well informed about their health and about healthcare services. Self-help and holistic healthcare are becoming more central to healthcare and the goal of achieving effective participation by consumers in their healthcare is widespread, requiring health professionals to diminish their decision-making authority and involve their clients actively in clinical decision making where possible (Fish and De Cossart, 2019; Matthias et al., 2013).

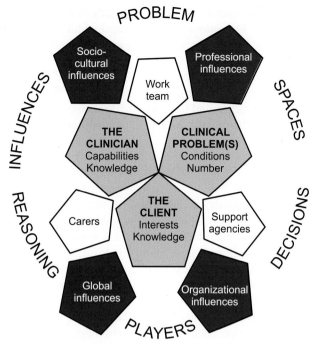

Fig. 5.1 ▪ Clinical reasoning spaces from the inside out.

Increasingly, clients' choices, rights and responsibilities in relation to their health are changing. For some time, people have advocated client involvement in decision making about the management of their health and well-being. Using understanding of their clients' rights and responsibilities, clinicians need to develop their own approaches to involving the client in reasoning and decision making. Mutual decision making requires not only a sharing of ownership of decisions but also the development of skills in establishing rapport, exploring the impact of problems on the client's life, empathy, explanation and negotiation (Frankel and Stein, 1999; Jones et al., 2022; Matthias et al., 2013) to facilitate shared understanding and decision making. Professional autonomy becomes redefined from being clinician-centred to a shared expertise across the players involved (within a teamwork context) including the client who has specialized knowledge about their problem(s), their personal circumstances, their goals and their healthcare preferences. An important aspect

of involving patients or clients in clinical decision making is determining and facilitating their appropriate level of participation and responsibility. A level of participation in clinical reasoning appropriate for the individual has been demonstrated to contribute to the client's sense of control (Edwards et al., 2004; Stacey et al., 2017).

Practitioner Spaces

Practitioners bring their personal and professional selves to the task of clinical decision making; these selves frame their problem space. As well as functioning within their personal frames of reference, practitioners operate within their professional frameworks (e.g. the ethical and competency standards/requirements of their profession, formal relationships with other health professionals, approaches to examination and management within a profession and area of practice) and within a broader context of professionalism. The term *health professional* implies a qualified healthcare provider who demonstrates professional autonomy, competence and accountability. Professional status incorporates the responsibility to make unsupervised and accountable clinical decisions and to implement ethical, competent and person-centred practice. This requires health professionals to consider the client's problem space, as described earlier, and to make decisions with the client about the client's level of involvement.

The Collaborative Problem Space of the Team

Most health professionals work in collaboration with other team members, either directly or indirectly via referral. This includes work across mainstream and complementary and alternative medicine. Grace and colleagues (2006) identified an increasing preference in clients with chronic health problems, particularly those dissatisfied with mainstream medicine, for practices that directly integrate complementary and alternative medicine with general practice; such models, they found, worked best for clients when both practitioners worked in collaboration.

The level of collaboration in clinical decision making in these settings varies considerably. Practitioners may make decisions separately and report decisions to others (e.g. via client records); they may refer clients to others to take over client care or to receive advice; they may operate as a decision-making team making decisions on behalf of their clients; or they may work with clients as members of the decision-making team. Croker and Higgs (2016) reminded us that practitioners are often members of multiple teams with different agendas and modes and roles of decision making.

REFLECTION POINT

Working at a solo level can be different to operating on a team basis.
- How does your practice vary when working at these levels (e.g. reliance on your own knowledge versus seeking input of others)?

The Problem Space of the Workplace and the Local System

Clinicians frequently face ill-defined problems, goals that are complex and outcomes that are difficult to predict clearly. Many aspects of the workplace influence clinical decision making, particularly levels of available human, material and economic resources.

The Knowledge-Reasoning Space of Clinical Decision Making

Three considerations are pertinent in considering this knowledge-reasoning space. First, professional judgement and decision making within the ambiguous or uncertain situations of healthcare is an inexact science (Kennedy, 1987). Checkland (1981) referred to 'soft systems' (such as healthcare systems) as those in which goals may be unrecognizable and outcomes ambiguous; these are typically social rather than physical world focussed. In such contexts reasoning and judgement are highly valued and essential: simple answers that neatly fit the given situation are rarely pre-learnable. Second, reasoning involves the three core elements of cognition, knowledge and meta-cognition. Third, judgement is referential rather than absolute.

The Problem Space of the Global Healthcare System With Its Discourse, Knowledge and Technology

Many factors of the wider healthcare environment need to be taken into consideration in clinical reasoning. Health professionals need to develop a broad understanding of the environment in which they work, including knowledge of the contextual personal and environmental factors influencing health. In addition, they need to understand how the information age has impacted on healthcare demands, provision and expectation. They need to be able to work confidently and effectively with an increasing body of scientific, technical and professional knowledge. Developing a sound individual understanding of clinical reasoning and a capacity to reason effectively will facilitate the clinician's ability to manage complex and changing information.

Errors

Avoiding errors in clinical reasoning requires attributes of skilled critical thinking, including open-mindedness, consideration of other perspectives, awareness and critique of assumptions, as well as more deliberate analysis as a backup of quick first impression judgements often based on fixed clinical patterns and habitual practice. Rather than unquestionably accepting information, skilled critical thinking within clinical reasoning fosters a sort of healthy scepticism that appraises information for its accuracy, precision, completeness and relevance to facilitate understanding and identification of solutions. Errors in the cognition of clinical reasoning (e.g. information perception, interpretation, analysis) can be linked to the various forms of human bias evidenced in health- and non–health-related human judgement. The priming influence of prior information (e.g. diagnosis provided in a referral, imaging findings, influence of a recent publication or course) and the tendency to attend to and collect data that confirm existing hypotheses (i.e. confirmation bias) are two classic examples. These errors are commonly associated with habits of thinking and practice, which themselves are a potential risk of inaccurate pattern recognition. That is, in adopting a pattern recognition approach the novice or unreflective practitioner might focus too much on looking for the presence or absence of specific patterns and overlook other potentially important information, or might find it difficult to see anything outside the most familiar patterns. Patterns can become rigid, making it difficult to recognize variations or alternatives.

Within the changing face of healthcare and the trend towards more biopsychosocial practice that values qualitative information of the client's experience alongside quantitative biomedical measures, there is a need to look beyond the cognitive processes and cognitive errors of the clinician. Errors in psychosocial or narrative-focussed reasoning can be manifest as having no consideration of psychosocial factors or engaging in superficial assessment based on insufficient information.

Errors of reasoning can be reduced through greater understanding of clinical reasoning generally and greater understanding and critique of your own clinical reasoning. The risks of uncritical pattern recognition can be offset by strategies that minimize the assumptions frequently underpinning pattern recognition. Such error avoidance strategies include screening to ensure information is not missed or inaccurate, qualifying clients' meanings, consideration and, if justified, testing for competing hypotheses and openly subjecting and comparing your reasoning to others' reasoning.

REFLECTION POINT

- What strategies could you use to ensure that any habits you may have are sufficiently justified and avoid errors?

CLINICAL REASONING STRATEGIES

Table 5.1 presents an overview of key models, strategies and interpretations of clinical reasoning. These have been divided into two groups: cognitive and interactive models. These are based on historical work of researchers such as Arocha et al. (1993), Barrows et al. (1978), Bordage and Lemieux (1991), Boshuizen and Schmidt (1992a, 1992b), Costanzo et al. (2019), Coulter and Collins (2011), Edwards et al. (1998), Elstein et al. (1978), Jones (2019), Kahneman (2011), Lipton (2004), Loftus (2006), Marcum (2012), Mattingly and Fleming (1994), Neufeld et al. (1981) and Patel et al. (1988).

Although it should be possible to justify clinical reasoning in professional and public discourse, how the strategy is implemented cannot be prescribed beyond discipline-specific agreements regarding the breadth of scope and range of appropriate strategies. The strategies and processes described in Table 5.1 feature to some extent across most health professions represented in this book.

Hypothetico-deductive reasoning (HDR) in the health professions traditionally refers to the process of formulating hypotheses based on specific features in the client's presentation and linked to established criteria (i.e. premises) for a type of clinical judgement (e.g. diagnosis or problem classification). Formal testing of initial hypotheses is said to occur through the collection of additional information such that when the judgement criteria are fulfilled the health professional can deduce a specific hypothesis is confirmed or at least supported. Although diagnosis is perhaps the category of clinical judgement most researched and described in the literature, other categories of judgement where profession-specific criteria exist similarly use this process, for example clinical judgements regarding the need for caution in

		TABLE 5.1	
		Models and Interpretations of Clinical Reasoning	
View	Model	Related Terms	Description
CR as cognitive process	Hypothetico-deductive reasoning	Procedural reasoning Diagnostic reasoning Induction-related probabilistic reasoning	The generation of hypotheses based on clinical data and knowledge and testing of these hypotheses through further inquiry. It is used by novices and in problematic situations by experts. Hypothesis generation and testing involve both inductive reasoning, i.e. moving from a set of specific observations to a generalization, to generate hypotheses and slower detailed deductive reasoning, i.e. moving from a generalization (if) to a conclusion (then) in relation to a specific case, to test hypotheses. Procedural reasoning identifying the client's functional problems and selecting procedures to manage them.
	Pattern recognition	Pattern interpretation Inductive reasoning Categorization Mental representations	Expert reasoning in nonproblematic situations resembles pattern recognition or direct automatic retrieval of information from a well-structured knowledge base. New cases are categorized, that is, similarities are recognized (signs, symptoms, treatment options, outcomes, context) in relation to previously experienced clinical cases. Through the use of inductive reasoning, pattern recognition/interpretation is a process characterized by speed and efficiency, albeit with risk for error if relied on in the absence of adequate knowledge and experience. With increasing experience, clinicians move through three kinds of mental representations, from basic mechanisms of disease to illness scripts of clinical features and semantic qualifiers to exemplars derived from experience.
	Forward reasoning Backward reasoning Abductive reasoning	Inductive reasoning Deductive reasoning Inference to the best explanation	Forward reasoning describes inductive reasoning in which data analysis results in hypothesis generation or diagnosis, utilizing a sound knowledge base. Backward reasoning is the re-interpretation of data or the acquisition of new clarifying data invoked to test a hypothesis. Forward reasoning is more likely to occur in familiar cases with experienced clinicians and backward reasoning with inexperienced clinicians or in atypical or difficult cases. Abductive reasoning, also called inference to the best explanation, refers to theorizing, typically regarding causal mechanisms, clinicians engage in when confronted with unexpected or unfamiliar information that cannot be deduced from established or accepted prior knowledge. It is an unproven, creative explanatory hypothesis for an area of clinical judgements when clear deductions are not available.
	Knowledge reasoning integration		Clinical reasoning involves the integration of knowledge, reasoning and metacognition. Clinical reasoning requires domain-specific knowledge and an organized knowledge base. With experience, clinical reasoning and the associated knowledge drawn on may progress through stages culminating in both exemplars and memory of specific client instances.
	Intuitive reasoning	Instance scripts Inductive reasoning Heuristics Pattern matching	'Intuitive knowledge' is related to 'instance scripts' or past experience with specific cases that can be used unconsciously in inductive reasoning. Intuition may be associated with the use of advanced reasoning strategies or heuristics. Such heuristics include pattern matching and listing (or listing items relevant to the working plan).

Continued

		TABLE 5.1	
		Models and Interpretations of Clinical Reasoning—cont'd	
View	Model	Related Terms	Description
CR as interactive process	Multidisciplinary reasoning	Interprofessional reasoning Team decision making	Members of a multidisciplinary team working together to make clinical decisions for the client about the client's condition, e.g. at case conferences, multidisciplinary clinics.
	Conditional reasoning	Predictive reasoning Projected reasoning	Used by practitioners to estimate client responses to treatment and likely outcomes of management and to help clients consider possibilities and reconstruct their lives after injury or the onset of disease.
	Narrative reasoning		Reasoning associated with understanding the client's narrative (i.e. story) with respect to their pain, illness and/or disability experiences incorporating the client's personal perspectives on their experiences.
	Interactive reasoning		Reasoning guiding the purposeful establishment and ongoing management of client–clinician rapport important to understanding the client's perspective and overall outcome.
	Collaborative reasoning	Mutual decision making	The shared decision making between client and clinician (and others) as a therapeutic alliance in the interpretation of examination findings, setting of goals and priorities and implementation and progression of treatment.
	Ethical reasoning	Pragmatic reasoning	Reasoning underpinning the recognition and resolution of moral, political and economic ethical dilemmas that impinge upon the patient's ability to make decisions concerning their health and upon the conduct of treatment and its desired goals.
	Teaching as reasoning		Reasoning associated with the planning, execution and evaluation of individualized and context-sensitive teaching, including education for conceptual understanding (e.g. diagnosis, disability, management options), education for physical performance (e.g. rehabilitative exercises) and education for behavioural change.

CR, Clinical reasoning.

the examination and management, the need for referral for further medical consultation and judgements regarding prognosis.

Pattern recognition occurs in situations where features in the client's presentation are sufficiently familiar to the practitioner to enable recognition of a clinical pattern so further testing through HDR is not essential. Pattern recognition is most commonly associated with diagnostic clinical judgements; however, pattern recognition is part of all human perception and judgement (Kahneman, 2011; Kahneman et al., 2021) and examples will be evident across all health professions' areas of practice with differences perhaps more related to the extent they are relied on.

Some would argue that narrative- (or psychosocial-) focussed reasoning exists as the opposite pole to diagnostic-focussed reasoning with expert physiotherapists described as being able to move dialectically in their focus and reasoning between these two poles as unfolding client information requires. Like diagnostic-focussed reasoning that involves more than simply assigning a label to a problem, psychosocial-focussed reasoning incorporates assessment and analysis of multiple client factors (e.g. problem understanding, threat evaluation, distress, resilience, coping behaviours and strategies, goals, readiness, willingness and ability to change, social factors).

Since HDR can be applied to any reasoning that formulates and tests hypotheses, it is likely to manifest in every health profession and with all client types. As a slower analytical process, it is often associated with the novice who lacks sufficient knowledge and experience to recognize clinical patterns and hence must consider and test a broader list of hypotheses not required by the expert. Experts may revert to HDR in complex or unfamiliar cases. Use of HDR will therefore depend on the experience and knowledge of the practitioner, their familiarity with the clinical presentation, the nature of the clinical judgements they are called to make (e.g. diagnostic versus narrative) and, unfortunately perhaps, also the time they are allocated per client. However, even with narrative reasoning, knowledge and experience enable identification of typical features of potentially restricting or facilitating psychosocial factors that elicit further investigation. Ultimately a hypothesis is still formed. With all reasoning, the client should be given the opportunity to validate the clinician's understanding of their story or presentation, yet the clinician still forms a judgement of the psychosocial factors.

PROFESSIONAL DEVELOPMENT OF CLINICAL REASONING CAPABILITY

In pursuit of continuing professional development in relation to clinical reasoning, we could consider expertise in reasoning to be the ultimate goal. In a review of clinical reasoning literature in medicine, Norman (2005) suggested that there may not be a single representation of clinical reasoning expertise or a single correct way to solve a problem. He noted that 'the more one studies the clinical expert, the more one marvels at the complex and multidimensional components of knowledge and skill that she or he brings to bear on the problem, and the amazing adaptability she must possess to achieve the goal of effective care' (p. 426). In contrast, Kahneman et al. (2021, p. 6) highlight the 'scandalously high' extent of unwanted variability in human judgement or 'noise' across diverse real-world decisions including medicine, child custody, asylum applications, criminal sentencing and more.

Clinical reasoning and clinical practice expertise are a journey, an aspiration and a commitment to achieving the best practice that one can provide. Rather than being a point of arrival, complacency and lack of questioning by self or others, expertise requires both the capacity to recognize one's limitations and practice capabilities and the ability to pursue professional development in a spirit of self-critique. It is – or at least we should expect it to be – not only a self-referenced level of capability or mode of practice, but also a search for understanding of and realization of the standards and expectations set by the community being served and the profession and service organization being represented.

We have added the idea of expectations to this discussion to emphasize that any human construct is sociohistorically situated. Beyond a research-driven, science-based view of technical expertise there is a need for any professional, but particularly experts, with their claim to superior service and performance, to address the needs of society. There is a growing expectation of client-centred humanization (including cultural competence, information sharing, collaborative decision making, virtuous practice) of expert practice that turns health professional expertise into a collaborative professional relationship rather than an expert-empowered, technically superior, practitioner-centred approach. As highlighted in the research findings of Jensen et al. (2006), this client-centred approach is grounded in a strong moral commitment to beneficence or doing what is in the client's best interest. This manifests in therapists' nonjudgemental attitude and strong emphasis on client education, with expert therapists being willing to act as client advocate or moral agent in helping them be successful.

Box 5.1 demonstrates an evolution in thinking about expertise, beginning with the classic research by Glaser and Chi (1988) of expert attributes. In 2000 we added to this view ideas of client-centredness, collaboration, metacognition, mentoring, effective communication and cultural competence (Higgs and Jones, 2000). In 2008 we added a third group of characteristics for the third edition (Higgs and Jones, 2008). The fourth section reflects messages about the evolution of context and approaches to clinical reasoning.

BOX 5.1
CHARACTERISTICS, EXPECTATIONS AND EMERGING ABILITIES OF EXPERT PRACTITIONERS

a) *General characteristics of experts (Glaser and Chi, 1988)*
- Experts excel mainly in their own domains.
- Experts perceive large meaningful patterns in their domain.
- Experts are fast: they are faster than novices at performing the skills of their domain, and they quickly solve problems with little error.
- Experts have superior short-term and long-term memory.
- Experts see and represent a problem in their domain at a deeper (more principled) level than novices; novices tend to represent a problem at a superficial level.
- Experts spend a great deal of time analysing a problem qualitatively.
- Experts have strong self-monitoring skills.

b) *Characteristics and expectations of health professional experts (Higgs and Jones, 2000)*
- Experts need to pursue shared decision making between client and clinician if 'success' is to be realized from the client's perspective.
- Experts need to monitor and manage their cognitive processes (i.e. to use metacognition) to achieve high quality decision making and practice action.
- Experts critically use propositional and experience-based up-to-date practice knowledge to inform their practice.
- Expertise requires the informed use and recognition of patient-centred practice.
- Expert practitioners are mentors and critical companions (see Titchen, 2000) to less experienced practitioners.
- Experts are expected to communicate effectively with clients, colleagues and families and to justify clinical decisions articulately.
- Experts should demonstrate cultural competence.

c) *Further characteristics and expectations of expert professionals (Higgs and Jones, 2008)*
- Experts demonstrate information and communication literacy.
- Experts value and utilise the expertise of other team members.
- Experts own and embody their practice model.
- Expertise goes beyond technical expertise in pursuit of emancipatory practice.
- Expert practice is community-oriented.
- Expertise is informed by reflexive practice as well as research.

- Expert decision making is informed by the health and demographic trends in the communities they serve.
- Experts' behaviour demonstrates a strong moral commitment to beneficence through such behaviours as patient advocacy and non-judgemental attitudes.

d) *Emerging expectations of expert professionals*
- Experts are skilled critical thinkers that consider other perspectives.
- Experts have the intellectual humility to know what they don't know and seek further understandings.
- Experts retain creativity and imagination.
- Experts appreciate the value of wisdom in practice.
- Experts look beyond their professional backgrounds for ideas and strategies.
- Experts look into innovative spaces for practice.
- Experts learn to balance economics and entrepreneurship with professional practice.
- Experts demonstrate epistemological and ontological fluency.
- Experts survive and flourish in the face of difficult problems and situations.

We propose that clinical expertise, of which clinical reasoning is a critical component, be viewed as a continuum along multiple dimensions. These dimensions include clinical outcomes, personal attributes such as critical thinking embedded in professional judgement, technical clinical skills, communication and interpersonal skills (to involve the client and others in decision making and to consider the client's perspectives), a sound knowledge base combined with the intellectual humility to know one's limitations, an informed and chosen practice model and philosophy of practice, as well as cognitive and metacognitive proficiency.

A related concept to expertise is professional artistry, which 'reflects both high quality of professional practice and the qualities inherent in such artistic or flexible, person-centred, highly reflexive practice' (Paterson and Higgs, 2001, p. 2). Professional artistry reflects a uniquely individual view within a shared tradition involving a blend of practitioner qualities, practice skills and creative imagination processes (Higgs and Titchen, 2001). This idea was linked with clinical reasoning to develop the concept and practice of professional practice judgement artistry (Paterson and

Higgs, 2008). Similarly, 'practice wisdom' challenges our ideas of what it means to bring knowledge and wisdom, plus reasoning and judgement artistry, into the act of clinical decision making.

SUMMARY

We have portrayed clinical reasoning as a complex set of processes and interactions occurring within multiple and multidimensional problem spaces. The complexity of clinical reasoning in the health professions is evident in the scope of reasoning required to address the full range of biopsychosocial factors that can contribute to clients' health problems and experiences. Adding to this complexity, health professionals have at their disposal a broad range of clinical reasoning strategies to understand their clients and their clients' health problems to assist their collaborative management. Although these reasoning processes have relevance to all areas of health professions' practice, their use varies across professions. Greater understanding of the spaces in which clinical reasoning occurs and of the reasoning strategies that can be used will assist health professionals' understanding of their own clinical reasoning. Errors of reasoning are linked to different forms of human bias and can be reduced through greater understanding of clinical reasoning generally and greater understanding and critique of one's own clinical reasoning. Professional development is an essential part of ensuring the quality of clinical reasoning and the capability of professionals performing this key practice.

REFLECTION POINT

- Which clinical reasoning strategies can you identify in your own practice?
- How might you improve your clinical reasoning abilities?

REFERENCES

Arocha, J.F., Patel, V.L., Patel, Y.C., 1993. Hypothesis generation and the coordination of theory and evidence in novice diagnostic reasoning. Medical Decision Making 13, 198–211. https://doi.org/10.1177/0272989X9301300305 PMID: 8412548

Barrows, H.S., Feightner, J.W., Neufield, V.R., Norman, G.R., 1978. An analysis of the clinical methods of medical students and physicians (Report to the Province of Ontario Department of Health). McMaster University.

Bordage, G., Lemieux, M., 1991. Semantic structures and diagnostic thinking of experts and novices. Academic Medicine 66, S70–572. https://doi.org/10.1097/00001888-199109000-00045 PMID: 1930535.

Boshuizen, H.P.A., Schmidt, H.G., 1992a. Biomedical knowledge and clinical expertise. Cogn. Sci. 16, 153–184.

Boshuizen, H.P.A., Schmidt, H.G., 1992b. On the role of biomedical knowledge and clinical reasoning by experts, intermediates and novices. Cogn. Sci. 16, 153–184.

Checkland, P.B., 1981. Systems thinking: Systems practice. John Wiley and Sons.

Costanzo, C., Doll, J., Jensen, G.M., 2019. Shared decision making in practice. In: Higgs, J., Jensen, G., Loftus, S., Christensen, N. (Eds.), Clinical reasoning in the health professions, 3rd ed. Elsevier, pp. 181–190.

Croker, A., Higgs, J., 2016. Reinterpreting professional relationships in healthcare: The question of collaboration. In: Croker, A., Higgs, J., Trede, F. (Eds.), Collaborating in healthcare: Reinterpreting therapeutic relationships. Sense, pp. 3–16.

Coulter, A., Collins, A., 2011. Making shared decision-making a reality. No decision about me, without me. https://www.kingsfund.org.uk/sites/default/files/Making-shared-decision-making-a-reality-paper-Angela-Coulter-Alf-Collins-July-2011_0.pdf.

Edwards, I.C., Jones, M.A., Carr, J., et al. 1998. Clinical reasoning in three different fields of physiotherapy: A qualitative study. In Proceedings of the Fifth International Congress of the Australian Physiotherapy Association, Melbourne, VIC (298–300).

Edwards, I., Jones, M., Higgs, J., Trede, F., Jensen, G., 2004. What is collaborative reasoning? Advances in Physiotherapy 6, 70–83. https://doi.org/10.1080/14038190410018938

Elstein, A.S., Shulman, L.S., Sprafka, S.A., 1978. Medical problem solving: An analysis of clinical reasoning. Harvard University Press.

Fish, D., De Cossart, L., 2019. Clinical thinking, client expectations and patient-centred care. In: Higgs, J., Jensen, G., Loftus, S., Christensen, N. (Eds.), Clinical reasoning in the health professions. Elsevier, pp. 97–107.

Frankel, R.M., Stein, T., 1999. Getting the most out of the clinical encounter: The four habits model. The Permanente Journal 3, 79–88.

Glaser, R., Chi, M.T.H., 1988. Overview. In: Chi, M.T.H., Glaser, R., Farr, M.J. (Eds.), The nature of expertise. Lawrence Erlbaum, pp. xi–xxviii.

Grace, S., Higgs, J., Horsfall, D., 2006. Integrating mainstream and complementary and alternative medicine: Investing in prevention Proceedings of the University of Sydney From Cell to Society 5: Proceedings of the Health Research Conference, 9-10 November. The University of Sydney. 1–25.

Higgs, J., Jones, M., 2000. Clinical reasoning in the health professions. In: Higgs, J., Jones, M. (Eds.), Clinical reasoning in the health professions, 2nd ed. Butterworth-Heinemann, pp. 3–14.

Higgs, J., Jones, M., 2008. Clinical decision making and multiple problem spaces. In: Higgs, J., Jones, M., Loftus, S., Christensen, N. (Eds.), Clinical reasoning in the health professions, 3rd ed. Elsevier, pp. 3–17.

Higgs, J., Titchen, A., 2001. Towards professional artistry and creativity in practice. In: Higgs, J., Titchen, A. (Eds.), Professional practice in health, education and the creative arts. Blackwell Science, pp. 273–290.

Jensen, G.M., Gwyer, J., Hack, L.M., Shepard, K.F., 2006. Expertise in physical therapy practice, 2nd ed. Saunders-Elsevier.

Jones, M.A., 2019. Clinical reasoning: Fast and slow thinking in musculoskeletal practice. In: Jones, M.A., Rivett, D.A. (Eds.), Clinical reasoning in musculoskeletal practice, 2nd ed. Elsevier.

Jones, M., Hall, K., Lewis, J., 2022. Clinical reasoning, behavioral change, and shared decision-making. In: Lewis, J., Fernández-de-las Peñas, C. (Eds.), The shoulder, theory and practice. Handspring Publishing, Edinburgh, pp. 183–198.

Kahneman, D., 2011. Thinking, fast and slow. Allen Lane.

Kahneman, D., Sibony, O., Sunstein, C.R., 2021. Noise: A flaw in human judgment. William Collins.

Kassirer, J., Wong, J., & Kopelman, R. (2010). Learning clinical reasoning. Wolters Kluwer, Lippincott Williams & Wilkins.

Kennedy, M., 1987. Inexact sciences: Professional education and the development of expertise. Review of Research in Education 14, 133–168. https://doi.org/10.2307/1167311

Lipton, P., 2004. Inference to the best explanation, 2nd ed. Routledge.

Loftus, S., 2006. Language in clinical reasoning: Learning and using the language of collective clinical decision making [Doctoral dissertation, The University of Sydney]. http://ses.library.usyd.edu.au/handle/2123/1165

Marcum, J.A., 2012. An integrated model of clinical reasoning: Dual-process theory of cognition and metacognition. Journal of Evaluation in Clinical Practice 18, 954–961. https://doi.org/10.1111/j.1365-2753.2012.01900.x

Matthias, M.S., Salyers, M.P., Frankel, R.M., 2013. Re-thinking shared decision-making: Context matters. Patient Educ Couns 91, 176–179. https://doi.org/10.1016/j.pec.2013.01.006)

Mattingly, C., Fleming, M.H., 1994. Clinical reasoning: Forms of inquiry in a therapeutic practice. FA Davis.

Neufeld, V.R., Norman, G.R., Barrows, H.S., Feightner, J.W., 1981. Clinical problem-solving by medical students: A longitudinal and cross-sectional analysis. Medical Education 15. 315–22 https://doi.org/10.1111/j.1365-2923.1981.tb02495.x

Norman, G., 2005. Research in clinical reasoning: Past history and current trends. Medical Education 39, 418–427. https://doi.org/10.1111/j.1365-2923.1981.tb02495.x

Patel, V.L., Evans, D.A., Groen, G.J., 1988. Biomedical knowledge and clinical reasoning. In: Evans, D.A., Patel, V.L. (Eds.), Cognitive science in medicine: Biomedical modelling. MIT Press, pp. 49–108.

Paterson, M., Higgs, J., 2001. Professional practice judgement artistry CPEA Occasional Paper 3, The Centre for Professional Education Advancement. The University of Sydney.

Paterson, M., Higgs, J., 2008. Professional practice judgement artistry. In: Higgs, J., Jones, M., Loftus, S., Christensen, N. (Eds.), Clinical reasoning in the health professions, 3rd ed. Elsevier, pp. 181–189.

Stacey, D., Légaré, F., Lewis, K., et al., 2017. Decision aids for people facing health treatment or screening decisions. Cochrane Database Syst Rev 4, Cd001431. https://doi.org/10.1002/14651858.CD001431.pub5

Titchen, A., 2000. Professional craft knowledge in patient centred nursing and the facilitation of its development. Ashdale Press.

6

A CRITICAL SOCIAL SCIENCES MODEL FOR PRACTICE

JOY HIGGS ■ FRANZISKA V. TREDE

CHAPTER AIMS

The aims of this chapter are:

- to support a critical social science model as a basis for practice
- to encourage practitioners to develop, critically, their own practice models.

INTRODUCTION

Today's healthcare systems and practice models need to rethink their structures, policies and guidelines due to constant and profound disruptions. The global pandemic with social distancing imperatives and its long-term COVID-19 effects (Moynihan et al., 2021) are one such disruption. It is being taken over by rapid advances of generative artificial intelligence tools that promise to have impact on the way we practise in healthcare (Kung et al., 2023). In times of rapid and constant change, critical and ethical engagement with these influences is called for. Without a thoughtful and informed stance to practise under changing conditions, healthcare risks losing sight of what matters and instead constrains practitioners to be reactive and following change rather than being part of making change (Stetsenko, 2019). With this chapter we draw on well-established critical social sciences (CSS) perspectives that foreground critique and transformation and interpreted within the healthcare context encourage practitioners to become deliberate professionals who understand what matters, identify choices and act to improve those elements of practice that need change (Trede and McEwen, 2016b).

RECOGNIZING OUR PRACTICE CONTEXT AND INFLUENCES

Neither clinical reasoning nor professional practice as a whole occur in a vacuum. They occur in social contexts and are shaped by and shape values, interests, purpose, choices and decision-making practices. At the core of a CSS perspective is the question of purpose: *what matters here*? Questioning the purpose is an invitation to rethink outcomes and processes to achieving them. It is also a reminder that patients as social human beings matter. A CSS perspective places emphasis on critical understanding of current practices by situating the many levels of healthcare contexts from interpersonal to managerial, national and global with interests and values and with this, awareness enables changes.

Understanding and Valuing Interests and Priorities

Clinical practice is influenced by a complex interplay between different interests and priorities that can range from wanting to assert professional authority and control over healthcare situations, to wanting to negotiate common ground with clients and create meaning, to striving to learn, transform and change oneself and one's clients. This discussion is framed by Habermas' (1972) theory of knowledge and human interests, in which he argued that interests shape knowledge and actions. Here we explore the link between interests and the actions of clinical reasoning and clinical practice. Interests can be thought of as the motivation for wanting to think and act in certain ways. Such motivation can be internally driven by values, attitudes and desires, such as a humanistic perspective, valuing of rationality, or wanting to be patient-centred. Interests can also be shaped by external interests, such as pressures to adhere to the dominant healthcare practice model, system imperatives such as economic rationalism, society and peer expectations of professional behaviour, and trends and discourses in healthcare.

Health professionals are accountable and accept responsibility for their decisions and actions. What values, assumptions and reasons underpin and guide their thinking and decisions? Often such interests are subconscious and have been acquired through the pervasive and often osmotic process of professional socialization (Eraut, 1994) rather than being consciously learned and adopted through critical self-appraisal and informed choice of a desired model of practice. Once practitioners are aware of their interests and understand what motivates these interests, they are in a better position to make critically conscious choices as to how they seek to frame their clinical reasoning and consequent actions.

The Social and Historical Construction of Practice Approaches

When graduates enter healthcare professions, many practices already exist. Professional practice is socially and historically constructed (Higgs, 2016, p. 191): 'it comprises individual and shared activities and expectations across a community of practice; it is manifest in language, discourses and traditions; its conduct is linked to morality and ethical conduct; its standards and implementation are regulated and evaluated by individual practitioners as well as the practice community, external authorities and society; it is manifest in a range of levels of expertise development; and beyond all of this, practice is embodied through practical consciousness'. Deliberate professionals need this understanding of practice because they knowingly create their practice models and take responsibility for their clinical reasoning, decision making and ultimately, the outcomes of their practice actions.

The Shaping of Practice Models: The Place of Ideology

We tend to interpret and justify our clinical reasoning processes with theoretical knowledge and research findings without acknowledging the interests and assumptions that inform our practice. Practice is justified with theories, guidelines and professional training. The ideology behind these theories and training remains hidden. To bring the assumptions out of hiding and question our way of reasoning enhances our practice awareness and provides us with real choices about practising optimally in each given clinical context.

It would be simplistic and limiting for a profession to define its practice purely on the basis of technical knowledge and skills (Schön, 1987). This would reduce practice to the aspects that can be measured with empirico-analytical evidence only. What we observe and what we do is only the visible part of practising. The reasoning that has gone before the observable actions in practice needs to be interpreted to make sense for us and to be communicated to others. Measurements and numbers on their own are meaningless. We need to understand all the various measurements and knowledge and synthesize them through critical reasoning processes to enable purposeful decision making for each complex practice situation. Without this deliberate and autonomous reasoning process based on contributing to good and just decisions we run the risk that the dominant, routine or unreflected reasoning processes dominate to make up our minds for us (Arendt, 2003). Deliberate professionals choose this Arendtian action over mindless routines. As professions develop and mature they become more involved with questions of expertise development, knowledge growth and disciplinary boundary crossing. Higgs et al. (1999) claimed that a mature profession is one that enters into dialogue about its practices, is self-reflexive, and proactively transforms with global changes.

Workplace Influences

Trede's (2006) research on clinical practice approaches identified the importance and impact of external context factors on the preferred or existing practice model of the practitioners and the workplace. She found that the level of acceptability of the technical, biomedical model was high in situations where the environment was high-tech and healthcare delivery relied on advanced technology and in acute care or emergency situations where patients were very ill or required critical care. In such arenas there was an unchallenged focus on pathological diagnoses and biomedical intervention approaches, with the expectation of patient compliance. In less acute and less technology-dependent healthcare settings, participants in Trede's research considered that there was greater opportunity for patient-centred care that involved patient participation in clinical decision making. However, the notion of emancipatory practice was foreign to most of the participants. In early research discussions they considered that in their workplace situations with high workloads, time pressures, medical model frameworks, traditional approaches to professional hierarchies and an emphasis on evidence-based practice and cost efficiency, moves to treat patients on an equal footing in terms of clinical decision making were not particularly feasible, expected or needed.

Working Across and Within Different Practice Communities

Work by Croker (2011) into collaboration between health professionals and in teams identified the importance of understanding how different communities of practice influence workplace expectations of how professionals work and how they work together. Her research explored the ways practitioners often work across multiple practice communities including their direct work teams, their disciplines and their workplaces. Not only do they need to respond to the norms, expectations and practices of each community, but they may also be faced with challenges associated with each of these communities having different, and possibly contradictory, practice models. A practitioner could work in both a patient-centred palliative care unit and a protocol-driven cardiac surgery biomedical-model ward, yet desire to be a client collaborator who helps their clients conduct their own wellness narratives, in rejection of the restitution narrative (Alder, 2003).

In her research into practice models, Trede (2006) identified that practitioners unknowingly adopted their practice models. Much of their practice was unreflective and taken for granted. Most of these practitioners (physiotherapists) identified a preference for the biomedical practice model as the hegemonic system and educational model of the participants' workplaces and professional socialization. Most of these research participants claimed to be patient-centred but generally reverted to therapist-centred approaches based on technical interests. For a minority, the practice model preferred by the practitioner was so incompatible with the workplace model that the practitioner chose to leave that workplace.

Being Deliberate: Making Choices About Our Practice Models

Another key influence on our chosen practice model is how we consciously position and act in the world. As Arendt (1958) reminded us, practice or action is not a neutral activity. Inaction is also an action. When we do not understand the wider influences on us and choose how to position ourselves, to reason and to be in practice, others will choose it for us. Trede and McEwen, 2016a, p. 7) introduced the term deliberate professional to 'define ways of developing moral, thoughtful, purposeful and agentic stances that enable practitioners to counterbalance one-dimensional and instrumental practices'. Deliberate professionals are people who are informed by social justice consideration of self and others; they have the capacity and drive to promote positive changes through their professional practice. 'The deliberate professional is aware of complex and ever-changing relational dimensions in practice that shape the way practitioners think, talk and relate to self, others and the wider context around them; behave thoughtfully and courageously; resist unreflected conformity and notions of neutrality, repair and change conditions; and not disavow accepted practices, but rather acknowledge, appreciate, critique and change aspects of practices that need improving' (Trede and McEwen, 2016b, p. 22). Since, by definition, our practices are pursued deliberately, knowingly and informedly, practitioners need to realize and enact their practices within a coherent and deliberately owned practice model (Higgs, 2016).

REFLECTION POINT

- When we consider the global, national and local interests on how practice should be done, it could be assumed that practice models and clinical reasoning processes are predetermined and prescribed. Could you argue that your way of practising and reasoning is informed by the ideas of the deliberate professional as outlined previously?

MODELS OF PRACTICE

Models of practice are abstract ideas of what practice should look like if it followed a given framework. These frameworks comprise a variety of interests, criteria, norms, practice principles and strategies and behavioural expectations that inform clinical reasoning and practice. Models can be thought of as mental maps that assist practitioners to understand their practice. They serve to structure and to fine-tune practitioners' clinical reasoning. Whether they are learned, chosen or unconsciously acquired through professional socialization, practice models generate the principles that guide practice and create the standards practitioners strive towards and the behavioural expectations that determine performance.

Professional practice models can be categorized in a number of ways. One such categorization is based on the theory of knowledge and human interest (Habermas, 1972). According to this theory, there are three types of interest: technical, practical and critical, each of which generates a certain type of knowledge. Each interest directs the types of question that can be asked in practice, in turn dictating the type of knowledge that is generated and used in practice. These interests not only shape the professional practice we enact and determine which modes of practice we see as valuable, but they also influence the identity we adopt as professionals, how we see the role of patients, how we believe clinical decisions should be made and how we justify and argue our professional roles and actions. Table 6.1 presents the illness, wellness and capacity practice models and their inherent interests, based on

the three Habermasian interests. We argue that professional reasoning processes need to start with making explicit the purpose of what matters or what is at stake in a given practice situation, and continue with identifying probable, possible and impossible choices to then arrive at possibilities for decision making and action (Trede and McEwen, 2016b). Critically exploring values, purpose and desirable outcomes enables a kind of agency, a capacity to act that is transformative (Stetsenko, 2019). Agency underpinned by purpose is transformative because it boldly steers away from taken-for-granted reasoning processes towards searching for new possibilities.

Table 6.1 illustrates how interests shape practice models, knowledge and clinical reasoning in practice. Some aspects are of particular relevance in this discussion of clinical reasoning.

- The chosen focus and definition of health influences the healthcare goals pursued. When healthcare focuses on illness and biomedical pathology, the goal of care is limited to reducing deficit or merely helping patients cope with current situations. When health is seen as a potential, the focus of reasoning and healthcare is on building capacity. A capacity practice model transcends the dualism of the illness and wellness models.
- The relative power of the clinician and patient varies significantly across different practice models and is reflected in clinical reasoning strategies. For instance, in an emancipatory model collaboration, inclusiveness and reciprocal facilitation of responsibility are embedded in clinical decision making.
- The type(s) of knowledge that practitioners value is mediated through professional socialization. Practice knowledge is inclusive of dominant scientific (empirico-analytical) and psycho-sociocultural (ethnographic, phenomenological) constructs of knowledge. Being aware of different types of knowledges enables engagement with plurality of knowledges.
- The relative roles of practitioners and patients are significantly influenced by practice approaches, whether chosen or unconsciously adopted. Biomedical practice models speak of providers and recipients of practice. In an

			TABLE 6.1
		Three Frameworks for Professional Practice Models in Health	
Practice Model	**Illness Model**	**Wellness Model**	**Capacity Model**
Kind of interest	Technical	Practical	Emancipatory
Approach	Clinician-centred	Patient-centred	Patient-empowered
Philosophical paradigm	Empirico-analytical	Interpretive	Critical
Health definition	Reductionist	Holistic	Holistic
Focus of health	Technical	Practical	Political
Clinician has power	Clinician has power	Clinician may share some power	Equal power sharing
Patient power	Disempowered	Empowered	Empowered in a way that can be sustained
Practice knowledge	Propositional-technical	Propositional-technical and experiential	Propositional-technical, experiential and political
Stance towards status quo	Taking things for granted, accepting, reinforcing	Being aware of taken-for-granted things	Challenging status quo and changing frameworks
Role of patient	Passive, obedient, not asked to think for self	Interactive, participative but obedient, encouraged to think a bit for self	Interactive, participative, contributing, self-determining, learn to think for self
Role of clinician	Teacher/provider	Listener	Facilitator
Context of decision making	Out of context	Psychocultural context (definitely not political)	Historical-political context
Clinician as helper	Helping to survive	Helping to cope	Helping to liberate
Clinicians helping patients	To comply	To cope	To liberate
Clinician self-awareness	Unreflective	Reflective with the aim to empower	Reflective with the aim to transform

emancipatory/capacity model, patients and practitioners engage in dialogues and learn from each other, both accepting the roles of listening and negotiating. Professional roles shape and are shaped by organizational structures and cultures.

■ The level of critique and reflexivity that practitioners bring to their practice is grounded in practice and reasoning approaches. Critical self-awareness of professional or personal interests is the key to consciously choosing a practice model. Capacity for critique and change is a shared responsibility between structures and human agency.

Traditionally in orthodox Western medicine most practitioners acquire a biomedical science or medical practice model during their education and practice acculturation. This acquisition frequently occurs with limited critique or questioning of this model. Such practitioners are commonly unaware of their practice model because it represents the unquestioned norm and they are consequently unaware of how this model influences the way they reason. They reason within their adopted practice model without challenging the values and interests their practice model may entail. The key features of this model and reasoning are an emphasis on cure and the restitution of health, the role of the practitioner as professional authority in the decision-making process, and patients being regarded as 'the ones without expertise'. At times practitioners even disregard the patient's knowledge of self and their ability to participate in healthcare apart from being compliant and seeking cures. Reasoning in this model is largely performed by the expert/practitioner and is hypothetico-deductive in nature following the hypothesis generation and testing strategy of the hegemonic scientific model.

REFLECTION POINT

- The illness, wellness and capacity models outlined previously are theoretical constructs that do not exist in their purity in practice realities. However, what do you think are the benefits of this framework of conceptualizing professional practice models in health?
- How could you work with this framework in your teaching or clinical practice?

REASONING IN A CRITICAL SOCIAL SCIENCE MODEL FOR PRACTICE

To consider how a practitioner's chosen and enacted model of practice influences their clinical reasoning, we now turn to an in-depth interpretation of a particular model – the Critical Social Science (CSS) Model – as researched by Trede (2006). The primary goal of the research (Trede 2006; Trede and Higgs, 2003) was to understand how a CSS perspective, with its inherent emancipatory interests, might influence and transform healthcare practice. The development of the CSS model for practice resulted from four cycles of critical transformative dialogues based on critique and reflexivity and the pursuit of change that led to liberation. The dialogues involved two-way conversations with self and others (including other participants, patients, colleagues) using critical reasoning. The first dialogue described the status quo of the CSS and health-related literature and developed a conceptual approximation of a CSS model for healthcare practice. The second dialogue involved critique and interpretation of the related physiotherapy literature followed by a critical dialogue with the first group of physiotherapist participants to critique the status quo of physiotherapy practice. In the third dialogue, a group of practitioners trialled a CSS approach using action-learning strategies. The fourth dialogue, with another physiotherapy participant group, envisioned a CSS approach to practice.

In discussion of the status quo of practice, a few participants in Trede's (2006) study, either through dissatisfaction with their model or prompted by further education, consciously chose to adopt an alternative model based on humanistic philosophy or, less frequently, a CSS perspective. The more conscious the choice of practice model and the more this model differed from hegemonic practices, the more likely it was that the practitioners adopted a heightened level of awareness into their reasoning and behaviour. Instead of reasoning against scientific knowledge, evidence, established practice guidelines, or learned behaviour expectations set by their professions, workplaces or society at large, these practitioners sought to critically construct their own set of practice standards and ways of being in the world of practice and they monitored their behaviour against these standards. These participants, without theoretical understanding of CSS theory, had created a critical practice model.

A critical practice model starts with the assumptions that practice is complex, outcomes are uncertain and perceptions and interpretations of patient presentations are diverse. This means that a patient with an arthritic knee is not simply 'an arthritic knee' – an *object* of treatment. Instead, practitioners need to consider patients wholistically; this includes age, gender, attitude towards pain and physical activity, expectations of practitioners and themselves. Gaining a critical perspective means becoming aware of the interests that collide in practice and questioning these interests.

CSS is distinguished from the natural and social sciences in that it focusses on critique that leads to change and emancipation (Fay, 1987). Critique is raising awareness about interests that have arisen in the sociocultural, historical worlds that influence clinical reasoning and practice approaches. From a CSS perspective, critical thinking means being able to take a sceptical stance towards self, culture, norms, practices and institutions, as well as policy and regulations. Critical thinking questions the very roots of discipline-accepted knowledge and how it informs clinical reasoning (Brookfield, 2012; Trede and McEwen, 2015). During clinical reasoning this scepticism is both a conscious and a meta process; practitioners would explicitly challenge data, decisions and treatment alternatives and bring a heightened awareness of their own thinking and actions into the moments of practice, not just to posttreatment reflections.

CSS starts from the assumption that the influences listed earlier are human-made and therefore can be changed. Before these aspects of practice and reasoning are accepted and adopted they should be challenged and checked for their intentions and assumptions. CSS separates truth from ideology, reason from power and emancipation from oppression. The agenda of CSS is to critique, to engage in dialogue and to transform the status quo at an individual as well as a collective level, working towards transformation through professional development and maturity to become a self-aware and articulate professional who works with patients, policy and institutions that respect diversity and support social justice. The focus is on transforming unnecessarily constraining policies and oppressive practices that restrict workforce development as well as patient empowerment.

REFLECTION POINT

- With your peers identify where you already enact elements of a CSS model and where you could cultivate them more.

During Trede's (2006) research some of the participants trialled and experienced what it was like to transform their practice into (or towards) a critical practice model. This dialogue cycle included a preimplementation workshop, an action-learning phase and a critical appraisal workshop. Participants were informed about the findings from the first phase of the research investigating the status quo of physiotherapy practice models. They were educated about the dimensions of critique, power and emancipation of CSS and they were invited to critically discuss our critique of current practices. The findings from this phase indicated that the practitioners had varied levels of readiness (cognitive, emotional and pragmatic) to engage in practice reflection and change, and different perceptions of the value of CSS as a basis for practice. Different levels of engagement with CSS were identified. Some of the participants were happy to help with the research but persisted with their more traditional biomedical model approaches. Others practised a patient-centred model closely related to the emerging CSS model.

The CSS Model

The CSS model (Trede, 2006) for practice has two core dimensions.

(a) An emancipatory dimension

The emancipatory dimension entails recognition that to adopt a CSS or emancipatory model in a world

of practice where such practice is a minority view requires a journey of critical transformative dialogues of emancipation for the practitioner. The research identified five modes of engagement with CSS as a practice model. These were labelled:

1. *The Uninformed*   those who had not heard of CSS
2. *The Unconvinced*   those who trialled CSS but did not change their current practice, which remained in the biomedical model
3. *The Contemplators*   those who trialled CSS and thought that some aspects of CSS were convincing but encountered too many perceived barriers to transform their practice substantially
4. *The Transformers*   those who were convinced of CSS and were transforming aspects of their practice
5. *The Champions*   those who were convinced of the value of CSS and embodied CSS in their practice

Across these five levels only a few participants progressively engaged more deeply in transforming their practice towards a CSS approach and in learning more about CSS, came to value these principles and practices more deeply, and journeyed further away from their traditional practice knowledge base and practices. Table 6.2 details the interests, practices and characteristics of each of these modes. Of particular relevance here are the changing patterns of interaction, power use and reasoning approaches, ranging from therapist-centred and therapist-empowered decision making for patients to patient-centred and mutually empowered decision-making dialogues with patients.

REFLECTION POINT

- The prototypical categorization of how professionals engage with the CSS model is intended to help readers identify themselves where they fit and where they might possibly want to position themselves on the table. It can be used as a discussion starter in teams to clarify purposes of clinical reasoning processes.

TABLE 6.2
Five Prototypical Engagements with CSS

Practice Dimension	The Uninformed	The Unconvinced	The Contemplators	The Transformers	The Champions
Definition	Those who have not heard of CSS	Those who have trialled CSS but do not change their current practice	Those who have explored CSS in their practice and have chosen to adopt some aspects of CSS in their practice	Those who are convinced of critical practice and are transforming their practice to this model	Those who are convinced of the value of critical practice and advocate it
Practice model	Typically the biomedical model	Typically the biomedical model	Mixed biomedical and critical model	Approximating a critical practice model	Critical model
Interests	Technical/practical	Technical/practical	Practical/technical/ emancipatory	Emancipatory (plus technical/practical)	Predominantly emancipatory
Self-appraisal	Mastering technical application	Mastering technical application	Mastering technical application and acknowledging patients' interests	Acknowledging own assumptions and unreflected ideology	Seeking critical self-understanding, reflexive
Mode of critique	Critiquing practice from an empirico-analytical, technical perspective	Critiquing practice from an empirico-analytical, technical perspective	Critiquing practice from practical perspectives working within systems that are taken for granted or at least assumed unchangeable	Critiquing practice by starting with self-critique and awareness of system challenges	Being open, sincere, curious; avoiding making generalizations and unreflected judgements; paying attention to detail (rethinking practice dimensions through relational thinking)
Approach to reasoning	Linear, cause and effect, minimal contextual consideration	Linear, cause and effect, minimal contextual consideration	Appreciate critical reasoning without adopting it	Adopting critical reasoning in aspects of practice	Critical, dialogical reasoning
Approach to knowledge	Propositional-technical	Propositional-technical	Propositional-technical and experiential	Propositional-technical, experiential and critical	Propositional-technical, experiential and critical
Patient relationships	Therapist is the expert and dominates	Therapist is the expert and dominates	Therapist is the expert but acknowledges patient experience	Democratizing patient-therapist relationship	Dialogical, reciprocal relationship where expertise of therapist and patient is acknowledged
Power/authority	Owned by physiotherapist's propositional knowledge	Owned by physiotherapist's propositional knowledge	Owned by propositional knowledge and some nonpropositional knowledge	Shift from propositional to critical knowledge. System propositional knowledge dominant	Shared as critical knowledge

Continued

		TABLE 6.2—Cont'd			
		Five Prototypical Engagements with CSS			
Practice Dimension	**The Uninformed**	**The Unconvinced**	**The Contemplators**	**The Transformers**	**The Champions**
Context interpretation	Within biomedical domain	Within biomedical domain	Within biopsychosocial domain	Within cultural and biopsychosocial domain	Within critical cultural biopsychosocial domain
Professional identity and role	Technical and telling patients what they need	Technical and telling patients what they need	Technical, practical and empathic, guiding patients	Moving to a facilitating role of emancipatory learning in self Asking patients what they need	Moving to a role of facilitating emancipatory learning in self and patients and chosen and self-owned identity
Goals	Achievement of positive technical, biomedical outcomes	Achievement of positive technical, biomedical outcomes	Achievement of functional and practical outcomes	Achievement of negotiated outcomes	Emancipation of self, others and the system for enhancement of patient outcomes in a critical framework

CSS, critical social sciences.
From Trede, F.V., 2006. A critical practice for physiotherapy. Doctoral dissertation, The University of Sydney. https://ses.library.usyd.edu.au/handle/2123/1430

(b) A critical, lived dimension

In advocating consideration and adoption of a CSS practice model, we recognize that critical practice has variable relevance and potential across the range of practice contexts and that other models (as discussed earlier) may be preferable or more feasible in certain contexts. Critical practice is the practice model of choice in situations of emancipatory need, predilection and support. The ultimate value of critical practice is its capacity to enhance the quality of life of its protagonists through critical appraisal, respect, particularization, empowerment and constructive collaboration in shared vision and actions.

CSS practice is an accessible and acceptable choice when four situations coincide: (1) when there is a perceived need for patients and healthcare practitioners to collaborate in clinical decision making and to liberate practice; (2) when it is the preferred practice model of a patient or practitioner (or group) who is a champion of critical practice; (3) when other team members are supportive of this approach and keen to embody authentic critical practice; and (4) where management and organizational systems support rather than restrict critical approaches. These four situations create a facilitative and supportive environment for embedding a critical practice perspective in the existing discourse. Critical practice would then be the practice model of choice because marginalized voices of patients and practitioners are heard and acted upon in a system-based environment that is sensitive, supportive and responsive to critique and emancipation.

Practitioners bring their assumptions, values and prejudgements and professional experiences to the clinical situation. Practitioners with a critical perspective are aware of the interests that collide in practice and they question these interests. Practising in a CSS model involves engaging in critical transformative dialogues that enable practitioners to make practice model choices and living CSS in the everyday.

Practising and reasoning within a CSS model requires practitioners:

- to challenge models of practice, practice cultures and taken-for-granted practice interests
- to choose CSS as the overall practice framework for decision making and action
- to be accountable to self as well as to those influenced by their professional practice

- to analyse what type of practice knowledge is valuable and situationally applicable
- to exercise choice about courses of action critically and responsibly
- to engage patients (and carers) in transformative dialogue
- to plan a team CSS approach
- to make alternatives happen
- to be willing to rethink their sense of self, their professional identity and their chosen model of practice
- to appraise their reasoning critically and practice on a big picture level (is my practice model relevant and meaningful) and within the moments of reasoning and practice.

The relevance of CSS for health professional practice is that such a practice model:

- engages with increasingly complex health conditions and steers away from one-dimensional ideas for health
- builds the capacity of practitioners for critical self-reflection as a tool for practice development
- democratizes professional relations and ensures inclusive, appropriate and ethical practice that fosters self-determination of patients
- raises awareness of interests and values that inform clinical reasoning
- redefines professional identity within a constantly changing world to liberate practitioners from restrictive hegemonic practice rules
- encourages rethinking of the boundaries and inclusions of the practice context.

A critical practice model is challenging because it unsettles current power structures in healthcare at the macro level and at the personal professional level requires individuals to be vigilant and question self. But without critique there is little chance for the healthcare sector and practitioners to make the radical changes required now. And they start with professional development that focusses on awareness raising and capacity to act otherwise. These changes are needed because reacting and empathizing is no longer enough.

REFLECTION POINT

- How might you write a practice manifesto in your workplace that incorporates elements of a CSS model?

SUMMARY

In this chapter we have presented:

- the interdependence between reasoning and practice in the context of models of practice
- the implication of a critical social science practice model for practice and reasoning.

REFERENCES

Alder, S., 2003. Beyond the restitution narrative [Doctoral dissertation. University of Western Sydney. http://handle.uws.edu.au:8081/1959.7/22873]

Arendt, H., 1958. The human condition. University of Chicago Press, Chicago, II.

Arendt, H., 2003. Responsibility and judgment, with introduction from Jerome Kohn. Schocken Books, New York.

Brookfield, S., 2012. Teaching for critical thinking: Tools and techniques to help students question their assumptions. Jossey-Bass.

Croker, A., 2011. Collaboration in rehabilitation teams. [Doctoral dissertation, Charles Sturt University]. https://researchoutput.csu.edu.au/en/publications/collaboration-in-rehabilitation-teams-3

Eraut, M., 1994. Developing professional knowledge and competence. The Falmer Press. https://doi.org/10.4324/9780203486016

Fay, B., 1987. Critical social science. Cornell University Press. ISBN: 0801494583

Habermas, J., 1972. Knowledge and human interest (Translator J.J. Shapiro). Heinemann.

Higgs, J., 2016. Deliberately owning my practice model: Realising my professional practice. In: Trede, F., McEwen, C. (Eds.), Educating the deliberate professional: Preparing practitioners for emergent futures. Springer, pp. 189–203.

Higgs, J., Hunt, A., Higgs, C., et al., 1999. Physiotherapy education in the changing international healthcare and educational contexts. Advances in Physiotherapy. 1 (1), 17–26. https://doi.org/10.1080/140381999443528

Kung, T.H., Cheatham, M., Medenilla, A., Sillos, C., De Leon, L., Elepaño, C., et al., 2023. Performance of ChatGPT on USMLE: Potential for AI-assisted medical education using large language models. PLOS Digit Health 2 (2), e0000198. https://doi.org/10.1371/journal.pdig.0000198

Moynihan, R., Sanders, S., Michaleff, Z.A., et al., 2021. Impact of COVID-19 pandemic on utilisation of healthcare services: A systematic review. BMJ Open 11, e045343. https://doi.org/10.1136/bmjopen-2020-045343

Schön, D.A., 1987. Educating the reflective practitioner. Jossey-Bass.

Stetsenko, A., 2019. Radical-transformative agency: Continuities and contrasts with relational agency and implications for education. Frontiers Education vol 4. https://doi.org/10.3389/feduc.2019.00148

Trede, F., Higgs, J., 2003. Re-framing the clinician's role in collaborative clinical decision making: Re-thinking practice knowledge and the notion of clinician–patient relationships. Learning in Health and Social Care 2 (2), 66–73.

Trede, F., McEwen, C., 2015. Critical thinking for future practice. In: Davies, M., Barnett, R. (Eds.), Palgrave handbook of critical thinking in higher education. Palgrave Publishers, pp. 457–475.

Trede, F., McEwen, C., 2016a. Scoping the deliberate professional. In: Trede, F., McEwen, C. (Eds.), Educating the deliberate professional: Preparing practitioners for emergent futures. Springer, pp. 3–14.

Trede, F., McEwen, C., 2016b. Carving out the territory for educating the deliberate professional. In: Trede, F., McEwen, C. (Eds.), Educating the deliberate professional: Preparing practitioners for emergent futures. Springer, pp. 15–28.

Trede, F.V., 2006. A critical practice for physiotherapy [Doctoral dissertation, The University of Sydney]. https://ses.library.usyd.edu.au/handle/2123/1430

7

THE DEVELOPMENT OF CLINICAL REASONING EXPERTISE

HENNY P.A. BOSHUIZEN ■ HENK G. SCHMIDT

CHAPTER OUTLINE

CHAPTER AIMS

The aims of this chapter are:

- to examine the development of clinical reasoning expertise, particularly in medicine
- to answer the question of whether clinical reasoning can be taught to medical students
- to present approaches to clinical reasoning skills training building on the stage theory.

INTRODUCTION

The main objective of medical schools is to turn relative novices into knowledgeable and skilled professionals who are able to solve clinical problems and are aware of the reach of their knowledge and skills and what goes beyond their capacities. In this chapter, we seek to answer the question of whether clinical reasoning can be taught to medical students. We start by describing the development from novice in medicine to expert, providing a theoretical cognitive psychological framework. Several approaches to clinical reasoning skills training are then described and the implications of this theory are considered for the

way medical education can improve students' clinical reasoning. We end with some conclusions about the necessity of keeping knowledge up-to-date and the importance of a learning culture in the workplace.

A THEORY OF THE DEVELOPMENT OF MEDICAL EXPERTISE

For a long time, it has been thought that the human mind can be trained in logical thinking, problem solving or creativity and that these skills could transfer to all domains of daily and professional life. For this purpose, children are encouraged to play chess or to learn Latin in school. In the same vein, it was thought that experts in an arbitrary domain had trained their minds and had developed general problem-solving and thinking skills. This opinion has, however, been superseded, because research has shown that experts in a specific domain have not developed problem-solving skills that can be applied across domains. Instead, domain knowledge and the associated skills to use this knowledge in problem solving develop simultaneously and interdependently.

In medicine, research has shown that clinical reasoning is not a separate skill acquired independently of medical knowledge and other diagnostic skills. Instead, research suggests a stage theory of the development of medical expertise, in which knowledge acquisition and clinical reasoning go hand in hand (Boshuizen and Schmidt, 1992; Schmidt and Boshuizen, 1992; Schmidt et al., 1992; Schmidt et al., 1990). This theory of medical diagnosis is essentially a theory of the acquisition and development of knowledge structures upon which a student or a physician operates when diagnosing a case. Notable changes in problem solving or clinical reasoning are the result of structural changes in knowledge, whereas knowledge structure and quality are affected by the quality of the reasoning process that operates on the knowledge base. Clinical reasoning leaves its traces in the knowledge structure directly by strengthening or weakening links between concepts and indirectly as a result of concurrent or post hoc evaluation thereof and the knowledge actions of the learner – of every expertise level – that may follow from that.

During the first stage of expertise development, medical students acquire large amounts of knowledge about the biomedical basic sciences. They acquire concepts that are linked together in a semantic, knowledge network. Gradually, more concepts are added and refined and more and better connections are made. Knowledge accretion and validation are the students' main concerns in this period of their study. This process takes much more time than teachers might expect. In particular, the integration and integrated use of knowledge from different domains (e.g. the clinical sciences, biochemistry, pathophysiology and microanatomy) is not self-evident (Boshuizen and van de Wiel, 1998; Groothuis et al., 1998). During this stage, the clinical reasoning process is characterized by lines of reasoning consisting of chains of small steps commonly based on detailed biomedical concepts. An example of detailed reasoning is given in Table 7.1. It has been taken from a longer protocol in which a fourth-year medical student is dealing with a case of pancreatitis. His initial hypothesis set contained gall-bladder and pancreas disease. Apparently, this student is entertaining the hypothesis of biliary tract obstruction. First, he reasons whether the new finding about the patient's stools affects this hypothesis and decides that this is not the case. Next, three items later, he combines the information acquired and concludes that there is no inflammation (causing this obstruction) (step 1), hence no cholecystitis (step 2), hence the biliary tract must be obstructed by something else, a stone for instance (step 3) or a carcinoma (step 4), which might be the case because the patient has lost weight (step 5).

TABLE 7.1	
Lines of Reasoning by a Fourth-Year Medical Student	
Case Item (Number and Text)	**Think-Aloud Protocol**
31. (History) Defecation: paler and more malodorous stools according to the patient	... not so much undermines that idea ... er... their frequency... and their pattern compared with colour and the like... their smell er... yes... no problems with defecation, that means in any case no constipation, which you wouldn't expect with an obstruction of the biliary tract... well yes
32. (History) Last bowel movement was yesterday	...
32. (History) Temperature: 37°C at 6 p.m.	so no temperature
33. (Physical examination) Pulse rate: regular, 72 beats/min.	... er. yes ... the past two ... together. means that there's er no inflammation ... and that would eliminate an er ... an er. cholecystitis ... and would rather mean an ... er ... obstruction of the biliary tract ... caused by a stone, for instance ... or, what may be the case too, by a carcinoma, but I wouldn't ... although, it might be possible, lost 5 kilograms in weight ...

Note: Protocol fragment obtained from a fourth-year medical student working on a pancreatitis case showing detailed reasoning steps. See Boshuizen and Schmidt (1992) for a detailed description of the experiment.

By the end of the first stage of knowledge acquisition, students have a knowledge network that allows them to make direct lines of reasoning between different concepts within that network. The more often these direct lines are activated, the more these concepts cluster together and students become able to make direct links between the first and last concept in such a line of reasoning, skipping intermediate concepts. We have labelled this process 'knowledge encapsulation', a term that refers to the clustering aspect of the process and can account for the automatization involved (e.g. Boshuizen and Schmidt, 1992; Boshuizen et al., 2020; Schmidt and Boshuizen, 1993). Many of these concept clusters have (semi-)clinical names, such as *microembolism, aortic insufficiency, forward failure* or *extrahepatic icterus*, providing a powerful reasoning tool. Encapsulation of biomedical knowledge results in the next stage of development of clinical reasoning skills, in which biomedical knowledge has been integrated into clinical knowledge. At this stage, students' clinical reasoning processes no longer involve many biomedical concepts. Students tend to make direct links between patient findings and clinical concepts that have the status of hypotheses or diagnoses in their reasoning process. However, if needed, this encapsulated biomedical knowledge can be unfolded again, for instance when dealing with a very complicated problem. Van de Wiel et al. (2000) showed that experts' clinical knowledge structures subsumed biomedical knowledge. Rikers et al. (2005) demonstrated that in expert clinical reasoning, biomedical knowledge is also activated, operating in a sort of stand-by mode.

At the same time, a transition takes place from a network type of knowledge organization to a structure referred to as 'illness scripts'. Illness scripts have three components. The first component refers to enabling conditions of disease: the conditions or constraints under which a disease occurs. These are the personal, social, medical, hereditary and environmental factors that affect health in a positive or negative way or affect the course of a specific disease. The second component is the fault: the pathophysiological process that is taking place in a specific disease, represented in encapsulated form. The third component consists of the consequences of the fault: the signs and symptoms of a specific disease (also see Feltovich and Barrows, 1984, who introduced this theoretical notion). Contrary to

(advanced) novice knowledge networks, illness scripts are activated as a whole. After an illness script has been activated, no active, small-step search within that script is required; the other elements of the script are activated immediately and automatically, which results in a major cognitive advantage. While solving a problem, a physician activates one or a few illness scripts. The illness script elements (enabling conditions and consequences) are then matched to the information provided by the patient. Illness scripts not only incorporate matching information from the patient, but they also generate expectations about other signs and symptoms the patient might have. Activated illness scripts thus provide a list of phenomena to seek in history taking and in physical examination. In the course of this verification process, expected values are substituted by real findings, instantiating and further activating the script. Illness scripts that fail in this respect will become deactivated. The instantiated script yields a diagnosis or a differential diagnosis when a few competing scripts remain active.

An example of script activation by an experienced physician, dealing with the same clinical case as the student in Table 7.1, is given in Table 7.2. The information about the patient's medical past and psychosocial circumstances (summarized in the protocol), combined with the presenting complaint, activated a few competing illness scripts: pancreatic disease, liver disease and abdominal malignancy (which he considers implausible because of the patient's age), and stomach perforation. In addition, he thought of cardiomyopathy as an effect of excessive drinking. In the course of the think-aloud protocol, he seemed to monitor the level of instantiation of every illness script. Except for gallbladder disease, no new scripts were activated. So far, we have seen that expert and novice knowledge structures differ in many respects. As a consequence, their clinical reasoning differs as well. Medical experts, who have large numbers of ready-made illness scripts that organize many enabling conditions and consequences associated with a specific disease, will activate one or more of these illness scripts when dealing with a case. Activation will be triggered by information concerning enabling conditions and/or consequences. Expert hypothesis activation and testing can be seen as an epiphenomenon of illness script activation

TABLE 7.2	
Illness Script Activation by a Family Physician	
Case Item (Number and Text)	**Think-Aloud Protocol**
8. Complaint: Continuous pain in the upper part of the abdomen, radiating to the back	… well, when I am visiting someone who is suffering an acute … continuous – since when? – pain in his upper abdomen, radiating to the back, who had pancreatitis a year before … of whom I don't know for sure if he still drinks or not after that course of Refusal, but of whom I do know that he still has mental problems, so still receives a disability benefit, then I think that the first thing to cross my mind will be: well, what about that pancreas, … how's his liver … and also that – considering his age – eh it is not very likely that there will be other things wrong in his abdomen … eh … of a malign thing er nature … of course eh if he's taking huge amounts of alcohol there's always the additional possibility of a stomach eh problem, a stomach perforation … excessive drinking can also cause eh serious cardiomyopathy, which eh may cause heart defects mm I can't er judge the word 'continuous' very well yet in this context

Note: Protocol fragment obtained from an experienced family physician working on a pancreatitis case. Earlier, he had received information about enabling conditions such as mental problems and alcohol abuse. See Boshuizen and Schmidt (1992).

and instantiation. These are generally automatic and 'unconscious' processes. As long as new information matches an active illness script, no active reasoning is required. Only in cases of severe mismatch or conflict between activated scripts does the expert engage in active clinical reasoning. During this process either illness-script-based expectations are adjusted based on specific features of the patient or the expert reverts to pure biomedical reasoning, drawing on de-encapsulated biomedical knowledge. Our old-time favourite example of deliberate script adjustment was given by Lesgold et al. (1988). They described expert radiologists' interpretations of an enlarged heart shadow on an X-ray screen. These experts took into consideration the scoliosis of the patient's thoracic spine, which affected the position of the heart relative to the slide. Hence, they concluded that the heart was not actually enlarged.

Students, on the other hand, can rely only on knowledge networks, which are less rich and less easily activated than experts' illness scripts. They require more information before a specific hypothesis will be generated. Semantic networks must be reasoned through step by step. This is a time-consuming process and often requires active monitoring. Hence, contrary to illness scripts, the knowledge structures that students activate do not automatically generate a list of signs and symptoms that are expected. Active searching through their networks is needed to generate such a list that might verify or falsify their hypotheses. In general, students' clinical reasoning is less orderly,

less goal-oriented and more time consuming and it is based on less plausible hypotheses resulting in less accurate diagnoses than those of experts.

The differences described thus far were all investigated in the context of solving cases that did not require further data collection. This rather artificial task has the advantage that participants can devote all their time and attention to the cognitive processing of the information given. However, authentic clinical reasoning takes place during the action of data gathering and evaluation. Recently we investigated clinical reasoning of pathologists. Similar to radiologists, their material is mostly visual: pathological slides that are inspected under a microscope. Information must be extracted by inspecting the slides at several levels of magnification. Verbal data, combined with eye movement data, suggested that students described their 'findings' in rather perceptual terms such as form and colour and searched for cues they could interpret in pathological terms without being able to come to a satisfactory conclusion. Experts and intermediates (residents) differed in the number of specific pathologies mentioned (intermediates mentioned more) and in the way they checked alternative scripts: experts actively searched for alternatives of their diagnosis at the end of the inspection, while intermediates appeared to have more scripts open already in the beginning (Jaarsma et al., 2014).

A study by Wagenaar (2008) has shown that third-year students have great difficulty combining data collection and clinical reasoning. They are very dependent

				TABLE 7.3			
				Knowledge Restructuring, Clinical Reasoning and Levels of Expertise			
Expertise Level	Knowledge Representation	Knowledge Acquisition and (Re)-Structuring	Clinical Reasoning	Control Required In Clinical Reasoning	Demand on Cognitive Capacity	Clinical Reasoning in Action
Novice	Networks	Knowledge accretion and validation	Long chains of detailed reasoning steps through preencapsulated networks	Active monitoring of each reasoning step	High	Difficulty to combine data collection and evaluation and clinical reasoning
Intermediate	Network	Encapsulation	Reasoning through encapsulated network	Active monitoring of each reasoning step	Medium	…
Expert	Illness scripts	Illness script formation	Illness script activation and instantiation	Monitoring of the level of script instantiation	Low	Adjust data collection to time available and to verification/ falsification level of hypotheses

on the information the client volunteers and seem unable to reason in action. Instead, they try to collect as much information as possible and only after they have completed the interview do they review the information collected to formulate a diagnosis. Experts, on the other hand, think on their feet, adapting their data collection to the level of verification or falsification of their hypotheses and to the time available. Table 7.3 summarizes these differences between novices, intermediates and experts. The picture that emerges here is that novices and intermediates are handicapped in two ways: their knowledge is insufficient, and it requires extra cognitive capacity when solving problems. Both aspects negatively influence clinical problem solving; they also hinder learning.

REFLECTION POINT

- The quality of a clinical reasoning process depends on the quality of the knowledge it operates on; case, knowledge and regulation together determine the quality of the result.
- Knowledge networks are transformed into illness scripts as a consequence of dealing with real or simulated patients.

- Encapsulating concepts integrate biomedical and clinical knowledge; to play their role in the communication with colleagues, they need to have a shared meaning.
- Illness scripts are powerful cognitive structures that allow automatic processing; their validity deserves continuous attention.

TEACHING CLINICAL REASONING

Until this moment we have avoided defining the concepts of clinical reasoning and clinical reasoning skills, first giving attention to the knowledge structures upon which these reasoning processes operate. Nor have we explicitly addressed the question of whether clinical reasoning can be taught. Yet there is huge pressure on the profession to improve the quality of diagnosis and treatment, which is apparent from the numerous publications on medical error and patient safety (e.g. Baker et al., 2004) and evidence-based medicine (see for instance the rapidly growing number of COVID-19 reviews in the UNCOVER database Usher Institute, which contained 3566

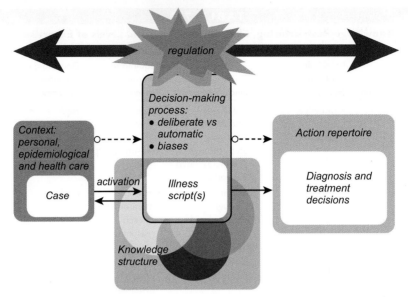

Fig. 7.1 ▪ The relationship between case, knowledge and regulation in expert clinical reasoning. The underlying knowledge structure can be further activated when no acceptable solution is found.

publications as of 26 December 2022). Generally, clinical reasoning equals the thinking process occurring when dealing with a clinical case. Most researchers who investigate teaching clinical reasoning differentiate between different phases in the clinical reasoning process (e.g. Bowen, 2006): beginning with hypothesis generation, inquiry strategy, data analysis, problem synthesis or diagnosis and finally ending with diagnostic and treatment decision making.

Clinical reasoning, its form and quality, is thus affected by the features of the case and the validity and structure of the knowledge base. Typical cases activate one illness script, plus maybe some alternatives one should always be aware of, not because of their plausibility but because of their severity (Custers et al., 1996). Atypical cases may activate several scripts that have to be sorted out by checking the script elements that are part of one but not of other scripts (Mamede et al., 2007) or that have to be further reasoned through by means of basic science knowledge (see Lesgold et al., 1988, example described earlier). Invalid knowledge jeopardizes the validity of the whole process. Apart from these two factors, a third factor plays a role in the quality of the reasoning process. This factor is the 'regulation of the decision-making process' itself,

which may vary between automatic and deliberate analytic processing (see Fig. 7.1).

Decision making as a general human information processing activity has a couple of features that can make it prone to biased reasoning and others that can protect against that. For instance, the speedy activation of one illness script may lead to confirmation bias (the tendency to confirm a diagnosis or to fill the open slots in an illness script instead of searching for information that might contradict that) or to premature closure (the tendency to accept a diagnosis before other relevant options have been excluded). Also priming of one illness script (e.g. as a result of recent exposure to a similar case or a presentation in the media) leads to easier activation of the same script at the cost of others, which in turn may lead to premature closure. In the medical literature, these biases have been frequently described as a cause of medical error (Croskerry, 2003). However, Norman et al. (2017) concluded that educational interventions focussing on recognition of bias in clinical reasoning did not result in a reduction of error.

Researchers have investigated whether information processing in 'careful mode' helps overcome such biases. It turned out that for residents this was indeed the case but not for students (Mamede et al., 2010) and for complex cases only (Mamede et al., 2008). In a later study, Mamede et al. (2012) found that fourth-year students performed worse when stimulated to process cases very carefully than in unreflective or in 'light' mode; however, after 1 week, careful processing led to better diagnostic scores compared with their own previous performance and with the other groups. Other studies (e.g. Schmidt et al., 2014) directed the participants' attention to their conclusions afterwards and so could override bias. Some of the manipulations studied had a positive effect on later case processing. A similar phenomenon was found by Grohnert (2017) in a very different domain, that is, auditing. Grohnert found that having made a certain kind of mistake before and *not* seeing a certain task as pure routine was beneficial for later performance.

The interventions in these studies all related to regulation of the process. The positive results related to the effects on present and future problem solving. Our conclusion from these studies is that thoughtful case processing by students as well as reflection on performance improves the quality of their knowledge structure. Norman et al. (2017) hypothesized an interaction between expertise level, case complexity and reflection. They concluded that 'to the extent that reflection is effective, it achieves these results by encouraging participants to identify and reconfigure their knowledge' (p. 27). Discussions on the process of clinical reasoning and its fallibilities may furthermore provide students with the vocabulary and metaknowledge that can help them reflect on their performance (Kassirer, 2010).

After this analysis, we return to the question of how clinical reasoning expertise can be stimulated and whether clinical reasoning skills can be taught and trained as such or whether other educational measures will be needed to improve students' clinical reasoning. It might be evident that our theory and previous experiences with direct training programmes suggest direct training of the different phases of clinical reasoning does not provide a general solution and that other measures are needed, as far as the reasoning component of the diagnostic process is concerned. What is more important, our theory suggests that to improve clinical reasoning, education must focus on

the development of adequate knowledge structures. Similar conclusions permeate publications such as Bowen (2006) and Lubarsky et al. (2015). Hence, teaching, training, coaching, modelling or supervising should adapt to the actual knowledge organization of the student. During the first stage in which knowledge accretion and validation take place, students should be given ample opportunity to test the knowledge they have acquired for its consistency and connectedness, to identify misconceptions, to correct concepts and their connections and to fill the gaps they have detected. Students will do many of these things by themselves if they are provided with stimuli for thinking and with appropriate feedback. This stuff for thinking does not necessarily have to consist of patient problems. Short descriptions of physiological phenomena (e.g. jet lag) that have to be explained should also be considered. Self-explanations (e.g. Chamberland et al., 2013) and mind-mapping (Daley et al., 2016) are powerful learning instruments for students to explore and validate their knowledge.

During the next stage of knowledge encapsulation, students should deal with more elaborate patient problems. As students go through the process of diagnosing a patient and afterwards explaining the diagnosis to a peer or supervisor, biomedical knowledge will become encapsulated into higher-level concepts. For instance, diagnosing a patient with acute bacterial endocarditis will first require detailed reasoning about infection, fever reaction, temperature regulation, circulation, haemodynamics and so on. Later, a similar case will be explained in terms of bacterial infection, sepsis, microembolisms and aortic insufficiency (Boshuizen, 1989). These problems are not necessarily presented by real patients in real settings. Paper cases and simulated patients will serve the same goal, sometimes even better. Especially during the earlier stage of knowledge encapsulation, when students have to do a great deal of reasoning, it might be more helpful to work with paper cases that present all relevant information. Reasoning through their knowledge networks to build a coherent explanation of the information available, students need not be concerned whether the information on which they work is complete and valid. Later in this stage, when knowledge has been restructured into a more tightly connected format, greater uncertainty can be allowed.

Finally, the stage of illness script acquisition requires experience with real patients in real settings. Research by Custers et al. (1996) suggests that at this stage, practical experience with typical patients (i.e. patients whose disease manifestations resemble the textbooks) should be preferred over experiences with atypical patients. With increasing knowledge, a confrontation with sets of related cases is helpful to learn about the possible manifestations of diseases, while a well-chosen combination of cases with similar signs and symptoms but different underlying diseases is essential to improve the knowledge structure (Custers, 2015; Huwendiek et al., 2013). There are no empirical data that can help to answer the question of whether illness script formation requires active dealing with the patient or whether observing a doctor–patient contact could serve the same goal. On the other hand, because encapsulation and script formation go hand in hand, especially earlier on in this stage, it is probable that 'hands-on' experience is to be preferred. Having to reason about the patient would result in further knowledge encapsulation, while direct interaction with the patient provides the opportunity for perceptual learning, adding 'reality' to the symbolic concepts learned from textbooks. During this phase, students might initially be overwhelmed by the information available in reality. They can easily overlook information when they do not know its relevance. This will especially affect their perception of enabling conditions. Therefore, it might be helpful to draw the student's attention to the enabling conditions operating in specific patients to make sure that their illness scripts are completed with this kind of information. Boshuizen et al. (1992) emphasize that in this stage of training a mix of practical experience and theoretical education is needed. They found that during clinical rotations students tend to shift towards the application of clinical knowledge, although it is not yet fully integrated in their knowledge base. A combination of the two ways of learning can help students to build a robust and flexible knowledge base.

Thus we see that working on problems and diagnosing and explaining authentic patient cases, applying biomedical knowledge and receiving feedback on their thinking might help students to form a knowledge system that enables efficient and accurate clinical reasoning that does not require all control capacity available (monitoring of reasoning on encapsulated concepts in a network requires less control than monitoring of reasoning on preencapsulated, detailed concepts; see Table 7.3). Van Merriënboer et al. (2003) have shown that good planning and design of the learning process, such that integration and automatization are fostered, are very important. Their 4C-ID model (van Merrienboer and Kirschner, 2017) provides an excellent scaffold for educational design in which working with cases plays an essential role, whereas Jossberger et al. (2022) presented their PETS model, a complementary format for learning in and from simulations.

Before we conclude, there is an interrelated cluster of three other aspects on the way to expertise that we claim is very important for the future physicians who are trained in our universities, hospitals and practices. They are learning from experience, are staying up-to-date and are prepared for change. Yet, as (clinical) teachers we have much less control over this part of their learning trajectory. The patient mix that interns are confronted with during training is neither under their control nor their supervisors' control or to a limited extent only. Based on these cases illness scripts will be refined. Ohlsson (2011) calls this 'monotonic change', which he considers the default, effortless way of learning. This adaptation is their strength in the case of routine problems and their weakness in the face of uncommon presentations and combinations. Non-monotonic learning in medicine can happen when a person notices that a proposed solution or an activated illness script does not sufficiently match the patient findings. Unfortunately, Ohlsson conjectures, non-monotonic learning is not under voluntary control. It can be triggered by multiple conditions, it happens to a person and it takes time. The process described by Ohlsson bares close similarity with 'gut feelings' in medical practice (Stolper et al., 2015) that just happen but are formed by previous learning. Mentors and supervisors can help interns analyse their gut feelings. Education can also prepare students by making them aware of how their professional knowledge has been shaped by the epidemiology and practices of the country, the city or the hospital in which they work. Change, small and large, is also a factor that can require non-monotonic learning. The case described by Brouwers (December 24–25, 2022, see Box 7.1) may illustrate that. The non-monotonic learning required here considers illness script on metabolic disease as

BOX 7.1
A RECONSTRUCTION OF A COURSE OF EVENTS

Uzair is a 4-year-old Afghan boy, who was evacuated with his parents and three brothers during the turbulent days that foreign troops, embassy personnel and their local helpers left the country. This boy had been sick since he was about 2 months old but due to the medical situation in Afghanistan the cause of his problems was not identified. Once in the Netherlands, his parents consulted a paediatrician in the nearby regional hospital, who gave priority to the child's low weight and referred him to the academic children's hospital for further diagnosis. In the reconstruction, this course of action resulted in an adverse event due to the child's underlying rare metabolic disorder. The boy gained weight on a diet high in proteins but further accumulated the neurotoxic metabolites he could not digest. Apparently, the physicians involved did not have an illness script that matched the child's symptoms, which can be attributed to the neonatal screening program that identifies these children, who can grow up normally with the right diet.

Brouwers, L., 2022, December, 24–25. Zorgenkind; Een reconstructie [Problem child; A reconstruction]. NRC-Weekend, 20–23

well as nonstandard patients who traverse the healthcare system in unknown ways. Education can prepare students by making them sensitive to the effects of change in the population, healthcare organization or disease expression.

The learning required for staying up-to-date is similar to pregraduation learning as it includes learning from text, presentations, demonstrations, video, etc. However, there is also a big difference, that is, the role of self-direction in choosing materials is much stronger, while the learners' goal is mostly inspired by patient problems (van de Wiel and Van den Bossche, 2013). This need of learning for the sake of patient care may be rooted in the same cognitive phenomena as the gut feelings discussed earlier. The same problem of not recognizing that there is a problem may also apply here. Van de Wiel and Van den Bossche plead for more attention in the healthcare organization for workplace learning. In line with the findings of Grohnert (2017) we wish to emphasize the importance of a positive learning culture in an organization and an open eye of the professional for the nonstandard elements of the patient situation to stay tuned to novelty and change.

REFLECTION POINT

Consider how these points relate to your practice:
■ Case processing in 'careful mode' does not necessarily lead to better outcomes.
■ Post hoc reflection on errors in clinical reasoning improves the knowledge structure and future clinical reasoning.
■ Teaching with cases requires a well-designed set of cases with similar features (but dissimilar fault) and dissimilar features (but similar fault); this improves the richness of illness scripts as well as the network they are part of.
■ Teaching with cases should be adapted to the level of expertise development of the students' knowledge networks, encapsulation or illness scripts.

SUMMARY

In this chapter we have presented:

■ a stage theory of development of medical expertise
■ differences in expert and novice knowledge structures
■ case examples to review the previous points
■ implications for teaching clinical reasoning.

REFERENCES

Baker, G.R., Norton, P.G., Flintoft, V., Blais, R., Brown, A., Cox, J., et al., 2004. The Canadian adverse events study: The incidence of adverse events among hospital patients in Canada. CMAJ. May 25;170 (11), 1678–1686. https://doi.org/10.1503/cmaj.1040498

Boshuizen, H. (1989). De ontwikkeling van medische expertise: Een cognitief-psychologische benadering. [Doctoral Thesis, Maastricht University]. Krips Repro. https://doi.org/10.26481/dis.19890224hb?

Boshuizen, H.P.A., Gruber, H., Strasser, J., 2020. Knowledge restructuring through case processing: The key to generalise expertise development theory across domains? Educational Research Review 29, 100310. https://doi.org/10.1016/j.edurev.2020.100310

Boshuizen, H.P.A., Hobus, P.M.M., Custers, E.J., Schmidt, H.G., 1992. Cognitive effects of practical experience. In: Evans, D.A., Patel, V.L. (Eds.), Advanced models of cognition for medical training and practice. Springer, pp. 337–348. https://doi:10.1007/978-3-662-02833-9_19

Boshuizen, H.P.A., Schmidt, H.G., 1992. On the role of biomedical knowledge in clinical reasoning by experts, intermediates and novices. Cognitive Science 16, 153–184. https://doi.org/10.1016/0364-0213(92)90022-M

Boshuizen, H.P.A., van de Wiel, M.W.J., 1998. Multiple representations in medicine: How students struggle with it. In: van

Someren, M.W., Reimann, P., Boshuizen, H.P.A., de Jong, T. (Eds.), Learning with multiple representations. Elsevier, pp. 237–262.

Bowen, J.L., 2006. Educational strategies to promote clinical diagnostic reasoning. New England Journal of Medicine 23, 2217–2225. https://doi.org/10.1056/NEJMra054782

Brouwers, L. (2022, December, 24–25). Zorgenkind; Een reconstructie [Problem child; A reconstruction]. NRC-Weekend, 20–23.

Chamberland, M., Mamede, S., St-Onge, C., Rivard, M.-A., Setrakian, J., et al., 2013. Students' self-explanations while solving unfamiliar cases: The role of biomedical knowledge. Medical Education 47, 1109–1116. https://doi.org/10.1111/medu.12253

Croskerry, P., 2003. The importance of cognitive errors in diagnosis and strategies to minimize them. Academic Medicine 78, 775–780. https://doi.org/10.1097/00001888-200308000-00003

Custers, E.J.F.M., 2015. Thirty years of illness scripts: Theoretical origins and practical applications. Medical Teacher 37 (5), 457–462. https://doi.org/10.3109/0142159X.2014.956052

Custers, E.J., Boshuizen, H.P., Schmidt, H.G., 1996. The influence of medical expertise, case typicality and illness script component on case processing and disease probability estimates. Memory and Cognition 24, 384–399. https://doi.org/10.3758/bf03213301

Daley, B.J., Durning, S.J., Torre, D.M., 2016. Using concept maps to create meaningful learning in medical education. MedEdPublish, 5. https://doi.org/10.15694/mep.2016.000019

Feltovich, P.J., Barrows, H.S., 1984. Issues of generality in medical problem solving. In: Schmidt, H.G., De Volder, M.L. (Eds.), Tutorials in problem-based learning: A new direction in teaching the health professions. Van Gorcum, pp. 128–142.

Grohnert, T., 2017. Judge|Fail|Learn. Enabling auditors to make high-quality judgments by designing effective learning environments. Maastricht University. https://cris.maastrichtuniversity.nl/ws/portalfiles/portal/12427484/c5660.pdf

Groothuis, S., Boshuizen, H.P.A., Talmon, J.L., 1998. Analysis of the conceptual difficulties of the endocrinology domain and an empirical analysis of student and expert understanding of that domain. Teaching and Learning in Medicine 10, 207–216. https://doi-org.ezproxy.elib11.ub.unimaas.nl/10.1207/S153280 15TLM1004_3

Huwendiek, S., Duncker, C., Reichert, F., et al., 2013. Learner preferences regarding integrating, sequencing and aligning virtual patients with other activities in the undergraduate medical curriculum: A focus group study. Medical Teacher 35, 920–929. https://doi.org/10.3109/0142159X.2013.826790

Jaarsma, T., Jarodzka, H., Nap, M., van Merrienboer, J.J.G., Boshuizen, H.P.A., 2014. Expertise under the microscope: Processing histopathological slides. Medical Education 48, 292–300. https://doi.org/10.1111/medu12385

Jossberger, H., Breckwoldt, J., Gruber, H., 2022. Promoting expertise through simulation (PETS): A conceptual framework. Learning and Instruction 82, 101686. https://doi.org/10.1016/j.learninstruc.2022.101686

Kassirer, J.P., 2010. Teaching clinical reasoning: case-based and coached. Academic Medicine 85, 1118–1124. https://doi.org/10.1097/acm.0b013e3181d5dd0d

Lesgold, A.M., Rubinson, H., Feltovich, P.J., Glaser, R., Klopfer, D., Wang, Y., 1988. Expertise in a complex skill: diagnosing X-ray pictures. In: Chi, M.T.H., Glaser, R., Farr, M.J. (Eds.), The nature of expertise. Erlbaum, pp. 311–342.

Lubarsky, S., Dory, V., Audétat, M., Custers, E., Charlin, B., 2015. Using script theory to cultivate illness script formation and clinical reasoning in health professions education. Canadian Medical Education Journal 6, e61–e70.

Mamede, S., Schmidt, H.G., Penaforte, J.C., 2008. Effects of reflective practice on the accuracy of medical diagnoses. Medical Education 42, 468–475. https://doi.org/10.1111/j.1365-2923.2008.03030

Mamede, S., Schmidt, H.G., Rikers, R.M., Custers, E.J.F.M., Splinter, T.A.W., van Saase, J.L.C.M., 2010. Conscious thought beats deliberation without attention in diagnostic decision-making: At least when you are an expert. Psychological Research 74, 586–592. https://doi.org/10.1007/s00426-010-0281-8

Mamede, S., Schmidt, H.G., Rikers, R.M., Penaforte, J.C., Coelho-Filho, J.M., 2007. Breaking down automaticity: Case ambiguity and the shift to reflective approaches in clinical reasoning. Medical Education 41, 1185–1192. https://doi.org/10.1111/j.1365-2923.2007.02921.x

Mamede, S., van Gog, T., Moura, A.S., de Faria, R.M.D., Peixoto, J.M., Rikers, R.M.J.P., et al., 2012. Reflection as a strategy to foster medical students' acquisition of diagnostic competence. Medical Education 46, 464–472. https://doi.org/10.1111/j.1365-2923.2012.04217.x

Norman, G.R., Monteiro, S., Sherbino, J., Ilgen, J., Schmidt, H.G., Mamede, S., 2017. The causes of error in clinical reasoning: Cognitive biases, knowledge deficits, and dual process thinking. Academic Medicine 92 (1), 23–30. https://doi.org/10.1097/ACM0000000000001421

Ohlsson, S., 2011. Deep learning: How the mind overrides experience. Cambridge University Press.

Rikers, R.M., Schmidt, H.G., Moulaert, V., 2005. Biomedical knowledge: Encapsulated or two worlds apart? Applied Cognitive Psychology 19, 223–231. https://doi.org/10.1002/acp.1107

Schmidt, H.G., Boshuizen, H.P.A., 1992. Encapsulation of biomedical knowledge. In: Evans, A.E., Patel, V.L. (Eds.), Advanced models of cognition for medical training and practice. Springer, pp. 265–282.

Schmidt, H.G., Boshuizen, H.P.A., 1993. On acquiring expertise in medicine. Educational Psychology Review 5, 205–221. https://doi.org/10.1007/BF01323044

Schmidt, H.G., Boshuizen, H.P.A., Norman, G.R., 1992. Reflections on the nature of expertise in medicine. In: Keravnou, E. (Ed.), Deep models for medical knowledge engineering. Elsevier, pp. 231–248.

Schmidt, H.G., Mamede, S., van den Berge, K., van Gog, T., van Saase, J.L.C., M., Rikers, R.M.J.P., 2014. Exposure to media information about a disease can cause doctors to misdiagnose similar-looking clinical cases. Academic Medicine 89, 285–291. https://doi.org/10.1097/ACM.0000000000000107

Schmidt, H.G., Norman, G.R., Boshuizen, H.P.A., 1990. A cognitive perspective on medical expertise: Theory and implications. Academic Medicine 65, 611–621. https://doi.org/10.1097/00001888-199010000-00001

Stolper, C.F., Van de Wiel, M.W.J., Hendriks, R.H.M., Van Royen, P., Van Bokhoven, M.A., Van der Weijden, T., et al., 2015. How do gut feelings feature in tutorial dialogues on diagnostic reasoning in GP traineeship? Advances in Health Science Education 20, 499–513. https://doi.org/10.1007/s10459-014-9543-3

van de Wiel, M.W.J., Boshuizen, H.P.A., Schmidt, H.G., 2000. Knowledge restructuring in expertise development: Evidence from pathophysiological representations of clinical cases by students and physicians. European Journal of Cognitive Psychology 12, 323–355. https://doi.org/10.1080/09541440050114543

van de Wiel, M.W.J., Van den Bossche, P., 2013. Deliberate practice in medicine: The motivation to engage in work-related learning and its contribution to expertise. Vocations and Learning 6, 135–158. https://doi.org/10.1007/s12186-012-9085-x

Van Merrienboer, J.J.G., Kirschner, P.A., 2017. Ten steps to complex learning: A systematic approach to four-component instructional design. Routledge.

Van Merriënboer, J.J.G., Kirschner, P.A., Kester, L., 2003. Taking the load off the learner's mind: Instructional design for complex learning. Educational Psychology 38, 5–13. https://doi.org/10.1207/S15326985EP3801_2

Wagenaar, A. (2008). Learning in internships: What and how students learn from experience. [Doctoral Thesis, Maastricht University]. Datawyse/Universitaire Pers Maastricht. https://doi.org/10.26481/dis.20081218aw

8

THE LANGUAGE OF CLINICAL REASONING

STEPHEN LOFTUS ■ JOY HIGGS

CHAPTER AIMS

The aims of this chapter are:

- to look at clinical reasoning and its communication through the frame of language
- to examine three key devices of language in relation to clinical reasoning: metaphor, narrative and rhetoric
- to consider the implications of using these devices on the acts, experience and sense making involved in clinical reasoning.

INTRODUCTION

In this chapter we examine the role of language in clinical reasoning. We consider that attention to this aspect of clinical reasoning can help all health professionals come to a deeper understanding of what clinical reasoning is. An awareness of how language works in practice can help novices master the intricacies of clinical reasoning. This awareness can also help teachers develop appropriate pedagogies that can assist students to develop mastery of clinical reasoning.

An immediate problem with an approach based on language use is that we need first to dispel a commonly held myth. In the Western world there is a widespread belief that language is nothing more than the representation of what is already 'out there' in the world. This is often called the representation view of language. This view oversimplifies things to the extent that it distorts how we can think about reality. Reality includes the clinical reality of our patients who come to us and expect us to understand their problems and deal with them.

A growing number of scholars have come to realize that language is far more complicated than the simple representation view. As Rorty once remarked, 'The world is out there, but descriptions of the world are not' (Rorty, 1989, p. 5). goes on to claim that we make up ways of describing the world that suit our particular purposes. For example, the way a clinical psychologist will use language to describe a patient with chronic pain will be quite different to the way that a physician will use language to describe the same patient, even though both are being scientific and objective. Representation is just one of the functions of language and there can be more than one valid way of representing something or someone. However, Wittgenstein (1958) pointed out there are many more functions of language besides representation that are just as important. For example, the following selection of 'language games' that Wittgenstein (1958) lists can all be relevant to the activity of clinical reasoning. They include describing the appearance of an object or giving its measurements, reporting an event, speculating about an event, or forming and testing a hypothesis. These are language activities that include and go beyond mere representation and they can all play a part in clinical reasoning. Wittgenstein's work has inspired other scholars, such as Gadamer (1989), who have deepened our understanding of how language works.

From the work of Gadamer (1989) we realize that language can also be about presentation and bringing things to our awareness in the first place. The ways in which we use language affect how we perceive the world around us and this is just as true of clinical reasoning (Loftus, 2012). This view of clinical reasoning is interpretive and contrasts with the current and more widespread view that clinical reasoning is, or should be, regarded as a phenomenon of computational logic and symbolic processing, combined with probability mathematics and statistics. This is not to say that the mainstream approaches to clinical reasoning, such as information processing, are wrong, but that there are alternative views that can be just as powerful and that can help us both theoretically and practically. This alternative view, based on language use, can sensitize us to important aspects of clinical reasoning that would otherwise be missed. One aspect of this view is how we regard thinking/reasoning.

Many have argued, following Aristotle (1983), that thinking is the internalization of talk we have with others and that in learning to think we learn to have conversations with ourselves (Bakhtin, 1984; Toulmin, 1979; Vygotsky, 1986). According to this argument we do not first have thoughts, which are then 'dressed up' in language. As Vygotsky (1986, p. 218) explained, 'Thought is not merely expressed in words: it comes into existence through them'. Language acts as a means of controlling what we think and how we communicate. To speak a particular language is to inhabit a particular 'way of being' (Wittgenstein, 1958). Language both shapes and limits how we construct our social realities (Higgs et al. 2004).

From this viewpoint, language is of primary importance for understanding the nature of thought. The underlying metaphors, the narrative formats and the persuasive ways in which we speak and write all play a role in our thinking and clinical reasoning. According to Vygotsky (1986), we learn at an early age to perceive the world as much through our language as through our eyes. Clinical reasoning is no exception. It is clear that language performs an integrative function. Other symbol systems and cognitive tools can have meaning because they are imbued with language and integrated within it. In the realm of clinical reasoning there are many symbol systems. These can include ECG traces, manual therapy symbols, dental notation, radiographs and MRI scans. Language, in Vygotsky's view, is the 'tool of tools' (Cole and Wertsch, 1996) that allows us to bring other symbol systems together into a meaningful whole. There are connections here with evidence-based medicine (EBM).

When Sackett et al. (1996) introduced EBM, they said that a good clinical decision integrates the best available scientific evidence with the experience and expertise of the practitioner together with the desires of the patient. It can be argued that most attention (and research funding) has been focussed on the first factor, the best available evidence. This is probably because most health professionals are familiar with the language (vocabulary and concepts) of the biomedical sciences. The biomedical sciences do not have the vocabulary to articulate expertise, experience and the desires of the people involved in the clinical encounter. This is why the humanities and social sciences should play a more important role in healthcare practice and education. These disciplines do have the language to articulate these issues. This is one way that attention to language can help us develop clinical reasoning that engages with patients as meaningful wholes rather than as collections of body parts (Loftus, 2021).

There are several ways of looking at language use in clinical reasoning. In this chapter we will focus on a few of the better known. One example of language use is metaphor.

METAPHOR

Lakoff and Johnson (1980) claimed that thought and language are fundamentally metaphorical. Metaphor is not simply an embellishment of language exploited by writers and poets. It can be argued that language and thought are intensely and inherently metaphorical and, because of this, metaphor use goes largely unnoticed because it is so completely natural to us. Metaphor is therefore a major means for constituting reality. The implication of this view is that we do not perceive reality and then separately interpret it and give it meaning. Once we acquire language we perceive reality immediately through the lens of language. As Foss observed:

> *Metaphor is a basic way by which the process of using symbols to construct reality occurs. It serves as a structuring principle, focusing on particular aspects of a phenomenon and hiding others; thus, each metaphor produces a different description of the 'same' reality.*
>
> *(2009, p. 268)*

In recent years there has been a growing recognition of the extent to which metaphor underlies scientific and medical practice and shapes the ways in which both health professionals and their patients conceptualize their health problems and how they can be addressed (e.g. Reisfield and Wilson, 2004). One example of how different metaphors have shaped

thinking in healthcare comes from the literature on the HIV/AIDS issue (Case Studies 8.1 and 8.2).

Metaphors shape the way we think about healthcare in general terms but they also shape the way health professionals think through the individual problems of patients as they reason their way towards a diagnosis and treatment plan.

REFLECTION POINT

- What metaphors underpin clinical reasoning in your health profession?
- How are these metaphors helpful?
- What do they ignore or miss?

NEW METAPHORS IN CLINICAL REASONING

In recent years there have been debates about other ways of reconceptualizing patient experiences; these debates include consideration of new metaphors that might be used to enrich our understanding of symptoms so that we can manage them better (Loftus, 2011). For example, pain has traditionally been regarded as a symptom but there have been calls to reconceptualize pain as a disease entity in its own right (Siddall and Cousins, 2004). This debate is essentially about two

---

CASE SUDY 8.1

Metaphors in the Area of HIV/AIDS

Sherwin (2001) looked at the metaphors used by various interest groups in the HIV/AIDS issue, revealing how certain metaphors favour distinctive ways of thinking and showing that there are ethical implications arising from using particular metaphors. Sherwin argued that at one time epidemiologists favoured the metaphor 'AIDS is a lifestyle disease'. This encouraged them to pursue certain sorts of scientific practices such as looking for a multifactorial disease model, attending to some social conditions such as sexual orientation and patterns of drug use. However, the metaphor discouraged other lines of inquiry such as investigating homosexual behaviour in men who considered themselves to be heterosexual. The epidemiologists also resisted for some time the suggestion that

a single causal virus might be responsible for AIDS. High-risk groups therefore became the focus of attention, instead of high-risk behaviour. Sherwin's opinion was that the underlying metaphor discouraged the epidemiologists from considering other ways of thinking about AIDS and because they were so dominant in the field there was some delay before the medical establishment eventually accepted the viral cause of AIDS. The ethical implication is that the metaphors used might have resulted in unnecessary suffering of AIDS patients and infection of people who might otherwise have been alerted earlier to the dangers they faced. Another way of representing this is that the different metaphors encouraged health professionals to tell particular stories/narratives about AIDS.

CASE STUDY 8.2

Metaphors in Pain Management

Metaphors used in pain management can show how metaphor use affects clinical reasoning. A key metaphor underlying the biomedical model is 'the body is a machine'. This metaphor shapes the way many health professionals think and is so widespread that many patients in Western societies also use this metaphor when thinking about their bodily problems (Hodgkin, 1985). The implication of this metaphor is that we can always, in principle at least, repair a broken machine. In acute care this metaphor could be appropriate. For example, a patient with toothache can go to a dentist who can provide a technical 'fix' in the form of fillings, root canal treatments or extractions. From this viewpoint the body's technical problem is repaired and the patient can go about their business. However, the metaphor frequently falls down in the chronic situation where repeated attempts at repair fail, resulting in frustration and disappointment for both patients and health professionals. Often such patients are 'discarded' by the system as failed patients (Alder, 2003). This metaphor can also confuse health professionals when they try to make sense of phenomena such as the placebo effect.

The placebo effect occurs when a beneficial effect is produced by a mechanism that is known to be technically ineffective. A well-known placebo example is pain relief from pills with no active ingredient. For health professionals who restrict themselves to thinking with 'the body is a machine' metaphor this makes little sense (Loftus, 2011). It is as if we took a malfunctioning car to a mechanic who used tools that do not work and we then discover that the ineffective tools have repaired the problem. A way to understand what is happening in the placebo effect is to use different metaphors to conceptualize what is going on. Perhaps a more useful metaphor here would be 'pain is interpretation'. It is now widely accepted that pain is a subjective interpretation and that restricting ourselves to mechanistic thinking misses this interpretive element. Moerman (2002) spoke of the meaning effect. Placebos can work because of what they subjectively mean to us as people. Purely technical thinking prevents us from seeing that what experience means to us can profoundly alter how we perceive experiences such as pain. This takes us back to the point made by Foss (2009) that metaphors can emphasize some aspects of a phenomenon but at the expense of hiding other aspects. The 'body is a machine' metaphor hides away the people who come to us as patients and seduces us into thinking of them only as machines to be mended.

metaphors we can use to think about pain; the older metaphor is representing pain as a symptom, the newer metaphor is representing pain as a disease. Changing metaphors like this provides a 'reframing' in which the new metaphor offers a different way for interpreting and understanding patients and the problems they have. Conventionally, pathologies are seen as causes that produce effects that are called symptoms, such as pain. Following the 'body is a machine' metaphor, health professionals have been taught that it is far more important to deal with the cause of a mechanistic problem rather than the effects. Once the root cause of a mechanistic problem is dealt with, the effects tend to disappear. Because pain is seen as a 'mere' effect, it is often ignored while health professionals focus their attention on finding and dealing with the causal pathology. As Siddall and Cousins (2004) point out, the result is that pain management is still very poor in the Western world. By trying to depict pain as a disease entity (a cause/effect mechanism in its own right) they are trying to reconceptualize pain as something that is more likely to attract the attention of health professionals and be dealt with much more effectively.

Much of the debate in the literature has been about which metaphors are closer to the 'truth'. In a sense this debate is irrelevant. Metaphors cannot be true or false but they can be more or less useful. What really matters in these debates is which metaphors are more useful and for whom. The overriding question is: what works for patients? How can we improve our clinical reasoning so that we get better results for patients? These questions emphasize the difference between medical science and medical practice. Medical practice is based on medical science but the two are not identical. Whereas medical science, like all science, is concerned with the 'truth', medical practice is concerned with what works for patients. As Elliott (1999) reminds us, health professionals are not scientists, they are pragmatists. It is worth remembering the words of Rorty:

> *Human beings, like computers, dogs and works of art, can be described in lots of different ways, depending on what you want to do with them—take them apart for repairs, reeducate them, play with them, admire them and so on for a long list of alternative purposes. None of these descriptions is closer to what human beings really are than any of the others. Descriptions are tools invented for particular purposes, not attempts to describe things as they are in themselves, apart from any such purposes.*
>
> *(Rorty, 1998, p. 28)*

REFLECTION POINT

As we have seen, different metaphors provide the foundations for different descriptions. What matters is how well the descriptions (and their underlying metaphors) serve the purposes for which they are used. If the purpose is encouraging health professionals to manage pain better, then describing pain as a disease or vital sign may well serve the purpose better than thinking of pain as a nerve signal or symptom. In this sense the truth is irrelevant. The various descriptions health professionals make of patients' problems are often in the form of narratives.

NARRATIVE

A major aspect of clinical reasoning is the construction of a narrative about a patient within the conceptual framework of a health profession and the specific context of the patient and the workplace. There is a growing realization of the importance of narrative in therapeutic encounters (e.g. Charon et al., 2017). The construction of a clinical narrative occurs in a manner that not only takes account of the past and present but also suggests the narrative trajectory that the patient's story might follow in the future, predisposing towards particular decisions about management. Such narratives can be diagnostic, prognostic and therapeutic (Case Studies 8.3 and 8.4).

CASE STUDY 8.3
Patient Narrative in Dentistry

A patient in her late teens presents to a dentist with a story of toothache at the back of the mouth that comes and goes spontaneously, is becoming more frequent and lasts longer each time it occurs. The dentist assesses the patient and reinterprets the patient's story in the professional discourse of dentistry and surgery. The reinterpreted narrative might then become a story of impacted wisdom teeth. This new story can be substantiated with scientific evidence in the form of radiographs that show the offending teeth in their impacted position. The scientific evidence is given its meaning and importance by being integrated into the story of this patient's impacted wisdom teeth (Loftus and Greenhalgh, 2010). A major advantage of this professional reinterpretation is that the dentist's version has a narrative trajectory into the future. This narrative trajectory gives meaning to the whole episode.

CASE STUDY 8.4
Patient Narrative in Rehabilitation

Sometimes the meaning given by this narrative trajectory can be crucial. One of the best examples of this comes from the work of a rehabilitation centre in which a patient recovering from a head injury is introduced to the centre by an occupational therapist and shown where the various therapeutic activities will take place (Mattingly, 1994). The therapeutic activities, however, are not introduced simply as activities. As Mattingly points out, there is a deliberate effort by the occupational therapist to outline to the patient how the activities can be used so that he can eventually leave and move on to a life beyond therapy. Mattingly's point is that without this narrative trajectory there is a risk that the patient would find the therapy meaningless and might not collaborate with treatment. This is another situation in which the meaning of the clinical situation can have a dramatic effect on what happens and how well patients do. It is also clear from this example that the health professional has to persuade the patient to accept this narrative trajectory.

REFLECTION POINT

- What kinds of stories does your health profession use?
- How do these stories help your clinical reasoning?

RHETORIC

Rhetoric is the art of persuasive speaking or writing. A great deal of clinical reasoning is concerned with persuasion. Health professionals need to persuade other people, such as funders, patients and their families, and other clinicians, that a particular assessment and proposed course of action is both legitimate and sound. Above all, health professionals have to persuade themselves. One medical student reflected on the importance of this issue when discussing how to cope with an inadequate clinical report from a colleague:

It's just being able to say what you find, and be able to say that … this person is in very dire straits. It's not making up stuff, but it's being able to present it in a convincing and competent manner that they [senior doctors] can say, 'All right, this requires my attention'.

(Loftus, 2006, p. 190).

Another medical student described the feedback he received after reporting on a complex patient assessment conducted under exam conditions. The setting was an exam and the two senior clinicians hearing the student's report knew exactly what was wrong with the patient, along with all the comorbidities and how they complicated management. They told the student: 'you're very organised but you've got to get to the point now and tell us where you want to go. You should be a bit more specific' (Loftus, 2006, p. 154).

Reflecting on this exchange, the student realized that the examiners wanted him to be more persuasive and lead them more convincingly to a definitive diagnosis and course of action. They wanted to hear a more persuasive story that worked towards a clear goal at the end. This is an important aspect of medical practice. In many countries senior doctors cannot physically see all the patients nominally in their care. They rely on junior doctors doing assessments and giving reports. The senior doctors want to be able to make decisions based on these reports and therefore they depend on junior doctors persuading them that the assessment has been done thoroughly and can be relied on. Senior doctors themselves confirm this insight.

The trainees [junior doctors] need to learn that [they have to] cut down the amount of information to a manageable summary for your colleagues … and for yourself because … at the end of the day … you have to be able to isolate them [important findings] and make a decision on them.

(Loftus, 2006, p. 193).

This ability is both a narrative and a rhetorical skill. In constructing a clinical report, a health professional is justifying a claim about a patient. The justification is supported by arguments that depend on the context of that patient, and that will stand up to reasonable criticism. As Perelman (1982, p. 162) argued, 'As soon as a communication tries to influence one or more persons, to orient thinking … to guide their actions, it belongs to the realm of rhetoric'.

There is frequently uncertainty in clinical reasoning, uncertainty that is associated not with self-doubt or the inability to make sound decisions but rather with the 'greyness' or complexity of practice situations, the variability of patient's or client's needs and the presence in many situations of various acceptable solutions (e.g. management strategies). When there is uncertainty, judgements must be made in light of all the information available for that case. This is not done mathematically or statistically but persuasively and argumentatively. This is the essence of rhetoric and of pragmatism; not the abandonment of logic or professional judgement but the incorporation of these into the intensely practical and human world of healthcare.

Consider the use of language devices in reasoning using Case Study 8.5.

CASE STUDY 8.5

Joe's Story

Joe was getting used to working as a physiotherapist in an interprofessional pain management clinic. He wrote quickly as he summarized the assessment of his last patient. Although the assessment had taken an hour and the patient had lots of problems, he knew that he would only get about a minute to report on this patient at the case conference with the other health professionals who had also seen the patient that day. He was mastering the art of confining his report to the key findings that the rest of the team would find useful. He realized that there would be some overlap with the doctor's report and he would need to avoid repetition. On reflection, he realized that the rest of the team questioned him now far less than they did when he first started work there. They were clearly learning to trust his judgement.

One of his key findings was that the patient strongly believed that her ongoing pain meant that there was continuing injury. This was why the patient was so reluctant to move. If their management was to be successful, it would need to include a strong educational element in the treatment plan. They would need to persuade the patient to think about the pain differently. He realized just how much his own thinking had changed through working in the clinic. Most of the therapy they offered was designed to get patients to move away from thinking of their bodies as broken machines and instead to work on ways of managing their chronic pain. The underlying message of the therapy was that 'life is a journey' and they could provide patients with the means of moving on with that life, despite chronic pain.

REFLECTION POINT

- Does Joe's story reflect your experience of framing and presenting your reasoning?
- What sort of language devices do you use to make sense of your reasoning and communicate it?

SUMMARY

Using language as a theoretical lens allows us to see clinical reasoning in a very different way compared with the mainstream views such as hypothetico-deductive reasoning, information processing or evidence-based practice. This is not to deny the importance of the mainstream views but to point out that we can integrate them into a more coherent and more cohesive whole by seeing the role they play in the overall language game of clinical reasoning. The information from the evidence base, like all relevant information about a patient, has to be integrated into the narratives we construct about our patients and this is done persuasively.

REFLECTION POINT

- How can we use the ideas in this chapter to improve the teaching of clinical reasoning to students?

REFERENCES

Alder, S., 2003. Beyond the restitution narrative (Doctoral dissertation, University of Western Sydney). University of Western Sydney. http://handle.uws.edu.au:8081/1959.7/22873

Aristotle, 1983. Aristotle's physics i, ii. Oxford University Press. (Original work published c 400 BC).

Bakhtin, M., 1984. Problems of Dostoevsky's poetics. University of Minnesota Press.

Charon, R., DasGupta, S., Hermann, N., Irvine, C., Marcus, E.R., Colon, E.R., et al., 2017. The principles and practice of narrative medicine. Oxford University Press.

Cole, M., Wertsch, J.V., 1996. Beyond the social-individual antimony in discussions of Piaget and Vygotsky. Human Development 39 (5), 250–256.

Elliott, C., 1999. A philosophical disease: Bioethics culture and identity. Routledge.

Foss, S.K., 2009. Rhetorical criticism: Exploration and practice, 4th ed. Waveland Press.

Gadamer, H.-G., 1989. Truth and method (2nd ed.). Continuum.

Higgs, J., Andresen, L., Fish, D., 2004. Practice knowledge: Its nature, sources and contexts. In: Higgs, J., Richardson, B., Abrandt Dahlgren, M. (Eds.), Developing practice knowledge for health professionals. Butterworth-Heinemann, pp. 51–69.

Hodgkin, P., 1985. Medicine is war: And other medical metaphors. British Medical Journal 291 (6511), 1820–1821. https://doi.org/10.1136/bmj.291.6511.1820

Lakoff, G., Johnson, M., 1980. Metaphors we live by. University of Chicago Press.

Loftus, S., 2006. Language in clinical reasoning: Learning and using the language of collective clinical decision making (Doctoral dissertation, The University of Sydney). The University of Sydney. http://ses.library.usyd.edu.au/handle/2123/1165

Loftus, S., 2011. Pain and its metaphors: A dialogical approach. Journal of Medical Humanities 32 (3), 213–230. https://doi.org/10.1007/s10912-011-9139-3

Loftus, S., 2012. Rethinking clinical reasoning: Time for a dialogical turn. Medical Education 46, 1174–1178. https://doi.org/10.1111/j.1365-2923.2012.04353.x

Loftus, S., 2021. Goethe and embodiment in professional education and practice. In: Loftus, S., Kinsella, E.A. (Eds.), Embodiment and professional education: Body, practice, pedagogy. Springer, pp. 135–147. https://doi.org/10.1007/978-981-16-4827-4_10

Loftus, S., Greenhalgh, T., 2010. Towards a narrative mode of practice. In: Higgs, J., Fish, D., Goulter, I., Loftus, S., Reid, J., Trede, F. (Eds.), Education for future practice, pp. 85–94. Sense.

Mattingly, C., 1994. The concept of therapeutic "emplotment". Social Science and Medicine 38 (6), 811–822. https://doi.org/10.1016/0277-9536(94)90153-8

Moerman, D., 2002. Meaning, medicine and the placebo effect. Cambridge University Press.

Perelman, C., 1982. The realm of rhetoric (W. Kluback, Trans.). Notre Dame University Press.

Reisfield, G.M., Wilson, G.R., 2004. Use of metaphor in the discourse on cancer. Journal of Clinical Oncology 22 (19), 4024–4027. https://doi.org/10.1200/JCO.2004.03.136

Rorty, R., 1989. Contingency, irony and solidarity. Cambridge University Press.

Rorty, R., 1998. Against unity. Wilson Quarterly, 22(1), 28–39. http://archive.wilsonquarterly.com/sites/default/files/articles/WQ_VOL22_W_1998_Article_01_2.pdf

Sackett, D.L., Rosenberg, W.M.C., Muir Gray, J.A., Haynes, R.B., Richardson, W.S., 1996. Evidence based medicine: What it is and what it isn't. British Medical Journal 312, 71. https://doi.org/10.1136/bmj.312.7023.71

Sherwin, S., 2001. Feminist ethics and the metaphor of AIDS. Journal of Medicine and Philosophy 26 (4), 343–364. https://doi.org/10.1076/jmep.26.4.343.3011

Siddall, P., Cousins, M., 2004. Persistent pain as a disease entity: Implications for clinical management. Anesthesia & Analgesia 99 (2), 510–520. https://doi.org/10.1213/01.ANE.0000133383.17666.3A

Toulmin, S., 1979. The inwardness of mental life. Critical Inquiry 6, 1–16. https://www.jstor.org/stable/1343082

Vygotsky, L.S., 1986. Thought and language (A. Kozulin, Trans.). MIT Press. (Original work published 1962)

Wittgenstein, L., 1958. Philosophical investigations (3rd ed.) (G.E.M. Anscombe, Trans.). Prentice Hall. (Original work published 1953)

9

EXPERTISE AND CLINICAL REASONING

GAIL M. JENSEN ■ RAINE OSBORNE ■ AMY M. HADDAD

CHAPTER AIMS

The aims of this chapter are:

- to describe why expertise is essential but not sufficient for providing excellent healthcare
- to discuss the critical importance of the integrative bridge across the concepts of expertise and clinical reasoning
- to illustrate the concept of adaptive expertise and provide considerations for teaching and learning strategies
- to propose considerations for novice development of analytical and humanistic thinking.

INTRODUCTION

Our challenge in professional education is how to prepare learners who can engage in analytical thinking, skilful practice and wise judgements, often in uncertain conditions. As Schön (1987) argued, we are preparing professionals to practice in that *swampy lowland of practice*. In all professions, there are individuals who perform exceptionally well and who are held in high regard by their colleagues and their patients – in other words, experts. Experts are also engaged in shared decision making and collaborative practice (Bowen et al., 2022). A core assumption in our chapter is that we must not separate expert knowledge from expert activity including the development of clinical reasoning and deliberate action. This is an interactive and integrative relationship in which knowledge development, analysis and action each influence the others (Woods and Mylopoulos, 2015; Mylopoulos et al., 2017). There is continued focus on the argument that expertise is much more of a process or continuum of development than a static state resulting from a cluster of attributes such as knowledge and problem-solving skills or high-level performance (Bereiter and Scardamalia, 1993; Cooke et al., 2010). The process of moving towards expertise is not based merely on years of experience, but there is something central about the continued development of the learner. Ideally, an enhanced understanding of what distinguishes novices from experts should facilitate learning strategies for more effective professional education. We know that experience alone does not lead to more expertise, but it is the reflection on that experience that is critical for the learner (Trowbridge et al., 2015; Musolino and Jensen, 2020).

We begin this chapter with a 'deconstruction of the interrelated concepts of expertise and clinical reasoning' through a brief, analytical overview of key domains of theory and research. Next, we argue that the integration of context is inherent in clinical reasoning and an essential element in adaptive expertise. From this review, we generate a working list of attributes that we believe need to be considered when talking about clinical reasoning and decision making. In the final section of the chapter, we engage in a discussion of strategies for facilitating learning and novice development in clinical reasoning that focuses on developing essential habits of mind and development and integration of ethical comportment. The goal of understanding expertise and clinical reasoning is, first, to promote effective reasoning in practice and, second, the translation of understanding about good reasoning into more effective teaching and student learning and ultimately the delivery of the highest-quality care.

DECONSTRUCTING THE INTERRELATED CONCEPTS OF EXPERTISE AND CLINICAL REASONING

Expertise as Mental Processing and Problem Solving

Expertise is a complex, multidimensional concept that has captured the interest of researchers for over 50 years (Ericsson, 2009, 2015; Rikers and Paas, 2005). The early work in this area came from cognitive psychology and accepted a tradition of basic information-processing capabilities of humans. Initial work in expertise concentrated on mental processing or, more simply, the conceptualization of problem solving. In deGroot's (1966) well-known work with chess players, he began to look at differences among chess players with varying levels of expertise. He found that chess masters were able to recognize and reproduce chess patterns more quickly and accurately than novice

players. Subsequent studies in areas such as chess (Chase and Simon, 1973) and physics (Chi et al., 1981) revealed that expertise depended not only on the method of problem solving but also on the expert's detailed knowledge in a specific area, ability to memorize and ability to make inferences.

One of the most fundamental differences between experts and novices is that experts will bring more and better organized knowledge to bear on a problem. In medicine, the ability to determine the proper patient diagnosis was discovered to be highly dependent on the physician's knowledge in a particular clinical specialty area, called case specificity (Rikers and Paas, 2005; Schwartz and Elstein, 2008). Case specificity implies that a successful reasoning strategy in one situation may not apply in a second case, because the practitioner may not know enough about the area of the patient's problem. Identification of case specificity focussed attention on the role of knowledge in expertise. Both clinician experience and the features of the case are factors that affect the problem-solving strategy that is used. Experts appear to have not only methods of problem solving but also the ability to combine these methods with knowledge and an understanding of how the knowledge necessary to solve the problem should be organized (Trowbridge et al., 2015; Brandsford et al., 2000; Chi et al., 1988). Experts can make connections or inferences from the data by recognizing the pattern and links between clinical findings and a highly structured knowledge base. This explains why experts tend to ask fewer more relevant questions and perform examinations more quickly and accurately than novices. Novices and intermediate subjects tend to use hypothetico-deductive processes that involve setting up hypotheses and gathering clinical data to prove or disprove them (Schwartz and Elstein, 2008). Thus, less experienced clinicians tend to ask patients more questions (and in the same order) than do experts, regardless of their relevance to the case (Jones and Rivett, 2019).

Expertise as Skill Acquisition

Moulton et al. (2007) argue that there has been far too much focus on diagnostic performance and the role of experience. For health professions in which diagnosis is not the predominant decision point, there has been perhaps no more influential work in expertise than that by Patricia Benner in nursing (Benner, 1984; Benner et al., 1996, 2010, 2011). In her original work, Benner applied a model of skill acquisition developed by Hubert Dreyfus, a philosopher, and Stuart Dreyfus, a mathematician and system analyst (Dreyfus and Dreyfus, 1980). Dreyfus' work came out of a reaction to the cognitive psychology tradition that intelligent practice is not just the application of knowledge and rules for instrumental decision making. A central premise in this work is that human understanding is a skill akin to knowing how to find one's way about the world, rather than knowing a lot of facts and rules for relating them.

Dreyfus' conception of expertise is much more focussed on the context of actual practice. Several critical elements emerged from the Dreyfus and Dreyfus model (1980, 1996): (1) expertise is more about 'knowing how' (procedural knowledge, knowing how to do things) rather than knowing what (declarative knowledge, knowing information and facts); (2) expert knowledge is embedded in the action of the expert rather than propositional knowledge; (3) experience is a critical factor in the development of expertise; (4) much of expert performance is automatic and nonreflective (but when a situation is novel, experts engage in deliberation before action) and (5) intuition of experts or the knowing how to do things is both experiential and tacit.

The principles of the Dreyfus and Dreyfus Model of Skill Development (Table 9.1) remain a useful framework for facilitating learner skill development and assessment of competencies used across the health professions (Carraccio, 2008; Cutrer et al., 2020; Englander et al., 2013.).

TABLE 9.1		
Aligning Teaching Strategies With Key Concepts From the Dreyfus and Dreyfus (1980, 1996) Model of Skill Acquisition		
Stage	**Key Concepts**	**Teaching Strategies**
Novice	Factual, rule driven, relies on others Cannot see whole situation	Point out meaningful diagnostic information Eliminate irrelevant information and highlight discriminating evidence Encourage learners to work with multiple hypotheses
Advanced beginner	Objective facts Begins to use intuition in concrete situations Uses both analytic reasoning and pattern recognition	Build what the learner knows, and work from common ground to uncommon ground Facilitate learners' ability to verbalize thinking and differentiation of diagnoses and treatments
Competent	Can devise new rules based on the situation Sees the big picture Better use of pattern recognition with common problems	Balance supervision with autonomy in decision making Expose learners to breadth and depth of cases Identify learners' developmental stage as may not be in the competent category across all areas
Proficient	Is comfortable with evolving situations Intuitive behaviours replace reasoned responses Can tolerate uncertainty	Expose learners to a balance of cases, not all complex Learners have to know when to trust intuition and when to slow down and be more analytical Facilitate learners' ability to self-regulate and know when they do not know
Expert	Can align thought, feeling and action into intuitive problem recognition Where intuition is not developed, reasoning is applied	Keep experts challenged with complex cases Apprentice expert to a master who models the skills of a true reflective practitioner
Master	Demonstrates practical wisdom Sees the big picture Reflects in, on and for action Demonstrates moral agency	Master clinician is self-motivated and engages in lifelong learning Challenged by complex cases and habitually engaged in learning more

Source: Adapted from Benner, P. (1984). From novice to expert: Excellence and power in clinical nursing practice. Addison-Wesley; Carraccio, C., Benson, B., Nixon, J., et al. (2008). From the educational bench to the clinical bedside: Translating the Dreyfus Developmental model to the learning of clinical skills. *Academic Medicine*, 83, 761–767.

Key Elements in Expertise and Adaptive Expertise

Although there has been prolonged debate and controversy in expertise research on the acquisition of expert characteristics, there continues to be strong agreement on the characteristics of experts (Box 9.1) (Ericsson, 2009).

Although these characteristics of experts maintain consistency, educators are deeply interested in the development of the learner. How does expertise develop? What does expert practice look like? Education researchers have taken their understandings of expert processes and applied these to learners and learning. This has resulted in a distinction between routine expertise and adaptive expertise.

The argument is that routine experts possess mastery of knowledge in their domain and can apply that knowledge effectively and efficiently to well-known problems, but they are challenged by novel problems. A key premise in adaptive expertise is the experts' ability to break away from the routines and be adaptable as they practice in what is called the 'optimal adaptability corridor' (Mylopoulos and Woods, 2009; Cutrer et al., 2016). There is a need to balance the efficiency of routine expertise with the ability to innovate and to engage in progressive problem solving. A major criticism of professional education is that we overemphasize the efficiency dimension of learning and practice. We place major emphasis on certainty and right answers and little focus on how the learner can manage uncertainty (Irby et al., 2010; Shulman, 2004).

How do we facilitate the development of expert-like learners who can engage in progressive problem solving and are on a path towards the development of adaptive expertise? Adaptive expertise requires: (1) an openness to reflecting on practice, (2) metacognitive reasoning skills to recognize that a routine approach to the problem will not work, (3) critical thinking to challenge current assumptions and beliefs and (4) the ability to reconstruct the problem space (Cutrer et al., 2016). Although relatively new in the context of health professions, education strategies that focus on preparation for future learning (PFL) are known to support development of adaptive expertise (Mylopoulos et al., 2018a). PFL is 'the ability to learn new information, make effective use of resources, and invent new procedures in order to support learning and problem solving in practice' (Mylopoulos et al., 2016). Strategies that support PFL emphasize understanding over performance, expose learners to meaningful variations of a problem, encourage struggle and risk taking in the learning process, and provide immediate feedback or instruction to make sure the struggle results in the desired learning outcomes (Mylopoulos et al., 2018b). Other commonly studied strategies to develop adaptive expertise include: (1) early exposure to abstract materials, (2) helping learners integrate their existing knowledge with new conceptual models, (3) guiding learners through the process of problem solving and hypothesis testing to uncover new discoveries and (4) being aware and intentional in coaching learners through a metacognitive learning process (Kua et al., 2021).

The major components of a metacognitive learning process, also termed the master adaptive learner process (Cutrer et al., 2016), include the following activities:

- *Planning*: Identify a gap between what is and what should or could be; select an opportunity for learning; search for resources for learning.
- *Learning*: Engage in learning; critically appraise different sources for learning; move beyond traditional learning strategies such as rereading or highlighting to more effective strategies such as spaced repetitions, elaboration and concept integration.
- *Assessing*: Try out what is learned; engage in informed self-assessment that uses external feedback.

BOX 9.1
CHARACTERISTICS OF EXPERTS

- Experts mainly excel in their domain of expertise.
- Experts are faster than novices in performing skills.
- Experts can solve problems more quickly and with little error.
- Experts have superior short-term and long-term memory.
- Experts can see the problem in their domain at a deeper more principled level than novices, who have a more superficial representation of the problem.
- Experts spend more time trying to understand the problem and experts have strong self-monitoring skills.

- *Adjusting*: Incorporate what is learned into daily routines; reexamine new learning and consider opportunities and barriers needed to adjust practice; determine individual versus system implementation.

In summary, we know that experts are knowledgeable because they have extensive, accessible, well-organized knowledge and that they continue to build their practical knowledge base through a repertoire of examples, images, illness scripts and understanding that has been learned through experience (Boshuizen et al., 2004). We also see elements of the critical importance of adaptive learning as experts learn from experience by using reflective inquiry or metacognitive strategies to think about what they are doing, what worked and what did not work (Cutrer et al., 2016). Creating a learning environment that supports learners' development of creative exploration and adaptive expertise is also critical for the health professions (see Case Study 9.1).

CASE STUDY 9.1
Encouraging Adaptive Learning

You have an experienced student, with an exceptional academic record, completing their last clinical rotation in your clinic. The student demonstrates generally good judgement and always seems to be the first to respond with routine cases. Now you want to develop their ability to solve more complex and ambiguous clinical problems. Here are some things that you can do to facilitate adaptive learning. Model a complex case from your own case load and do a think aloud as you highlight where you struggled with the case. Try focussing your questions on reflection by framing the case as follows: 'Most cases are more complex than they initially appear. If they seem too simple, ask "What am I missing – where are my gaps?" "What else could be going on?"' Challenge the student about how a routine approach to this case will not work: so now what? Have the student share the assumptions they have made about the patient. Collaborate with the interprofessional team and ask the student to compare and contrast how each profession conceptualizes the case.

EXPERTISE AND CLINICAL REASONING IN EVERYDAY PRACTICE

Qualitative research methods have been central tools in investigative, grounded theory work done in several applied professions such as nursing (Benner, 1984; Benner et al., 1996, 2010, 2011; Uemura and Kido, 2022), teaching (Berliner, 1986; Sternberg and Horvath, 1995; Tsui, 2003), occupational therapy (Fleming and Mattingly, 2000; Mattingly and Fleming, 1994; Robertson et al., 2015) and physical therapy (Reilly et al., 2022; Black et al., 2010; Edwards et al., 2004; Jensen et al., 2000, 2007; Resnik and Jensen, 2003; Shaw and DeForge, 2012). These are all professions in which human interactions and care are central aspects of practice. In these studies, we find that clinical reasoning has to include both an analytical and a narrative approach as the focus of care extends beyond the identification of a diagnosis. The clinical reasoning process is iterative and ongoing. Knowing a patient, understanding their story, fitting the patient's story with clinical knowledge and collaborating with the patient to solve problems are the kinds of integral components of clinical reasoning that emerge from these studies.

In analysis of nursing practice, Benner found that much of expert performance in nursing emphasizes individual perceptions and decision-making abilities rather than just the performance of the skill. Benner et al. used observations and narrative accounts of actual clinical examples as primary tools for understanding the everyday clinical and caring knowledge and practical reasoning that were used in nursing practice. Clinical skills were identified as an overall approach to professional action that includes both perception and decision making, not just what we would think of as technical skill or technique (Benner, 1984; Benner et al., 1996, 2010, 2011). It is the integration of the knowledge with skilled know-how (i.e. knowing how to perform a skill in its real setting), along with ethical comportment, that was foundational to expertise in practice. Ethical comportment, simply stated, is the ability to engage in ethical reflection to discern moral dilemmas. This is more fully described in 'Clinical reasoning and novice development: Balancing the analytical model of thinking and humanistic thinking' of the chapter on habits of mind.

In physical therapy, Jensen et al. developed a grounded theory of expert practice (Jensen et al., 2000, 2007). This model of expertise in physical therapy is a combination of multidimensional knowledge, clinical reasoning skills, skilled movement and virtue. All four of these dimensions (knowledge, reasoning, movement and virtue) contribute to the therapist's philosophy of practice. For novices, each of these core dimensions of expertise may exist, but they do not appear to be as well integrated. As novices continue to develop, each of the dimensions may become stronger, yet they may not be well integrated for proficient practice. When the expert therapist has fully integrated these dimensions of expertise, this in turn leads to an explicit philosophy of practice (Fig. 9.1) (Jensen et al., 2007).

Subsequent work by Resnik and Jensen (2003) corroborated the presence of a patient-centred approach to care in collaborative clinical reasoning and promotion of patient empowerment. At the foundation of the patient-centred approach, this research identified an ethic of caring and a respect for individuality, a passion for clinical care and a desire to learn and improve continually. The primary goals of empowering patients, increasing self-efficacy beliefs and involving patients in the care process are facilitated by patient–therapist collaborative problem solving and enhanced through attentive listening, trust building and observation. The patient-centred approach is exemplified by the therapist's emphasis on patient education and by strong beliefs about the power of education. This approach alters the therapeutic relationship and enhances patients' abilities to make autonomous choices. Resnik and Jensen (2003) reported that these efforts not only promoted patient empowerment and self-efficacy but also resulted in greater continuity of services, more skilful care and more individualized plans of care and ultimately better outcomes.

Although experts in that study possessed a broad, multidimensional knowledge base, Resnik and Jensen (2003) discovered that (many) years of clinical experience and specialty certification did not appear to be mandatory in achieving expertise. This seemed to challenge a basic assertion of the Dreyfus model that (ongoing) experience is a critical factor in development of expertise. In Resnik and Jensen's (2003) study, this was not observed and, in fact, some therapists classified as experts were relatively new physical therapists

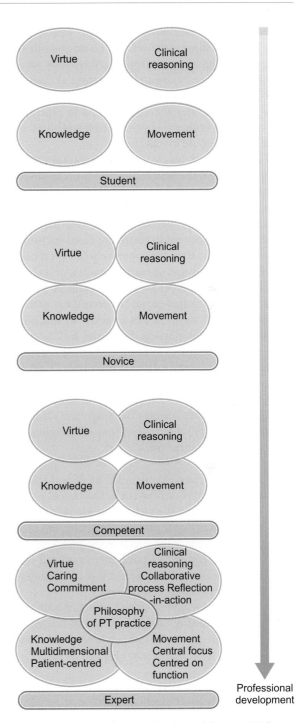

Fig. 9.1 ■ Model of expertise in physical therapy. (With permission from Jensen, G.M., Gwyer, J., Hack, L.M., Shepard, K.F., 2007. Expertise in physical therapy practice, 2nd ed. Saunders-Elsevier, St. Louis.)

or perhaps expert-like novices (see also Resnik and Hart, 2003). In these instances, the researchers theorized, knowledge acquisition was facilitated by work and life experience before attending physical therapy school, by being in a work environment that offered access to pooled collegial knowledge and by practitioners' values and virtues of inquisitiveness and humility, which drove their use of reflection.

In-depth ethnographic work by Edwards et al. (2004) on expert physical therapists' clinical reasoning strategies has further revealed an interplay of different reasoning strategies in every tasks of clinical practice (e.g. interactive reasoning, diagnostic reasoning, narrative reasoning, ethical reasoning, reasoning about teaching). Rather than contrasting the cognitively based rational models of reasoning and interactive models of reasoning, Edwards et al. (2004) proposed a dialectic model of clinical reasoning that moves between the cognitive and decision-making processes required to diagnose and manage patients' physical disabilities and the narrative or communicative reasoning and action required to understand and engage patients and careers. Critical reflection is required with either process.

In their classic ethnographic study of clinical reasoning in occupational therapy, Mattingly and Fleming (1994) originally proposed three types of reasoning in their 'theory of the three-track' mind:

1. *Procedural reasoning* (similar to hypothetical-propositional reasoning but in the case of occupational therapy the focus is on identifying the patient's functional problem and selecting procedures to reduce the effects of the problem)
2. *Interactive reasoning* (active interaction and collaboration with the patient are used to understand the patient's perspective)
3. *Conditional reasoning* (based on social and cultural processes of understanding and is used to help the patient in the difficult process of reconstructing a life that is now changed by injury or disease)

   A fourth form of reasoning, narrative reasoning (Fleming and Mattingly, 2000; Mattingly and Fleming, 1994), was subsequently identified.
4. *Narrative reasoning* is used to describe the storytelling aspect of patient cases. Often therapists use narrative thinking and telling of a kind

---

BOX 9.2
CONSIDERING SIMILARITIES ACROSS REASONING STUDIES

■ Hypothetico-deductive reasoning is used for specific procedural issues.
■ The patient is a respected and central aspect of the work.
■ Collaboration with the patient is a critical strategy in clinical reasoning and decision making.
■ Metacognitive skill (reflection) is an integral aspect of patient care.
■ Narrative is a critical tool for understanding the clinical situation including patient, carers and the clinical knowledge that is part of the story.
■ Moral agency and deliberate actions are essential elements of what it means to be 'good' at one's work (it is difficult to separate clinical and ethical reasoning).

---

of 'short story' in coming to understand or make sense of the human experience (Furze et al., 2019).

REFLECTION POINT

■ What do these examples of investigative work centred on everyday practice tell us about clinical reasoning and development of adaptive expertise?

Across these studies, we see striking similarities that emerge from understanding the contextual factors that are essential in the clinical reasoning process (Box 9.2). Specifically, the integration of knowledge and context is critical for understanding and facilitating expertise. It is the human or relationship side of practice that emerges as a central component of clinical reasoning and, we would argue, part of progressive problem solving that is part of adaptive expertise.

CLINICAL REASONING AND NOVICE DEVELOPMENT: BALANCING THE ANALYTICAL MODEL OF THINKING AND HUMANISTIC THINKING

If understanding and integrating context are so critical in the clinical reasoning process and in models of adaptive expertise, then finding ways to facilitate habits of mind is essential. The university setting does well in training the analytic 'habits of mind', but it does far less in developing practical skills and capacity for professional judgement (Colby and Sullivan, 2008). Although expert practitioners bring scientific evidence, analysis and problem-solving skills to the clinical situation, they also bring the skills of practical reasoning as they listen to patients and reflect on and make meaning of what they hear. It is this narrative understanding and practical reasoning that are informed by scientific knowledge but guided by concern for human well-being that are central to expertise. The challenge for professional education is finding the balance between the dominant analytic model of thinking with narrative thinking that can result in skilful practice and wise judgement. How do we go about developing habits of mind in our students? We argue that the relationship between patient and practitioner is a critical element of skilful ethical comportment and is foundational in expert work. Ethical comportment requires the skilful embodiment of the moral standards of practice that includes the development of 'soft skills' (empathy, humility, respect, etc.), which are really not soft skills but essential skills (Benner and Purtilo, 2019; Blanton et al., 2020). Therefore, the focus on the patient and practitioner relationship is an essential foundation for novice development.

The choice of the metaphor of *foundation* is important in that it emphasizes the supportive nature of ethical comportment. A foundation allows something, in this case expert work, to stand on a solid base. If something is lacking in a foundation or is shakily built, it will not be strong enough to withstand the stresses encountered in clinical practice. Skilful ethical comportment draws on at least three basic approaches to ethics: principled reasoning, virtue and a care orientation. A solid moral foundation includes all these approaches because an expert needs to understand moral norms and theories and to be adept at using such tools to examine moral problems and practices. However, 'General norms are usually only starting points for more specific norms of conduct suitable for contexts such as clinical medicine [all health professions] and biomedical research' (Beauchamp and Childress, 2019, p. 2). An expert must also possess the virtues or character to do the right thing. If a clinician knows the correct moral action but lacks the courage or

compassion to act, the knowledge is of little significance. Lastly, a solid foundation in ethics includes the ability to discern what is worth caring about in healthcare practice. A care orientation considers what values should be pursued, nurtured or sustained and, conversely, what should be disvalued. Approaches that include only abstract principles or duties often lead to conclusions that minimize the particulars of individual circumstances that are considered morally relevant to care orientation.

Within the realm of expert practice, the emotions of compassion, sympathy and empathy have a central place in our understanding of humane and ethical treatment of patients. Beyond these basic expressions of care, patients expect a range of emotional responsiveness from healthcare professionals that is appropriate to context. For example, in an emergency situation, most patients would prefer quick and competent action to save their lives rather than heartfelt empathy. However, it is clear that in certain cases, the emotional tone matters deeply. It is the life work of healthcare professionals to recognize those situations and adapt their emotional response to the particular needs of the patient at that time. One way to bring emotions to the forefront of the discussions around expressions of care is to focus on the health humanities. 'The health humanities generally have an underlying moral function that helps students question their own unrealized assumptions, values, and behaviours' (Haddad, 2019, p. 84; Klugman, 2017). Additionally, Kumagai (2022) emphasizes, 'art also offers a way to explore the challenges and triumphs of providing care to those in need and to explore the meanings, feelings, and experiences of living and dying' (p. 1116).

The processes of self-reflection, reflecting together between novice and expert at the moment of a clinical encounter, or small-group discussion on the identification and understanding of emotions are steps in strengthening novices' capacity to hold onto and name their emotional experiences. Rather than novices being told what they should feel or should have felt (such as empathy and compassion) when interacting with patients or others, opportunities should be provided to let novices interact with simulated patients or real patients in clinically complex situations and then reflect on their experiences in their own words.

Although emotions are sometimes seen as a somewhat fragile platform upon which to build such heavy obligations as moral duty or care, by attending to emotions we can see that they highlight certain aspects of a situation, serve as a mode of communication, lead to deeper self-knowledge and provide insight into motivation. Grounding and naming emotions in specific examples from novices' and experts' experiences in clinical practice begins to create a framework that legitimizes this component of the self in one's professional role. Novices can then examine, question and develop their skills in emotional sensitivity; this is an important part of ethical comportment and caring for others.

It is essential that novices have multiple opportunities to act on ethical judgements in a safe environment and reflect not only on the reasons for a particular action or set of actions but also on the thinking and responses that led up to the action. Novices need to hear experts 'think out loud' after a particularly difficult exchange with a patient or colleague so that the process of arriving at a sound decision becomes more transparent. The habit of reflecting on what is going on ethically in a situation, what should be done about it and the meaning for the broader professional and public community *can and must* be fostered throughout professional education Case Study 9.2.

CASE STUDY 9.2

Consider a review of a 'routine' clinical activity such as an interdisciplinary patient care meeting in which there are different views among team members on how to proceed. Create a case in which a treatment or diagnostic test is viewed as futile by one of the members of the team. After a role play, ask participants to make a list of demonstrations representing the use of power during the care meeting, i.e. degrees/education level, expertise, gender, seniority, institutional title, control of resources. Make another list of how patients were referred to in the care meeting and if patients and family members were included, how they were addressed and whether they participated. Use the lists for individual reflection or small group discussion. Examine how people are addressed and how they acknowledge each other's contributions. What does this tell you about power differentials and expressions of care with patients? What is the role of analytical thinking and humanistic thinking in your clinical reasoning process?

REFLECTION POINT

- How does this discussion fit in with your previous ideas on expertise and clinical reasoning?
- What are the implications for your practice, teaching and facilitating learner development?

SUMMARY

- Expertise is not a static state, a list of specific attributes or something that is obtained through years of experience but a continuum of development and a dynamic process in which critical reflection and deliberate action are central components.
- Adaptive expertise requires: (1) an openness to reflecting on practice, (2) metacognitive reasoning skills to recognize that a routine approach to the problem will not work, (3) critical thinking to challenge current assumptions and beliefs and (4) the ability to reconstruct the problem space.
- Clinical reasoning is a complex process in which critical analysis and reflection take place in the context of the action and interaction with the patient.
- Experts demonstrate their patient-centred focus through a consistent commitment to knowing the patient, intense listening that leads to a rich understanding of the patient's perspective and character to do the right thing.
- The challenge in professional education is to teach the complex ensemble of analytic thinking, skilful practice and wise judgement that is required in the health professions. This skilful ethical comportment based on principled reasoning, virtue and a care orientation is the foundation of expertise.

REFERENCES

Beauchamp, J., Childress, J., 2019. Principles of biomedical ethics, 8th ed. Oxford University Press. https://doi.org/10.1016/j.dcn.2020.100861

Benner, P., 1984. From novice to expert: Excellence and power in clinical nursing practice. Addison-Wesley. https://doi.org/10.1002/nur.4770080119

Benner, P., Hooper-Kyriakidis, P., Stannard, D., 2011. Clinical wisdom and interventions in acute and critical care, 2nd ed. Springer Pub.

Benner, P., Sutphen, M., Leonard, V., et al., 2010. Educating nurses: A call for radical transformation. Jossey-Bass.

Benner, P., Tanner, C.A., Chesla, C.A., 1996. Expertise in nursing practice. Springer Press.

Benner, P., Purtilo, R., 2019. In: Jensen, G., Mostrom, E., Hack, L., Nordstrom, T., Gwyer., J. (Eds.), Educating for professional responsibility: Integration across habits of head, hand, and heart. *Educating physical therapists*. Slack Inc., pp. 211–222. (2019).

Bereiter, C., Scardamalia, M., 1993. Surpassing ourselves: An inquiry into the nature and implications of expertise. Open Court Press.

Berliner, D., 1986. In pursuit of the expert pedagogue. Education Research 15, 5–13.

Black, L., Jensen, G.M., Mostrom, E., et al., 2010. The first year of practice: An investigation of the professional learning and development of promising young novice physical therapists. Physical Therapy 90, 1758–1773. https://doi.org/10.2522/ptj.20100078

Blanton, S., Greenfield, B., Jensen, G., Swisher, L., Kirsch, N., Davis, C., et al., 2020. Can reading Tolstoy make us better physical therapists? The role of the health humanities in physical therapy. Physical Therapy 100, 885–889. https://doi.org/10.1093/ptj/pzaa027

Boshuizen, H., Bromme, R., Gruber, H., 2004. Professional learning: Gaps and transitions on the way from novice to expert. Kluwer Academic. https://doi.org/10.1007/1-4020-2094-5

Bowen, J., (annotated by Parsons, A., Rencic, J., Bowen, J., Abdulnour, R.), 2022. Educational strategies to promote clinical diagnostic reasoning. New England Journal of Medicine 355, 2217–2229. https://doi.org/10.1056/nejmra054782

Brandsford, J., Brown, A., Cocking, R., 2000. How people learn: Brain mind, experience and school. National Academy Press.

Carraccio, C., Benson, B., Nixon, J., et al., 2008. From the educational bench to the clinical bedside: Translating the Dreyfus Developmental model to the learning of clinical skills. Academic Medicine 83, 761–767. https://doi.org/10.1097/acm.0b013e31817eb632

Chase, W., Simon, H.A., 1973. Perception in chess. Cognitive Psychology, 455–481. https://psycnet.apa.org/doi/10.1016/0010-0285(73)90004-2

Chi, M.T., Feltovich, P.J., Glaser, R., 1981. Categorization and representation of physics problems by experts and novices. Cognitive Science (Hauppauge) 5, 121–152.

Chi, M.T., Glaser, R., Farr, M., 1988. The nature of expertise. *Lawrence Erlbaum*. https://doi.org/10.1207/s15516709cog0502_2

Colby, A., Sullivan, W., 2008. Formation of professionalism and purpose: Perspectives from the preparation for the professions program. University of St Thomas Law Journal, 5, 404–426.

Cooke, M., Irby, D., O'Brien, B., 2010. Educating physicians. Jossey-Bass.

Cutrer, W.B., Miller, B., Pusic, M., et al., 2016. Fostering the development of master adaptive learners: A conceptual model to guide skill acquisition in medical education. Academic Medicine 92, 70–75. https://doi.org/10.1097/acm.0000000000001323

Cutrer, W., Pusic, M., Gruppen, M., Santen, S., 2020. The master adaptive learner. Elsevier.

deGroot, A., 1966. Perception and memory versus thought. In: Kleinmuntz, B. (Ed.), Problem solving research, methods and theory. Wiley Press, pp. 19–50.

Dreyfus, H.L., Dreyfus, S.L., 1980. Unpublished report supported by the Air Force of Scientific Research (AFSC), USAF (Contract F49620-79-C-0063). A five stage model of the mental activities involved in directed skill acquisition. University of California.

Dreyfus, H.L., Dreyfus, S.E., 1996. The relationship of theory and practice in the acquisition of skill. In: Benner, P., Tanner, C.A., Chesla, C.A. (Eds.), Expertise in nursing practice. Springer Press, pp. 29–48.

Edwards, I., Jones, M., Carr, J., et al., 2004. Clinical reasoning strategies in physical therapy. Physical Therapy 84, 312–335. https://doi.org/10.1093/ptj/84.4.312

Englander, R., Cameron, T., Ballard, A.J., Dodge, J., Bull, J., Aschenbrener, C.A., 2013. Toward a common taxonomy of competency domains for the health professions and competencies for physicians. Academic Medicine 88(8), 1088–1094. https://doi.org/10.1097/ACM.0b013e31829a3b2b

Ericsson, K. (Ed.), 2009. Development of professional expertise. Cambridge University Press. https://psycnet.apa.org/doi/10.1017/CBO9780511609817

Ericsson, K., 2015. Acquisition and maintenance of medical expertise: A perspective from the expert-performance approach with deliberate practice. Academic Medicine 90, 1471–1486. https://doi.org/10.1097/acm.0000000000000939

Fleming, M.H., Mattingly, C., 2000. Action and narrative: Two dynamics of clinical reasoning. In: Higgs, J., Jones, M. (Eds.), Clinical reasoning in the health professions, 2nd ed. Butterworth-Heinemann, pp. 54–61. https://doi.org/10.1080/09593985.2018.1472686

Furze, J., Greenfield, B., Barr, J., Geist, K., Gale, J., Jensen, G., 2019. Clinical narratives in residency education: Exploration of the learning process. Physiotherapy Theory and Practice 35, 1202–1217.

Haddad, A., 2019. Shine a light here, dig deeper over there. Integrating the health humanities in online bioethics education. In: Banner, O., Carlin, N., Cole, T. (Eds.), Teaching health humanities. Oxford University Press, pp. 75–88.

Irby, D., Cooke, M., O'Brien, B., 2010. Calls for reform of medical education by the Carnegie Foundation for the Advancement of Teaching: 1910–2010. Academic Medicine 85, 220–227. https://doi.org/10.1097/acm.0b013e3181c88449

Jensen, G.M., Gwyer, J., Hack, L.M., et al., 2007. Expertise in physical therapy practice, 2nd ed. Saunders-Elsevier.

Jensen, G.M., Gwyer, J., Shepard, K.F., et al., 2000. Expert practice in physical therapy. Physical Therapy 80, 28–43. https://doi.org/10.1093/ptj/80.1.28

Jensen, G., Mostrom, E., Hack, L., Nordstrom, T., Gwyer, J., 2019. Educating physical therapists. Slack Inc.

Jones, M., Rivett, D., 2019. Clinical reasoning in musculoskeletal practice, 2nd ed. Elsevier.

Klugman, C., 2017. How the health humanities will save the life of the humanities. Journal of Medical Humanities 38, 419–430. https://doi.org/10.1007/s10912-017-9453-5

Kua, J., Lim, W.S., Teo, W., Edwards, R.A., 2021. A scoping review of adaptive expertise in education. Medical Teacher 43 (3), 347–355. https://doi.org/10.1080/0142159x.2020.1851020

Kumagai, A., 2022. The powers of the fish: Clinical thinking, humanistic thinking and different ways of knowing. Academic Medicine 97, 1114–1116. https://doi.org/10.1097/ACM.000000000000468

Mattingly, C., Fleming, M.H., 1994. Clinical reasoning: Forms of inquiry in a therapeutic practice. FA Davis.

Moulton, C., Regehr, G., Mylopoulos, M., et al., 2007. Slowing down when you should: A new model of expert judgment. Academic Medicine 82, S109–S116. https://doi.org/10.1097/acm.0b013e3181405a76

Musolino, G., Jensen, G., 2020. Clinical reasoning and decision-making in physical therapy. Slack Inc.

Mylopoulos, M., Woods, N., 2009. Having our cake and eating it too: Seeking the best of both worlds in expertise research. Medical Education 43, 406–413. https://doi.org/10.1111/j.1365-2923.2009.03307.x

Mylopoulos, M., Kulasegaram, K., Woods, N.N., 2018a. Developing the experts we need: Fostering adaptive expertise through education. Journal of Evaluation in Clinical Practice 24 (3), 674–677. https://doi.org/10.1111/jep.12905

Mylopoulos, M., Steenhof, N., Kaushal, A., Woods, N.N., 2018b. Twelve tips for designing curricula that support the development of adaptive expertise. Medical Teacher 40 (8), 850–854. https://doi.org/10.1080/0142159x.2018.1484082

Mylopoulos, M., Brydges, R., Woods, N.N., Manzone, J., Schwartz, D.L., 2016. Preparation for future learning: A missing competency in health professions education. Medical Education 50 (1), 115–123. https://doi.org/10.1111/medu.12893

Mylopoulos, M., Borschel, D., O'Brien, T., Martinmianakis, S., Woods, N., 2017. Exploring integration in action: Competencies. Academic Medicine 92, 1794–1799. https://doi.org/10.1097/acm.0000000000001772

Resnik, L., Hart, D., 2003. Using clinical outcomes to identify expert physical therapists. Physical Therapy 83, 990–1002. https://doi.org/10.1093/ptj/83.11.990

Resnik, L., Jensen, G.M., 2003. Using clinical outcomes to explore the theory of expert practice in physical therapy. Physical Therapy 83, 1090–1106. https://doi.org/10.1093/ptj/83.12.1090

Reilly, M., Furze, J., Black, L., Knight, H., Niski, J., Peterson, J., et al., 2022. Development of a clinical reasoning blueprint: A guide for teaching, learning, and assessment. Journal of Physical Therapy Education 36, 43–50. https://doi.org/10.1097/JTE.0000000000000217

Rikers, R., Paas, F., 2005. Recent advances in expertise research. Applied Cognitive Psychology 19, 145–149. https://doi.org/10.1002/acp.1108

Robertson, D., Warrender, F., Barnard, S., 2015. The critical occupational therapy practitioner: How to define expertise? Australian Occupational Therapy Journal 62, 68–71. https://doi.org/10.1111/1440-1630.12157

Schön, D., 1987. Educating the reflective practitioner. Jossey-Bass.

Schwartz, A., Elstein, A.S., 2008. Clinical reasoning in medicine. In: Higgs, J., Jones, M., Loftus, S. (Eds.), Clinical reasoning in the health professions, 3rd ed. Elsevier, pp. 223–234.

Shaw, J., DeForge, R., 2012. Physiotherapy as bricolage: Theorizing expert practice. Physiotherapy Theory and Practice 28, 420–427. https://doi.org/10.3109/09593985.2012.676941

Shulman, L., 2004. The wisdom of practice. Jossey-Bass.

Sternberg, R.J., Horvath, J.A., 1995. A prototype view of expert teaching. Education Research 24, 9–17. https://doi.org/10.3102/0013189X024006009

Trowbridge, R., Rencic, J., Durning, S. (Eds.), 2015. Teaching clinical reasoning. American College of Physicians. ISBN: 9781938921056

Tsui, A., 2003. Understanding expertise in teaching. Cambridge University Press.

Uemura, Y., Kido, K., 2022. Clinical reasoning process of novice and expert using consensual qualitative research in observational situations of postpartum mothers and newborns. International Journal of Nursing Education 14, 171–178. https://doi.org/10.37506/ijone.v14i3.18375

Weiner, S., 2022. Contextualizing case: An essential and measurable clinical competency. Patient Education and Counseling 105, 594–598. https://doi.org/10.1016/j.pec.2021.06.016

Woods, N., Mylopoulos, M., 2015. On clinical reasoning research and applications: Redefining expertise. Medical Education 49, 542–544. https://doi.org/10.1111/medu.12643

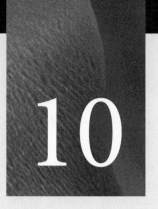

10

EMPOWERMENT AND CLINICAL REASONING

CATHERINE MAITLAND ■ RICK FLOWERS

CHAPTER OUTLINE

CHAPTER AIMS

The aims of this chapter are:

- to present a model of social justice-oriented clinical reasoning that is underpinned by a feminist relational approach to care, an ethics of vulnerability and an ethics of listening
- to draw on narratives of people with intellectual disability to provoke reflection about traditional approaches to social justice and empowerment within clinical practice.

INTRODUCTION

Three Schools of Social Justice-Oriented Theorizing About Care

One school of social justice-oriented theorizing (critical disability studies) strongly contests the concept of care, regarding it as a historically oppressive act that misrecognizes and misrepresents people, particularly those who are marginalized. In this view, **benevolent** care fails to challenge the systemic and institutional influences that define and negatively impact the experiences of people receiving care (Bond-Taylor, 2015; Fine, 2005; Watson et al., 2004). Another school of social justice-oriented theorizing (critical emancipatory practice) calls for patients or clients to aspire not to be dependent, but to be agentic, autonomous and emancipated. However, Fraser (1990) argues that while participation of individuals in public deliberation and decision making is essential for promoting empowerment and agency, marginalized people experience multiple barriers to participation. In this chapter, we argue for a third school of social justice-oriented theorizing: relational practice.

Relational approaches to clinical reasoning, in which people become interconnected in relationships where they feel the positive support of another, foster a sense of belonging and opportunity rather than limitation. This may seem like common sense. But orthodox emancipatory approaches to communicative action, as theorized by Habermas (1970a; 1970b), imply that interconnection may leave clients vulnerable, dependent and excluded (Clifford, 2012). A relational approach, by contrast, accepts that interdependency can be productive. It involves:

- decentring a behaviourist and biomedical model of practice;
- listening to, and learning from, historically silenced 'voices' or, another way of putting it: deploying a phenomenological approach to connecting with clients (Ajjawi and Higgs, 2007).

REFLECTION POINT

- We invite readers to reflect on this question before reading further:
  Empowerment for people means having a voice in decisions that affect their lives, as well as how support is provided and by whom. What types of care and clinical reasoning can facilitate this?

JOAN TRONTO'S FRAMEWORK OF CARE AND DEMOCRACY

Behaviourist perspectives reproduce care practices as transactional and reparative, which 'perpetuates rather than challenges paternalism and ableism' (Maitland, 2022, p. 105). This chapter begins by presenting a framework of care that was developed over 30 years ago by Joan Tronto, political scientist at the University of Minnesota. She advocates to recognize care as a fundamental human need (2015; Tronto and Fisher, 1990), thus disrupting the notion of dependency as a limitation. Tronto's framework, a cycle of action and reflection, initially included four principles:

- **caring about**: attentiveness to identifying care needs;
- **caring for**: taking on the responsibility of providing personalized assistance;
- **care giving:** providing competent care;
- **care receiving:** responsive listening to care recipients' subjective experiences and feelings in order to evaluate the care provided from the perspectives of those who receive care and to identify new or unmet care needs so that the cycle of care begins again (Kittay, 2001a; Tronto, 1993;

2015; Tronto and Fisher, 1990; Sevenhuijsen, 2003).

Tronto (2015) subsequently added a fifth phase:

- **caring with**: a democratic ideal of contributing and receiving care over a lifetime.

Practising care that is relational and democratic is, of course, deeply challenging. Tronto's initial framework has been criticized for inadequately focussing on the perspectives of care recipients (Fine, 2007; Keyes et al., 2015), and for focussing on the 'maintenance quality' of care (Simplican, 2018, p. 1). Nevertheless, her later work spotlighting democratic care (2015) emphasizes the importance of building trust and solidarity between givers and receivers of care, eschewing hierarchical relationships that frequently produce a one-way stream of authority, which results in the care receiver telling the care provider what they think they want to hear. Democratic care, Tronto (2015) argues, opens up the way for a truly just society, where everyone may live as well as possible, giving and receiving care as needed.

Social justice thus requires us to '**care about**' people, not just in the politics of everyday interactions, but also at the political level, where services that people need are identified and decisions are made about how they are provided.

CATHERINE MAITLAND'S TYPOLOGY OF CARE

In order to help practitioners examine their own practice and their part in perpetuating or disrupting paternalistic, transactional care, we next present a typology of care developed by the first author, grounded in empirical data from her doctoral research (Maitland, 2022). The typology of care, a grounded analysis of experiences of care from multiple perspectives, suggests ways of prompting reflexivity by care practitioners, managers and policy makers.

Maitland's typology seeks to synthesize analytically the full spectrum of care from the perspectives of people who receive care and people who provide it. Care is not inherently good or positive; it can be harmful and domineering (Steele, 2020). Maitland goes beyond focussing on caring practices that are inclusive; she troubles the uncritical acceptance of the ontology of disability as inherently deficit. When care practitioners are reflexive about the ways in which power and control are exercised, they may better realize the negative impacts of their practice on the subjectivities of care recipients. Such critical recognition of unequal power, oppression and marginalization paves the way to a more equal and just engagement.

KEY TERMS

Transactional care: care needs are determined and provided by the caregiver.

Controlling care: paternalistic support practices that subjugate a person's local knowledges.

Relational care: goes beyond practical and physical 'care for' by recognizing the practical and emotional dependency on care that everyone has.

Relational autonomy: through a process of interaction, listening and collaboration, choices and decision are made within a web of relationships.

Relational solidarity: collective, mutually empowering partnerships, built on shared understanding, that challenge oppression (Maitland, 2022).

Radical mutuality: care that transcends dominant disempowering discourses; it is based on **relational solidarity** that encompasses fairness, equality and democracy.

Reflexivity: a critical focus on personal biases, social position and social forces that have shaped a person's beliefs.

Subjectivity: a sense of a person's 'self' which may be deeply affected by power imbalances.

Four 'Moves' of Care

The four metaphorical moves in Maitland's typology of care depict the struggle against reproducing dominant deficit discourses and offer a way to navigate the ethical and moral dilemmas implicit in care work. Crucial to the four moves is critical recognition of unjust social relations, even within notions of solidarity and mutuality where misrepresentation may occur (hooks, 1994; Walters and Butterwick, 2017).

Stand Over

'Standing over' is about controlling care practices. The expression 'stand over' originated from a disability

support worker, Graham, who said: 'I believe it's not good enough to be standing over and observing [people]' *(Maitland, 2022, p. 313).*

Care work is often controlling and has to be sometimes in order to ensure health and safety. Furthermore, Maitland's research found that people with intellectual disability may be subjected to a controlling environment in the interests of making a care worker's job easier. But Graham is more interested in a form of care that is relational rather than controlling where he learns by interacting, listening and collaborating with the people he is supporting (Maitland, 2022).

Stand Back

There are two types of standing back. The first is a positive move: when workers deliberately stand back in order to make space for people who receive care to act and speak for themselves. The workers remain attentive. The second is a negative move, when workers are inattentive, sometimes to the point of neglect, to the thoughts, feelings and actions of people in their charge (Maitland, 2022).

Stand With

This type of care is about workers being advocates who act in solidarity with, not for, the people they support. 'Standing with' is a move that encompasses recognition of democratic citizenship that includes all people, not only those who are rational and self-regulating (Tronto, 2015). It embraces our shared need to experience a sense of belonging and relating and opens up the possibilities for relational rather than individual autonomy within care practices.

It is easy to claim that a person is standing with. But there is an implicit risk of smothering and speaking for the 'other', which results in a practice of standing over. To mitigate that risk, it is necessary to build a relationship reflexively in order to try to find out how people navigate their personal world in their own way, for example, their unique communication style (Maitland, 2022).

Stand Up

We may also disrupt the broader contexts that impact on care recipients' lives, by 'standing up': speaking out to challenge structural oppression. Standing up is about forming a mutually agreed partnership between worker or practitioner and care recipient, in which the former realizes that sometimes they, as well as the system, are complicit with oppression and subjugation of othered knowledges (Maitland, 2022). 'Standing up' is built on freely shared knowledge and is grounded in the lived experience of the lives of people who are routinely controlled and coerced. To build trust is when both 'helper' and 'helped' speak up as allies without speaking for, or about, the other. This is radical mutalitly (Maitland, 2022).

KEY TERMS

Phenomenological accounts: are based on lived experiences and understandings that people have formed about themselves, rather than those, often oppressive, that are imposed upon them.
Ontological injustice: Ontology refers to the philosophical study of being. It is unjust to conceive the being of intellectual disability through a normative lens as Other.
Epistemic injustice: Epistemology refers to the study of knowledge. People with intellectual disability are perceived, even by people with physical and sensory disability, to be at the bottom of the social hierarchy and their knowledge is excluded (Deal, 2003).

WHAT SOCIAL JUSTICE ISSUES ARE HIGHLIGHTED THROUGH ANALYSIS OF CARE PRACTICES IN THE INTELLECTUAL DISABILITY SPACE?

We have chosen to illustrate the aims of the chapter with examples from the lived experiences of people with intellectual disability. We believe that phenomenological accounts of disability highlight and disrupt the ontological and epistemic injustices that are enacted upon people with intellectual disability. They are wronged by entrenched imbalances of power and exclusion from political processes that construct people with intellectual disability as deficit and passive (Chappell, 1998; Goodley, 2001). We argue that these wrongs effectively silence them far more than any 'inherent' disability does.

We consider Maitland's (2022) typology of care, along with Narratives 10.1 and 10.2 from the first author's doctoral research, in order to provoke reflection by health practitioners on their practice and their part in perpetuating dominant and disempowering discourses. Maitland's typology of care, in its four metaphorical moves, reframes speaking up for people with intellectual disability as the critical recognition of the diverse subjectivities of people with intellectual disability.

Grand Narratives of Disability

KEY TERMS

Biomedical approach to disability: a discourse that dominates management of the body, excluding embodied experiences and knowledges.
Social model of disability: In the 1970s, activists, led by Mike Oliver and Vic Finkelstein, began arguing that disability is a social construct (Oliver, 1990). They were concerned with externally imposed oppression rather than inherent impairment.

In a biomedical approach, disability is perceived only as a physical construct. Nondisabled clinicians plan therapeutic interventions. Hegemonic ableist views (Titchkosky, 2007) misrepresent people with disability as 'wrong' (Michalko, 2001) and reinforce the invisibility of the embodied experience (Ghai, 2002).

But although the social model of disability has been used by disability activists to organize for social and political change since the 1970s (Thomas, 2004b), it is not a viable model to refute deficit ontologies and epistemologies of individualized incompetence and pathology. This is because first, the social model of disability represents disabled people as a homogenous group with similar experiences of oppression (Hughes, 2014; Hughes and Paterson, 1997; Paterson and Hughes, 1999) and, as feminists in particular have argued, denies personal experiences of impairment, such as pain, which endure even when social and environmental barriers are removed (Morris, 1991). Second, people with intellectual disability were excluded from the social model of disability because they were regarded as inferior by disability activists, who mainly had physical or sensory impairment (Chappell, 1998; Goodley, 2001). Because of this discrimination, even by disability activists, people with intellectual disability have historically been excluded from collective resistance and action.

Narrative 10.1: James

James was diagnosed with an intellectual disability as a child and is now experiencing physical health issues as he ages. He is described by the disability support service manager, to his face, as a 'walking time bomb' due to his very high blood pressure and diabetes type 2. Although the manager is concerned, she believes that the day programme staff do not have responsibility for James's health. She says that the support service where he lives should look after all medical matters. However, she knows that, since his mother died several years ago, James has lived alone, semi-independently, with minimal drop-in support, and does not receive any support to attend medical appointments.

Nevertheless, James attends a Diabetes Centre regularly on his own. He recounts that doctors and diabetes nurse educators frame the various health problems as his own personal failings. He says the nurses 'nag' and 'pick on' him as they try to persuade him to do more exercise and eat more healthily. They describe the negative effects of his current lifestyle on his health. James, scared that he will die of heart and kidney failure, as his mother did, tells the diabetes nurse: 'I don't want to hear that'. But 'they', as James refers to health professionals and support workers, respond with further threats, telling him that he'll end up in a coma in hospital and what will he do then?

James is worried by their threats that he will be on his 'death bed' soon and says that his anxiety about dying stays with him for a long time after leaving the Diabetes Centre. To James, the health professionals' notion of 'care' practice is to tell him what to do and to threaten him with the consequences of non-compliance. James says that he feels blamed for not doing what they expect him to do; he feels 'wrong' much of the time, in the face of professionals believing that they are right.

James has thus internalized a negative sense of self by being made to feel wrong much of the time.

Narrative 10.2: Fiona

It is 11 a.m. on a Thursday morning and Fiona has been ready to go out since before 9 a.m. Every Thursday is her 'treat day' when she has one-to-one support instead of going to a day programme.

Fiona is keen to start the day, but first she has to wait for the support worker to complete various tasks, have a cup of tea and chat with the other support workers about operational matters. To pass the time, Fiona walks outside and sits waiting in the van. On this occasion, as the time edged closer to noon, 3 hours after the 'treat day' was supposed to start, Fiona reentered the kitchen, picked up a bowl of cooked rice that was sitting on the kitchen bench and threw it into the sink.

Fiona has been living in a Supported Independent Living home (SIL) for several years with three other people with intellectual disability. None of them had any say in choosing where they lived or who with. Fiona loves classical music and she has a boyfriend. But even on her 1 day per week of individualized support, she has no say in what she does. If she did, she might choose to go to a classical music concert every week or visit her boyfriend Ron. But instead, a support worker takes her out to lunch every week.

The SIL manager and support staff at the SIL home say that Fiona cannot express herself or make choices and decisions because she is nonverbal, has autism and an intellectual disability. They believe that their job is to understand and 'manage' the effects of autism on her behaviour.

The SIL manager explains that Fiona has to have certain things happening in a particular order, otherwise she becomes confused and then frustrated. When asked, the manager says that she does not believe that Fiona is frustrated by the staff not making an effort to understand her communication styles.

Although Fiona can use sign language, none of the staff know how to. She has a 'compix' communication book of pictures that represent a word or concept, but the book is upstairs in her bedroom and the SIL manager remarked that she has only seen Fiona use the book once in several years.

A speech pathologist recently performed a clinical assessment of Fiona's capacity for learning to use another form of communication aid, such as an iPad, and reported that it was feasible. But according to the SIL manager, there are many other issues to deal with before that can happen, such as working with a psychologist on Fiona's behaviours of concern – like throwing a bowl of rice into the sink in frustration at the 3-hour delay in starting what is supposed to be a treat day for her of one-to-one support.

Following the manager's lead, the SIL staff believe that Fiona does not understand much about what is going on around her and therefore they hardly engage in conversation with her. They apply behaviour modifications that, far from understanding Fiona as a person, aim to guide her to become compliant with their schedules and plans. One of the behaviour management strategies is a 'social story', written by support workers with the guidance of a behaviour support professional. Developed by Carol Gray in 1990, social stories are meant to provide a learning experience for people with autism that engenders physical, emotional and social safety, by supporting them to know what to expect in a particular situation, in order to reduce confusion and increase predictability (Gray, 2023).

But the SIL staff describe the social story that they have written for Fiona as a proactive measure that informs Fiona what is expected of her in certain situations. The story lists the activities that are going to take place and the behaviour that is expected. They diligently read the story to Fiona twice every day.

This use of social stories written in this way suggests that the staff do not value trying to explore, with Fiona, her authentic expressions of lived experience. They are working on her, to manipulate and modify her behaviour so that it aligns with normative expectations. The staff do not perceive that there is anything amiss in writing the story about Fiona and using it as a mechanism of control.

REFLECTION POINT

Traditional pillars of medical ethics

1. Respect for patients' autonomy to make decisions about their own treatment;
2. Beneficence on the part of health professionals to act in the best interests of their patients and their well-being;
3. Nonmaleficence: the obligation to cause no harm to patients;
4. Justice: the obligation to treat all patients in a fair and equitable way, without discriminating on factors such as race, gender or socioeconomic status (Beauchamp and Childress, 2013).

REFLECTION POINT

We invite you to reflect on the following questions that relate to James (Narrative 10.1):

1. What can health professionals who adopt a relational approach do to help James in his decision making about managing his health?
2. The manager is 'standing back' and the nurse is 'standing over' (see Maitland's typology of care). The support workers provide inconsistent, tokenistic support to James with regard to exercise and diet. What are other more empowering ways to help James improve his health? For example, a warm referral could be made to a local 'Walking Group' and accessible information (in Easy Read) about healthy eating choices could be provided.
3. How can health professionals prevent exacerbating James' feelings that they make him feel he always gives the wrong answer or makes a wrong decision? How might they work to dispel that feeling and instead promote James' sense of agency and lay the groundwork to build trust?
4. What needs to be done at a systemic level to improve public health outcomes for patients like James?

REFLECTION POINT

We invite you to respond to the following questions relating to Fiona (Narrative 10.2):

1. What is the root cause of Fiona's frustration?
2. The social story that is used to change Fiona's behaviour is an example of trying to make Fiona control herself in certain situations and thus overcome the behaviour that is perceived negatively by staff as a symptom of autism. In what ways could Fiona be empowered to express her frustration at controlling staff practices? And how would staff enact that support on a daily basis?

In addition, unlike professionally qualified care providers, such as allied health practitioners, the everyday provision of care of people with intellectual disability has historically been a gendered, poorly resourced, low-status position. Such caregivers are subject to multiple oppressions themselves, whether care is paid for or provided invisibly – usually by women – within the family home (Kittay, 1999). Recent Australian research suggests that disability support workers feel devalued and unheard due to their low status (Robinson et al., 2020; Quilliam et al., 2018). Their work is under-theorized and not 'well circumscribed' like that of a doctor or teacher, and yet direct care workers play a valuable role as the 'sustainers' who implement professionally prescribed interventions (Kittay, 1999, p. 40).

UNSETTLING TRADITIONAL MEDICAL ETHICS AND PREVAILING ORTHODOXY ABOUT EMPOWERMENT AND EMANCIPATORY PRACTICE

In order to unsettle the dominant discourses in clinical reasoning, which are largely based on the traditional pillars of medical ethics (Beauchamp and Childress, 2013), this chapter proposes that an additional set of ethics be considered. This is informed by a feminist ethic of care, buttressed by an ethics of vulnerability and an ethic of listening. We illustrate such ethics with Narratives 10.1 and 10.2 from the first author's doctoral research and propose her typology of care (Maitland, 2022) to aid practitioners in reflecting upon their clinical reasoning in order to promote empowerment and social justice at individual and systemic levels.

Empowerment and Individual Autonomy (Going Beyond Traditional Pillar of Medical Ethics 1)

The first pillar of traditional medical ethics (see the second reflection point box) rests on the principle of individual autonomy. However, our start and end points in life are different (Tronto, 2015) and we should not assume that we all aspire to the same kind of autonomy, nor that all experiences, needs and perspectives are homogenous (Maitland, 2022). An intellectual disability standpoint helps us to see that, for example, an intervention that increases empowerment and personal control for one person may lead to social isolation and disengagement for another (Cummins and Lau, 2005). Moreover, behaviourist techniques that are intended to bestow empowerment – or

rather a 'bounded frame of empowerment' that may be revoked at any time – have not resulted in increased feelings of empowerment by people with intellectual disability (Jingree and Finlay, 2008, p. 719). On the contrary, such approaches have reinforced inadequacy and deficit as an individualized problem, thereby discouraging individual and collective empowerment (Dowse, 2007).

Emancipatory Practice and the Neo-Liberal Prized Independent Citizen (Going Beyond Pillar 1)

The Australian National Disability Insurance Scheme (NDIS) appears emancipatory. But while it is designed to give clients choice and control, this alone does not necessarily lead practitioners to value embodied experiences and insider knowledges of people with intellectual disability (Davy, 2019). Underpinned by converging discourses of ableist normativity and neo-liberalism, it is assumed that clinical reasoning and care in NDIS should strive to facilitate choice for participants. Maitland writes (2022, p. 294):

> *The irony and injustice is that the majority of NDIS participants cannot actually exercise choice—for example, by leaving a particular service and selecting one that suits their particular needs better—because they rely on regular support (Thill, 2015) or they lack confidence to make a move (Mavromaras et al., 2018). Or indeed, they lack access to the information and support required to make an informed decision about who they want to deliver their care. The result is that, perceived as lacking capacity to exercise the key tenets of independence—'choice and control'— they are re-confirmed as deficit and dependent and without further analysis or dialogue, are provided with care; but it is the 'booby prize' (Barnes, 2011, p. 160) of care in its oppressive guise as a mechanism of protection and remedial intervention.*

KEY TERMS

Ableist normativity: the practice of measuring humanness against the ideological benchmark of ability (Campbell, 2009; Siebers, 2008).

Neo-liberalist ideology of care: care as a commodity that is based on competitive market growth, privatization and profit (Connell, 2011).

Acting in Best Interests Through a Relational Lens (Going Beyond Pillar 2)

To act in the best interests of people with intellectual disability is not straightforward (Kelly, 2011). It could end up as 'standing over' or 'standing with' (as in Maitland's typology of care). To 'stand with' requires recognizing that we are all dependent on others and share the need for interdependence (Maitland, 2022). As Jackie Leach Scully claims:

> to be so involved in social relations that choice and action are possible at all is at the same time to be dependent on people and institutions
>
> **(2014, p. 213).**

Alongside Scully's argument that dependency thus becomes an intrinsic part of autonomy, not a threat to it, sits the warning from Catriona Mackenzie (2014, p. 47) that 'objectionably paternalistic' social policy interventions lead to pathogenic vulnerability (Fig. 10.1).

We suggest that a relational approach that values listening and recognition of insider perspectives protects, in an emancipatory sense, against domination and inequality.

KEY TERMS

Dependency: perceiving dependency as an individual failing stigmatizes and marginalizes recipients of care. However, the concept of dependency is used by feminist ethic of care theorists to spotlight that different perspectives and interests are served in a care relationship (Barnes, 2012), thereby enabling the fostering of relationships of trust and mutuality, which protect against domination (Held, 2006).

Interdependency: interdependent relationships acknowledge our ongoing or occasional shared dependency on others across our lifespan and generate nondominating forms of relational rather than individual autonomy (Kittay, 2001b).

Relational autonomy: autonomy is traditionally based on human rights, while a feminist ethic of care claims that people become autonomous – making decisions, challenging inequality and pursuing social justice goals – within a care relationship (Barnes, 2006; Bond-Taylor, 2015; Mackenzie and Stoljar, 2000; Tronto, 2015).

Relational practice: the practice of supporting the development of relational autonomy through 'standing with' as in Maitland's typology of care (Maitland, 2022).

Misrecognition as a Site of Harm (Problematizing Pillar 3)

Maitland's research (2022) found that people with intellectual disability are misrecognized by nondisabled people who pathologize idiosyncratic expressions of communication, resistance and frustration, which, they claim, deviate from the norms of acceptable

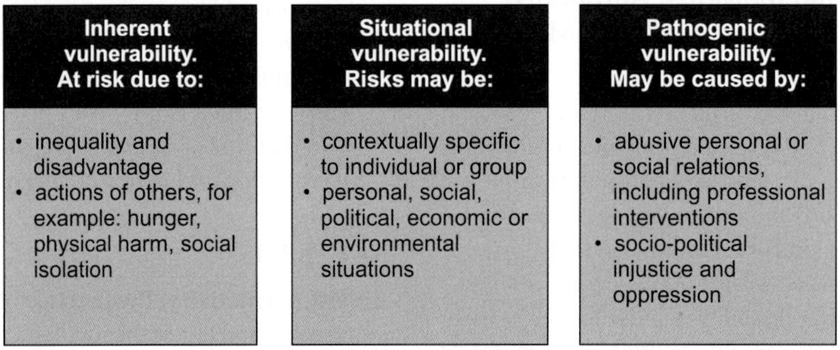

Inherent vulnerability. At risk due to:	Situational vulnerability. Risks may be:	Pathogenic vulnerability. May be caused by:
• inequality and disadvantage • actions of others, for example: hunger, physical harm, social isolation	• contextually specific to individual or group • personal, social, political, economic or environmental situations	• abusive personal or social relations, including professional interventions • socio-political injustice and oppression

Fig. 10.1 ■ Taxonomy of vulnerability. Modified with permission from Mackenzie, C., 2014. The importance of relational autonomy and capabilities for an ethics of vulnerability. In: Mackenzie, C., Rogers, W., Dodds, S., (Eds.), Vulnerability. New essays in ethics and feminist philosophy (pp. 33–59). Oxford University Press, Oxford; and Mackenzie, C., Rogers, W., Dodds, S., 2014. Introduction: What is vulnerability and why does it matter for moral theory? In: Mackenzie, C., Rogers, W., Dodds, S., (Eds.), Vulnerability. New essays in ethics and feminist philosophy (pp. 1–32). Oxford University Press, Oxford.

behaviour, and must therefore be managed and reha-bilitated, rather than recognized as nascent agency. As Robinson et al.'s research (2020) claims, this kind of misrecognition is harmful to people with intellectual disability, as well as exacerbating pathogenic vulner-ability to further harm (Fig. 10.1).

Elaborating How a Feminist Ethic of Care Is Alternative to Justice (Going Beyond Pillar 4)

This pillar evokes American philosopher John Rawls' theory of justice that focusses on equity and fairness (1971). Feminist ethic of care philosopher Eva Feder Kittay is critical of Rawls' assertion that equality and social stability depend on a person being rational, independent and reasonable (1999) and argues that no one is fully functioning throughout their entire life and that all humans need care in times of dependency, for example, newborn babies and frail elderly people. Thus, along with Martha Nussbaum (1999), Kittay (1999) claims that justice relies not just on equity but also on care. Maitland (2022) claims that, unlike a tra-ditional justice perspective:

> a care perspective pays attention [not only] to the maintenance and repair of relationships; it values personal narrative, and is sensitive to contexts when making moral judgements
>
> *(Maitland, 2022, p. 102)*.

Carol Gilligan, in her gendered analysis of care, suggests that hierarchies of relationships are mascu-linist and women are interested in nonhierarchical interconnections (1982). There are critics who point to a tendency to romanticize dependency and ignore exploitation of people with disability (Meekosha and Shuttleworth, 2009). For example, domestic violence towards people with disability is still rife and minors are forced to undergo sterilization. The best way to illustrate the response to this criticism is to describe and discuss, respectively, an ethics of vulnerability and listening.

Ethics of Vulnerability

An ethics of vulnerability draws attention to where vulnerability lies, what has caused it and who decides which vulnerabilities are taken for granted. Some pop-ulations have less power and control over their lives

and so are more susceptible to harm and exploitation. Catriona MacKenzie distinguishes between three dif-ferent types of vulnerability (Fig. 10.1). The signifi-cance of this theorizing is to get us to avoid labelling people with disability as inherently vulnerable, because that results in their being seen as 'other', dependent and burdensome, in other words, politically invisible (Scully, 2014).

Kittay (1999) claims that dependency and victim-hood are frequently contained in the rubric of vul-nerability. Being dependent on external supports, whether that be health professionals or family mem-bers, exacerbates the vulnerability of people with intellectual disability to the actions of others. Hence the importance of an ethics of vulnerability and a feminist ethic of care theorizing in developing the possibility of a relational approach that 'challenge[s] the thinking that defines dependency and concomi-tant vulnerability as incompatible with full autonomy' (Maitland, 2022, p. 114).

Ethics of Listening and Epistemic In/Justice

A standard part of person-centred communication skills for clinicians includes active listening (Barratt, 2019). Gerard Goggin distinguishes, however, between active listening and 'listening as if disability mattered' (Goggin, 2009, p. 499). It is one thing to listen actively, it is another to have an epistemological commitment to valuing the knowledge of people with intellectual disability. Campbell (2009) claims that ableist listen-ing practices tend to result in subordinate responses. Maitland (2022) describes the oppression of being unheard:

> As disability justice activist Mia Mingus (2018) asserts, many people do not tell their stories because there is no-one there to listen and under-stand the complex, intersectional, embodied nature of disability; and that opens the way for others to speak for them. Because their marginalised position is not valued or respected, their voices go unheard, even though phenomenological understand-ings – their insider perspectives – about disability often provide a clearer view of injustices and their solutions
>
> *(Maitland, 2022, p. 302)*.

Ethical listening shifts the focus away from simply giving voice. It draws attention to challenging the taken-for-granted narrative of 'overcoming' disability: a dominant hierarchical discourse which is often perpetuated by health workers, and even people with disability themselves if they grow up learning that their disability must be 'overcome' (Michalko, 2002, p. 182).

Internalized oppression may take hold with alarming ease when a construction of self is imposed by others who have taken control of the subject position of people with intellectual disability. Internalization of a sense of 'the wrong way of being in the world' (Titchkosky, 2007) is seen in Narrative 10.1:

James claimed that he felt that he always gave the 'wrong answer', not the 'right' answer that 'they' (people who exercised control over him) wanted to hear. Reeve (2014, p. 95) names this 'psycho-emotional disablism' that arises from relationships that people with disability have with other people, and from the relationship that they develop with themselves as a result of controlling encounters

(Maitland, 2022, p. 301).

In contrast, Maitland argues that:

the feeling of safety and security that comes from knowing that they will be listened to and believed, rather than belittled and controlled, is an important part of empowerment, positive development of the self, and agency

(2022, p. 94; see also Schormans, 2015; Thill, 2015).

SUMMARY

This chapter has presented a reflexive model of social justice-oriented, relational practice. There are no blueprints or checklists to guide practitioners in clinical reasoning because care is experienced subjectively and embedded in particular contexts and settings. Socially just care must be accessible, equitable and empowering and to that end we have argued for a relational practice underpinned by a feminist ethic of care, an ethics of listening and an ethics of vulnerability, and enacted by means of Maitland's typology

of care. A disability standpoint has enabled us to go beyond traditional theorizing about empowerment to disrupt misrecognition and dismissal of 'difference', whatever the particular axes of difference, as out of step with normative expectations and therefore in need of remediation.

REFERENCES

Ajjawi, R., Higgs, J., 2007. Using hermeneutic phenomenology to investigate how experienced practitioners learn to communicate clinical reasoning. Qualitative Report 12 (4), 612–638. http://hdl.handle.net/10536/DRO/DU:30081266

Barnes, M., 2006. Caring and social justice. Palgrave Macmillan. https://doi.org/10.1007/978-1-137-05193-6

Barnes, M., 2011. Abandoning care? A critical perspective on personalisation from an ethic of care. Ethics and Social Welfare 5 (2), 157–167. https://doi.org/10.1080/17496535.2010.484265

Barnes, M., 2012. Care in everyday life: An ethic of care in practice. Policy Press. https://doi.org/10.1332/policypress/9781847428233.001.0001

Barratt, J., 2019. Developing clinical reasoning and effective communication skills in advanced practice. Nursing Standard 34 (2). https://doi.org/10.7748/ns.2018.e11109

Beauchamp, T., Childress, J., 2013. Principles of Biomedical Ethics, 7th ed. OUP.

Bond-Taylor, S., 2015. Tracing an ethic of care in the policy and practice of the Troubled Families Programme. Getting with the Programme Workshop, Durham.

Campbell, F.A.K., 2009. Contours of ableism: The production of disability and ableness. Palgrave McMillan. https://doi.org/10.1057/9780230245181

Chappell, A., 1998. Still out in the cold: People with learning difficulties and the social model of disability. In: Shakespeare, T. (Ed.), The disability reader: Social science perspectives. Cassell.

Clifford, S., 2012. Making disability public in deliberative democracy. Contemporary Political Theory 11 (2), 211–228. https://doi.org/10.1057/cpt.2011.11

Connell, R., 2011. Southern bodies and disability: Re-thinking concepts. Third World Quarterly 32 (8), 1369–1381. https://doi.org/10.1080/01436597.2011.614799

Cummins, R.A., Lau, A.L.D., 2005. Empowerment versus quality of life – a perspective based on subjective wellbeing homeostasis. In: O'Brien, P., Sullivan, M. (Eds.), Allies in emancipation, shifting from providing service to being of support. Thomson Dunmore Press.

Davy, L., 2019. Between an ethic of care and an ethic of autonomy. Negotiating relational autonomy, disability and dependency. Angelaki. Journal of the theoretical humanities 24 (3), 101–114. https://doi.org/10.1080/0969725X.2019.1620461

Deal, M., 2003. Disabled people's attitudes toward other impairment groups: A hierarchy of impairments. Disability & Society 18 (7), 897–910. https://doi.org/10.1080/0968759032000127317

Dowse, L., 2007. 'Stand up and give 'em the fright of their life'. A study of intellectual disability and the emergence and practice of self-advocacy, [PhD thesis], University of New South Wales. https://doi.org/10.26190/unsworks/17251

Fine, M., 2005. Dependency work: A critical exploration of Kittay's perspective on care as a relation of power. Health Sociology Review 14 (2), 146–160. https://doi.org/10.5172/hesr.14.2.146

Fraser, N., 1990. Re-thinking the public sphere: A contribution to the critique of actually existing democracy. Social Text 25/26, 58–80.

Ghai, A. (2002). Disability in the Indian context: Post-colonial perspectives. In: Corker, M., Shakespeare, T. (Eds.), Disability/postmodernity: Embodying disability theory (pp. 88–100). Continuum.

Gilligan, C., 1982. In a different voice: Psychological theory and women's development. Harvard University Press.

Goggin, G., 2009. Disability and the ethics of listening. Continuum: Journal of Media and Cultural Studies 23 (4), 489–502. https://doi.org/10.1080/10304310903012636

Goodley, D., 2001. 'Learning difficulties', the social model of disability and impairment: Challenging epistemologies. Disability & Society 16 (2), 207–231. https://doi.org/10.1080/09687590120035816

Gray, C., 2023. Carol Gray Social Stories. Retrieved 13 April 2023, from https://carolgraysocialstories.com/social-stories/what-is-it/

Habermas, J., 1970a. Toward a rational society. Beacon Press.

Habermas, J., 1970b. On systematically distorted communication. Inquiry 13 (1-4), 205–218. https://doi.org/10.1080/00201747008601590

Held, V., 2006. The ethics of care: Personal, political and global. Oxford University Press.

hooks, b., 1994. Teaching to transgress. Routledge. https://doi.org/10.3366/para.1994.17.3.270

Hughes, B., 2014. Disability and the body. In: Swain, J., French, S., Barnes, C., Thomas, C. (Eds.), Disabling barriers - Enabling environments. Sage.

Hughes, B., Paterson, K., 1997. The social model of disability and the disappearing body: Towards a sociology of impairment. Disability & Society 12 (3), 325–340. https://doi.org/10.1080/09687599727209

Jingree, T., Finlay, W.M.L., 2008. 'You can't do it…it's theory rather than practice': Staff use of the practice/principle rhetorical device in talk on empowering people with learning disabilities. Discourse and Society 19 (6), 705–726. https://doi.org/10.1177/0957926508095890

Kelly, C., 2011. Making 'care' accessible: Personal assistance for disabled people and the politics of language. Critical Social Policy 31 (4), 562–582. https://doi.org/10.1177/0261018311410529

Keyes, S.E., Webber, S.H., Beveridge, K., 2015. Empowerment through care: Using dialogue between the social model of disability and an ethic of care to redraw boundaries of independence and partnership between disabled people and services. ALTER, European Journal of Disability Research 9, 236–248. https://doi.org/10.1016/j.alter.2015.05.002

Kittay, E.F., 1999. Love's Labor. Essays on women, equality and dependency. Routledge.

Kittay, E.F., 2001a. When caring is just and justice is caring: Justice and mental retardation. Public Culture 13 (3), 557–579. https://doi.org/10.1215/08992363-13-3-557

Kittay, E.F., 2001b. A feminist public ethic of care meets the new communitarian family policy. Ethics 1 (1), 523–547. https://doi.org/10.1086/233525

Mackenzie, C., 2014. The importance of relational autonomy and capabilities for an ethics of vulnerability. In: Mackenzie, C., Rogers, W., Dodds, S. (Eds.), Vulnerability. New essays in ethics and feminist philosophy. Oxford University Press, pp. 33–59.

Mackenzie, C., Rogers, W., Dodds, S., 2014. Introduction: What is vulnerability and why does it matter for moral theory? In: Mackenzie, C., Rogers, W., Dodds, S. (Eds.), Vulnerability. New essays in ethics and feminist philosophy. Oxford University Press, pp. 1–32.

Mackenzie, C., Stoljar, N. (Eds.), 2000. Relational autonomy: Feminist perspectives on autonomy, agency and the social self. Oxford University Press.

Maitland, C., 2022. Ontological politics of intellectual disability: Where do you stand? "We'll figure it out.", University of Technology Sydney. http://hdl.handle.net/10453/162781

Mavromaras, K., Moskos, M., Mahuteau, S., Isherwood, L., Goode, A., Walton, H., et al., 2018. Evaluation of the NDIS. Final report. National Institute of Labour Studies, Flinders University. https://www.dss.gov.au/sites/default/files/documents/04_2018/ndis_evaluation_consolidated_report_april_2018.pdf

Meekosha, H., Shuttleworth, R., 2009. What's so 'critical' about critical disability studies? Australian Journal of Human Rights 15 (1), 47–75. https://doi.org/10.1080/1323238X.2009.11910861

Michalko, R., 2001. Blindness enters the classroom. Disability & Society 16 (3), 349–359. https://doi.org/10.1080/09687590120045923

Michalko, R., 2002. Estranged-familiarity. In: Corker, M., Shakespeare, T. (Eds.), Disability/postmodernity. Continuum.

Mingus, M., 2018. DIS 2018 Keynote. Massachusetts Institute of Technology. Retrieved 12 May 2022, from https://www.disabilityintersectionalitysummit.com/mia-mingus-dis-2018-keynote/

Morris, J., 1991. Pride against prejudice: A personal politics of disability. Women's Press.

Nussbaum, M., 1999. Conversing with the tradition: John Rawls and the history of ethics. Ethics 109 (2). https://doi.org/10.1086/233901

Oliver, M., 1990. The politics of disablement. Macmillan Education. https://doi.org/10.1007/978-1-349-20895-1

Paterson, K., Hughes, B., 1999. Disability studies and phenomenology: The carnal politics of everyday life. Disability & Society 14 (5), 597–610. https://doi.org/10.1080/09687599925966

Quilliam, C., Bigby, C., Douglas, J., 2018. Staff perspectives on paperwork in group homes for people with intellectual disability. Journal of Intellectual & Developmental Disability 43 (3), 264–273. https://doi.org/10.3109/13668250.2017.1378315

Rawls, J., 1971. A theory of justice. Harvard University Press.

Reeve, D., 2014. Psycho-emotional disablism and internalised oppression. In: Swain, J., French, S., Barnes, C., Thomas, C. (Eds.), Disabling barriers - Enabling Environments, 3rd ed. Sage, pp. 92–98.

Robinson, S., Graham, A., Fisher, K., Neale, K., Davy, L., Johnson, K., et al., 2020. Understanding paid support relationships: Possibilities for mutual recognition between young people with disability and their support workers. Disability & Society 36, 1423–1448. https://doi.org/10.1080/09687599.2020.1794797

Schormans, A.F., 2015. People with intellectual disabilities (visually) re-imagine care. In: Barnes, M., Branelly, T., Ward, L., Ward, N. (Eds.), Ethics of care: Critical advances in international perspective. Policy Press.

Scully, J.L., 2014. Disability and vulnerability: On bodies, dependence and power. In: Mackenzie, C., Rogers, W., Dodds, S. (Eds.), Vulnerability. New essays in ethics and feminist philosophy. Oxford University Press, pp. 204–221.

Sevenhuijsen, S., 2003. The place of care: The relevance of the feminist ethic of care for social policy. Feminist Theory 4 (2), 179–197. https://doi.org/10.1177/14647001030042006

Siebers, T., 2008. Disability theory. University of Michigan Press. https://doi.org/10.3998/mpub.309723

Simplican, S.C., 2018. Democratic care and intellectual disability: More than maintenance. Ethics and Social Welfare 12 (2), 1–16. https://doi.org/10.1080/17496535.2018.1452954

Steele, L., 2020. Submissions on redress to Royal Commission into violence, abuse, neglect and exploitation of people with disability. Australian Government. https://disability.royalcommission.gov.au

Thill, C., 2015. Listening for policy change: How the voices of disabled people shaped Australia's National Disability Insurance Scheme. Disability & Society 30 (1), 15–28. https://doi.org/10.1080/09687599.2014.987220

Titchkosky, T. 2007. *Reading and writing disability differently: The textured life of embodiment*. University of Toronto Press. https://doi.org/10.3138/9781442683839

Tronto, J., 1993. Moral boundaries: A political argument for an ethic of care. Routledge.

Tronto, J., 2015. Who cares? How to reshape a democratic politics. Cornell Selects. https://doi.org/10.7591/cornell/9781501702747.001.0001

Tronto, J., Fisher, B., 1990. Towards a feminist theory of caring. In: Abel, E.K., Nelson, M.K. (Eds.), Circles of care: Work and identity in women's lives. State University of New York Press.

Walters, S., Butterwick, S., 2017. Moves to decolonise solidarity through feminist popular education. In: Forging solidarity. Brill Sense. pp. 27–28. https://doi.org/10.1007/978-94-6300-923-2_3

Watson, N., McKie, L., Hughes, B., Hopkins, D., Gregory, S., 2004. (Inter)Dependence, needs and care: The potential for disability and feminist theorists to develop an emancipatory model. Sociology 38 (2), 331–350. https://doi.org/10.1177/0038038504040867

PART 3

The Context of Emerging Clinical Reasoning

This part of the book brings together the context of emerging clinical reasoning. Underpinned by the stance that clinical reasoning is not performed out of context, this section of the book explores the many contemporary influences and shifts that play into clinical reasoning. The nine chapters in this part discuss how clinical reasoning is being transformed and advanced by spotlighting various contexts including global population migration, policies and guidelines, evidence-based practice, liquid times, the humanities and the arts, ethics and advances in technology.

This third section celebrates clinical reasoning as being complex, interrelated and contextual by blending global, national and local contexts with social, cultural, ethical and technical ways of knowing. It decentres essentialist, monodisciplinary views and moves to a space where different perspectives come together and where broader or new perspectives are created. Bringing multivocal perspectives together can be thought of as the space in-between, or hybrid space. In a hybrid space, clinical reasoning is not performed from one perspective alone and it no longer belongs to one stakeholder alone. According to Bhabha (2004), theoretical ideas of hybridity emphasize many voices and highlight their interdependence. It rejects binary thinking and advocates for redressing the balance away from medical dominance. There is potential for co-creation of new ways of conceptualizing clinical reasoning practices.

Here are some examples from this section that invite the reader to think of clinical reasoning existing in a hybrid space. Due to migrations, populations change and with it individual clinical presentations change. Policies and guidelines no longer provide safety or assurance of good practices. The biophysical model of health is being expanded to include ideas of well-being and healing models. The place of practice is being broadened to digital online spaces through advances in telehealth.

What this hybridity crystallizes is that capabilities for emergent clinical reasoning require a foundation based on respect, human rights, ethics and social justice. By blending or hybridizing clinical reasoning, possibilities open up for culturally safe practices, deep patient histories, shared responsibilities and accurate diagnostics. This section proposes an emphasis on storytelling, subjectivities and narrative medicine, bringing humane conditions into relief with biomedical stories. Authors propose inclusive ways of knowing from biophysical evidence to narratives, using shared decision-making approaches to flatten hierarchies and reduce power imbalances.

New capabilities include critical thinking, reflexivity and an awareness of self and others. There is a greater need to uncover biases, assumptions and taken-for-granted thinking. This section indirectly touches on the very essence of the clinical professional identity because it decentres clinical dominance, privilege and expertise.

In times of rapid and relentless disruptions, clinical reasoning needs to embrace working with uncertainty, navigating ethical dilemmas based on respect. Students and clinicians need to ask the questions: what reasoning processes are pursued, who speaks, who makes the decisions, who benefits and what are the wider impacts?

REFERENCE

Bhabha, H.K., 2004. *The location of culture*. Routledge, Abingdon.

11

CHANGING DEMOGRAPHIC AND CULTURAL DIMENSIONS OF POPULATIONS
Implications for Healthcare and Decision Making

JASON A. WASSERMAN ■ STEPHEN LOFTUS

CHAPTER AIMS

The aims of this chapter are:

- to articulate how shifts in the composition and character of populations promote greater complexity in diagnosis and treatment
- to elaborate how greater complexity in the diagnostic and treatment processes challenges traditional forms of clinical reasoning
- to use the examples of ageing and increasing race/ethnic diversity to underscore the ways that demographic shifts confound traditional clinical reasoning
- to consider the characteristics that need to attend clinical reasoning to navigate these new complexities, including the incorporation of reflexive logics and the recognition of intersubjective processes.

INTRODUCTION

Clinical reasoning is not practised in a vacuum. Rather, it takes place against the backdrop of any number of different social contexts. One of these contexts is the composition and characteristics of different populations of patients and the dramatic shifts these can sometimes undergo. Even though a healthcare professional is usually dealing at any given time only with one patient, the influence of population demographics on clinical reasoning is often overlooked. In this chapter, we draw attention to the importance of understanding demographics and their profound influences on clinical reasoning.

Social changes, including shifts in the composition and character of populations, affect clinical reasoning through a variety of mechanisms. Ways of thinking about health are themselves nested in cultural beliefs, attitudes and ways of knowing. This is true not just of the patient population but also of the professionals who provide healthcare. A simple example is the traditional (and wrong) belief that both infants and older persons do not feel as much pain as the rest of the population (Buchbinder, 2015; Maxwell et al., 2019; Sierra and Kohanski, 2016). This myth probably emerged because these age groups could not express pain easily, yet it took root in ways that dramatically affected clinical reasoning. For example, those who believed this myth were unlikely to take the need for pain management sufficiently into consideration for these patients.

Such examples underscore that clinical reasoning is not simply something the healthcare professional does in isolation. Instead, clinical reasoning occurs within a dialogical relationship between the healthcare professional and the patient (at the individual level) – a relationship that is, in turn, nested in a social structural arrangement, including the social contract between medicine and society. In this way, the clinical relationship is bidirectional, sometimes called intersubjective. Of course, the scientific basis of healthcare remains highly influential, but it is important to remember that social norms, beliefs, behaviours and attitudes of social groups place demands on healthcare that affect how that science is translated into practice. For example, different beliefs and values about contraception and abortion may profoundly affect the clinical reasoning surrounding fertility and family planning. The controversies in this example are not dependent on scientific facts but on the values of all those involved and, moreover, the comingling of their perspectives as they interact in a clinical dialogue. Healthcare and clinical reasoning, therefore, are not value-free activities. The personal and professional values of the healthcare provider and the values of the patient, and significant others, play important roles. Moreover, the values that patients and providers hold are partly individual but are also shaped by the wider society and especially the social groups with which they identify. Our focus in this chapter concerns the way in which many of these wider social groups have recently experienced dramatic change.

We now live in an increasingly globalized world, where the pluralism of cultural norms and attitudes can affect clinical reasoning and healthcare decision making. The coming together of diverse populations with varied beliefs about the body, disease, expectations of health and normative practices places demands on the exercise of clinical reasoning. Everywhere, we encounter greater social complexity than in the past and, like other areas of social life, clinical reasoning must shift accordingly. In what follows, we first briefly describe key social changes that affect clinical practice, particularly through introduction of those new complexities. We also underscore the challenges of adapting how healthcare professionals think about disease and their roles in the diagnosis and treatment process with diversifying populations. We conclude with some theorizing about the future direction of these trends.

CHANGING POPULATIONS

Providing a comprehensive description of demographic shifts in populations in various countries around the world is beyond the scope of this chapter. Instead, we focus on a few key demographic shifts that highlight how increased complexity in disease epidemiology dramatically affects clinical reasoning (something elaborated later). Among many important demographic shifts, we find that a particularly instructive examination concerns how the changing age structure and the cultural diversification that attend globalization and mass migration are significantly disruptive to traditional forms of clinical reasoning.

Industrialized countries around the world have, for over a century or more, witnessed marked increases in the life expectancy of their populations. Despite recent data suggesting a small decline in the United States from 78.9 years in 2014 to 78.8 years in 2015 (Xu et al., 2016), as well as the effects of the COVID-19 pandemic, long-standing trends towards greater longevity represent greater complexity for healthcare and society at large.

Although we usually think of ageing as something experienced by individuals, aggregate increases in longevity can be thought of as the ageing of society. As people live longer, the average age of a population increases, meaning that older people make up a greater percentage of the population. This is particularly important because social systems, including healthcare, often tier social support in a way that assumes healthy, working persons will care for both the young and old. At its simplest, this means that primary caregivers within family units are likely to be caring for more older family members than they did in the past. At the societal level, social service programmes are funded by contributions from those in the workforce to support those who are not. As populations age, the foundations of this system of support will be more heavily stressed, a phenomenon that is already occurring in developed countries around the world and projected to increase dramatically into the future.

Data from the European Commission in the European Union (EU) show striking degrees of population ageing (EU, 2015). Between 2005 and 2015, the percentage of the EU population 65 years of age and older increased by 2.3% (EuroStat, 2016). Projections find the life expectancy for men increasing from 77.6 years in 2013 to a projection of 84 years by 2060. Similarly, women in the EU lived an average of 83.1 years in 2013 but are projected to live an average of 89.1 years by 2060. Importantly, this means that the relative proportion of workers will decline by nearly 10% in light of dramatic increases in the population older than 65 years of age. In fact, individuals 65 to 79 years of age made up 13.3% of the EU population in 2013 but are projected to make up 16.6% by 2060. More striking still, individuals older than 80 years of age made up only 5.1% of the population in 2013 but are projected to make up 11.8% of the population by 2060. This is associated with significant costs, with the percentage of GDP represented by healthcare increasing from 6.9% to 7.8% and long-term care from 1.6% to 2.7%. Although these may seem like comparatively small increases, the problem represented by an ageing population is exacerbated by the declining number of workers relative to pensioners, which was 4:1 in 2013 but is projected to be 2:1 in 2060. This means that far fewer workers will support these costlier populations in the not-so-distant future.

Trends from Australia and the United States parallel those of the EU. The percentage of Australians 65 years of age and older is expected to increase from 13% to 25% by 2042, representing an additional 4 million individuals in that age group (Commonwealth of Australia, 2004). Although in 2002 there were over 5 workers for every person older than 65 years of age in Australia, just as in the EU, by 2042 this number will decline to 2.5. In the United States, the percentage of the population 65 years of age and older increased

from about 8% in 1950 to about 14% in 2013 (Martin et al., 2015). As mirrored in other Western nations, the US birth rate in the two decades after the Second World War was significantly elevated compared with the preceding decades and those that followed. Members of this baby boomer cohort are currently entering retirement, representing a population bubble that will have to be supported by a relatively small number of people in the workforce.

One clinical challenge in ageing societies concerns the complexity of geriatric health. Older persons frequently have several chronic health conditions, each with its own treatment that carries potential for adverse interactions. Ageing populations pose challenges for healthcare professionals on an individual level but also at the societal level where questions about funding, capitation and rationing emerge. However, ageing is not the only demographic challenge to healthcare and clinical reasoning.

Increasing cultural diversity also presents new forms of complexity that challenge clinical care. This occurs not only as a result of shifting internal demographics of different nations but also because of the interlinked nature of a global society. Although there are many different, often value-laden, definitions of globalization, here we are primarily concerned with it as the increasingly dynamic and rapid flow of populations and their characteristics (e.g. values, beliefs and customs) across national borders. New technologies, along with increasingly interwoven economic systems, have promoted greater laxity in national boundaries and a corresponding increase in cultural diversity within countries that, historically, were more culturally homogenous. For example, 20 EU countries experienced increases in the percentage of foreign-born population between 2009 and 2015; 13 of those saw increases of more than 10% in that period. Australia also witnessed a marked increase in net overseas migration (Australian Bureau of Statistics, 2016). In the United States, increasing cultural diversity is being driven by increases in the populations of minority groups and migration patterns, particularly of immigrating Hispanic populations. Pol and Thomas (2013, p. 87) write that 'Current figures reveal an America that is becoming less "white", while African American, Asian American and American Indian/Alaskan Native populations are becoming proportionately larger'.

The increasing diversity of cultural groups in most developed countries holds significance for clinical reasoning that must match a patient's presentation of symptoms to a diagnosis and a treatment plan. The diagnosis and treatment plan need to fit with the patient's values, because the patient (and often their family) must agree to comply with any treatment. Each stage of this process can be significantly affected by the cultural and social norms of the patient.

CHANGING POPULATIONS AND CLINICAL REASONING

The foundations of clinical reasoning in the Western world are grounded in modernist forms of rationality tracing back to Cartesian thought. This means that ideas such as the logic of cause and effect are largely taken for granted. It is also often assumed that the body is a biological machine where disease is a technical problem to be solved. Moreover, there is an implicit assumption that the 'disease problem' can always be solved if we have sufficient scientific data and the technological capacity to intervene. In this model, healthcare professionals are also assumed to be technicians who can act on the body and solve those problems (Scott, 2013). However, the demographic changes we are currently witnessing challenge this worldview.

One reason for this concerns the growing incidence of chronic diseases. Acute conditions may fit well in a model that conceptualizes disease as a biophysical technical problem to be fixed once and for all. But with chronic conditions, problems often cannot be solved but instead must be managed over long periods of time. Well-known examples involve chronic pain and diabetes. Over time, chronic disease management often has to be adjusted and may become more complex. Individuals with diabetes can slowly deteriorate over the years, even with the best care. Patients with chronic pain can acquire other health problems that may complicate palliative care. In these situations, patients need to have significant input into the clinical reasoning of the physician, not just provide information as part of the history-taking process. Even the many well-intentioned attempts at patient-centred care often utilize strategies of relationship building simply for the purpose of getting better diagnostic information from patients. There

is a need to go beyond these approaches that can be seen as paternalistic and condescending. Patients, especially those with chronic conditions, need to be involved in the decisions made about their care. Clinical relationships need to be seen more as true partnerships and 'shared decision making' needs to involve more than simply the clinician leading the patient towards agreement. Instead, the clinical encounter should centre on a robust dialogue that is open, at least at the outset, to a pluralistic set of options, and then collaboratively navigates towards the options that fit best with the patient's beliefs, values and preferences. As the social landscape grows increasingly diverse, the goals of the clinical encounter will probably need to entertain a greater range of possibilities which may deviate significantly from the historical norms of Western medical practice.

In an age where epidemiological and demographic complexity are increasing, there is a need to have a good understanding of this complexity and how it affects clinical reasoning. We next take a closer look at this issue of complexity and how it manifests in both ageing and increasingly diverse populations.

Epidemiological Complexity, Ageing and Clinical Reasoning

In the later decades of the 20th century, developed nations experienced an epidemiological shift in which chronic illnesses surpassed acute illnesses as the most significant mortality threats (Hinote and Wasserman, 2020; Omran, 1971). As a class of ailments, acute conditions can be successfully treated using a relatively simple causal model. Infectious disease, for example, can be understood in terms of an agent (microbe or virus) infecting a host (a person or, more specifically, an organ, tissue, blood, etc.). The miracles of modern medicine developed around disrupting the causal pathways within that paradigm, either by eliminating the pathogen from the host (antisepsis) or by steeling the host against the pathogen to prevent infection (vaccination). As notions of public health took a more significant role throughout the 20th century, the role of environment was incrementally added to create the 'epidemiological triad', but it remained conceptualized in a relatively limited way, focussing primarily on the contexts of contagion (Dubos, 1965). Importantly, this model becomes insufficient for complex chronic diseases (at least without significant reformulation of what is traditionally meant by 'environment').

Chronic diseases represent a paradigm shift in complexity in at least two ways. The first is ontological; that is, chronic illnesses are paradigmatically different kinds of diseases compared with acute illnesses. Chronic diseases are different kinds of entities and the clinical reasoning required to address them needs to be different. Although infectious diseases typically involve agents that are foreign to and distinct from the human body, most chronic illnesses involve not the presence of something foreign but elevated or depleted levels of things endemic to the human body (e.g. cholesterol or blood sugar that is too high). The targets of treatment for chronic illnesses are therefore less discrete and are natural and necessary to the body itself. Second, chronic illnesses emerge not from acute moments of contagion but frequently from thousands of decisions across a person's life course, each of which is nested within different social contexts (e.g. culture, class, community, neighbourhood). Well-known examples of such decisions include smoking, alcohol use, lack of exercise and diets high in fat and sugar. These decisions are not always freely made. For example, low-income families may not have access to affordable or fresh food and a poor diet may be the only realistic option. Thus values, beliefs, purchasing power, proximity to healthy or unhealthy opportunities and other social factors are fundamental causes of disease that can no longer be excised from our thinking about disease management (Link and Phelan, 1995).

Put another way, rather than intervening in a single causal pathway (i.e. between agent and host), the multifactorial nature of chronic illness necessitates drawing together understandings of physiology and biochemistry on the one hand and sociological and psychological insights on the other. Insofar as traditional forms of clinical reasoning were able to disregard much of that information, clinical reasoning now needs to be just as multifactorial and wide ranging as the causes of disease in the contemporary epidemiological landscape.

As populations age, the proportion of chronic illnesses increases. In one US study, for example, nearly 87.6% of adults 65 years of age and older had at least one chronic condition and 63.7% had two or more (Boersma et al., 2020). The successes of modern healthcare have presented new complexities that cannot be met with an old logic and the demand on healthcare now concerns its attentiveness to a larger case narrative inclusive of social and psychological features of a patient's illness experience.

The increasing focus on patient-centred care over the last several decades might be read as an implicit recognition of the salience of this growing complexity. However, a fully delineated corresponding form of clinical reasoning has yet to take root in any widespread way. Still, efforts at elaborating and promoting narrative medicine (Charon et al., 2017; Loftus and Greenhalgh, 2010) and schemas for inductive logics inclusive of the humanistic aspects of disease today (Wasserman, 2014) suggest that attending to new forms of illness complexity and their attendant social and humanistic elements is entirely possible. Patient narratives can be read for insights into aspects of illness complexity. These include, for example, patient values or the challenges posed by contexts in which they get sick, experience illness and carry out treatment, such as their families and neighbourhoods. Utilizing such information, not just to make the patient feel more 'accompanied' by the physician but rather by fully integrating different kinds of complex information into the diagnostic and treatment processes, will be a key task for clinical practice over the coming decades. However, the nature of disease in ageing populations and growing diversity suggest doing so is necessary.

In the chronic illness era, seeking a single biomedical diagnosis on the basis of pathophysiological signs and symptoms alone is frequently no longer sufficient. For some years now, there have been calls to replace the biomedical model of clinical reasoning with a biopsychosocial model that takes social and psychological factors into account (Engel, 1977). However, even the biopsychosocial model has been critiqued as not going far enough. Morris (1998) has called for a biocultural model of healthcare that puts more emphasis on sociocultural factors. We would argue that this biocultural model can be part of a more relationship-centred approach to clinical reasoning that allows insights about the nature of disease and the direction of treatment to be genuinely co-created by physician and patient, but this requires the healthcare professional to abandon some simplistic assumptions about definitions of disease and their role as a paternalistic practitioner. Other calls to amend the biopsychosocial model point to a similar impulse about clinical care, e.g. biopsychosocial-spiritual and the biopsychosocial-existential.

Only from a basis of greater epistemological freedom – where clinicians are free to rethink traditional assumptions of clinical science to better collaborate with their patients' ways of thinking – can healthcare professionals and patients co-create an understanding of illness truly grounded in patients' experiences and values and develop a treatment plan best fitting to each patient's life. This is especially true among ageing populations where value-driven decisions related to cost and quality of life may call for a fundamental reconsideration of a traditionally unquestioned drive to treat all 'problems' (see Case Study 11.1).

REFLECTION POINT

- For Case Study 11.1, articulate the various ways that this case entails different aspects of complexity (in terms of how the patient became ill, the providers who must treat her illnesses, the contexts in which she faces those illnesses and treatments, the personal values she might bring to the experience, how her age might affect her treatment goals and/or those of her providers and so on).
- What challenges does each of these complexities pose for clinical reasoning?

The increasingly complex and pluralistic world in which practitioners meet patients today would seem to include new more reflexive forms of clinical reasoning. By 'reflexive', we mean forms of clinical reasoning that are more dialogical and intersubjective.

Reflexivity in clinical reasoning gives permission to go beyond thinking only with simplistic cause-and-effect mechanisms, for example, by recognizing that cause and effect can be linked together in multifaceted ways in complex relationships that persist over time. This is the reality of chronic disease where complex long-term relationships need to be maintained and developed over months or years (Tasker et al., 2017). For example, in Case Study 11.1, a reflexive reconsideration of what is the best course of treatment calls us to ask whether we ought to treat the problem at all, interrogating the underlying values and goals of treatment. Building on this idea, it could even be argued that we need a form of clinical reasoning that thinks about the nature of clinical reasoning itself at the outset of each patient encounter, rather than carrying a universalized clinical logic into each encounter.

Reflexive thinking brings social and psychological features of a patient's life into consideration but also considers other important issues. The increasing complexity of healthcare that comes with an ageing population stresses health systems such that values-based decisions become more important, which also can affect clinical reasoning. Healthcare resources are finite and consideration of who gets them and who does not stretches the boundaries of the single case narrative to include the larger social context. In the early 1970s, there was both a cultural upswing in individualism and rapid scientific advances that promoted new capacities for extending life. For example, once medical science could keep someone alive on a ventilator and/or feeding tube, new questions emerged about whether it should do so and under what conditions. Similarly, as the complex

---

CASE STUDY 11.1

Mattie is an 83-year-old woman with a history of chronic obstructive pulmonary disease (COPD) and diabetes. Because of her diabetes, she has a very difficult time healing when she is scraped or cut and has been prone to infection of even minor skin contusions. She has discussed her end-of-life wishes with her primary care physician and signed a do-not-resuscitate order. On a routine visit to her pulmonologist, she notes that she's begun having palpitations in her heart. She's referred to a cardiologist, who recommends a catheter ablation, which involves the insertion of catheter wires into the groin or neck that are sent to the heart and which intentionally destroy the tissue causing the palpitations. The cardiologist tells Mattie and her son Mitch that the procedure is routine. Mitch insists that she needs to consent to the procedure, but Mattie is hesitant. She consults with her primary care provider.

illnesses of ageing populations present resource challenges at the clinical, institutional and national levels, decisions about what to treat, when to treat and how to treat inevitably must account not only for the values of the patient but also the institution and the broader society in which they are made. Put another way, modernist clinical reasoning traditionally was underpinned by an assumption that if an intervention could be performed, it should be performed. Today, that assumption and others must be interrogated with a new more complex form of reflexive clinical reasoning.

Cultural Complexity, Race/Ethnic Diversification and Clinical Reasoning

The traditional paradigm of clinical reasoning – a Cartesian process of diagnosis using a differential logic applied to pathophysiological symptoms (Scott, 2013) – inherently discourages reflexivity, particularly in regard to value-laden assumptions of healthcare. Perhaps most generally, there is an implicit assumption that disease should always be treated (as underscored in Case Study 11.1). However, the success of modern medicine and the tacit crises that have emerged from these successes only amplify the problems associated with the value-laden nature of clinical science. Increasingly, in the era of chronic illness and long-term care, science may supply the information and the technology needed to intervene, but sometimes it is inappropriate to do so. With respect to these issues, our clinical reasoning needs to make use of perspectives from disciplines such as philosophy, anthropology, sociology and psychology. Shifting cultural demographics further complicate such value questions because cultural experiences shape the value orientations of different groups in ways that might not align with the traditional practices of modern healthcare. A moving account of how different value systems can collide in healthcare is the tragic story of a child with epilepsy from southeast Asia being raised in an immigrant family in the United States (Fadiman, 2012).

This situation is further complicated by the mass movement of people between countries as immigrants and refugees. In the first few months of 2022, for instance, the number of forcibly displaced persons worldwide reached a record high of more than 100 million. Healthcare professionals may increasingly have to cope with not only enculturated ways of thinking about health and the body, but also a variety of physical and psychological traumas associated with migration as well as what may seem to them like exotic physiological conditions they may have not previously encountered (see Case Study 11.2).

REFLECTION POINT

- For Case Study 11.2, articulate the various ways that these cases entail different aspects of complexity (in terms of how the patients became ill, the providers who must treat these illnesses, the cultural values that both patient and provider bring to the encounter, the contexts in which the patient faces those illnesses and treatments, the cultural lens through which each patient might view and experience illness, the personal and cultural values each might bring to the experience and so on).
- What challenges does each of those complexities pose for clinical reasoning?

Cultural diversity forces reconsideration of commonly held ethical practices, and thus of clinical decisions, in a number of ways. First, Western orientations towards clinical ethics and medical decision making focus squarely, and often exclusively, on the individual patient. Take, for example, the notion of truth-telling, which has, since the 1970s, been a staple of ethical practice in most Western societies. It is taken for granted that patients must be autonomous and fully informed to exercise that autonomy. However, in other countries, including many Eastern and Middle Eastern cultures (e.g. China and Japan), the orientation towards collectivities making decisions, especially in terms of the family, undercuts the individualism of Western ethics (Zahedi, 2011). As healthcare professionals treat patients from increasingly diverse backgrounds, they may need to be more reflexive about the assumptions built into their communication and their ethical decision making.

Whether to disclose an illness, who serves as the primary communicator and decision maker (the patient or a family member), the terms used in the discussion – all of these affect how the relationship between the patient and the healthcare professional proceeds. These sociocultural considerations are

CASE STUDY 11.2

An Australian medical student (George) in his final year was doing an elective study in the emergency department of a hospital in a major American city with a large immigrant population from many parts of the world. The demographic mixture brought a number of challenges that stretched his clinical reasoning ability.

'I had a gentleman that I saw in the emergency department in the United States who came in with seizures and lots of neuro signs. So I went through the history, and he's a young guy, would've been about 18 and so I was thinking epilepsy, brain tumour. Ran through everything quite well, obviously ordered a CT scan and it came back cysticercosis … now I would never have thought of that diagnosis in a million years. I'd never heard of it, but I was able to work through the process and do the appropriate investigations' (Loftus, 2006, p. 201).

Cysticercosis is an infection by *Taenia solium*, the pork tapeworm, acquired by eating raw or undercooked pork containing the larval form of the worm. The larvae can migrate to the brain and cause epilepsy. George's patient was an immigrant from Mexico where he had presumably contracted the disease.

George also described a patient with koro. 'He [the patient] was standing in the doorway of the room, clutching himself. The registrar thought he had to go to the toilet. So he indicated the toilet and he [the patient] said "No, no", and he's pointing and indicating, and we have no idea what's going on, absolutely no idea, and eventually got a Laotian interpreter and from there it became quite obvious. He said "It's going to crawl back up inside me and I'm gonna die". No matter what clinical reasoning skills that I had there I don't think I would've been prepared for it.' (Loftus, 2006 p. 208).

Koro is described in South East Asia, although cases have been reported in Africa. It is the morbid fear that one's genitals are retracting into one's body and will bring about a rapid death when they do so. Sufferers have been known to go to extreme lengths to prevent what they see as their imminent demise, such as impaling the offending member or cutting it off. George's patient was, apparently, seriously considering these options.

(Note: Koro should not be confused with kuru. Kuru is a neurodegenerative disorder, a form of Creutzfeldt-Jakob disease, caused by infection by a prion. It was described in parts of Papua New Guinea in regions where cannibalism was practised. It was contracted by eating the brains of one's close relatives as part of a funerary practice.)

---

relatively new challenges in the process of clinical reasoning, and they become even more pressing as the race/ethnic and cultural composition of various societies becomes more diverse. Other kinds of complexity regarding values decisions may take on greater import as race/ethnic and cultural diversity increases. The diagnoses and prognoses made by healthcare professionals are, at least ideally, based on scientific evidence and a scientific logic. But other orientations may reject altogether the validity of the scientific perspective or define core understandings of things such as hope and futility in radically different ways. For example, cultural or religious orientations towards life may reject definitions of futility based on neurological activity, favouring the idea that the soul resides in the body as long as the heart is still beating. If this is the case, questions about discontinuing artificial nutrition and hydration in a neurologically devastated or even brain-dead patient must contend not only with questions about physiological futility but also broader notions about the meaning of life. It may no longer be sufficient, at least from a functional perspective, to anchor clinical reasoning solely around pathophysiological data and evidence-based science to the exclusion of the social and religious values that patients and their families bring to bear. Deciding what kinds of interventions are futile can be fraught with complexity on pathophysiological grounds alone, but considering different orientations towards the meaning of life makes it all the more complex. There are yet other challenges facing clinical reasoning in this changing world.

CLINICAL REASONING IN A POSTINDUSTRIAL WORLD

In the preceding section, we discussed the challenges to clinical reasoning faced at the nexus of science and values in a postindustrial and globalizing world, characterized by greater complexity not only with respect to social, cultural and religious pluralism, but in terms of the causal profile of illness itself. This has given rise to efforts to change the way medicine and healthcare are practised. There is a general push towards a warmer and more engaged patient-centred care that can offset or conflict with the cold, calculating objectivity of modern science. In recent decades, different strategies designed to 'meet the patient where they are' have become popular, but there has been little thought given to how clinical reasoning fits this approach. This is particularly true where clinical reasoning is traditionally seen as a rather deductive process involving the straightforward computation of medical facts. It can be argued that demographic shifts and their attendant complexities now require healthcare professionals to function as scientists in what might be called a post-truth environment. That is, healthcare professionals must not only attend to the medical evidence in a classic process of diagnosis and prognosis, but at the same time they must weave all this together with a socially sensitive and individualized understanding of who the patient is and how they see the world.

This more complex view of clinical reasoning is not new; it has simply been ignored nearly altogether. The pioneers of evidence-based medicine recognized this when they stated that good decision making required the integration of not only the best available evidence and the expertise of the professional but also the views, values and desires of the patient (Sackett et al., 1996). Many health professions have paid attention only to gathering the best available evidence and have ignored the other two components. This is probably a result of the grounding of the health professions in the biomedical sciences. Healthcare professionals are comfortable discussing and working with the best scientific evidence, but many are poorly equipped to talk about personal expertise and the values of patients. However, the medical humanities and social sciences do have vocabularies that can enable healthcare professionals to engage these neglected components of clinical reasoning. The huge demographic and social changes we now face mean that clinical reasoning will require social science and humanities discourses to adequately address not only the social and emotional aspects of patient care but also its diagnostic and treatment functions. This clearly provides a warrant for more significant inclusion of the social sciences and humanities, something we are beginning to witness in evolving medical, nursing and allied health curricula, and on gateway examinations into these programmes (e.g. the MCAT in the United States).

Clinical reasoning will have to become more reflexive. It will no longer be sufficient to apply the modernist form of deductive logic to medical problems. The case studies in this chapter underscore how the challenge to our clinical reasoning is growing. In this environment of complexity, clinical reasoning becomes a negotiation, not just about what to do, where the healthcare professional tries to get the patient closest to what is in their own 'best interest', but where there are no longer a priori criteria for determining what that best interest might be. Instead, healthcare professionals in a postindustrial world must not only think about the relationship of symptoms to diagnosis but must also reflect on their own thinking about these things. This will require an unprecedented form of openness about the nature of healthcare, its goals and our roles as healthcare professionals (e.g. curing versus helping people die; helping the patient versus keeping the family whole).

CONCLUSION

In this chapter, we have chosen to focus on two demographic shifts common to most Western nations that underscore the core problem of changing demographics vis-à-vis clinical reasoning. The ageing of the population and increasing cultural diversity represent growing complexity at both the medical and sociological levels. Modern clinical reasoning emerged to match a set of observable pathophysiological factors to an underlying disease process, but it is poorly equipped to manage the complexity of multiple morbidities and pluralistic value systems. Reshaping it to match the challenges of postindustrial complexity will represent an enormous change in how healthcare professionals think.

SUMMARY

In this chapter, we have outlined:

- how shifts in the composition and character of populations amplify the complexity of disease and its treatment, which in turn affects clinical reasoning
- how the ageing of populations brings about new complexities with respect to comorbid disease processes that are difficult to navigate within clinical medicine, which has high degrees of specialization
- how mass migration and resulting cultural diversity challenge may not only present clinicians with unfamiliar diseases but also bring the relevance of values and beliefs in the diagnosis and treatment processes into sharp relief
- how the new terrain of disease complexity that results from demographic shifts calls for new more reflexive and intersubjective forms of clinical reasoning.

REFLECTION POINT

- Why are chronic diseases such a challenge for clinical reasoning?
- Consider not only how traditional forms of clinical reasoning are mismatched to the complexity of contemporary disease but also how the increased specialization of clinical medicine confounds treatments of comorbid diseases and so on.
- Consider how other demographic shifts might affect clinical reasoning (e.g. the feminization of medicine, rising social inequality in some countries).

REFERENCES

Australian Bureau of Statistics. (2016). Australia today. http://www. abs.gov.au/ausstats/abs@.nsf/mf/2024.0

Boersma, P., Black, L.I., Ward, B.W., 2020. Prevalence of multiple chronic conditions among US adults, 2018. Prev Chronic Dis 17, 200130. http://doi.org/10.5888/pcd17.200130external icon

Buchbinder, M., 2015. All in your head: Making sense of pediatric pain. University of California Press.

Charon, R., DasGupta, S., Hermann, N., Irvine, C., Marcus, E.R., Colsn, E.R., et al., 2017. The principles and practice of narrative medicine. Oxford University Press.

Commonwealth of Australia. (2004). Australia's demographic challenges. http://demographics.treasury.gov.au/content/discussion.asp

Dubos, R., 1965. Man adapting. Yale University Press.

Engel, G., 1977. The need for a new medical model: A challenge for biomedicine. Science 196, 129–136. https://doi.org/10.1126/science.847460

European Union, 2015. The 2015 aging report: Projected demographic changes in the European Union. http://ec.europa.eu/economy_finance/graphs/2015-05-12_ageing_report_en.htm

EuroStat, 2016. Population age structure by major age groups: 2005 and 2015 (% of the total population). http://ec.europa.eu/eurostat/statistics-explained/index.php/File:Population_age_structure_by_major_age_groups,_2005_and_2015_(%25_of_the_total_population)_YB16.png

Fadiman, A., 2012. The spirit catches you and you fall down: A Hmong child, her American doctors, and the collision of two cultures. Farrar, Strauss and Giroux.

Hinote, B., Wasserman, J., 2020. Social and behavioral *science for health professionals*, 2nd ed. Rowman & Littlefield.

Link, B., Phelan, J., 1995. Social conditions as fundamental causes of disease. J. Health Soc. Behav, 35 (extra issue), 80–94. https://doi.org/10.1177/0022146510383498

Loftus, S., 2006. Language in clinical reasoning. [Doctoral dissertation, The University of Sydney]. http://hdl.handle.net/2123/1165

Loftus, S., Greenhalgh, T., 2010. Towards a narrative mode of practice. In: Higgs, J., Fish, D., Goulter, I. (Eds.), Education for future practice. Sense, pp. 85–94.

Martin, J.A., Hamilton, B.E., Osterman, M.J.K., et al., 2015. Births: Final data for 2013. National Vital Statistics Reports, 64. National Center for Health Statistics. http://www.cdc.gov/nchs/data/nvsr/nvsr64/nvsr64_01.pdf

Maxwell, L.G., Fraga, M.V., Malavolta, C.P., 2019. Assessment of pain in the newborn: An update. Clinics in Perinatology 46, 693–707. https://doi.org/10.1016/j.clp.2019.08.005

Morris, D., 1998. Illness and culture in the postmodern age. University of California Press.

Omran, A.R., 1971. The epidemiologic transition: A theory of the epidemiology of population change. Milbank Mem. Fund. 49 (4), 509–538. PMID: 5155251

Pol, L., Thomas, R., 2013. The demography of health and healthcare, 3rd ed. Springer.

Sackett, D., Richardson, S., Rosenberg, W. (Eds.), 1996. Evidence- based medicine: How to practice and teach EBM. Churchill Livingstone.

Scott, J., 2013. Complexities in the consultation. In: Strumberg, J., Martin, C. (Eds.), Handbook of systems and complexity in health. Springer, pp. 257–278.

Sierra, F., Kohanski, R. (Eds.), 2016. Advances in Geroscience. Springer International Publishing.

Tasker, D., Higgs, J., Loftus, S. (Eds.), 2017. Community-based healthcare: The search for mindful dialogues. Sense.

Wasserman, J., 2014. On art and science: An epistemic framework for integrating social science and clinical medicine. J. Med. Philos. 39, 279–303. https://doi.org/10.1093/jmp/jhu015

Xu, J., Murphy, S., Kochanek, K., Arias, E., 2016. Mortality in the United States: 2015, NCHS data brief no. 267. Centers for Disease Control and Prevention.

Zahedi, F., 2011. The challenge of truth telling across cultures: A case study. J. Med. Ethics Hist. Med 4, 11. PMID: 23908753; PMCID: PMC3713926.

12

MULTIPLE CONTEXTS OF HEALTHCARE

MOHAMMAD S. Y. ZUBAIRI ■ MARIA MYLOPOULOS ■ MARIA A. MARTIMIANAKIS

CHAPTER OUTLINE

CHAPTER AIMS

The aims of this chapter are:

- to discuss the effect of neo-liberal policies and globalization on education and practice in the health professions
- to identify how a changing context influences socialization, professional identity development and the application of expertise
- to introduce critical reflexivity as a mechanism to think beyond the clinical encounter.

INTRODUCTION

This section of the book deals with the changing context of clinical practice and clinical reasoning. In this chapter, we use a case exemplar to explore several key movements and trends emerging from contemporary neo-liberal policies and globalization more broadly. We further explore the effect of these trends on knowledge and reasoning, practice models and expectations of health professions education. Other chapters will address other influences, including the effect of the information evolutions, and changes in clients' expectations and input to decision making.

REFLECTION POINT

In Case Study 12.1, there are actual and perceived differences between the parents and the paediatrician that can be assumed to affect their interaction.
- What about situations in which differences between patient/families and carers are not clearly evident?
- Is the verbatim message subject to influences by any sociocultural interpretation that may take place in the conversations between patient and interpreter?

The discourse of neo-liberalism promotes ideas and practices that prioritize and value free markets. It is often linked to globalization and the amplification of the movement of services, ideas and people across borders (Spring, 2008). This variably leads to diversification and standardization across many domains including health and education. With the increased

CASE STUDY 12.1

A Canadian-trained paediatrician, who identifies as a White Anglo-Saxon man, is working with a junior resident who completed her medical school in Ethiopia. He wants to discuss a case he has encountered. He tells the resident about a 4-year-old boy who just started school and whose family is originally from Bangladesh. They migrated to Canada a little over 3 years ago just before the COVID-19 pandemic. The boy's father is an engineer, his mother stays at home and his primary language exposure in the household up until the start of school was Bengali. The boy has slowly picked up some single words in English, but the teachers are concerned about language delay even as he interacts with other Bengali-speaking children in the classroom. His parents speak enough English for the paediatrician to communicate with them, but he finds that the typical strategies he might use (i.e. humour or talking about popular culture) don't work either with the parents or the child. As a result, developing rapport has been difficult. He has worked with visibly and linguistically Bangladeshi families before and tells the resident that he is trying to approach the case the same way as with others.

The paediatrician goes on to tell the resident that he struggles with explaining particular developmental diagnoses, such as autism or global developmental delay, when a language barrier is present and when cultural differences are perceived. Although this family speaks English, he wonders about the use of an interpreter particularly when time comes to give feedback to the family. He tells the resident 'If I have an interpreter, at least I know the verbatim message is getting across, and I am being culturally sensitive'.

---

mobility of people, numerous healthcare professionals are now studying and/or practising beyond the physical borders of their individual nation states. These trends have spurred the sharing of curricula and educational practices, with the goal of attaining greater standardization in the quality of training of healthcare professionals and the delivery of health services (Timmermans and Almeling, 2009). One such standard of care is interprofessionalism, perceived to improve the integration of expertise from across professions at the point of care. Globalization has spurred the uptake of this approach, witnessed in the proliferation of interprofessional, patient-centred and person-centred care models across the world calling for stronger collaborative interactions with patients (Haddara and Lingard, 2013; Pluut, 2016).

Through such movement of people, practices and ideas, across the world there are healthcare professionals who have trained outside the context in which they practice, commonly referred to as internationally educated health professionals (IEHPs). Despite assumptions that healthcare training is portable, the lived experience of IEHPs exposes serious challenges in integrating a diversely trained set of health professionals into new work contexts and requires further

attention (Paul et al., 2017). This is highlighted in the initial interactions between the resident trainee in Case Study 12.1 and the paediatrician.

Although discourses of globalization perpetuate the notion that the training of healthcare professionals and the object of medical practice can be standardized (Schwarz and Wojtczak, 2002; Timmermans and Epstein, 2010), the realities of being trained elsewhere make visible how knowledge as a commodity underpins contemporary healthcare educational practices. For instance, IEHPs experience exhaustive licensure requirements in contrast to those who have trained locally. Such requirements more often than not end up leaving them outside the workforce (Paul et al., 2017; Yen et al., 2016). In many jurisdictions within the global north, the COVID-19 pandemic expedited the credentialing of IEHPs in response to emergent needs, bringing into focus many barriers (Bell and Katz, 2021). Additionally, the perceived differences in how IEHPs orient to the delivery of care often evoke client safety concerns and added surveillance. Thus, IEHPs who do make it into the workforce often experience marginalization and a devaluing of their expertise (Mickleborough and Martimianakis, 2021).

Relatedly, the phenomenon of medical tourism, spurred by ideas of standardization of healthcare delivery, along with broader immigration and refugee trends, affects patient demographics across the world. As a result, healthcare professionals are frequently exposed to patients and colleagues with cultures, values, histories and beliefs related to health and illness that are different from their own (McKimm and McLean, 2011; Perfetto and Dholakia, 2010; Seeleman et al., 2009; World Health Organization, 2010). Healthcare professional educators are starting to report the challenges of applying curricula, pedagogies and educational tools across different healthcare contexts (Ho et al., 2011, 2012; Giuliani et al., 2021), drawing attention to how these differences affect how we operationalize 'competence' as a construct, particularly in relation to clinical reasoning (Hodges and Lingard, 2012).

SHIFTING CONTEXTS AND IDENTITIES

Although the tensions discussed earlier are amplified by growing resource constraints and efficiency mandates, globalization has conceptually and materially blurred our understanding of what constitutes context (the social, political, cultural circumstances that surround an event). This has implications for how we think about learning, expertise and clinical reasoning. Whether homogeneity or heterogeneity is the outcome, the interconnected movement of ideas and people across borders challenges contemporary healthcare professional educators to be attentive to knowledge flow and politics. Specifically, the types of knowledge that come to be valued and/or emerge as dominant in clinical contexts affect how healthcare professionals conduct their work and how patients and their families experience healthcare (Bleakley et al., 2008; Hodges et al., 2009; Martimianakis and Hafferty, 2013). As one example, the physician can play several different roles in the globalized context (Box 12.1). In our case, the paediatrician, to some extent, exemplifies the 'culturally versed global physician'. While working in Canada he acknowledges that the patient, a new immigrant, may be bringing into the encounter cultural experiences of illness that would complicate the interaction. The strategies he

---

BOX 12.1
DISCOURSES OF THE GLOBAL PHYSICIAN

UNIVERSAL GLOBAL PHYSICIAN

This global physician is someone who can be trained anywhere in the world using a set of universally applicable standards of competency.

CULTURALLY VERSED GLOBAL PHYSICIAN

This global physician is someone who has acquired culturally specific knowledge and training through exposure and experience. This knowledge can be applied in culturally specific contexts (locally or internationally).

GLOBAL PHYSICIAN ADVOCATE

This global physician is a socially minded individual trained to understand the economic, cultural and political determinants of health. Global physicians promote global health and use their positions of authority to advocate for marginalized populations.

Martimianakis, M. A., Hafferty, F. W., 2013. The world as the new local clinic: A critical analysis of three discourses of global medical competency. Soc. Sci. Med. (1982), 87, 31–38.

---

has tried thus far to build rapport typically work with patients who are native to Canada, but they do not seem to be working with this family. His decision to work with an interpreter is an attempt to close the distance with the patient, to travel closer to their context. However, in this example, the cultural context of the patient is perceived to interfere with the diagnosis and management of the case. It is not used to make sense of symptoms or illness experiences. Nor does it become a starting point for thinking about alternative approaches to care. The patient is acknowledged as different and in the process is othered in a system that still functions on the premise that healthcare is universal because illness is purely biological.

Contemporary educators face tensions and challenges associated with reconciling competing mandates of standardization and diversification. These challenges provide researchers with a unique opportunity to clarify and critique emergent definitions of clinical reasoning. Specifically, quality control on the one hand and attunement to patient and learner needs on the other bring into focus competencies that may be at odds with one another (Gregg and Saha, 2006; Koehn and Swick, 2006).

As a result, there is a rethinking of how people, including healthcare professionals, are socialized into their profession and within a particular work context. This has implications for the positions we take in relation to clinical reasoning and expert development. Although multidirectional healthcare professional interactions and patient-centred approaches to care are by no means universal and may often be limited to Western contexts, clinical reasoning is generally agreed to be a core standard component of practice in the health professions. The proliferation of Western models of care has affected notions of what make a 'good' healthcare professional and how clinical reasoning is executed. Trainees in the health professions around the world are routinely first taught a standard mix of basic science and clinical approaches, frequently algorithmic, through combinations of didactic lectures and small-group learning. They then have the opportunity to interact with patients they see as part of their education. Finally, they may become members of teams. This sequence in and of itself is quite standardized and has been implemented in medical schools, for example, around the world (Waterval et al., 2015).

The adoption of similar approaches to clinical practice has not resulted in sameness in how health is experienced and healthcare is provided. The complexity of what healthcare professionals engage with may be influenced by structures, processes and belief systems that did not evolve or emerge from the same context as their training. This is further complicated by interprofessional models of care, which call for knowledge sharing and team problem solving. We cannot assume that everyone has been socialized into healthcare in the same way. Given that clinical reasoning informs a large component of a practitioner's identity, it is extremely important to consider how such an identity engages with the identities of other team members, administrators and patients (Frost and Reghr, 2013; Rummens, 2003). When the identities of the latter are different from one's own or change as a result of globalization and exposure to other health contexts, we should expect a corresponding change in how clinical reasoning occurs in day-to-day practice.

Clinical reasoning in the globalized workforce can be conceptualized as an ongoing negotiation of the discrepancies in knowledge, attitudes and practices stemming from cultural differences in what constitutes 'good care', because more likely than not there are marked differences between where healthcare professionals are currently located and where they originally trained (Hodges et al., 2009). It is not unreasonable, then, to speculate that healthcare professionals find themselves challenged by such discrepancies in their daily practice, as in the example of our case (Case Study 12.2) and they may over time resort to choosing one way to practice (most likely the dominant way in the context of their current work) as a way to adhere to notions of quality and standardization. Clinical care guidelines are facilitative mechanisms for such standard setting, where standardization of process becomes a proxy for quality care. However, what happens when clinical care guidelines call for attention to culture and differences? How is clinical reasoning affected by growing demands to attend to sociocultural differences?

REFLECTION POINT

- How and when do race and culture factor into encounters with patients?
- How would one distinguish whether the challenges experienced by the White physician are related to cultural differences?

CLINICAL REASONING: VALUING EVIDENCE

In contrast to dominant models of expertise, clinical reasoning is defined as the 'creative and open-ended exploration of a (clinical) problem that aims to develop an understanding of a situation … (and where) a diagnosis can be a valuable aid to reasoning, but it does not define the entirety of the reasoning process … converging (only) on an answer that is either right or wrong' (Ilgen et al., 2016, p. 436) (see Mylopoulos and Woods, 2017). This process is closely related to case formulation, which may involve making a diagnosis as the paediatrician, in our case, prioritizes. However, his understanding and/or explanation of the patient's presentation only superficially address context and the perspectives available to him (including those of the parents and resident trainee from Ethiopia).

CASE STUDY 12.2

The paediatrician, introduced in Case Study 12.1, tells the resident that there are very clear guidelines in establishing a diagnosis of autism or global developmental delay, and although there may be some cultural differences in how such diagnoses may be understood, 'a diagnosis is a diagnosis is a diagnosis, and there are standardized ways to come to that diagnosis, such as intelligence testing, or using tools such as the autism diagnostic observation schedule, better known as the ADOS'. The resident, aware that she had limited training in developmental disorders in Ethiopia, has read up on autism ahead of her current placement. She quickly points out that in some cultures people do not look people directly in the eye and in others, how and what a child plays with may be different. However, diagnostic criteria for autism, grounded in a biomedical model, do not capture this variability.

The paediatrician reminds the resident that 'they've come to me as the doctor, so although there is some room for negotiation, I need to make sure I get the diagnosis right (implying there can only be one right diagnosis) to support the child best'. The resident wonders what is meant by 'negotiation' in the clinical setting and is confused about how to think about cultural variance in diagnostic criteria.

The paediatrician goes on to tell the resident that he makes an extra effort to ensure that families who are new to Canada and 'who don't speak much English' or 'who don't quite know the system yet' get connected with culturally appropriate resources. He wants to be able to meet with the child's extended family (if available) but often does not have the time and even has less time to connect with agencies directly, including those that provide therapy and the schooling. He gives a diagnosis and plans to see the family again in 4 to 6 months. The resident walks away asking herself 'does that mean that culture and race only affect communication in health encounters?'

In this regard, clinical reasoning, as a process of exploring problems emerging from and being influenced by globalization, becomes greater than the individual practitioner, team or organization. Although clinical reasoning could be described as application of specific algorithms and thinking very categorically about patients and their diseases (Norman, 2005), as our case highlights, globalization is challenging such a categorical and algorithmic approach. As one example, related to the developmental difficulties that children may face, it is important to consider that some diagnostic categories such as those of attention deficit hyperactivity disorder or autism may not have the same uptake as diagnoses in particular parts of the world.

This has implications for how diverse patients interact with healthcare professionals in contexts where such diagnostic categories do matter. Simultaneously, how clinical reasoning may be taught to trainees in countries where such categories do not matter also needs to be addressed, given how complex and multidimensional globalization is and how local and global needs may vary (Rashid, 2022). Curricular strategies, diagnostic criteria and treatment algorithms developed in one context may not apply in other contexts or vice versa (Bleakely et al., 2008). Such differences are increasingly seen as important in the provision of patient-centred care models. A good example of this might be guidelines related to management of diabetes, and similarly some guidelines around end-of-life care may pose unique challenges in places where death and dying are governed by religious and cultural norms. In our case, a difference in eye contact and play is invoked by the resident highlighting the situated nature of knowledge.

Expertise in a traditional sense, therefore, is very much a product of utilizing expert knowledge. In many contexts, clinical experts are predominantly situated within the biomedical model. Lawlor (2010, p. 169) challenges this notion of expertise by asking 'What if expertise were considered to be more multiply located or distributed? Perhaps even more radically, what if the expertise of parents or children and adults with [specific disease] were foregrounded or privileged over other sources of knowledge … Strengthening reflections on the nature of expertise and domains of local knowledge will generate more deliberate attempts to examine multiple perspectives on understandings and events in which expertise is enacted'.

Drawing from the medical education literature, on the one hand, healthcare professionals hold all power of knowing, and on the other, knowing is strategically co-constructed and distributed between the practitioner and patient (Kawamura et al., 2014). With the latter, it becomes relevant to identify, incorporate and consider all elements, including those that are non-human, symbolic and discursive, at multiple levels, including the individual, organization, community and beyond (Zubairi et al., 2016). Such a reframing of expertise, to which clinical reasoning is fundamental, challenges both the definitions of the reified 'single expert' and what it means to make meaning of complex situations. In an evidence-based world, this creates an opportunity to expand what is valued as evidence in clinical reasoning (Mylopoulos et al., 2017; Chaudhary et al., 2019).

Specifically, the emergence and continual proliferation of evidence-based medicine (EBM) have created challenges in identifying and addressing context-specific pockets of cultural, religious and social knowledge pertinent in the delivery of patient-centred care. Some of our own work has demonstrated how objective diagnostic formulations and treatment recommendations are determined at the expense of broader considerations that are patient-specific, including race, class and gender (Zubairi et al., 2016). As a result, 'good' healthcare professionals in today's context may be the ones who are best at practising EBM, but using said scientific evidence runs the risk of perpetuating inequities when sociocultural knowledge related to the patient is ignored. At the same time, there are frequent 'intercultural exchanges where hybridity has become significant in healthcare encounters, because this is where the culture of medicine collides with patients' ways of knowing and being' (Nielsen et al., 2015, p. 2).

Such varying contextual factors may challenge the practitioner to think differently about a case and influence their decision to take into account (or not) such elements as culture or socioeconomic differences, religion and sexual orientation. More specifically, this can challenge a healthcare professional's comfort with more standardized biomedical approaches that they would have learnt through education and an emphasis towards a specific diagnosis. There is evidence to suggest that although some practitioners draw more and more strictly on EBM, there are others who still rely on experience and context (Peters et al., 2017).

CRITICAL REFLEXIVITY AND 'NEGOTIATION'

It has been suggested that educating healthcare professionals to be able to orient themselves to different forms of knowledge requires the practice of critical reflexivity (Ng et al., 2015). Critical reflexivity is the process by which healthcare professionals think about their practice in deeper ways, evaluating their own beliefs, values and context within the boundaries of their clinical practice, which are socially and systematically drawn. There is potential for practitioners to identify how they are exercising or activating the power that rests within their work (Frambach and Martimianakis, 2017). The voice of the patient has become more dominant and it continues to collide with the historical dominance of the healthcare professional. In the context of person- or patient-centred care, there is the potential for greater awareness of the hierarchies of knowledge and a relative flattening of such hierarchies. Different contexts around the world have differential attitudes to hierarchy and power among practitioners and different attitudes around avoiding uncertainty in the practice of clinical reasoning (Findyartini et al., 2016).

Although there may be multiple social negotiations taking place between providers and patients who come to an encounter with different ideologies and knowledge, in the absence of an awareness of the power differentials, there may be perpetuation of racism and discrimination (Bleakley et al., 2008). The spaces for negotiations and co-construction of knowledge are those 'grey' spaces where the pendulum continues to swing between how practitioners define their own roles in clinical encounters and how their engagement with patients is defined.

It is in these spaces where neo-liberal constructs designed to be taught and/or measured, such as 'cultural competency', run the risk for 'othering' the patients, as in our case example (Betancourt, 2006; Pon, 2009; Wear, 2003) while separating clinical reasoning from important contextual factors such as illness experiences and alternative approaches to care that patients may have encountered elsewhere. Cultural competency as practised currently in North American contexts standardizes how care is delivered and develops efficiencies in the health system. However, in the process, culture can become reduced in clinical encounters to a limited number of situations, for example when (1) it is visible from the perspective of the practitioner, (2) evidence and guidelines isolate culture as a variable, perpetuating race-based stereotypes, and (3) physicians use their power to treat culture as secondary to diagnostic considerations (Zubairi et al., 2016). As we have argued, reflexivity on the part of the healthcare provider allows for a reconceptualization of the role of culture, opening the door to a more fulsome appreciation of context and its potential contributions to clinical reasoning, in a globalized world.

SUMMARY

In this chapter we have outlined:

- how neo-liberal policies and globalization intersect with one another to influence clinical reasoning in current models of practice and education in healthcare
- how shifting contexts influence identities and affect the types of knowledge that are valued and made dominant
- how practitioners can begin to reflect on the challenges and opportunities that emerge as a result of multiple trends in healthcare.

REFLECTION POINT

- The healthcare professional may assume different roles such as being the expert (and keeper of knowledge) versus a resource to the client/family or somewhere in between.
- Additionally, the differences that emerge between a professional and patient and the family/caregiver can become points of tension or conflict that can be used as starting points for ongoing reflection.

REFERENCES

Bell, D.L., Katz, M.H., 2021. Modernize medical licensing, and credentialing, too—Lessons from the COVID-19 pandemic. JAMA Internal Medicine 181 (3), 312–315. https://doi.org/10.1001/jamainternmed.2020.8705

Betancourt, J.R., 2006. Eliminating racial and ethnic disparities in health care: What is the role of academic medicine? Academic Medicine: Journal of the Association of American Medical Colleges 81 (9), 788–792. https://doi.org/10.1097/00001888-200609000-00004

Bleakley, A., Brice, J., Bligh, J., 2008. Thinking the post-colonial in medical education. Medical Education 42 (3), 266–270. https://doi.org/10.1111/j.1365-2923.2007.02991.x

Chaudhary, Z.K., Mylopoulos, M., Barnett, R., Sockalingam, S., Hawkins, M., O'Brien, J.D., et al., 2019. Reconsidering basic: Integrating social and behavioral sciences to support learning. Academic Medicine: Journal of the Association of American Medical Colleges, 94(11S Association of American Medical Colleges Learn Serve Lead: Proceedings of the 58th Annual Research in Medical Education Sessions), S73–S78. https://doi.org/10.1097/ACM.0000000000002907

Findyartini, A., Hawthorne, L., McColl, G., Chiavaroli, N., 2016. How clinical reasoning is taught and learned: Cultural perspectives from the University of Melbourne and Universitas Indonesia. BMC Medical Education 16, 185. https://doi.org/10.1186/s12909-016-0709-y

Frambach, J.M., Martimianakis, M.A., 2017. The discomfort of an educator's critical conscience: The case of problem-based learning and other global industries in medical education. Perspectives on Medical Education 6 (1), 1–4. https://doi.org/10.1007/s40037-016-0325-x

Frost, H.D., Regehr, G., 2013. "I am a doctor": Negotiating the discourses of standardization and diversity in professional identity construction. Academic Medicine: Journal of the Association of American Medical Colleges 88 (10), 1570–1577. https://doi.org/10.1097/ACM.0b013e3182a34b05

Giuliani, M., Martimianakis, M.A.T., Broadhurst, M., Papadakos, J., Fazelzad, R., Driessen, E.W., et al., 2021. Motivations for and challenges in the development of global medical curricula: A scoping review. Academic Medicine: Journal of the Association of American Medical Colleges 96 (3), 449–459. https://doi.org/10.1097/ACM.0000000000003383

Gregg, J., Saha, S., 2006. Losing culture on the way to competence: The use and misuse of culture in medical education. Academic Medicine: Journal of the Association of American Medical Colleges 81 (6), 542–547. https://doi.org/10.1097/01.ACM.0000225218.15207.30

Haddara, W., Lingard, L., 2013. Are we all on the same page? A discourse analysis of interprofessional collaboration. Academic Medicine: Journal of the Association of American Medical Colleges 88 (10), 1509–1515. https://doi.org/10.1097/ACM.0b013e3182a31893

Ho, M.J., Lin, C.W., Chiu, Y.T., Lingard, L., Ginsburg, S., 2012. A cross-cultural study of students' approaches to professional dilemmas: Sticks or ripples. Medical Education 46 (3), 245–256. https://doi.org/10.1111/j.1365-2923.2011.04149.x

Ho, M.J., Yu, K.H., Hirsh, D., Huang, T.S., Yang, P.C., 2011. Does one size fit all? Building a framework for medical professionalism. Academic Medicine: Journal of the Association of American Medical Colleges 86 (11), 1407–1414. https://doi.org/10.1097/ACM.0b013e31823059d1

Hodges, B.D., Lingard, L. (Eds.), 2012. The Question of Competence. Cornell University Press, Ithaca, NY.

Hodges, B.D., Maniate, J.M., Martimianakis, M.A., Alsuwaidan, M., Segouin, C., 2009. Cracks and crevices: Globalization discourse and medical education. Medical Teacher 31 (10), 910–917. https://doi.org/10.3109/01421590802534932

Ilgen, J.S., Eva, K.W., Regehr, G., 2016. What's in a label? Is diagnosis the start or the end of clinical reasoning? Journal of General Internal Medicine 31 (4), 435–437. https://doi.org/10.1007/s11606-016-3592-7

Kawamura, A.A., Orsino, A., Mylopoulos, M., 2014. Integrating competencies: Exploring complex problem solving through case formulation in developmental pediatrics. Academic Medicine: Journal of the Association of American Medical Colleges 89 (11), 1497–1501. https://doi.org/10.1097/ACM.0000000000000475

Koehn, P.H., Swick, H.M., 2006. Medical education for a changing world: Moving beyond cultural competence into transnational competence. Academic medicine: Journal of the Association of American Medical Colleges 81 (6), 548–556. https://doi.org/10.1097/01.ACM.0000225217.15207.d4

Lawlor, M.C., 2010. Autism and Anthropology? Ethos (Berkeley, Calif.) 38 (1), 167–171. https://doi.org/10.1111/j.1548-1352.2009.01086.x

Martimianakis, M.A., Hafferty, F.W., 2013. The world as the new local clinic: A critical analysis of three discourses of global medical competency. Social Science & Medicine (1982) 87, 31–38. https://doi.org/10.1016/j.socscimed.2013.03.008

Mickleborough, T.O., Martimianakis, M.A.T., 2021. (Re)producing "Whiteness" in health care: A spatial analysis of the critical literature on the integration of internationally educated health care professionals in the Canadian workforce. Academic Medicine: Journal of the Association of American Medical Colleges 96 (11S), S31–S38. https://doi.org/10.1097/ACM.0000000000004262

McKimm, J., McLean, M., 2011. Developing a global health practitioner: Time to act. Medical Teacher 33 (8), 626–631. https://doi.org/10.3109/0142159X.2011.590245

Mylopoulos, M., Borschel, D.T., O'Brien, T., Martimianakis, S., Woods, N.N., 2017. Exploring integration in action: Competencies as building blocks of expertise. Academic Medicine: Journal of the Association of American Medical Colleges 92 (12), 1794–1799. https://doi.org/10.1097/ACM.0000000000001772

Mylopoulos, M., Woods, N.N., 2017. When I say … adaptive expertise. Medical Education 51 (7), 685–686. https://doi.org/10.1111/medu.13247

Ng, S.L., Kinsella, E.A., Friesen, F., Hodges, B., 2015. Reclaiming a theoretical orientation to reflection in medical education research: A critical narrative review. Medical Education 49 (5), 461–475. https://doi.org/10.1111/medu.12680

Nielsen, L.S., Angus, J.E., Howell, D., Husain, A., Gastaldo, D., 2015. Patient-centered care or cultural competence: Negotiating palliative care at home for Chinese Canadian immigrants. The American Journal of Hospice & Palliative Care 32 (4), 372–379. https://doi.org/10.1177/1049909114527338

Norman, G., 2005. Research in clinical reasoning: Past history and current trends. Medical Education 39 (4), 418–427. https://doi.org/10.1111/j.1365-2929.2005.02127.x

Paul, R., Martimianakis, M.A.T., Johnstone, J., McNaughton, N., Austin, Z., 2017. Internationally educated health professionals in Canada: Navigating three policy subsystems along the pathway to practice. Academic Medicine: Journal of the Association of American Medical Colleges 92 (5), 635–640. https://doi.org/10.1097/ACM.0000000000001331

Perfetto, R., Dholakia, N., 2010. Exploring the cultural contradictions of medical tourism. Consumption Markets & Culture 13, 399–417. https://doi.org/10.1080/10253866.2010.502417

Peters, A., Vanstone, M., Monteiro, S., Norman, G., Sherbino, J., Sibbald, M., 2017. Examining the influence of context and professional culture on clinical reasoning through rhetorical-narrative analysis. Qualitative Health Research 27 (6), 866–876. https://doi.org/10.1177/1049732316650418

Pluut, B., 2016. Differences that matter: Developing critical insights into discourses of patient-centredness. Medicine,l Health Care and Philosophy. 19, 501–515. https://doi.org/10.1007/s11019-016-9712-7.

Pon, G., 2009. Cultural competency as new racism: An ontology of forgetting. Journal of Progressive Human Services 20, 59–71. https://doi.org/10.1080/10428230902871173

Rashid, M.A., 2022. Hyperglobalist, sceptical, and transformationalist perspectives on globalization in medical education. Medical Teacher 44 (9), 1023–1031. https://doi.org/10.1080/0142159X.2022.2058384

Rummens, J.A., 2003. Conceptualising identity and diversity: Overlaps, intersections, and processes. Canadian Ethnic Studies Journal 35, 10.

Schwarz, M.R., Wojtczak, A., 2002. Global minimum essential requirements: A road towards competence-oriented medical education. Medical Teacher 24 (2), 125–129. https://doi.org/10.1080/01421590220120740

Seeleman, C., Suurmond, J., Stronks, K., 2009. Cultural competence: A conceptual framework for teaching and learning. Medical Education 43 (3), 229–237. https://doi.org/10.1111/j.1365-2923.2008.03269.x

Spring, J., 2008. Research on globalization and education. Review of Educational Research 78 (2), 330–363. https://doi.org/10.3102/0034654308317846

Timmermans, S., Almeling, R., 2009. Objectification, standardization, and commodification in health care: A conceptual readjustment. Social Science & Medicine (1982) 69 (1), 21–27. https://doi.org/10.1016/j.socscimed.2009.04.020

Timmermans, S., Epstein, S., 2010. A world of standards but not a standard world: Toward a sociology of standards and standardization. Annual Review of Sociology 36, 69–89. https://doi.org/10.1146/annurev.soc.012809.102629

Waterval, D.G.J., Frambach, J.M., Driessen, E.W., Scherpbier, A.J.J.A., 2015. Copy but not paste: A literature review of crossborder curriculum partnerships. Journal of Studies in International Education 19 (1), 65–85. https://doi.org/10.1177/1028315314533608

Wear, D., 2003. Insurgent multiculturalism: Rethinking how and why we teach culture in medical education. Academic Medicine: Journal of the Association of American Medical Colleges 78 (6), 549–554. https://doi.org/10.1097/00001888-200306000-00002

World Health Organization. (2010, August). How health systems can address health inequities linked to migration and ethnicity. https://apps.who.int/iris/handle/10665/345463

Yen, W., Hodwitz, K., Thakkar, N., Martimianakis, M.A., Faulkner, D., 2016. The influence of globalization on medical regulation: A descriptive analysis of international medical graduates registered through alternative licensure routes in Ontario. Canadian Medical Education Journal 7 (3), e19–e30.

Zubairi, M., Kawamura, A., Mylopoulos, M., 2016. The cultural encounter in developmental paediatrics Unpublished MRP. Ontario Institute for Studies in Education. University of Toronto, Canada.

13

NEXT-GENERATION CLINICAL PRACTICE GUIDELINES

STEPHEN LOFTUS ▪ JANINE MARGARITA DIZON

CHAPTER OUTLINE

CHAPTER AIMS

The aims of this chapter are:

- to update views on Clinical Practice Guideline development
- to update views on the implementation of Clinical Practice Guidelines
- to review future directions for Clinical Practice Guidelines.

INTRODUCTION

In this chapter, we provide an update on Clinical Practice Guideline (CPG) development and implementation in real-world practice. CPGs are developed based on the evidence and provide recommendations across a wide range of topics or conditions. Various methods in CPG use are recommended based on the need for answers to guide practice. However, there can be problems with the use of CPGs. These include limited guidance in undertaking practical assessment of barriers to implementation in the local context. In this chapter, we focus on identifying real-world questions related to clinical reasoning and finding the right answers from CPGs together with other issues confronting the use of CPGs.

SEEKING GUIDANCE IN PRACTICE: ASKING THE QUESTIONS

There is no 'one size fits all' approach in managing patients' health. It is common knowledge that although health professionals can devote years to their education and clinical practice, there are clinical scenarios that will challenge their clinical reasoning and decision making. They will be faced with uncertainties in practice that will prompt them to seek answers from several sources of information because each patient is different. Before we go into these uncertainties, it is important to clear up terminology. Table 13.1 summarizes common terms used in this context and that may be confused with CPGs.

Health professionals can be faced with clinical reasoning questions that are directly about the health management of patients or service delivery questions that relate to the adequacy and efficiency of the health service. Examples of questions about health management include:

TABLE 13.1	
Summary of Pertinent Terminology and Definitions	
Term	**Definition**
Practice standard	Minimum desired and achievable level of clinical practice as defined by a professional society
Clinical Practice Guideline	Systematically developed documents created with a validated methodology, which includes identifying the literature on specific clinical question(s), characterized by explicit methods of searching, selection and grading the available evidence. This is followed by development and grading the strength of the recommendation(s)
Consensus statement	Recommendations developed based on a collective opinion or consensus of the convened expert panel
Practice advisory	Synonymous with consensus statement
Position statement or paper	Comprehensive document that elucidates, justifies and recommends a particular approach to a clinical problem
Practice alert	Short statement that is developed in response to a time-sensitive clinical issue that requires immediate action

Based on Joshi,, G.P., Benzon, H.T., Gan, T.J., Vetter, T.R., 2019. Consistent definitions of Clinical Practice Guidelines, consensus statements, position statements, and practice alerts. Anesth. Analg. 129 (6), 1767–1770. https://doi.org/10.1213/ANE.0000000000004236.

- What is the optimal time to perform a swallow screen test for adults suffering from stroke?
- What are the most effective rehabilitation interventions for managing nonspecific low back pain?

Examples of health service delivery questions include:

- Who is the best allied health professional to perform a swallow screen test in the absence of a speech pathologist?
- What are the barriers that are important to consider in implementing an intervention?

Regardless of the question type, it is important that the right questions are identified, questions are clear and specific and include such details as patient population, to find the most appropriate answers. For this to be possible, health professionals and other key stakeholders, such as managers and policy-makers, should be consulted during the early stages of the CPG development process. Knowing the type of questions that clinicians might need help with can provide useful insights for those who are tasked with developing CPGs.

DEVELOPING CPGs

There are now thousands of CPGs and thousands of guideline development groups. There are also many guidelines available for developing CPGs (e.g.

Guidelines International Network https://g-i-n.net). CPGs can reduce inappropriate practice variation. They can also be used to improve the translation of research into practice, as well as improving healthcare quality and safety. CPGs have also been used to develop performance measures for physicians and hospitals. The data gathered from these measures have provided consumers with information on the quality of different healthcare providers. It has also been claimed that CPGs provide physicians and hospitals with an economic incentive to improve the quality of the care they provide.

However, many health professionals, consumer groups and other stakeholders have been concerned with the quality of the processes supporting development of CPGs (e.g. Steinberg et al., 2011). This has raised questions about the resulting validity of many CPGs and CPG-based clinical performance measures. There are several good reasons for these concerns, such as:

- Limitations in the scientific evidence base
- Limitations in the systematic review process
- Lack of transparency of development groups' methodologies
- Failure to convene multistakeholder and multidisciplinary development groups
- Conflicts of interest among guideline development group members and funders
- Reconciliation between conflicting guidelines.

For example, a limitation in the guideline development process is that many CPGs have failed to include evidence affecting subpopulations of patients such as those with comorbidities, the socially and economically disadvantaged and patients with rare conditions. In response to these challenges, there has been a move to develop standards for CPG development. For example, a widely adopted tool for grading the quality of evidence and making recommendations is the GRADE framework (Grading of Recommendations, Assessment, Development, and Evaluations). There is now a large series of GRADE publications (for a comprehensive list see https://www.jclinepi.com/content/jce-GRADE-Series). Using the GRADE framework, a clinical question is first specified that includes the population that the question will be applied to. The quality of evidence is then rated before a recommendation is made. GRADE uses four certainty ratings: very low, low, moderate and high. It is accepted that there is some subjectivity in each decision, but it is claimed that GRADE provides a reproducible and transparent framework for grading certainty in evidence (Mustafa et al., 2013).

According to the GRADE framework, certainty in the evidence can be rated down according to the following factors (Guyatt et al., 2008):

- Risk of bias
- Imprecision
- Inconsistency
- Indirectness
- Publication bias

Evidence can be rated upwards according to the following factors:

- Large magnitude of effect
- Dose-response gradient
- All residual confounding would decrease magnitude of effect (in situations with an effect)

In the GRADE framework, the quality of the evidence can lead to recommendations that can be strong or weak in favour or against an intervention. A strong recommendation implies that most people would select a particular option. A weak recommendation implies that there can be important variations in the decision that an informed person might take and shared decision making with all people involved is important.

Steinberg et al. (2011) recommend particular attributes that should characterize all CPGs:

Validity

CPGs can be valid if they lead to the health and cost outcomes they project. The development process can include a prospective assessment and consider projected health outcomes and the costs of alternative courses of action. Questions to be asked focus on the relationship between evidence and recommendation, the quality of evidence and how the evidence has been evaluated.

Reliability/Reproducibility

CPGs can be considered reliable and reproducible if there are satisfactory answers to the following questions. If another set of experts considered the same evidence and used the same guideline development process, would they produce the same CPGs? Can the CPGs be interpreted and applied consistently by health professionals? What are the outcomes of independent external reviews and pretests of CPGs?

Clinical Applicability and Flexibility

Do the CPGs specify which patient populations they apply to? Do the CPPGs identify exceptions to their recommendations?

Clarity

Do the CPGs use unambiguous language and easily followed modes of presentation?

Multidisciplinary Process

Are key affected groups included in CPG development?

Scheduled Review

Do the CPGs include statements about when they are to be reviewed? Fast changing fields are likely to need regular and frequent review.

Documentation

Documentation should include the procedures followed in the development process, participants and the analytic processes used.

One recent, and promising, approach to developing CPGs is to start with the kinds of clinical questions that health professionals need help with. These are the sorts of questions where they are likely to turn to CPGs to seek guidance and many of these questions directly concern clinical reasoning. These questions then become a key aspect of CPG development (Chakraborty et al., 2020).

How to Formulate Clinically Relevant Questions for CPGs

An example of a relevant question format is the PICO format for intervention or effectiveness questions (P-population, I-intervention, C-comparator, O-outcome). In these questions, there is a need to specify, in as much detail as possible, each component of the format. What are the characteristics of the patient? Young, and otherwise healthy, patients from prosperous socioeconomic backgrounds are going to be very different from elderly patients with many co-morbidities who have suffered from poverty for most of their lives. What precisely is the intervention being considered? Is this an increase in dosage of an existing drug that the patient is already receiving or a completely new treatment? What is the intervention being compared with? Is this, for example, a new drug being compared with an old drug. What outcome is desired? This could range from complete cure to providing some alleviation in a chronic condition. A variation is the PACO format for diagnostic accuracy questions (P-population, A-assessment, C-comparator, O-outcome).

A best practice approach to develop clinically relevant questions has been proposed in the literature by Chakraborty and colleagues (Chakraborty et al., 2020). This protocol consists of seven essential steps to develop clinically relevant questions based on several CPG methodologies but mainly informed by WHO and NICE (National Institute for Health and Care Excellence) (Table 13.2).

This protocol was developed based on literature reviews, interviews with stakeholders and end-users and clinical reasoning case studies based on patient scenarios. What this approach highlights is the use of different methods in question formulation and especially using qualitative methods with inductive thematic analysis.

Questions to be answered by CPGs can be generated using different methods such as surveys as well as the focus groups used by Chakraborty et al. (2020). There can be multiple iterations to clarify and formulate the questions. More in-depth discussions may be needed for some difficult clinical scenarios. The final list of questions should be agreed upon by the members of the development team before the search for evidence to answer them commences. One approach to developing the clinical reasoning aspect of CPGs is to consider patient pathways.

REFLECTION POINT

Health professionals can be faced with difficult or challenging patient scenarios that will trigger questions about best practice. These questions could either be clinical questions that relate to diagnosis and treatment of patients or health service delivery questions that relate to the efficiency and adequacy of management of patients. What kinds of questions can you come up with from your own practice? For example, different categories of question could include the following:

- What is the reliability or validity of a particular diagnostic test?
- How can you compare the clinical effectiveness of different options for management?
- How is the clinical effectiveness of a management option assessed?
- What is the cost-effectiveness of different management options?

The Importance of Patient Pathways

What Are Patient Pathways?

A patient pathway is the route that a patient takes from the first contact with a health professional, through to the completion of treatment (Tshivhase, 2019). A patient pathway or care pathway is a 'complex intervention for the mutual decision making and organization of care processes for a well-defined group of patients during a well-defined period' (Vanhaecht et al., 2010, Schrijvers et al., 2012). Patient pathways are also known as integrated care pathways, anticipated recovery pathways, multidisciplinary pathways of care and critical care pathways (Johnson, 2016). Patient pathways can be specific to primary care, secondary care, tertiary care and community care and

TABLE 13.2

Steps in Developing Clinically Relevant Questions in Clinical Practice Guidelines

Step	Description
Step 1: Define the rationale for the guideline	Undertake a detailed needs analysis of patient outcomes, clinical practice, relevant policy and other research evidence to explain the need for a guideline
Step 2: Use qualitative research methods to determine the initial list of key questions based on the clinical challenges faced by target end users	Present clinical scenarios (case vignettes) to target end users and other key stakeholders
	Utilize an inductive thematic analysis approach to identify areas of clinical concern
	Map areas of clinical concern against a Clinical Reasoning Framework
	Generate an initial list of questions based on results from the qualitative study and extend these findings with research evidence about existing clinical challenges
Step 3: Convert the initial list of questions	Convert the initial list of questions developed in Step 2 into a population, intervention, comparator, outcome (PICO) format
Step 4: Specify all relevant outcomes for each possible question	This includes not only those specified in PICO but other positive and negative outcomes
Step 5: Review and revise draft key questions	Review and revise draft key questions, in light of the specific outcomes identified in Step 4
Step 6: Rate the outcomes in order of importance for clinical decision making	As part of this step, the Guideline Development Group may consider whether advice (in the form of high-quality clinical guidelines) already exists to answer the clinical challenges that were revealed during the qualitative study
Step 7: Decide on the final list of questions	Final questions are to be decided upon based on resource availability, which can be difficult to anticipate; specifically, the resource requirements for undertaking systematic literature reviews

From Chakraborty, S., Brijnath, B., Dermentzis, J., Mazza, D., 2020. Defining key questions for Clinical Practice Guidelines: A novel approach for developing clinically relevant questions. *Health Res Policy Syst, 18*(1), 113, pp. 4 and 9. https://doi.org/10.1186/s12961-020-00628-3.© The Author(s). 2020 Open Access This article is distributed under the terms of the Creative Commons Attribution 4.0 International License (http://creativecommons.org/licenses/by/4.0/).

even palliative care, or can span across all types of care. Patient pathways aid in ensuring adequacy, efficiency and coordination of healthcare to optimize healthcare benefits. In the patient pathway, consideration includes not only the health professionals who are involved with the patient and their families, but also the managers, providers and policy makers.

Mapping the Questions Against Typical Patient Pathways

Developing a 'typical' patient pathway is a substantial component in CPG development and implementation to answer questions faced by health professionals. The 'typical' patient pathway assists in providing a comprehensive understanding of what can happen to patients as they enter the healthcare continuum in a specific context (Grimmer et al., 2019). Developing the 'typical' patient pathway is undertaken by the same guideline development group that developed the questions needing answers. Similar to the question development, the methods used are surveys and focus group discussions. Usually, it takes more than one iteration of the 'typical' patient pathway before it can be finalized by the guideline development group.

The challenges faced by the health professionals that prompt them to seek answers are usually related to at least one point in the typical patient pathway. Therefore, it is reasonable to map the questions identified by the guideline development group against the typical patient pathway. By mapping the questions to the typical patient pathway, a better understanding of the questions and answers to inform practice throughout the pathway is achieved, especially in consideration of the local context.

An example of a patient pathway is presented in Fig. 13.1, extracted from the South African Contextualised

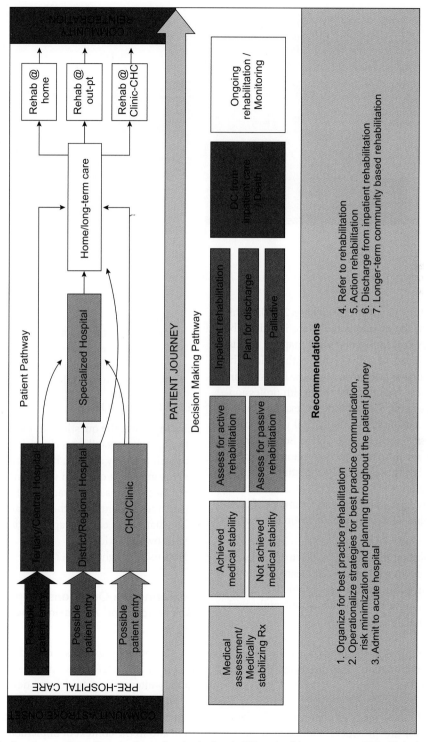

Fig. 13.1 ■ 'Typical' patient pathway for a stroke patient in the South African healthcare system. *CPG*, Clinical practice guideline. (From Grimmer, K., Louw, Q., Dizon, J.M., van Niekerk, S.M., Ernstzen, D., Wiysonge, C., 2018. Standardising evidence strength grading for recommendations from multiple clinical practice guidelines: A South African case study. Implement Sci, 13(1), 117.)

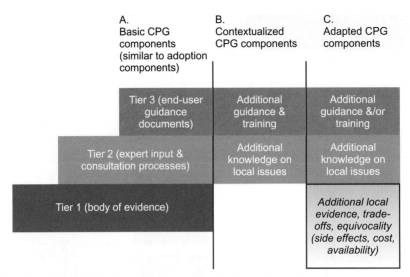

Fig. 13.2 ■ The clinical practice guideline tier approach. *CPG,* Clinical practice guideline.

Stroke Rehabilitation Guideline (Tshivhase, 2019). In this guideline project, the questions that were identified by the guideline development group were mapped against the typical stroke patient pathway in South Africa. The questions were further categorized into the levels of care and the key clinical decisions that the health professionals need to make along the pathway. For example, at the point where the patient enters the typical patient pathway and the possible entry points in the South African context are tertiary hospitals, district/regional hospitals or community health centres. The questions mapped against these points were those about medical assessments and achieving medical stability. Examples of questions from the guideline development group team were:

1. What education should be provided to allied health providers about multidisciplinary team building?
2. What education should be provided to medical and nursing professionals about multidisciplinary allied health teams?

Another example is at the point of patient referral to in-patient rehabilitation. The questions that were mapped against these were:

1. What is the best form of communication with other healthcare providers about allied health rehabilitation?

2. What factors are associated with safe commencement of rehabilitation?
3. What are the elements of comprehensive rehabilitation assessment?
4. Which outcome tools should be used?

REFLECTION POINT

Thinking about the questions in the context of patient pathways facilitates clinical reasoning skills. A patient pathway allows a better understanding of the reasons why a question was identified and the other mechanisms or interactions that need to be considered in identifying the right answers.

■ To what extent can you apply patient pathways to your own practice?
■ How useful might they be?

Answering the Questions: Applying the ACA Model and Assessing Local Context

ACA Model

The Adopt, Contextualise or Adapt (ACA) model (Dizon et al., 2016) was introduced and discussed among alternative guideline development methods that consider implementation (Fig. 13.2). In this update, the ACA model will be discussed in more detail and in the context of implementing the evidence to guide clinical decisions and direct future policies.

CPG adoption refers to a straightforward application of the CPG and/or its specific recommendations in practice. This does not require any change to implement in practice.

CPG contextualization refers to applying the evidence or the recommendations in practice but in consideration of the local context needs and barriers. The evidence or the recommendations do not need to change but how it will be applied, who will apply the evidence, what additional resources are needed and what policies or funding will cover the application of evidence, need to be determined for the evidence or the recommendation to work in practice.

CPG adaptation refers to changing something to suit different conditions or a different purpose. Adapting recommendations from a CPG should occur where the CPG recommendation cannot be delivered in its current form in the local situation and additional local research is needed.

REFLECTION POINT

CPGs are being developed by international and local groups. A number of CPGs on clinical conditions can be international, country specific or profession specific. The ACA model is a useful guide in determining the most relevant approach in applying the evidence recommendations from the CPGs to local practice.

- How does your own local clinical practice vary from practice elsewhere?
- How might this affect your use of CPGs?

Assessing Local Context: What Needs to Be Considered to Make the Evidence Work in Practice?

The importance of context was highlighted in the evidence-informed practice model (Satterfield et al., 2009). Decision making happens in consideration of the best available research evidence, clinical expertise and patient and population characteristics, based on the concept of evidence-based practice, and more importantly, within the larger environmental and organizational context. Understanding the context is key in making evidence-based decisions in healthcare, especially when there is immense variability in treatment options, resources, clinical skills and patient responses.

Context is defined as 'a set of characteristics and circumstances that surround the implementation effort' (Pfadenhauer et al., 2015, p. 104). Common context considerations include availability of resources (equipment and staffing), skills of health professionals, policies in place, organizational support and many more (Tshivhase, 2019). Assessing local context barriers is necessary to understand the next steps in applying the evidence.

A framework to assess local context considerations to implement recommendations for practice was developed as part of the South African Contextualised Stroke Rehabilitation Guideline Project (Tshivhase, 2019). The framework included elements related to the organization, service delivery, communication and clinical care barriers (Table 13.3). The elements identified were based on local discussions with end-users that include policy-makers, allied health professionals, patient representatives and family members, who are knowledgeable and experienced on the issues characterizing the local context. The framework is extracted from the South African Contextualised Stroke Rehabilitation Guideline.

This framework was used to prompt discussions about the local issues that need to be addressed. These local issues range from the minimum standards of care that might be available in settings as varied as community clinics or metropolitan hospitals, to the education that might be needed for best practice to be applied. For example, one of the recommendations to answer the question 'What education should be provided to allied health providers about multidisciplinary team building?' Is: Establish best practice multidisciplinary allied health stroke rehabilitation teams at all points of entry to the healthcare system. This is a consistent recommendation that comes from multiple CPGs.

In some contexts, such as metropolitan settings in high-income countries (HICs) and lower middle-income countries (LMICs), this recommendation can be readily adopted as there are existing facilities, resources and trained health professionals who comprise the multidisciplinary teams and can undertake comprehensive management in all stages of care (the higher standards of care in the framework described). However, in some contexts such as regional and remote areas in HICs and in most settings in LMICs, this recommendation needs to be contextualized to be applied. A multidisciplinary stroke team may not always be

TABLE 13.3			
Broad Barrier Prompts for Contextualisation Discussions			
	What Is Required to Affect change?	**In Minimum Standard of Care**	**In Higher Standard of Care**	**Training Required? If so What, and for Whom?**
Organization ▪ Resource (Grimmer et al., 2019, pp. 50–59) ▪ Type of workforce	Responses should identify and address specific local issues	In the least resourced environment for care provision (e.g. community clinics)	In a well-resourced environment for care provision (e.g. metropolitan tertiary hospital)	Who requires additional training to implement each recommendation? What training is required, and how should it be delivered?
Service delivery ▪ Legislative responsibilities/ constraints ▪ Availability of workforce	Responses should identify and address specific local issues	In the least resourced environment for care provision (e.g. community clinics)	In a well-resourced environment for care provision (e.g. metropolitan tertiary hospital)	Who requires additional training to implement each recommendation? What training is required, and how should it be delivered?
Communication ▪ People ▪ Resources ▪ (phone, internet, fax)	Responses should identify and address specific local issues	In the least resourced environment for care provision (e.g. community clinics)	In a well-resourced environment for care provision (e.g. metropolitan tertiary hospital)	Who requires additional training to implement each recommendation? What training is required, and how should it be delivered?
Clinical care ▪ Availability of workforce ▪ Type of workforce ▪ Capacity of workforce ▪ Available equipment ▪ Other available resources	Responses should identify and address specific local issues	In the least resourced environment for care provision (e.g. community clinics)	In a well-resourced environment for care provision (e.g. metropolitan tertiary hospital)	Who requires additional training to implement each recommendation? What training is required, and how should it be delivered?

From Grimmer, K., Louw, Q., Dizon, J. M., Brown, S. M., Ernstzen, D., Wiysonge, C. S., 2019. A South African experience in applying the Adopt-Contextualise-Adapt Framework to stroke rehabilitation clinical practice guidelines. Health Res. Policy. Syst., 17 (1), p. 56. https://doi.org/10.1186/s12961-019-0454-x. © The Author(s). 2019 Open Access This article is distributed under the terms of the Creative Commons Attribution 4.0 International License (http://creativecommons.org/licenses/by/4.0/).

available. At best, the setting may only have a doctor, a nurse and a physiotherapist, thus only the minimum standard of care is available. There may be lack of manpower resources to deliver other allied health services and possibly limited equipment. Therefore, there is a need to discuss how other medical and allied health services can be made available to a patient with a stroke. In the context where this question was raised and based on the assessment of the local context, the following was agreed upon (Tshivhase, p. 37).

Barrier to the Multidisciplinary Allied Health Stroke Rehabilitation

Not all levels of care have access to a multidisciplinary team consisting of doctors, nurses, physiotherapists, *occupational therapists, speech and language therapists, social workers, dieticians, clinical neuropsychologists/ clinical psychologists.*

Suggestions to Overcome This Barrier

The available member of the multidisciplinary team should assess a stroke patient to determine whether there is a need to be seen by a dietician, clinical neuropsychologist and/or clinical psychologist. If there is a need, a referral pathway should be in place to allow all stroke patients to have access to the specific member of the multidisciplinary team, at a facility where such a service is available.

A similar scenario was investigated in a study conducted in Africa (Pierpoint & Pillay, 2020). The barrier in this case was that there was no speech pathologist immediately available to conduct swallow screen testing for acute stroke patients. If the swallow screen test is not performed at the optimal time, there is a risk of aspiration occurring. Therefore, to apply the recommendation, nurses were trained to perform a specific swallow screen test for acute stroke patients, called the Gugging Swallowing Screen. This resulted in reduced pneumonia rates in the hospital and improved quality of the services provided. Performing this test was normally beyond the role and scope of the nurses' practice, but with the training provided, best available evidence was applied and optimum care for the patient with stroke was delivered.

These examples are useful in informing future planning and policy making in stroke management. If additional staff members cannot be employed, endorsements can be made to provide additional training to available health professionals, especially if there are increasing number of patients with stroke being admitted to the facility or if adverse events are occurring due to lack of other critical services. These endorsements can be backed up with reports such as those previously described and are an example of adapting CPGs to local context.

REFLECTION POINT

Assessing local context barriers is crucial in identifying effective and efficient strategies to implement the evidence despite the barriers. Local context considerations need to be part of the GDG discussions, which can be mapped back to the 'typical' patient pathway.

- Can you think of ways that your local context can be adapted with the aid of CPGs?

Artificial Intelligence and Clinical Practice Guidelines

Another major influence on the ways that CPGs can be used lies in the development of Artificial Intelligence (AI). Encouraging health professionals to accept and implement CPGs has long been recognized as a problem. Training and performance monitoring have been the traditional approach to encourage uptake (Cormican et al., 2023). As we have seen, adapting CPGs to the local context so that there are local protocols is one way to encourage their uptake in a critical

manner. In recent years, CPGs have been provided digitally and can be integrated into medical management systems, such as electronic health records. One important development in this field is the emergence of computer-interpretable guidelines. This means that health professionals can be alerted to relevant CPGs and can gain easy access to them. In this way they become more like decision support systems that can assist clinicians directly at the bedside (Oliveira et al., 2013). More recently, rapid advances in AI offer new possibilities (Rajpurkar et al., 2022). It is feasible that, in the near future, as a patient's information is entered into the system, an AI could proactively notify a health professional of the sections of different CPGs that are relevant for that patient and the AI could even offer a summary of the various CPGs and a critique where there are conflicts. AI may become a powerful tool in the implementation and monitoring of CPGs.

AI in medical practice is not new. There have been so-called expert systems for many years. The first expert system in healthcare was probably MYCIN (Davis et al., 1977). Expert systems have a limited ability to explain how they reach their decisions and the rules used can be made available to the user. In theory this makes them useful as teaching tools. The novice can follow the decision path taken and see how information was combined and analysed. A major problem with programmes such as MYCIN is that it takes a lot of work to develop them and they are strictly limited to narrow domains of knowledge. MYCIN, for example, was very good at prescribing antibiotics for septicaemia but could do nothing else. Modern AI systems work in very different ways.

Artificial neural networks attempt to simulate brain function. They often work with probabilities. Significant progress has been made in recent years because of improvements in processing power and the availability of vast amounts of data for machine learning. Their 'learning' ability is one of the most distinguishing features of modern AI systems, especially because learning can now occur very quickly. However, there are potential problems. It is a common observation that the machine learning of an AI is only as good as the data it is provided to learn from. If there are significant biases in the data, the AI is likely to reproduce these. This is, of course, the same problem that has confronted the developers of CPGs from the start. Poor quality evidence will result in poor quality CPGs. There is a possibility that AI can be used by CPG development groups to assist in the gathering and evaluation of evidence as CPGs evolve. For more on the practicalities of developing AI within CPGs see Oliveira et al. (2013) and Rajpurkar et al. (2022). Ethical aspects of integrating AI into CPG development and usage will continue to be a challenge.

Seng (2020) points out that many organizations have ethical principles and statements that are supposed to guide the development of AI. However, they are often vague and difficult to implement in any practical sense. Another ethical problem is that ethical/moral principles can contradict and conflict with each other. Ethical problems are also often insoluble from a purely rational perspective as there can be many conflicts and contradictions, together with a great deal of ambiguity. Within the field of bioethics there has never been any agreement on a moral theory that is useful under all circumstances. Utilitarianism, for example, may be useful as a moral theory when developing public health policy but is completely inadequate when making end-of-life decisions for an individual patient in palliative care (Beauchamp and Childress, 2009). As Seng (2020) points out, ethical debates need 'complex reflection of moral circumstances, valid argumentation, and rational justifications' (p. 168). It is clear that AI has great potential in healthcare in general and the development and implementation of AI in CPGs in particular also has great promise. However, there are many problematic details that have yet to be worked out in the next few years.

SUMMARY

CPGs have been used to assist clinical reasoning for some decades now. There are now thousands of CPGs available. They have not been without controversy for several reasons. These reasons include being developed with evidence from particular populations that distort the recommendations being made so that they do not apply to all patients. CPGs were originally seen as aids to clinical practice but they are sometimes used to monitor clinical performance. In this chapter, we have looked at some of these issues, focussing on attempts

to adapt CPGs for local contexts. We have also looked at trends in CPG development and usage, such as the influence that advances in AI may have on CPG development and implementation.

REFERENCES

Beauchamp, T.L., Childress, J.F., 2009. Principles of biomedical ethics, 6th ed. Oxford University Press, USA.

Chakraborty, S., Brijnath, B., Dermentzis, J., Mazza, D., 2020. Defining key questions for clinical practice guidelines: A novel approach for developing clinically relevant questions. Health Res Policy Syst 18 (1), 113. https://doi.org/10.1186/s12961-020-00628-3

Cormican, A., Hirani, S.P., McKeown, E., 2023. Healthcare professionals' perceived barriers and facilitators of implementing clinical practice guidelines for stroke rehabilitation: A systematic review. Clin Rehabil 37 (5), 701–712. https://doi.org/10.1177/02692155221141036

Davis, R., Buchanan, B., Shortliffe, E., 1977. Production rules as a representation for a knowledge-based consultation program. Artificial Intelligence 8 (1), 15–45.

Dizon, J.M., Machingaidze, S., Grimmer, K., 2016. To adopt, to adapt, or to contextualise? The big question in clinical practice guideline development. BMC Res Notes 9 (1), 442. https://doi.org/10.1186/s13104-016-2244-7

Guyatt, G.H., Oxman, A.D., Vist, G.E., Kunz, R., Falck-Ytter, Y., Alonso-Coello, P., et al., 2008. GRADE: An emerging consensus on rating quality of evidence and strength of recommendations. BMJ 336 (7650), 924–926. https://doi.org/10.1136/bmj.39489.470347.AD

Grimmer, K., Louw, Q., Dizon, J.M., Brown, S.M., Ernstzen, D., Wiysonge, C.S., 2019. A South African experience in applying the Adopt-Contextualise-Adapt framework to stroke rehabilitation clinical practice guidelines. Health Res Policy Syst 17 (1), 56. https://doi.org/10.1186/s12961-019-0454-x

Johnson, S., 2016. Pathways of care: What and how? Journal of Managed Care 1 (1), 15–17. https://doi.org/10.1177/136395959700100106

Mustafa, R.A., Santesso, N., Brozek, J., Akl, E.A., Walter, S.D., Norman, G., et al., 2013. The GRADE approach is reproducible in assessing the quality of evidence of quantitative evidence syntheses. Journal of Clinical Epidemiology 66 (7), 736–742. https://doi.org/10.1016/j.jclinepi.2013.02.004.e735

Oliveira, T., Novais, P., Neves, J., 2013. Development and implementation of clinical guidelines: An artificial intelligence perspective. Artificial Intelligence Review 42 (4), 999–1027. https://doi.org/10.1007/s10462-013-9402-2

Pfadenhauer, L.M., Mozygemba, K., Gerhardus, A., Hofmann, B., Booth, A., Lysdahl, K.B., et al., 2015. Context and implementation: A concept analysis towards conceptual maturity. Z Evid Fortbild Qual Gesundhwes 109 (2), 103–114. https://doi.org/10.1016/j.zefq.2015.01.004

Pierpoint, M., Pillay, M. (2020). Post-stroke dysphagia: An exploration of initial identification and management performed by nurses and doctors. South African Journal of Communication Disorders 67 (1), a625. https://doi.org/10.4102/sajcd.v67i1.625

Rajpurkar, P., Chen, E., Banerjee, O., Topol, E.J., 2022. AI in health and medicine. Nat Med 28 (1), 31–38. https://doi.org/10.1038/s41591-021-01614-0

Satterfield, J.M., Spring, B., Brownson, R.C., Mullen, E.J., Newhouse, R.P., Walker, B.B., et al., 2009. Toward a transdisciplinary model of evidence-based practice. Milbank Q 87 (2), 368–390. https://doi.org/10.1111/j.1468-0009.2009.00561.x

Schrijvers, G., van Hoorn, A., Huiskes, N., 2012. The care pathway: Concepts and theories: an introduction. Int J Integr Care, 12(Spec Ed Integrated Care Pathways):e192. https://doi.org/10.5334/ijic.812. PMID: 23593066; PMCID: PMC3602959.

Seng, L., 2020. Current challenges in ethics of artificial intelligence or: Old wine in new bottles. In: Göcke, B.P., Rosenthal-von der Pütten, A. (Eds.), Artificial Intelligence: Reflections in philosophy, theology, and the social sciences. Brill Mentis, pp. 159–172.

Steinberg, E., Greenfield, S., Wolman, D.M., Mancher, M., Graham, R., 2011. Clinical practice guidelines we can trust. National Academies Press.

Tshivhase, M., 2019. South African-contextualised Stroke Rehabilitation Guideline (SA-cSRG). Stellenbosch University, Cape Town, South Africa. http://www.sun.ac.za/english/faculty/healthsciences/health-rehabilitation-sciences/Documents/Completed%20stroke%20guidelines_May2019.pdf

Vanhaecht, K., Panella, M., van Zelm, R., Sermeusand, W., 2010. 'What about care pathways?', in John Ellershaw, and Susie Wilkinson (eds), Care of the Dying: A pathway to excellence, 2nd edn (Oxford, 2010; online edn, Oxford Academic, 17 Nov. 2011), https://doi.org/10.1093/acprof:oso/9780199550838.003.0001, accessed 12 Aug. 2024.

14

EVIDENCE-BASED PRACTICE AND CLINICAL REASONING
How Are the Two Related?

ALIKI THOMAS ■ MEREDITH YOUNG

CHAPTER OUTLINE

CHAPTER AIMS

The aims of this chapter are:

- to explore relationships and differences between clinical reasoning and evidence-based practice
- to consider the implications of adopting different perspectives to understanding these relationships
- to consider why and how this relationship may be important in practice.

INTRODUCTION

Evidence-based medicine (EBM) and clinical reasoning are distinct but interrelated concepts and have evolved in relatively parallel literatures. Several definitions of EBM have emerged over the years sparked largely by differences in disciplinary and professional perspectives. One of the earliest and most commonly used definitions of EBM described 'the conscientious, explicit, and judicious use of current best evidence in making decisions about the care of individual patients. The practice of evidence-based medicine means integrating individual clinical expertise with the best available external clinical evidence from systematic research' (Sackett et al., 1996, p. 71). In parallel to an evolution of the concept of EBM, we have also seen an evolution in language surrounding the concept: professions such as nursing and rehabilitation have adopted terms such as evidence-based practice (EBP) (Bennett and Bennett, 2000) or evidence-based healthcare (EBHC) (Hammell, 2001) to reflect a broader application of this concept across health professions. For the purposes of this chapter, we will use the term EBP to reflect the multiple dimensions of the concept.

The EBP process has traditionally been reflected in the following five steps also called the '5 As of EBP': (1) ASK: consists of posing a clinical question; (2) ACQUIRE: is about searching and selecting relevant literature; (3) APPRAISE the literature using critical appraisal tools; (4) APPLY: consists of considering and using the research evidence in clinical decision making; (5) ASSESS: consists of reviewing and assessing the procedure and outcome of the EBP process on patient care (Sackett et al., 1996; Sackett et al., 2000) (Fig. 14.1). In parallel, many scholars have written about the attributes of EBP, that is, the skills that are required to enact EBP (Salbach et al., 2013; Shaneyfelt et al., 2006; Shi et al., 2014). Findings from an extensive body of

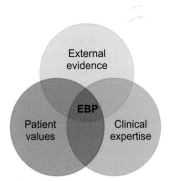

Fig. 14.1 ■ What is evidence-based medicine? (Adapted with permission from Sackett, D.L., Rosenberg, W.M., Gray, J.A., Haynes, B.R., Richardson, S.W., 1996. Evidence based medicine: What it is and what it isn't. BMJ 312, 71–72.)

research suggest that positive attitudes, knowledge and self-efficacy, as well as support from managers and affordances in the practice context, are necessary to support EBP (Albarqouni et al., 2018; Al Zoubi et al., 2018; Thomas et al., 2021).

Conceptualizations and ensuing refinements of the concept of EBP have evolved to include consideration for the sociohistorical, political, professional, economic and institutional contexts (Banningan and Moores, 2009) (Fig. 14.2). Further considerations can include explicit integration of the mandate of the healthcare organization, a role for community involvement and potential limitations imposed by organizational and resource constraints. This apparent evolution in what EBP is or represents is in large part a result of decades of debate about the merits of the EBP approach to decision making (Dijkers et al., 2012; Greenhalgh et al., 2015). A number of debates have been centralized around disagreements regarding the meaning and significance of evidence and the implications associated with clinical decision making based on evidence

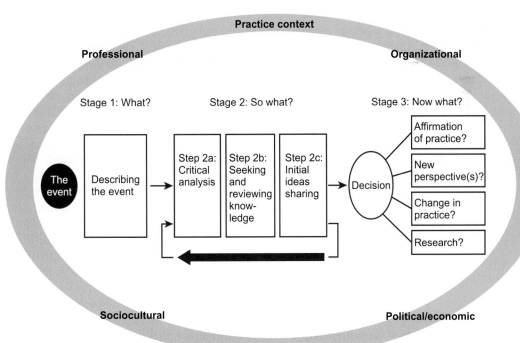

Fig. 14.2 ■ Model of professional thinking. (With permission from Banningan, K., Moores, A., 2009. A model of professional thinking: Integrating reflective practice and evidence based practice. Can. J. Occup. Ther. 76, 345.)

in contrast to clinical decisions informed by evidence (Greenhalgh et al., 2015; Mercuri and Baigrie, 2018).

The literature has been rich with discussions regarding the value of EBP and its corresponding epistemological foundations (Bennett et al. 2003; Djulbegovic et al., 2009; Hammell, 2001). It is beyond the scope of this chapter to delve into or preferentially support one particular viewpoint over another. The disputes and deliberations notwithstanding, EBP is regarded as an integral and necessary component of clinical decision making (Sackett et al., 2000; Salmond, 2013).

Clinical reasoning carries its own set of definitional challenges. There is an abundance of literature on clinical reasoning across disciplines, professions and methodological traditions, and clinical reasoning is considered core to the practice of health practitioners (Higgs et al., 2008; Schell, 2009). Though not as overtly contentious as the definition of EBP, there is little agreement about how to define the term clinical reasoning or what it entails (Durning et al., 2013; Young, Thomas et al., 2018; Young et al., 2020). Considered to be the backbone of professional practice (Higgs et al., 2008; Mattingly, 1991), clinical reasoning has been variably considered through the lens of outcomes (i.e. reasoning is 'seen' by the decisions made by a practitioner – whether through accuracy (Monteiro and Norman, 2013; Graber, 2013), as an individual cognitive process (i.e. reasoning is the process by which a decision is made by a clinician) (Eva, 2005), as a negotiated patient- or client-centred process (i.e. shared decision making or patient-as-partner (Braddock et al., 1999)), as a socially and healthcare-team embedded activity (i.e. team-based reasoning (Graber et al., 2017)), or as a general means by which healthcare providers generate a diagnosis, treatment or management plan (Cook et al., 2018; Eva, 2005).

REFLECTION POINT

■ To you, is clinical reasoning an outcome, a process, a means to an end, or something else?

Clinical reasoning and EBP have, for the most part, existed in parallel bodies of literature attempting to describe the practice of health professionals and suggest areas of improvement. Both literatures house independent debates regarding how a clinician should 'best solve' a clinical case, discuss areas for better patient outcomes, and how best to support clinical decisions. Increasingly scholars are exploring the relationship between the two and questioning whether there are areas of similarity or overlap. Though these have been historically siloed areas of work, important questions remain. Here, we propose to delve into three different ways of thinking about the relationship between EBP and clinical reasoning. The purpose of this chapter is not to provide a right answer to these questions, but rather, to explore these different ways of thinking about the interrelationship between clinical reasoning and EBP and the potential implications for how we think about, teach and study these central phenomena. In this chapter, we summarize appropriate frameworks or theories relevant to the relationship between EBP and clinical reasoning, consider potential unintended consequences of adopting any one of the relationships described, to discuss how these different interplays between EPB and clinical reasoning might manifest in clinical practice and to identify areas rich for future research.

The chapter is organized in three sections, each representing a different stance regarding the relationship between clinical reasoning and EBP. Within each section we pose a series of questions for reflection. The first section explores *EBP as one form of clinical reasoning*. Drawing from the literature on the theoretical and philosophical tenets of EBP, we present circumstances in which EBP is one likely way in which clinical reasoning unfolds or manifests and potential downstream consequences of this conceptualization. Then we discuss implications for health professionals who may be situated within this perspective and present unanswered questions for reflection and future research.

In the second section, we explore the premise that *Evidence-based Practice is the way one should reason clinically*. In this section, we draw primarily from the clinical reasoning literature to highlight how this relationship may or may not hold true depending on the chosen theoretical perspective informing clinical reasoning. We conclude the section with potential downstream consequences, implications for practitioners and future areas for research.

In the final section we consider the proposition that *EBP and clinical reasoning are distinct but related concepts*. We begin this section by presenting the multiple possible conceptualizations of evidence and propose that evidence is more than knowledge generated through empirical research. As with the first two sections, we explore potential downstream consequences of this approach and what this may mean for a practising health professional with a focus on issues of professional autonomy and discuss avenues for future research.

SECTION 1: EBP IS ONE FORM OF CLINICAL REASONING

Clinical reasoning has been proposed to encompass all cognitive and environmental factors that lead to, support and shape a final decision – whether about a diagnosis or treatment plan (Durning et al., 2013). If clinical reasoning reflects an overarching set of approaches or processes that are a means to an end, it stands to reason that EBP could be considered within the 'laundry list' of approaches or processes that lead to, support or shape a final clinical decision. As mentioned in the introduction to this chapter, there is an abundance of literature that converges on the notion that EBP is an approach to clinical decision making. It is considered an approach but not the only approach (Haynes, 2002). Whether one is referring to Sackett's earlier definition of EBP (Sackett et al., 1996) or conceptualizes EBP as per the transdisciplinary model by Banningan and Moores (2009) where we find new external frames containing the environment and the organizational factors likely to affect evidence-based decision-making, EBP emphasizes the interaction of three main factors within complex contexts: the best available evidence, input from the patient regarding their care and the clinician's experience and professional expertise (Craik and Rappolt, 2003; Thomas and Law, 2013). Fig. 14.1 is a traditional representation of EBP and in this Venn diagram, the clinical decision making lies in the middle: it is a result of the contribution of, and the interactions between, its three main components. There is no implied weight or size associated with each component, leaving one to presume that a clinical decision is the result of equal interdependent contributions from each of the three components. Though this equitable balance of sources of information may be the case in some clinical situations, there is a paucity of research to substantiate such an interpretation.

REFLECTION POINT

■ How does this interpretation align with your view of the relationship between EBP and clinical reasoning?

The notion of balancing multiple sources of information (Yousefi-Nooraie et al., 2007) puts the onus and focus on the reasoning of the individual clinician. Much of the debate surrounding the EBP movement has been attributed to the implicit value judgement that an evidence-based approach to any clinical decision is only as good as the clinician who is responsible for balancing the multiple sources of evidence and of evaluating the available scientific evidence, considering it in light of the patient's personal and unique circumstances and balancing the unique expertise of the clinician.

Haynes et al. (2002) have suggested that evidence on its own does not make decisions, that people make decisions. If one accepts this premise, it follows that most, if not all clinicians who find themselves in a situation of having to deliberately and consciously combine formal research evidence, patient preferences and a knowledge base derived from their own experience, are engaging in a particular form of clinical reasoning. The use of and reliance on information is predominantly for the end goal of making a clinical decision.

Combining various sources of data, making sense of the evidence, considering the patient's unique situation and goals for treatment would require that the clinician engage in clinical reasoning. In the absence of a reasoning process, it would seem reasonable to suggest that the various knowledge sources are discrete pieces of information without a unifying purpose and with limited meaning. If one accepts that clinical reasoning is a large collection of approaches and strategies used to reach a clinical decision (Young et al., 2020; Young et al., 2019), it follows that EBP represents one approach to reaching that decision and is one strategy amongst other strategies or approaches such as nonanalytic reasoning (Kulatunga-Moruzi et al., 2001), reliance on heuristics (Kahneman, 2011), mobilization of illness scripts (Charlin et al., 2007) and reflective practice (Kinsella, 2007).

Studies of experienced clinicians in rehabilitation contexts who embrace and apply EBP have shown that the patient is at the centre of all decisions (Craik and Rappolt, 2006; McCluskey et al., 2008; Thomas and Law, 2013; Thomas et al., 2012; Thomas et al.

(Forthcoming)). Although the available scientific evidence is used to inform assessment choices and treatment interventions, findings from these studies suggest that the reasoning involved in the decision-making process is largely influenced by a deep desire and motivation to improve patient outcomes (Thomas et al., 2012; Thomas et al., 2023). The scientific evidence in these circumstances is one tool in a clinician's repertoire. If EBP is one approach to clinical reasoning and formal scientific evidence is one component of that process, it follows that other component pieces such as clinical experience, patients' wishes, organizational mandates and professional culture are likewise significant and valued contributors to the reasoning process. In this conceptualization of EBP as one way of reasoning and evidence as a contributor to the process, these components are equally valued, recognized and rewarded.

If we adopt the view that EPB is one among many forms of clinical reasoning, several downstream consequences may become apparent (Box 14.1).

REFLECTION POINT

A medical scholar has been described in the CanMeds framework (Frank et al., 2015, p. 24) as 'physicians who demonstrate a lifelong commitment to excellence in practice through continuous learning and by teaching others, evaluating evidence, and contributing

to scholarship' and the medical expert described 'as a physician who provides high-quality, safe, patient-centred care, physicians draw upon an evolving body of knowledge, their clinical skills, and their professional values'.

- What would happen to the role of the medical scholar given this first perspective (i.e. that EBP is one form of clinical reasoning)?
- If we accept that EBP is one way, not the way, of engaging in clinical reasoning, how do we simultaneously encourage and promote the development of the scholarly practitioner?

AREAS FOR FUTURE RESEARCH

Accepting that *EBP is one form of clinical reasoning*, we are left with questions that we hope will stimulate discussion among our colleagues in the scholarly and clinical communities and present these as suggestions of areas for future research.

1. We need to understand better how evidence and other forms of knowledge are used and/or mobilized during the clinical reasoning process. It is possible that the process of evoking the evidentiary base for a clinical decision has become

---

BOX 14.1
DOWNSTREAM CONSEQUENCES OF THE VIEW THAT EBP IS ONE FORM OF CLINICAL REASONING

- EBP is 'one among many', not 'first amongst equals'. Therefore, it is not the 'best' way of reasoning, only one of many approaches to reasoning.
- If EPB is not the best kind of reasoning, but rather only one kind of reasoning, how do we decide what the best way to treat someone is? How do we develop decision algorithms or practice guidelines for best practice if EBP is just one way of reasoning?
- EBP may undervalue evidence that is not generated through empirical research. If EBP is only one potential approach to reasoning, what would the downstream consequences be for health professions education?
- The perspective that EBP is one potential approach to clinical reasoning may be both empowering and validating for clinicians. It supports the notion that there is a multiplicity of information and knowledge sources, factors that influence the reasoning process

and different 'means to an end'. This perspective allows recognition of the value of professional experience and clinicians' ability to make thoughtful decisions, some informed by best available scientific evidence, others not. Further, this perspective aligns well with what it means to be a health professional. Healthcare professionals have the autonomy to exercise judgement about how they make decisions (Cruess and Cruess 2008), what information sources they draw from in order to come to those decisions and under what circumstances they will resort to scientific evidence to support a clinical decision.

- Finally, this perspective suggests that complex health issues experienced by human beings with unique backgrounds and lived experiences cannot ultimately be reduced to problems that can and must be solved with the application of the best available scientific evidence.

automatic. If so, a clinician would not necessarily be engaging in the traditional evidence-based approach to practice with its corresponding five steps. In other words, EBP would not manifest as typically represented in the EBP literature. Is the practitioner still engaging in EBP? Or are they engaging in nonanalytic reasoning? What are the implications for education and continuing profession development, both in terms of process and practice change?

2. If we consider that *using or invoking the evidence* is, or can be, an automatic process, this may necessitate some conceptual reframing of the traditional understanding of EBP and the coordination with other clinical reasoning concepts such as nonanalytic reasoning.

3. What is the relative contribution of the scientific evidence to clinical reasoning, regardless of nomenclature? Some work has suggested the role of basic science in reasoning through novel problems (Woods et al., 2006); however, little is known regarding the extent to which clinicians evoke the evidence in a conscious or a more automatized process during decision making. In what kind of clinical situations would relying only on scientific evidence be most effective? How should this be communicated to learners and novice clinicians who, for the most part, have been trained in an era of formalized and stepwise EBP?

SECTION 2: EVIDENCE-BASED PRACTICE IS THE WAY ONE SHOULD REASON CLINICALLY

The assumption underlying this conceptualization is that EBP is how clinical reasoning should happen. It suggests that ideal clinical reasoning takes the form of EBP and, as such, is an integral part of clinicians' decision-making process. This conceptualization also assumes that all clinical decisions are, or ought to be, based on evidence. Thus, evidence of good clinical reasoning is through the 'doing' of EBP. In this case, if one accepts that EBP leads to better patient care, improves transparency, accountability and value, as has been suggested in the literature (Emparanza et al., 2015), then EBP is the way we should make decisions

about clinical care. Consequently, if clinical reasoning is best manifested as EBP, it should not be 'one of the ways to do it' but rather a 'first among equals' way of reasoning.

Consider three distinct instances of decision-making: a physician must order and justify the use of a series of diagnostic tests for acute onset of abdominal pain; a healthcare team must decide if a patient arriving in the emergency room with debilitating headaches needs immediate hospitalization; an occupational therapist considers how to provide psychosocial support for a young mother newly diagnosed with multiple sclerosis who is caring for her 3-month-old infant. Existing scientific evidence has informed the development of care algorithms or contributed to practice guidelines concerning the most appropriate use of health resources. Does the stepwise separation of scientific evidence from practice-based tools such as guidelines automatically divorce the enactment of these decisions from a frame of evidence-based tools? If good clinical reasoning is embodying the spirit (rather than solely the stepwise approach) of EBP, reliance on guidelines for good practice or care algorithms could be considered a manifestation of EBP. We reflect on this stance in Case Study 14.1.

What are the possible downstream consequences of this view of EBP (Box 14.2)?

Areas for Future Research

If we accept that EBP is the way one should reason clinically (i.e. clinical reasoning is enacted through EBP), we propose the following questions for discussion and future research:

1. Are there particular conceptualizations of clinical reasoning (Young et al., 2020) that are more amenable to the valuing of evidence and the consideration for EBP as a means to enact clinical reasoning? If such a conceptualization does not exist, could the health professions' education community benefit from multidisciplinary efforts towards developing one?

2. Do we need to understand *the balancing* of different sources of (potentially conflicting) evidence? If this is how clinicians 'should' reason, should we try to understand EBP as an overarching process or frame for clinical reasoning?

BOX 14.2

DOWNSTREAM CONSEQUENCES OF THE VIEW THAT EBP IS THE WAY ONE SHOULD REASON CLINICALLY

- If EBP is the means by which clinical reasoning should unfold, what happens to the concept of clinical reasoning in the absence of a concrete final decision? Does clinical reasoning need the decision-making framework of EBP to exist or to manifest itself? If one answers yes, how do we avoid a potential slippery slope whereby every decision, made under every possible circumstance, for all patients, in all contexts must by definition be made as a result of consulting or evoking the scientific evidence of some kind to be considered the result of good clinical reasoning? This perspective suggests that without a decision being made, or without an evidence base to draw from, there is no evidence of clinical reasoning. Anything that is not EBP is suboptimal or inadequate clinical reasoning. If EBP is manifested in a less than ideal manner, is enacted ineffectively or leads to the wrong decision for a given patient in a given situation and context, is this evidence of poor clinical reasoning?

- EBP, as defined in the literature and taught in many health professions' education programmes, is a deliberate, conscious process. If we accept the view that EBP is how clinical reasoning unfolds, it follows that understanding, valuing and teaching reasoning modes that are not perfectly conscious, structured, reportable and teachable become challenging at best and likely become devalued as reasoning processes.

- If we accept a broad definition of EBP in which scientific evidence, experiential knowledge and patient preferences are valued, the assumed necessary reasoning processes include the collection of evidence, the interpretation of that evidence and the balancing of that evidence across the three components of Fig. 14.1. If this is the interpretation of EBP being adopted, we assume that the framework of EBP is how reasoning should unfold and applying an EBP frame to the study of clinical reasoning may actually provide a more concrete structure through which to study the relatively nebulous concept of clinical reasoning.

- Finally, one could speculate that a consequence of disregarding contributors other than EBP approaches to clinical reasoning could result in devaluing professional expertise, which in turn can lead to professional dissatisfaction and clinician resentment towards efforts aimed at promoting EBP. Indeed, there are many lessons learned from earlier studies exploring attitudes towards EBP. Earlier studies showed clinicians less than favourable perceptions of and attitudes towards EBP were in part a result of an overemphasis on scientific evidence to the detriment of professional experience and expertise and the role that clinical reasoning plays in decision making (Dubouloz et al., 1999).

---

3. If EBP is how clinical reasoning should unfold, what are the implications for other theories or models of clinical reasoning across the health professions? Do they become actively discouraged? Does EBP then become distanced from its roots in order to become the accepted *stand in* for what makes for good and defensible clinical reasoning?

REFLECTION POINT

- How does this interpretation match your view of the relationship between EBP and clinical reasoning?

SECTION 3: EBP AND CLINICAL REASONING ARE DISTINCT BUT RELATED CONCEPTS

Are EBP and clinical reasoning different approaches to understanding decision making in clinical settings? In

this last stance regarding the relationship between the two processes, we propose that both clinical reasoning and EBP are approaches to understanding clinical decision making; that they are both means to arriving at a clinical decision. The EBP literature explores how a practitioner combines the scientific evidence with patients' input and their clinical experience when making a final decision. The clinical reasoning literature explores how the process of generating a clinical decision unfolds across a variety of care contexts. Both centre on the critical decisions that are made by healthcare providers, but these different literatures apply different theories and different approaches to research and focus on different components of the processes that generate a clinical decision.

Clinical reasoning, though a fragmented literature, has also been discussed as a means to an end, a process used to establish a diagnosis in order to decide and implement the best possible course of action (Eva, 2005). Although clinical reasoning has been informed

CASE STUDY 14.1

Julie is a physiotherapist working in an inpatient rehabilitation centre specializing in musculoskeletal conditions. She is asked whether Mrs. Jones, her 79-year-old recently widowed patient with a new onset of falls, is a suitable candidate for an outpatient falls prevention programme offered in the community. Knowing that Mrs. Jones lives alone, that she has limited social support and is at risk of recurrent falls, Julie discusses the benefits of the programme with Mrs. Jones and suggests that they look into transportation services. In this example, Julie is not formally searching for scientific research, not engaging in the 'stepwise' approach to EBP, nor is she appraising papers for their quality or relevance to Mrs. Jones' situation. She is, however, drawing from her practice knowledge of the effectiveness of fall prevention programmes to help her in suggesting and promoting the programme to her patient. Most importantly, her clinical decision is very much influenced by her in-depth knowledge of the lived experience and situation that her patient finds herself in. She knows that a recently widowed older adult with limited social support may isolate herself by fear of being a burden on her family or putting herself at greater risk of falling by venturing out of her home more often. Yet Mrs. Jones refuses to participate. Her decision to forego the fall prevention programme is further justified given her limited access to transportation services to the community centre where the programme is being offered.

This sophisticated and presumably rapid decision-making process rests upon Julie's extensive knowledge base of: the effectiveness of fall prevention interventions for community dwelling seniors, the functional outcomes following falls and injuries and the typical developmental features of the ageing process. Could Julie's decision about recommending the fall prevention programme be made without evoking the scientific literature? In other words, could Julie conclude through a process of clinical reasoning that this would be a beneficial programme for her patient without having to go through the full formal EBP stepwise process?

We suggest that it is indeed possible, particularly given the more modern broad definitions of EBP, and we posit that this situation occurs frequently. This scenario suggests that Julie is balancing various sources of knowledge and evidence when reasoning. She is, therefore, engaging in EBP and is likely to be demonstrating good clinical reasoning. This reflects the notion that EBP is the way in which clinical reasoning does, or should, unfold.

---

by a variety of theories, stances and perspectives, a common theme amongst these approaches has been the notion that clinical reasoning produces diagnoses, management plans or investigative plans. In other words, it is a process that ends in a decision (Durning et al., 2013; Eva, 2005; Young, Thomas et al., 2018). Viewed in this way, clinical reasoning and EBP are both processes or approaches used to come to a decision, whether that decision is about a diagnostic test, a discharge date, about admitting a patient to hospital or about assessing an older adult's competence to care for themselves. Although the components or nature of these processes are not trivial or inconsequential given that they likely contribute to the end goal (i.e. clinical decisions), they may take a backseat to the actual decision.

Alternatively, clinical reasoning and EBP could be two different families of approaches to the study of how clinical decisions are made, with different areas of focus, importance and value stances as to what are important contributors to the process of generating a clinical decision and shaping the research within each field. Clinical reasoning and EBP have emerged from different disciplinary areas; clinical reasoning emerging primarily from cognitive science and psychology and EBP from epidemiology, and as such, may have concretized different areas of focus or importance for the same set of processes. Although this interpretation remains speculative, and probably contentious, it is an area for future research. Consider the downstream consequences of this view (Box 14.3).

REFLECTION POINT

■ How does this interpretation match your view of the relationship between EBP and clinical reasoning?

BOX 14.3

DOWNSTREAM CONSEQUENCES OF THE VIEW THAT EBP AND CLINICAL REASONING ARE DISTINCT BUT RELATED CONCEPTS

- Accepting this view suggests that the component processes are less important than the quality of the eventual outcome as long as a decision is made, how the individual 'got there' is not as important. We propose that this has potentially precarious implications for teaching and assessment, particularly given the increasing attention to assessing process of learning as well as outcomes (Bransford et al., 2000; National Research Council, 2001).
- If EBP and clinical reasoning are indeed two different ways of understanding clinical decision making but remain largely in different research silos, we are not advancing the knowledge base, nor well situated to move our field(s) forward. We may actually be failing to clarify concepts that may reflect linguistic differences rather than conceptual ones.

Areas for Future Research

If we agree that EBP and clinical reasoning are distinct but related concepts, we propose the following questions for reflection and discussion:

1. The research community should find areas of overlap, similarity and differences across these bodies of work in order to deepen understanding of these key principles.
2. What main messages do we want to send to educators and scholars who teach, assess and study decision making in and out of the classroom about how best to teach or assess EBP or clinical reasoning?
3. If EBP and clinical reasoning both focus on decision-making processes, what cues would be available to see 'high quality reasoning or decision making' whether labelled as clinical reasoning or EBP?
4. How can we best design teaching, assessment and continuing professional development activities to align with and to promote both?

SUMMARY

This chapter presented three different stances regarding the relationship between clinical reasoning and EBP. We have deliberately not chosen to privilege one of these views. Rather we have presented them critically, considering practice, education and research implications. We invite readers to reflect on their own stance to the relationship, areas of overlap and areas of differentiation between these two concepts.

REFLECTION POINT

- Do the arguments presented in this chapter reflect your current stance on the relationship between EBP and clinical reasoning?
- Do they prompt you to consider a new stance?
- What implications arising from this discussion might lead you to make a change in your practice?

REFERENCES

Albarqouni, L., Hoffmann, T., Straus, S., Olsen, N.R., Young, T., Ilic, D., et al., 2018. Core competencies in evidence-based practice for health professionals: Consensus statement based on a systematic review and Delphi survey. JAMA Network Open vol. 1 (no.2), e180281. https://doi.org/10.1001/jamanetworkopen.2018.0281

Al Zoubi, F., Mayo, N., Rochette, A., Thomas, A., 2018. Applying modern measurement approaches to constructs relevant to evidence-based practice among Canadian physical and occupational therapists. Implementation Science 13 (1), 152. https://doi.org/10.1186/s13012-018-0844-4

Banningan, K., Moores, A., 2009. A model of professional thinking: Integrating reflective practice and evidence based practice. Canadian Journal of Occupational Therapy 76 (5), 342–350. https://doi.org/10.1177/000841740907600505

Bennett, S., Bennett, J.W., 2000. The process of evidence-based practice in occupational therapy: Informing clinical decisions. Australian Occupational Therapy Journal 47 (4), 171–180. https://doi.org/10.1046/j.1440-1630.2000.00237.x

Bennett, S., Tooth, L., McKenna, K., Rodger, S., Strong, J., Ziviani, J., et al., 2003. Perceptions of evidence based practice: A survey of occupational therapists. Australian Occupational Therapy Journal 50, 13–22. https://doi.org/10.1046/j.1440-1630.2003.00341.x

Braddock, C.H., III, Edwards, K.A., Hasenberg, N.M., Laidley, T.L., Levinson, W., 1999. Informed decision making in outpatient practice time to get back to basics. JAMA 282 (24), 2313–2320. https://doi.org/10.1001/jama.282.24.2313

Bransford, J.D., Brown, A., Cocking, R., 2000. How people learn: Brain, *mind, experience, and school.* National Academy Press.

Charlin, B., Boshuizen, H.P., Custers, E.J., Feltovich, P.J., 2007. Scripts and clinical reasoning. Medical Education 41 (12), 1178–1184. https://doi.org/10.1111/j.1365-2923.2007.02924.x

Cook, D.A., Sherbino, J., Durning, S.J., 2018. Management reasoning: Beyond the diagnosis. JAMA 319 (22), 2267–2268. https://doi.org/10.1001/jama.2018.4385

Craik, J., Rappolt, S., 2003. Theory of research utilization enhancement: A model for occupational therapy. Canadian

Journal of Occupational Therapy 70 (5), 266–275. https://doi.org/10.1177/000841740307000503

Craik, J., Rappolt, S., 2006. Enhancing research utilization capacity through multifaceted professional development. American Journal of Occupational Therapy 60, 155–164. https://doi.org/10.5014/ajot.60.2.155

Cruess, R.L., Cruess, S.R., 2008. Expectations and obligations: Professionalism and medicine's social contract with society. Perspectives in Biology and Medicine 51 (4), 579–598. https://doi.org/10.1353/pbm.0.0045

Dijkers, M.P., Murphy, S.L., Krellman, J., 2012. Evidence-based practice for rehabilitation professionals: Concepts and controversies. Archives of Physical Medicine and Rehabilitation 93 (Suppl. 8), S164–S176. https://doi.org/10.1016/j.apmr.2011.12.014

Djulbegovic, B., Guyatt, G., Ashcroft, R., 2009. Epistemologic inquiries in evidence-based medicine. Cancer Control 16 (2), 158–168. https://doi.org/10.1177/107327480901600208

Dubouloz, C.J., Egan, M., Vallerand, J., von Zweck, C., 1999. Occupational therapists' perceptions of evidence-based practice. The American Journal of Occupational Therapy 53 (5), 445–453. https://doi.org/10.5014/ajot.53.5.445

Durning, S.J., Artino Jr, A.R., Schuwirth, L., van der Vleuten, C., 2013. Clarifying assumptions to enhance our understanding and assessment of clinical reasoning. Academic Medicine 88 (4), 442–448. https://doi.org/10.1097/ACM.0b013e3182851b5b

Emparanza, J.I., Cabello, J.B., Burls, A.J., 2015. Does evidence-based practice improve patient outcomes? An analysis of a natural experiment in a Spanish hospital. Journal of Evaluation in Clinical Practice 21 (6), 1059–1065. https://doi.org/10.1111/jep.12460

Eva, K.W., 2005. What every teacher needs to know about clinical reasoning. Medical Education 39 (1), 98–106. https://doi.org/10.1111/j.1365-2929.2004.01972.x

Frank, J., Snell, L., Sherbino, J., 2015. CanMEDS 2015 physician competency framework. Royal College of Physicians and Surgeons of Canada.

Graber, M.L., 2013. The incidence of diagnostic error in medicine. BMJ Quality and Safety 1 (suppl. 22), ii21–ii27. https://doi.org/10.1136/bmjqs-2012-001615

Graber, M.L., Rusz, D., Jones, M.L., Farm-Franks, D., Jones, B., Gluck, J.C., et al., 2017. The new diagnostic team. Diagnosis 4 (4), 225–238. https://doi.org/10.1515/dx-2017-0022

Greenhalgh, T., Snow, R., Ryan, S., Rees, S., Salisbury, H., 2015. Six 'biases' against patients and carers in evidence-based medicine. BMC Medicine 13 (1), 200. https://doi.org/10.1186/s12916-015-0437-x

Hammell, K.W., 2001. Using qualitative research to inform the client-centered evidence-based practice of occupational therapy. British Journal of Occupational Therapy 64, 228–234. https://doi.org/10.1177/030802260106400504

Haynes, R.B., 2002. What kind of evidence is it that evidence-based medicine advocates want healthcare providers and consumers to pay attention to? BMC Health Services Research 2, 3. https://doi.org/10.1186/1472-6963-2-3

Haynes, R.B., Devereaux, P.J., Guyatt, G.H., 2002. Clinical expertise in the era of evidence-based medicine and patient choice. ACP Journal Club 136 (2), A11–A14. https://doi.org/10.1136/ebm.7.2.36

Higgs, J., Jones, M., Loftus, S., Christensen, N. (Eds.), 2008. Clinical reasoning in the health professions, 3rd ed. Elsevier.

Kahneman, D., 2011. Thinking, fast and slow. Doubleday.

Kinsella, E.A., 2007. Embodied reflection and the epistemology of reflective practice. Journal of Philosophy of Education 41 (3), 395–409. https://doi.org/10.1111/j.1467-9752.2007.00574.x

Kulatunga-Moruzi, C., Brooks, L.R., Norman, G.R., 2001. Coordination of analytic and similarity-based processing strategies and expertise in dermatological diagnosis. Teaching and Learning in Medicine 13 (2), 110–116. https://doi.org/10.1207/S15328015TLM1302_6

Mattingly, C. (1991). What is clinical reasoning? The American Journal of Occupational Therapy: Official Publication of the American Occupational Therapy Association, 45(11), 979–986. DOI: 10.5014/ajot.45.11.979

McCluskey, A., Home, S., Thompson, L., 2008. Becoming an evidence-based practitioner. In: Law, M., MacDermid, J. (Eds.), Evidence-based rehabilitation: A guide to practice, 2nd ed. Slack, p. 35.

Mercuri, M., Baigrie, B.S., 2018. What confidence should we have in GRADE? Journal of Evaluation in Clinical Practice 24 (5), 1240–1246. https://doi.org/10.1111/jep.12993

Monteiro, S.M., Norman, G., 2013. Diagnostic reasoning: Where we've been, where we're going. Teaching and Learning in Medicine 25 (Suppl. 1), S26–S32. https://doi.org/10.1080/10401334.2013.842911

National Research Council, 2001. Implications of the new foundations for assessment design. In: Pellegrino, J.W., Chudowsky, N., Glaser, R. (Eds.), Knowing what students know: The science and design of educational assessment. National Academy Press, pp. 176–219.

Sackett, D.L., Rosenberg, W.M., Gray, J.A., Haynes, B.R., Richardson, S.W., 1996. Evidence based medicine: What it is and what it isn't. BMJ 312, 71–72. https://doi.org/10.1136/bmj.312.7023.71

Sackett, D.L., Straus, S.E., Richardson, W.S., Rosenberg, W., Haynes, R.B., 2000. Evidence-based medicine: How to practice and teach EBM, 2nd ed. Churchill Livingstone.

Salbach, N.M., Jaglal, S.B., Williams, J.I., 2013. Reliability and validity of the evidence-based practice confidence (EPIC) scale. Journal of Continuing Education in the Health Professions 33 (1), 33–40. https://doi.org/10.1002/chp.21164

Salmond, S.W., 2013. Finding the evidence to support evidence-based practice. Orthopaedic Nursing 32 (1), 16–22. https://doi.org/10.1097/NOR.0b013e31827d960b

Schell, B.A.B., 2009. Professional reasoning in practice. In: Crepeau, E.B., Cohn, E.S., Schell, B.A.B. (Eds.), Willard and Spackman's occupational therapy, 10th ed. Lippincott Williams & Wilkins, pp. 314–327.

Shaneyfelt, T., Baum, K.D., Bell, D., Feldstein, D., Houston, T.K., Kaatz, S., et al., 2006. Instruments for evaluating education in evidence-based practice: A systematic review. Journal of the American Medical Association 296 (9), 1116–1127. https://doi.org/10.1001/jama.296.9.1116

Shi, Q., Chesworth, B., Law, M., Haynes, B.R., Macdermid, J.C., 2014. A modified evidence-based practice-knowledge, attitudes, behaviour and decisions/outcomes questionnaire is valid across multiple professions involved in pain management. BMC Medical Education 14, 263. https://doi.org/10.1186/s12909-014-0263-4

Thomas, A., Al Zoubi, F., Mayo, N., Ahmed, S., Amari, F., Bussières, A., et al., 2021. Individual and organizational factors associated with evidence-based practice among physical and occupational therapy recent graduates: A cross-sectional national study. Journal of Evaluation in Clinical Practice 27 (5), 1044–1055. https://doi.org/10.1111/jep.13518

Thomas, A., Amari, F., Mylopoulos, M., Vachon, B., Menon, A., Rochette, A., 2023. Being and becoming an evidence-based practitioner: Occupational therapists' journey towards expertise. The American Journal of Occupational Therapy 77 (5), 7705205030. https://doi.org/10.5014/ajot.2023.050193

Thomas, A., Law, M., 2013. Research utilization and evidence-based practice in occupational therapy: A scoping study. The American Journal of Occupational Therapy: Official Publication of the American Occupational Therapy Association 67 (4), e55–e65. https://doi.org/10.5014/ajot.2013.006395

Thomas, A., Saroyan, A., Lajoie, S.P., 2012. Creation of an evidence-based practice reference model in falls prevention: Findings from occupational therapy. Disability and Rehabilitation 34 (4), 311–328. https://doi.org/10.3109/09638288.2011.607210

Woods, N.N., Neville, A.J., Levinson, A.J., Howey, E.H., Oczkowski, W.J., Norman, G.R., 2006. The value of basic science in clinical diagnosis. Academic Medicine: Journal of the Association of American Medical Colleges 81 (10), 124–127. https://doi.org/10.1097/00001888-200610001-00031

Young, M., Dory, V., Lubarsky, S., Thomas, A., 2018. How different theories of clinical reasoning influence teaching and assessment. Academic Medicine 93, 1415. https://doi.org/10.1097/ACM.0000000000002303

Young, M.E., Thomas, A., Gordon, D., Gruppen, L., Lubarsky, S., Rencic, J., et al., 2019. The terminology of clinical reasoning in health professions education: Implications and considerations. Medical Teacher 41 (11), 1277–1284. https://doi.org/10.1080/0142159X.2019.1635686

Young, M.E., Thomas, A., Lubarsky, S., Ballard, T., Gordon, D., Gruppen, S., et al., 2018. Drawing boundaries: The difficulty in defining clinical reasoning. Academic Medicine 93 (7), 990–995. https://doi.org/10.1097/ACM.0000000000002142

Young, M.E., Thomas, A., Lubarsky, S., Gordon, D., Gruppen, L., Rencic, J., et al., 2020. Mapping clinical reasoning literature across the health professions: A scoping review. BMC Medical Education 20 (1), 107. https://doi.org/10.1186/s12909-020-02012-9

Yousefi-Nooraie, R., Shakiba, B., Mortaz-Hedjri, S., Soroush, A.R., 2007. Sources of knowledge in clinical practice in postgraduate medical students and faculty members: A conceptual map. Journal of Evaluation in Clinical Practice 13 (4), 564–568. https://doi.org/10.1111/j.1365-2753.2007.00755.x

15

COLLABORATIVE DECISION MAKING IN LIQUID TIMES

FRANZISKA V. TREDE ■ JOY HIGGS

CHAPTER AIMS

The aims of this chapter are:

- to consider the importance of our liquid times for decision making
- to support critical social science as a basis for collaborative decision making
- to encourage practitioners to develop, critically, their own collaborative decision-making practices.

INTRODUCTION

Healthcare practice has changed significantly in recent years with rapid advances in technology. Healthcare practitioners can more easily share information and patients are more literate about their health conditions. Due to the social distancing orders during the COVID-19 pandemic, telehealth practices have received amplified attention. However, challenges to collaborating in decision making are persisting between practitioners, across healthcare disciplines and between clients and practitioners.

The way we practise, communicate and relate to each other is relentlessly changing and with it the way we make decisions. Decision making in healthcare practice is an important clinical reasoning process and issue. It has impact on efficiency and consequences for effectiveness and patient well-being.

In a simple (science-driven) world, healthcare practitioners would make expert decisions based on scientific empirico-analytical evidence, which promises the best health outcomes. In this world, patients would concur with the expert decision and carry out the behaviours required. This vision portrays decision making from a biomedical model perspective where the roles of patients and healthcare practitioners are clearly defined.

Decision making affects not only patients, their families and carers but also healthcare teams and services. Furthermore, decision making occurs within sociopolitical and economic contexts. Decisions about postsurgery treatment in a developed country with free healthcare looks different from that of developing countries with limited resources. The decision-making process needs to include economic, educational, cultural, ethical and material considerations. We have seen in the COVID-19 pandemic the huge impact of bed shortages. Whose interests prevail? What role is played by hospital budgets, bed occupancy, views about good health and the pursuit of a quality life? What else should be included that enables responsible, morally justifiable, productive and effective decisions? In this chapter we focus on collaborative decision making and explore the new conditions of decision-making processes in liquid times (or times of rapid change where the only real constant is change itself), discuss conceptual perspectives and principles of collaborative decision making and accentuate an agentive, critical practice perspective on collaborative decision making.

NEW CONDITIONS OF DECISION-MAKING PROCESSES IN LIQUID TIMES

Decision making is part of everyday healthcare practice. Many decisions can be made in a largely routine manner and require little conscious effort such as how to greet a patient, position oneself in relation to a patient, read progress notes and so on. However, sharing decision-making processes with patients and others was not routinely part of traditional healthcare. Today, in thinking about shared decision making, a number of additional considerations arise. What questions should be asked? How can we encourage patients to reveal their expectations, hopes and fears? What label should be used to describe a diagnosis? What treatment options should be discussed? All these questions relate to providing a social context and boundaries for shared discussions.

The way decisions are made impacts patients' motivation, persistence with treatment, sense of ownership, control and perceptions of healthcare outcomes. The more patients participate in the decision-making process, the more likely they are to be well informed, involved, satisfied and feel valued (Trede and Higgs, 2003). It is equally likely that healthcare practitioners who enable collaboration come to understand their

patients better, practise person-centred care more deeply and role model respect and curiosity more authentically.

Many factors support the case for collaboration in decision making and these factors have been well documented (Elwyn et al., 2012; Lin and Fagerlin, 2014; Matthias et al., 2013). These include ethical issues related to quality of life, end-of-life decisions, legal issues regarding informed consent, patients' rights for self-determination, patient safety, culturally appropriate care and valuing of diversity. Many patient complaints about healthcare relate to dissatisfaction with communication aspects of healthcare including poor communication skills of healthcare practitioners and breakdown in communication. Potentially, collaborative decision-making processes could be a means of overcoming some of the causes of poor communication. Collaboration and communication are considered as important as delivering quality healthcare. These expectations are influenced by such factors as changing attitudes to health and patients' rights, increasing cultural diversity of concepts of what constitutes good health, advocacy of community support and patient groups, increasing litigiousness, improved patient education, increased access to healthcare information via the Internet, and organizing self-help groups online.

The world of healthcare practices and systems has been evolving over the centuries and continues to do so. However, over the last decade and with the arrival of mobile technology, advances in artificial intelligence and telehealth, possibilities and conditions for practising and collaborating in healthcare have changed radically. As Floridi (2015, p. 131) argued, our thinking, doing and relating 'is fluidly changing in front of our eyes and under our feet, exponentially and relentlessly'. The new ways of practising that are fast, public and open, made possible by digital and mobile technologies, have made the old ways of doing things redundant because they no longer suit these new conditions. These changes bring with them the increasing contestation of the notion and superiority of 'the knowledge expert'. The role of privileged and restricted knowledge owned by individuals and professional groups that underpinned decision making (performed by experts for their clients) needs to be rethought. We live in transitional times where it remains unclear what knowledge, practices and structures will be redundant, what will persist and what will emerge as new. In short, we live in uncertain, ambiguous times.

Bauman (2012) coined the concept of 'liquid times' to give expression to the current times we live in. He makes two key points about his term 'liquid times'. The changes we are experiencing are much more fundamental and rapid than ever before. The term liquid times describes how the concept of time has quickened. Knowledge, practice and structures liquefy before they have had time to solidify. Bauman (2012) explains that old, solidified ways of doing are no longer working, but new ways of doing have not yet been established and there is no clarity about where new directions lead. The focus is now on immediacy, on short-term outcomes and instant impact. Holding on to old ideas and long-term commitments can be seen as being outdated. Thus, standing still or slowing down is seen as a risk in liquid times. In this context, long-term thinking and long-term goals have collapsed and have been replaced by strategies that focus on being agile and keeping up with the latest developments.

The second assertion Bauman makes is his observation of a separation between power and politics. Regard for knowledge is decreasing, giving way to feeling. We live in postfactual times where it is increasingly difficult to distinguish between real and fake news. The idea of hard facts is changing to notions of fluid facts where new insights are generated more rapidly. The lifespan of knowledge is shortening more than ever before. We need to rethink how we interact with knowledge and news. This weakens certainty, control and authority. It also can undermine agency and confidence. The rapid developments in digital and mobile technologies provide a clear illustration of Bauman's argument. With digital and mobile technologies, boundaries are blurring between professions and laity, between personal and professional, and between producer and consumer of services.

In this context, predictability and certainty are increasingly unattainable. We have given up on modernity – the quest for certainty and control – and now live in liquid modernity – the acknowledgement of the need to align with complexity, diversity and ambiguity. Bauman (2012) describes liquid modernity as a world where '[e]verything could happen yet nothing can be done with confidence and certainty'. Liquid times remind us to stay humble. Yet, it is important to be mindful that not everything is liquid. Liquidity on its own would be meaningless. It becomes meaningful only in an interdependent relationship with solidity, where one without the other could not exist (Bauman, 2012). Without understanding and appreciating the role of solidity it would be impossible to understand and appreciate liquidity. Both provide opportunities and barriers and weighing up both enables deliberate, professional decision making.

Liquid times can be threatening but there are positive effects to living and working in liquid times, especially when it comes to collaborating in decision making. Liquid times make collaboration an imperative. In an increasingly complex and diverse healthcare landscape, collaborative decision making seems a desirable and productive way to proceed. It brings people together and engages with diversity. Healthcare models with strong and closed borders and rigid roles are no longer conducive to timely, safe and effective healthcare delivery. Instead, complex and global health problems and rich human diversity are in a state of constant growth, which cannot rest secure in the context of a single discipline, one healthcare model or one school of thought alone, as such rigidity cannot provide the answers and solutions. Instead, interdisciplinary, collaborative decision-making practices are needed in liquid times.

REFLECTION POINT

- How have you experienced liquid times?
- What changes and disruptions have you encountered in the last 12 months in your healthcare practice and more specifically in decision making?

CONCEPTUAL PERSPECTIVES AND PRINCIPLES OF COLLABORATIVE DECISION MAKING

Readiness for Collaborative Decision Making Is Not a Given

It cannot be taken for granted that patients (and clients) will be ready for and agree to participating in clinical decision-making processes or share in the responsibilities for clinical decision-making outcomes. Therefore, practitioners need to check on patients' readiness and willingness to collaborate in decision making about their healthcare.

Patients enter healthcare situations with a wide range of preparedness for the events that will unfold during their journey of ill-health or disability and limited preparedness (usually) for the processes and opportunities for decision making they will encounter. They may or may not have had time to investigate the nature of their condition or its medical management, to prepare mentally, physically or emotionally for the health situation they are facing, and to develop a position on what they want or hope their health outcome to be. In addition, they commonly do not have the relevant medical knowledge or expertise to understand adequately the nature of the condition, its treatment options and potential health outcomes.

Agreement to Participate in Collaborative Decision Making Needs to Be Checked via Informed Consent

Agreements (to participate and agreements about outcomes) need to be checked because patients may only indicate implicit agreement through apparent compliance with treatment or healthcare programmes. Practitioners need to consider whether agreements are real rather than apparent, and genuinely collaborative rather than a matter of compliance in the face of unbalanced power. To do this, practitioners need to ensure an authentic collaborative decision-making process is enabled, taking complex factors into consideration.

Many Factors Influence Patients' Agreements About Decisions – Yes May Not Mean (Informed) Yes

When it comes to the point of agreeing with a health professional or healthcare team in decision making, the patient's agreement could be influenced by many 'entry' factors. Any agreement or otherwise could also be influenced by factors within the communication or interaction, such as the relationship built up with the practitioner(s), language or cultural familiarity or barriers, aspects of behaviour such as intentions, motivations and practitioners' practice models (e.g. biomedical, biopsychosocial and emancipatory models). In addition, decision-making processes are influenced by professional authority, professional roles and expectations held by professional groups and the community.

Agreement May Be Apparent and Unchallenged Rather Than Genuine and Empowered

When clinicians and patients share the same values, intentions and interests, agreement is more likely. However, agreement or compliance that is unarticulated or unquestioned may not be true agreement at all. It is tempting to assume that patients adopt the role that practitioners assign to them, without checking with patients either at the point of decision making or during subsequent treatment programmes whether these roles are acceptable in terms of both ability and choice. Are patients reporting honestly on their perceptions of progress or their pain levels? Considering a critical perspective to decision making reminds us that commonality of values and interests between patients and practitioners should not be taken for granted.

CONCEPTUAL MODELS OF SHARED DECISION MAKING

The traditional way of decision making which was entrusted to expert practitioners no longer fits the new conditions where patients are not only encouraged but frequently expected to participate in their treatment decisions (Lin and Fagerlin, 2014). Today is the time to reframe the notion of decision-making experts to include practitioners *and* patients. Most of the literature on decision making has a tendency to use the term shared decision making but then discusses a great diversity of decision-making processes that range from paternalistic to informed decision making (Lin and Fagerlin, 2014). Makoul and Clayman (2006), in a systematic review of the literature on shared decision making, found great fluidity in what was understood by the term, ranging from clinician-led decision making across a spectrum to patient-led decision making. The authors listed essential elements of shared decision making: defining the problem, presenting the options, identifying patient values and preferences as well as doctor knowledge, and clarifying understanding. This checklist reflects the transactional procedures in decision making. Although this is a useful start, it falls short of considering contexts and deep-rooted motivations for collaborating.

Matthias et al. (2013) argued that shared decision making cannot be discussed out of context and requires consideration of the entire patient encounter and particularly the nature of the patient-practitioner relationship. Mulley et al. (2012) asserted that excluding patients from decision making can be the reason for misdiagnoses. What the literature is pointing to is the importance of integrating various interests and motivations that influence the reasoning behind decision making. To this end it is useful to consider a series of questions that helps to clarify assumptions about decision making and how knowledge is generated (Edwards et al., 2004).

REFLECTION POINT

Clarifying assumptions about decision making:

- When is it appropriate to be practitioner-centred and when is it appropriate to be patient-centred?
- Who has permission to define the problem?
- Who is authorized to identify and legitimize all the options?
- How are patients invited and encouraged to share their values?
- Whose understanding needs clarification?
- What counts as knowledge and evidence?

The Primacy of Interests: A Critical Social Science Model for Collaborative Decision Making

Interests are the motivations, intentions and goals that guide behaviours. In his seminal book *Knowledge and human interest*, Habermas (1972) identified three broad categories of interests that have implications for which knowledge, values and worldviews influence decision making. Of these three interest categories (technical, practical and emancipatory) we see emancipatory interests as most relevant to the liberatory goals mentioned that are linked to genuine patient-collaborative clinical decision making. Fig. 15.1 illustrates the extreme ends of the various interests that shape practice models.

Many scholars have delineated the dualism between practitioner-centred and patient-centred care (e.g. Lin and Fagerlin, 2014), leaving the reader and practitioner appreciating differences between these terms but not helping them to communicate and transcend this dualism. A critical perspective in this context starts with critical self-awareness of what motivates professional bias, professional authority and professional

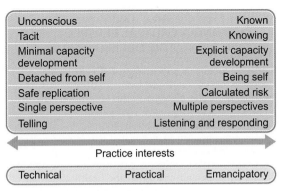

Unconscious	Known
Tacit	Knowing
Minimal capacity development	Explicit capacity development
Detached from self	Being self
Safe replication	Calculated risk
Single perspective	Multiple perspectives
Telling	Listening and responding

Practice interests

| Technical | Practical | Emancipatory |

Fig. 15.1 ■ Practice approaches.

roles, and it illuminates the various interests and interpretations underpinning practice approaches, especially those interests that pursue and drive power rather than reason. For example, adopting a critical perspective means seeking first to understand the historical and social factors and influences that have led practice to be accepted and valued the way it is (in a given context) and then to challenge and change this practice with the goal of emancipating those who are restricted or disempowered by it. Within this framework, practitioner-centred practice is typically practice that favours technical rationalism and privileges those in power (commonly the practitioners), whereas in truly (critical) patient-centred practice the practitioner seeks to share knowledge and power with the patient and to respect the input the patient can make to clinical decision making and healthcare management. Box 15.1 presents arguments in favour of adopting a critical perspective on collaborative decision making.

Collaboration is based on the conviction that inclusiveness and critical self-reflection produce better outcomes for patients than empirico-analytical precision. Collaborative decision making is based on inclusive evidence that entails embracing uncertainty and recognizing diversity of patients, clinicians and therapeutic environments (Jones et al., 2006). A critical approach helps practitioners to become conscious of their interests and choices in decision making because hidden agendas and bias are made explicit.

Collaborative decision making can be viewed as a strategy enabling practitioners to liberate themselves from unnecessary constraints to work authentically with patients, to empower patients to reclaim

BOX 15.1
ADOPTING A CRITICAL PERSPECTIVE IN COLLABORATIVE DECISION MAKING

When adopting a critical perspective in collaborative decision making, remember that:

- Not all parties involved in the decision-making process necessarily share the same values, intentions and interests about health beliefs and health behaviours. Decisions need to be negotiated free of coercion and power imbalances.
- Decision-making roles of practitioners and patients are dynamic and change as the health condition of patients progresses from acute, life-threatening to sub-acute and chronic conditions. Therefore, it is important to make conscious choices about which approach to decision making is appropriate.
- Patients are increasingly better informed and they (or at least many of them) want to know their options and be involved in decision making and self-management.
- Given appropriate opportunity and inclusive environments, most patients can be empowered to collaborate in decision making and have a say in their health management.

responsibility for their health, autonomy, dignity and self-determination. The intention of collaboration in critical practice is to engage in dialogue and to democratize roles. Collaboration starts with critique, scepticism and curiosity to deepen understanding and to identify the scope of common ground for change. In our work we have found that critique of decision making focussed on four closely interrelated dimensions:

- capacity for critical self-reflection
- rethinking professional roles
- rethinking professional power relations
- rethinking rationality and professional practice knowledge.

REFLECTION POINT

- Can you identify practice situations where collaborative decision making can be liberating for practitioners and patients?

OPERATIONALIZING COLLABORATIVE DECISION MAKING

There is not one way to operationalize collaborative decision making. There is scope for collaboration that amplifies one or all of the three human interests: technical collaboration, practical collaboration or critical collaboration. Interests are interdependent with the healthcare context, patient and practitioner willingness and capabilities for collaboration. In what follows, we focus on practitioners' collaborative decision-making practices using five prototypes (Trede, 2008). These prototypes (the uninformed, the unconvinced, the contemplators, the transformers and the champions) emerged from a research study that explored a critical practice model for physiotherapy. These prototypes can be applied to other healthcare disciplines. They are intended as a thinking tool and not as rigid professional identities to help make explicit the values and implications for nuanced, collaborative decision making.

The Uninformed

The *uninformed* are practitioners who are not aware of their own interests and how those interests influence their decisions; they know expertly about biomedical needs but are unsure and see as almost irrelevant what their patients really want and what their goals are. The uninformed group's practice interests are located in the technical, biomedical model. Practitioners do not think in terms of models or interests but react to presenting biophysical challenges. There seems to be a lack of reflexivity. The uninformed unknowingly adopt the mainstream approach to decision making. There is a tendency towards technical rather than emancipatory interests. One participant learned about collaborative decision making by reflecting upon a critical incident that made her question the way she tended to make clinical decisions (Box 15.2).

Seeing her patient mobilizing in a non-ideal way but with confidence and seeing him integrated into social community life helped this practitioner to question her goal-setting practices and her professional interests. Why should she make patients walk without a limp if all they wanted was to walk safely? This practitioner became aware of clashes between professional and patient goals. She was aware of peer expectations and she felt pressured to comply with the professional physiotherapy culture. Collaborative decision making is influenced not only by the stakeholders of decisions but also by the practice culture and the workplace environment.

BOX 15.2
BEING UNINFORMED

The penny dropped for me only after 10 years of clinical experience. I had [a patient with] an above-knee amputation and he had a prosthesis. He walked perfectly in the gym. I had him walk without a limp. I was really pleased with all this. Then I met him downtown in the shopping centre: he had his knee locked, he was walking on the inner quarter of his foot, foot stuck out at right angle and he was perfectly happy. I stood and looked at him and thought 'I can make you walk perfectly without a limp but you don't want to do that'. And you know when he came to treatment he would do it but obviously he wasn't feeling safe and he didn't want to do it that way and that is that. I think I wanted him to do what I wanted. I was trying to be a perfectionist. And it has also to do with all the other physiotherapists. They are checking on you that you are doing it all properly.

BOX 15.3
BEING UNCONVINCED

Giving the patients options is definitely making them feel more in control and you get a better response out of them. They don't just feel like sitting there having things done to them. They are having a bit more of a say about what is happening to them so it is good for both.

The Unconvinced

The *unconvinced* prototype are practitioners who equate collaboration with compliance. They feel that patients have to understand physiotherapy reasoning but they do not think that physiotherapists have to understand the way that patients reason. They do not challenge the biomedical interests that influenced the way they reach decisions (Box 15.3).

The unconvinced prototype experiences working in collaboration with patients as positive. However, their understanding of collaboration is narrowly defined because they limit the patients they choose to collaborate with. They notice that patients who share their values and expectations are more relaxed, which enables the unconvinced prototype to give them choice. These patients do not challenge unconvinced practitioners. They describe collaboration as patient compliance. With patients who question their practitioners they will choose to be more forceful.

The unconvinced categorize patients who do not agree as difficult people with stubborn personalities. It appeared that either patients work with the unconvinced or they will use professional power to get patients to comply. The unconvinced do not acknowledge their motivations and interests and they practise limited self-critique.

The Contemplators

The *contemplators* struggle with the concept of collaboration and patient emancipation. They interpret collaboration as allowing patients to dominate them and they reject this approach to decision making. However, they can see some benefits in trying to work with patients by 'making practice suitable to the patient's background, as much as their biomedical illnesses allowed'.

The contemplators understand collaborative decision making as persuading patients to adopt the physiotherapist's perspective. It is not based on egalitarian, equal terms; the biomedical perspective prevails unchallenged. Contemplators' practice values remain firmly grounded in the acute medical model despite appreciation of patients' individual fears and needs. They believe that once patients are familiar with their acute conditions they could be empowered to take more control and determine their own treatment routine in consultation (Box 15.4).

In Box 15.4 the pratitioner succinctly describes the attitude of the contemplators who see collaboration as optional and not suitable in some settings. The attitude is that practitioners have permission to assume professional power over their patients due to their professional status and knowledge. That is, they consider that professional relationships in the healthcare context start with uneven power relationships, where practitioners have more power than patients. Contemplators argue that patients have to be taken more seriously as people with a role to play in clinical decision making and self-management; however, they find it challenging to listen critically to patients and develop open dialogue with them.

The Transformers

The *transformers* are prepared to engage in democratizing their relationships with patients; they are willing to challenge their use of professional power. They

---

BOX 15.4
BEING A CONTEMPLATOR

'Doing-to' patients saves lives and prevents complications. 'Doing-to' is simple and straightforward. It means following my duty of care. In acute [settings], you focus on biomedical signs and you cannot always develop a relationship with the human being. In chronic settings you have time to develop a professional/personal relationship. In long-term rehabilitation you need to consider the human being more. It is more relaxing, working slower with patients.

BOX 15.5
BEING A TRANSFORMER

I could see that [this] patient was not interested in my plan. I thought this wasn't particularly functional [wanting to increase strength before increasing range of motion] but she was able to do everything: cook, clean, etc. The only thing she couldn't do was go shopping because she couldn't carry anything. So, that was really glaring in my face. This is what she wants to do. I am not sure if I always pick that up.

---

are attentive to interests and patients' expectations of physiotherapy. When patients have clear expectations and articulate what they want, the transformers are obliging (Box 15.5).

In Box 15.5, the practitioner appears to be comfortable with her patient's goals. Her decision was influenced by her patient's age. Had her patient been younger she might have insisted on improving range of motion as well. This practitioner made decisions in the context of her patient's age and function and with a critical stance to self. She was willing to reconsider. However, generally speaking, she was not content to allow patients to lead treatment plans unconditionally.

Transformers display a capacity for critical self-reflection in relation to their issues around professional authority and power relations (Box 15.6).

Transformers appreciate that they are not the only expert and that patients also have relevant knowledge. They reframe themselves as facilitators of collaborative decision making. They are operationalizing what they are learning from practice as a collaborative transformation.

The Champions

Champions operationalize collaborative decision making and endorse the values of inclusion and power-sharing. They are sceptical and critical of professional authority that is taken for granted and automatically assumed. Box 15.7 is a quote from a champion who identifies as a scientist, a critical self-reflector and a patient collaborator.

Champions integrate biomedical facts with patients' perceptions of their healthcare needs and condition. Their decision-making practice can be described as 'doing qualitative medicine'. They recognize that a collaborative approach to decision making does not exclude propositional or scientific knowledge but also requires nonpropositional knowledge to achieve emancipatory outcomes. Champions do not make decisions without continually checking their impact with individual patients; they regard patients as social, cultural and political human beings (Box 15.8).

BOX 15.6
BEING A TRANSFORMER

I want to learn from patients so that I can improve my own skills. I think that every treatment session is a learning session for me. I learn from my patients.

BOX 15.7
BEING A CHAMPION (1)

Is physiotherapy a social science? To me it is and my colleagues will hit me over the head. I think there are the arts and the sciences. It is somewhere between the two. You have to oscillate all the time to facilitate an outcome for the patient so I have this pulling force in me all the time. I value the scientific and searching for the evidence but I am worried about the patient.

BOX 15.8
BEING A CHAMPION (2)

You cannot tell a teenager to stop smoking. You need to look at their social issues. I practise physiotherapy like that. First [I consider] scientific knowledge and then social beliefs and patient knowledge.

In analysing the interviews with the champion group, a number of factors that indicated participants' capacity or inclination for participating in collaborative decision making were identified. These included:

- appreciating patients' perspectives (e.g. fear, lack of knowledge)
- becoming self-aware of personal bias
- actively providing opportunities for patients to participate
- being willing to reconsider treatment choices
- exploring options with patients
- establishing reciprocal relationships (by being open and enabling patients to be open)
- facilitating a reciprocal process of teaching and learning from each other
- recognizing clearly the values that inform decision making.

The champions in this study (Trede, 2008) used their human agency to facilitate change in their patients. They can be described as deliberate professionals (Trede and McEwen, 2016): they were aware of self, their patients and the context around them, they weighed up possibilities and made a decision together with their patients and shared responsibilities for the consequences of these decisions.

SUMMARY

In this chapter we:

- discussed the new conditions, diverse interests and fluid roles and contexts of practitioners and patients, as well as the complex processes that need to be meaningfully integrated in collaborative decision-making processes in these liquid times;
- identified a series of questions for clarifying assumptions about decision making;
- demonstrated the central importance of adopting a critical perspective on collaborative decision making;
- illustrated various operationalizations of collaborative decision-making practices.

REFLECTION POINT

- Can you see yourself as a practitioner in any of these prototypes?
- Where do you think students and experts fit into this set?
- What do you see as the implications for collaborative decision making?

REFERENCES

Bauman, Z., 2012. Liquid modernity. Polity Books.

Edwards, I., Jones, M., Higgs, J., Trede, F., Jensen, G., 2004. What is collaborative reasoning? Advances in Physiotherapy 6, 70–83. https://doi.org/10.1080/14038190410018938

Elwyn, G., Frosch, D., Thomson, R., Joseph-Williams, N., Lloyd, A., Kinnersley, P., et al., 2012. Shared decision making: A model for clinical practice. Journal of General Internal Medicine 27, 1361–1367. https://doi.org/10.1007/s11606-012-2077-6

Floridi, L., 2015. Hyperhistory and the philosophy of information policies. Philosophy and Technology 25 (2), 129–131. https://doi.org/10.1007/s13347-012-0077-4

Habermas, J., 1972. Knowledge and human interest (J.J. Shapiro, Trans.). Heinemann.

Jones, M., Grimmer, K., Edwards, I., Higgs, J., Trede, F., 2006. Challenges in applying best evidence to physiotherapy. The Internet Journal of Allied Health Sciences and Practice 4 (3). https://doi.org/10.46743/1540-580X/2006.1117

Lin, G.A., Fagerlin, A., 2014. Shared decision making: State of the science. Circulation: Cardiovascular Quality and Outcomes 7, 328–334. https://doi.org/10.1161/CIRCOUTCOMES.113.000322

Makoul, G., Clayman, M.L., 2006. An integrative model of shared decision making in medical encounters. Patient Education and Counseling 60 (3), 301–312. https://doi.org/10.1016/j.pec.2005.06.010

Matthias, M.S., Salyers, M.P., Frankel, R.M., 2013. Re-thinking shared decision making: Context matters. Patient Education Counseling 91, 176–179. https://doi.org/10.1016/j.pec.2013.01.006

Mulley, A.G., Trimble, C., Elwyn, G., 2012. Stop the silent misdiagnosis: Patients' preferences matter. BMJ 345, e6572. https://doi.org/10.1136/bmj.e6572

Trede, F.V., 2008. A critical practice model for physiotherapy: Developing practice through critical transformative dialogues. VDM Verlag Dr Müller.

Trede, F., Higgs, J., 2003. Re-framing the clinician's role in collaborative clinical decision making: Re-thinking practice knowledge and the notion of clinician–patient relationships. Learning in Health and Social Care 2 (2), 66–73. https://doi.org/10.1046/j.1473-6861.2003.00040.x

Trede, F., McEwen, C., 2016. Scoping the deliberate professional. In: Trede, F., McEwen, C. (Eds.), Educating the deliberate professional: Preparing for emergent futures. Springer.

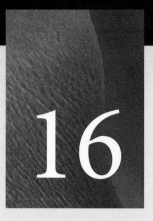

16

A MODEL FOR CLINICAL ETHICS REASONING IN ADULT AND PAEDIATRIC MEDICINE

ABRAM L. BRUMMETT ▪ MARK C. NAVIN ▪ ERICA K. SALTER

CHAPTER AIMS

The aims of this chapter are:

- to identify how the contemporary bioethics framework of principlism differs from the tradition of medical paternalism in moral reasoning
- to describe how principlism is operationalized in a standard model of decision making for both adult and paediatric medicine
- to reflect upon some ethical complexities that can arise when applying a standard model of clinical ethics reasoning.

INTRODUCTION

This chapter introduces clinicians to a model of clinical ethics reasoning that applies to adult and paediatric medicine. By understanding this model and its complexities clinicians will be better prepared to navigate ethical dilemmas and determine when it may be appropriate to seek consultation from a hospital clinical ethics service. The nature of clinical ethics services varies between hospitals. Some hospitals hire full-time clinical ethicists, others have committees or a small team of part-time or volunteer ethicists (Danis et al., 2021). The chapter begins with a brief history of the shift from medical paternalism to principlism in clinical ethics, describes a model of clinical ethics reasoning for adult and paediatric medicine in the United States and concludes by highlighting some complexities that invite further reflection. While this chapter is written from the perspective of authors in the United States, readers are invited to interpret the principles for application in their own unique healthcare contexts. Clinical cases are provided to stimulate reflection on key themes from the chapter.

FROM PATERNALISM TO PRINCIPLISM

We can contrast today's guidance for ethical clinical reasoning with the medical paternalism of previous generations. Medical paternalism placed decisions in the hands of the physician, guided solely by considering what *the physician* believed would produce the most benefit for the patient. A classic expression of paternalism can be found in an earlier version of the Hippocratic Oath, which reads, 'I will apply dietetic measures for the benefit of the sick *according to my ability and judgment*; I will keep them from harm and injustice' (Veatch and Guidry-Grimes, 2020, 269, emphasis added). Clinicians initially maintained a paternalistic orientation towards medicine in the face of 20th-century scientific advances that increased their abilities to intervene on patients, for example, the development of artificial ventilation and hemodialysis. Paternalism conflates technical expertise (e.g. that a particular intervention will produce certain effects) with moral expertise (e.g. that a particular intervention will be good for the patient) (Veatch, 2009). For example, the medical fact that chemotherapy could treat cancer supposedly generated the moral claim that a patient ought to undergo the treatment. It was believed that members of the profession that produced so many medical wonders were naturally best suited to decide which interventions sick patients should receive. In making decisions, physicians tended to presume the patient's health to be the highest good.

In the 1960s and 1970s, new legal and ethical conflicts challenged the role of medical paternalism in clinical reasoning and compelled clinicians to find other ways to make difficult decisions about patient care. For example, the invention of the indwelling shunt permitted patients to receive prolonged hemodialysis treatments, but the first hemodialysis center in Seattle possessed only 17 machines for the thousands of patients who needed them. Physicians with technical medical expertise about hemodialysis felt ill-equipped to make moral decisions about who ought to receive treatment. Instead, they created what came to be known as the Seattle God Squad, a seven-member committee composed of a minister, a lawyer, a housewife, a labour leader, a state government official, a banker and a surgeon that determined who would receive the life-saving treatment based on the dialysis candidate's employment status, children, education and professional achievements. The case of Dax Cowart offers another example. In 1973, this 25-year-old suffered severe burns over most of his body following a propane gas explosion. He was forcibly treated with painful chlorinated baths and bandage replacements for months despite repeatedly asking to be allowed to die, demonstrating how medical paternalism could run roughshod over a patient's refusal of medical treatment. A further example was the 1976 ruling of the New Jersey Supreme Court in the case of Karen Ann Quinlan. The court ruled in favour of her family's right to choose to have Karen's ventilator support be withdrawn and it suggested that hospitals establish ethics committees to address ethically complicated cases *before* they reach the courts (*In Re Quinlan*, 1976). These cases and many others like them occurred against the backdrop of important social movements that emphasized the moral importance of individual rights, such as the Civil Rights Movement and the Women's Liberation Movement. In the United States, attempts to establish clinical ethics consultation were bolstered by the passage of the Patient Self-Determination Act in 1991 and by the 1992 stipulation by the Joint Commission on Accreditation of Healthcare Organizations that member institutions must have a 'mechanism' for addressing moral uncertainty or conflict that arise during patient care (Joint Commission on Accreditation of Healthcare Organizations, 1993). However, the Joint Commission did not specify how the mechanism should be structured, for example, whether what was required was the intervention of an individual ethics consultant, a committee, or a small consultation team. Regardless of the particular forms that new kinds of clinical ethics work took, these developments were clearly motivated by values that were different from the paternalism of the Hippocratic Oath (Veatch, 2012).

The *Belmont Report*, which was published in 1978 by the National Commission for the Protection of Human Subjects of Biomedical and Behavioral Research, articulated three core moral principles for human research: respect for persons, beneficence and justice (Belmont Commission, 1979). In 1979, Tom Beauchamp (a primary author of the *Belmont Report*) and James Childress published *Principles of Biomedical Ethics*, which articulated four moral principles (beneficence, nonmaleficence, autonomy and justice). This book almost single-handedly created a new moral foundation for clinical ethical reasoning. It focussed on the obligation to benefit the patient and to avoid harming them, while also recognizing the importance of patient rights and considering the impact of medical decision making on others.

REFLECTION POINT

For Case Study 16.1, reflect on following:

- How Dr P's presentation of treatments to Mrs Z reflects a paternalistic approach.
- Why might Dr P feel that his omission of treatment options is justified in this case?
- Did Mrs Z agree to the surgery with all the relevant medical information?
- What nonmedical values might Mrs Z have that might be in tension with her medical values for good health?

A MODEL OF CLINICAL ETHICS REASONING IN ADULT AND PAEDIATRIC MEDICINE

Beauchamp and Childress's four principles (beneficence, nonmaleficence, autonomy and justice) have become operationalized into a standard model of moral decision making and versions of this model are commonly taught in medical education and elaborated upon in the clinical ethics literature (Berlinger et al., 2013, 43; Lo, 2013). Our version builds upon the models of Berlinger et al. (2013) and Lo (2013) and contains three steps. In step one, the medical team determines which treatments are medically appropriate to offer to the patient. In step two, the appropriate decision maker is identified. In the adult context, this typically falls to a singular person (often the patient or a surrogate), but the paediatric context can involve more than one decision maker (e.g. both parents). In step three, decision-making standards are applied to guide the decision maker. Importantly, key differences between the adult and paediatric contexts

---

CASE STUDY 16.1

A Paternalistic Approach

Dr P diagnoses Mrs Z with stage I breast cancer. Standard treatments include a mastectomy or a lumpectomy with radiation. However, Dr P believes the mastectomy will be in Mrs Z's best interests because it is the most effective treatment for eradicating the cancer and ensuring it will not recur. As a result, Dr P describes the mastectomy to Mrs Z as the 'only truly effective treatment' and Mrs Z agrees to the operation.

---

arise in steps two and three. This standard model does not apply in medical emergencies, where medical paternalism remains the dominant approach to decision making (Emanuel and Emanuel, 1992).

Step One: Clinicians Determine What Treatment(s) to Offer

Physicians should be guided by beneficence and nonmaleficence when determining which treatments (there may be more than one) are medically appropriate to offer patients. Beneficence requires that only beneficial treatments should be offered and nonmaleficence prohibits physicians from causing harm to their patients that will be disproportionate to the benefit patients receive. Nonmaleficence is not an obligation to refrain from causing *any* harm to patients, but only to providing *net* harmful interventions.

There are many ways to interpret the concepts of benefit and harm. For example, a patient might consider the best decision to be the one that prioritizes an aesthetic or religious value over a medical value. However, when determining which treatments will be sufficiently beneficial to offer and which of the offered treatments to recommend, physicians should prioritize medical values. Medical values are tied to the goals of medicine, which include preventing, curing or managing disease, promoting health, avoiding premature death and alleviating pain and suffering (Goals of Medicine Project, 1996). In most cases, this means physicians should prioritize treatments that will best control a patient's blood pressure, manage diabetes, restore their airway or numb their pain, etc. Other values the patient has (e.g. religious, aesthetic, financial, psychological, social, etc.) may be asserted at the subsequent stages of the standard model whereby the patient, or their surrogate, may decide to accept, delay or refuse the various treatments on offer (Veatch and Guidry-Grimes, 2020).

Once the physician has determined which treatments are medically appropriate, they may be limited in which treatments they can actually offer the patient due to justice considerations usually imposed from outside the doctor-patient relationship. For example, in times of scarcity, a scarce resource allocation protocol may restrict an individual patient's access to scarce medical goods. In developing these allocation protocols, a number of competing justice principles come into play, such as equity, need, benefit and social utility (Persad et al., 2009).

Step Two: Identify the Appropriate Decision Maker

Adult Context

Once the physician has determined which treatments should be offered, they should usually presume that an adult patient can give informed consent or refusal, in the absence of evidence to the contrary. Informed consent requires three components: disclosure, decision-making capacity and voluntariness (American Society for Bioethics and Humanities, 2015). Disclosure requires telling the patient about their diagnosis and prognosis, as well as information about the nature (e.g. invasive, iterative, etc.), risks and benefits of the treatment options, including the option for nontreatment. Information should be delivered at a level that is appropriate for the mental capacities of the patient and may need to be delivered repeatedly or spread out to aid patient processing.

Decision-making capacity requires that the patient can express a choice, understand the information about the diagnosis and treatment options, appreciate how the information applies to their life and reason comparatively about the various treatment options. Many patients can express a choice (e.g. 'no, don't bother'), but such an expression alone is not sufficient to demonstrate decision-making capacity. A patient will also need understanding, which can be evaluated by determining whether the patient has knowledge of key facts related to their diagnosis and treatment options. For example, a patient with diabetes can satisfy the understanding criterion by demonstrating basic knowledge of what diabetes is, how it can affect them if untreated and why certain treatments can be helpful. A patient will also need appreciation, which can be evaluated by determining whether the patient can reflect on how the facts apply to themselves. A patient can satisfy the appreciation criterion by acknowledging they have a disease and considering how a decision will impact their life (e.g. how will you manage the stairs in your home if you refuse this treatment?). Finally, a patient will also need reasoning, which can be evaluated by determining whether the patient has compared the risks and benefits of the various treatment options, including the option of nontreatment. A patient can satisfy the reasoning criterion by giving reasons why they made one decision as opposed to another

(e.g. 'I refused the dialysis because I can't stand needles') (Appelbaum, 2007). It is important to distinguish competency, which is determined by a judge, from decision-making capacity, which is determined by the treating physician. Also, decision-making capacity can fluctuate, is decision-specific and should not be presumed to be lacking merely because a patient has been diagnosed with a mental illness.

Voluntariness, the final criterion of informed consent, requires that the patient be free of controlling influences. A patient who has been given all the relevant information and has satisfied the criteria for decision-making capacity, but whose expressed preference is the result of coercion, has not given informed consent.

When an adult patient lacks decision-making capacity or is otherwise unable to provide informed consent or refusal for medical interventions, a surrogate must make decisions on their behalf. If such a patient still possesses the capacity to name their own surrogate – they can express a preference and show that they understand what a surrogate will do – then even patients who lack decision-making capacity for medical choices should be permitted to name their own surrogates. That is, even if a patient cannot understand or appreciate their medical condition or potential treatments to a sufficient degree to make informed choices about interventions, they may still be able to make an informed choice about their surrogate (Navin et al., 2021). If a patient is no longer able to name their own surrogate and if they have completed legally valid documents to appoint a surrogate decision maker, e.g. a durable power of attorney for healthcare decision making, that person should be empowered to make decisions. However, in the absence of either contemporaneous capacitated preferences or historical formal declarations, the medical team may need to work with family to identify an appropriate surrogate decision maker. Often the hierarchy of potential surrogates is addressed in state law (DeMartino et al., 2017). Usually, the law identifies spouses as having priority over other potential surrogates. Sometimes state laws further specify priority rankings for potential surrogates, for example, placing adult children before younger siblings. If state law does not resolve questions about the surrogate in a particular case, it can be useful to ask the family to appoint a primary spokesperson, though the authority to make decisions may still rest equally in all family members and require consensus. Surrogates must be available for conversations and meetings with members of the medical team and they must be willing to make decisions guided by the decision-making standards outlined later (known patient preferences, then substituted judgement, then best interests). Surrogates who are not fulfilling these duties can be replaced, although doing so may require going before a judge to request appointment of an alternative guardian.

Paediatric Context

In the paediatric context, it is not the patient, but the parents, who are given presumptive decisional authority. The presumption of parental decisional authority over children is a constitutionally-protected liberty right of parents, established by cases such as *Meyer v. State of Nebraska* (1923) and *Pierce v. Society of Sisters* (1925). There exist two notable legal exceptions to the presumption of parental authority wherein the child-patient is afforded decision-making authority. The *public health exception* permits minors to consent to medical services that address certain types of health issues (e.g. family planning, treatment of sexually transmitted diseases, mental health and substance abuse treatment, etc.) based on the public health interest of allowing citizens of any age to access these types of care. The *emancipated minor exception* permits minors to consent to all medical services based not on the type of service, but instead on the status of the minor (e.g. being married, being in the armed forces, graduating from high school, etc.). The *mature minor doctrine* is a third frequently cited exception to parental authority, wherein an adolescent with demonstrated or presumed decision-making capacity is given authority to make their medical decisions. This exception is not common, however; only 14 states have some version of a mature minor law, nine by state statute and five by judicial decision. These laws vary widely. Outside these exceptions, parents should be presumed to possess decision-making authority. Parental informed permission should include all the same elements of disclosure, understanding and voluntariness as informed consent for adult patients.

STEP THREE: STANDARDS FOR DECISION MAKING
Adult Context

Surrogates have a responsibility to make medical decisions that are guided by certain ethical standards. In the adult context, surrogates should first make decisions guided by the patient's *known preferences*, thereby extending a patient's right of self-determination into cases where contemporaneous capacitated decision making is unavailable. Advance directives are commonly used by patients to make their preferences known but have many important limitations. Very few patients have a written advance directive and even when they do, advance directives are often not available when they are needed. Further, patients completing advance directives may not be well informed, the directive itself may be vague or difficult to interpret and patients may change their minds about preferences, rendering their previous preferences irrelevant (Fagerlin and Schneider, 2004). Although advance directives may be useful in some cases, a written advance directive is not required to establish a patient's known preferences for medical treatment. When hospitalized, patients sometimes make statements to medical staff that are subsequently documented in the medical record. Family may also be able to report instances where the patient verbally expressed preferences for medical treatment. All these sources of known patient preferences should be used to guide surrogates when making decisions for the patient.

If the patient's preferences are unknown, the primary authority of a surrogate's medical decision making becomes *substituted judgement*. That is, their strongest claim to make decisions is that they are deciding in the way that the patient *would have decided* if the patient still possessed decision-making capacity. In this way, the surrogate exercises a kind of autonomous judgement on behalf of the patient. Their moral authority to make decisions is therefore based on the same value – autonomy – that is the basis for the authority of capacitated patients to decide. Accordingly, surrogates who are exercising substituted judgement should be allowed to select treatment options that are not in the patient's best interest. This is because capacitated patients are allowed to choose treatment options that are not in their best interests and because surrogates who exercise substituted judgment are exercising autonomy on behalf of patients.

Surrogates may use many different types of evidence to support both known preferences, claims and substituted judgement claims including both verbal statements, as well as values and preferences inferred from behaviour. Verbal statements range from direct and determinative (e.g. the patient said, 'If I were ever in a permanent coma, I would not want to kept alive') to the indirect and indeterminate (e.g. the patient said during the treatment of a loved one 'Uncle Chad should never have been kept alive that way. They should have let him die.') Behaviorally inferred values and preferences might include such observations as 'Dad consistently made decisions based on the financial interests of the family, even when it involved sacrifices to his own personal interests. I don't think this expensive experimental drug would be something he would choose.' Or 'Aunt Mary was always very diligent in pursuing the most advanced medical care available for her and her family. I think she'd be interested in giving this experimental therapy a shot.' Clinicians, themselves, may also have encounters with patients yielding evidence about a patient's preferences or values. These encounters might be used to inform or even corroborate substituted judgement claims made by surrogates.

Although the determinacy and helpfulness of the concept of 'best interests' has been debated (Salter, 2012), traditionally this decision-making principle instructs the decision maker to determine the net benefit of each treatment option (by weighting and adding benefits and weighting and subtracting burdens), and selecting the treatment option with the greatest net benefit. The factors accounted for in a best interest calculation are typically generic interests that most people would consider relevant to treatment decision making, including such factors as current and future physical and mental suffering, the chances of recovery, the nature of patient interaction with the environment and the chances of regaining function (Cantor, 2005). In addition to reflecting a general judgement about what most people would find important, this list of concerns also reflects clinical interests central to the goals of medicine (Berlinger et al., 2013). Thus, the task of the surrogate, with the help of the clinical team, is to 'replicate the now-incompetent patient's *likely* choices, as determined by what most people would want done for themselves' (Cantor, 2005).

Paediatric Context

Standards of surrogate decision making in the adult context aim first to protect and promote the patient's right to self-determination, as an autonomous agent, and second, to promote the patient's well-being, generally considered. Unlike surrogate decision making in the adult context, parental decision making is not exclusively informed by the patient's values and preferences. Rather, parental decision making is informed both by the interests and well-being of the patient (comparable to 'best interests' judgement in the adult context) and the values and interests of the family, which play a more robust and determinative role in paediatrics than in adult decision making (Buchanan and Brock, 1989). For example, parents are not obligated to choose the treatment option which maximizes medical benefit to the child patient if that option also bankrupts the family or requires the family to uproot and move. Further, while the child is rarely the authoritative decision maker, child-patients ought to be invited to participate to a degree that is developmentally appropriate (Katz et al., 2016). All children should be given the opportunity to voice concerns, questions or worries, even if they do not possess decisional authority. For a young child, participation may include using dolls or illustrations to describe an upcoming procedure or asking the child's preference for which scent of nitrous oxide to use. For older or more mature children, this may include more technical explanations of procedures and, in some situations, asking for the child's assent.

While the presumption of parental authority is wide-sweeping and well-justified, it is not unlimited. Third parties (typically the state) may justifiably intervene when a parental decision places the child at risk of harm (Buchanan and Brock, 1989; Diekema, 2004). The state's authority to intervene in decisions for children arises primarily from its constitutionally sanctioned *parens patriae* power to protect the health, welfare and safety of vulnerable citizens. The most widely-cited intervention principle for paediatrics is Douglas Diekema's Harm Principle, which asserts that the state is justified in intervening on parental decisions when a parental refusal of recommended treatment places the child at 'significant risk of serious harm' (Diekema, 2004). To assess whether a parental refusal does, in fact, cross this threshold, Diekema offers eight conditions that must be satisfied, including requirements that the harm must be imminent, the refused intervention must be of proven efficacy and necessary to prevent the serious harm, and the intervention be generalizable to other similar situations.

State intervention typically begins with a member of the clinical team making a report of potential medical neglect to the state agency charged with child protection, which is followed by an investigation by the state, which may culminate in either a dismissal of the case (thereby allowing parents to make their preferred decision), or a decision to intervene on parental decision making through either (a) a court order for recommended medical treatment or (b) a decision to remove the child from parental custody altogether. Because state involvement introduces new harms to both the child and the family, intervention should only be considered as a last resort to protect a child from significant harm (e.g. death, disability, severe suffering) and clinicians should look for every opportunity to explore alternatives and negotiate with parents before reaching this step.

REFLECTION POINT

For Case Study 16.2, reflect on whether Mr K has the decision-making capacity to refuse the replacement of the nasogastric feeding tube.

- Consider how the medical team might try to communicate further with Mr K to determine whether he has decision-making capacity. What sorts of questions might they ask?
- Additionally, how should the role of a surrogate decision maker be explained to the son?
- Finally, what should be a *first response* if another family member arrives at the hospital and disagrees with the son about what decision to make.

CASE STUDY 16.2
Decision-Making Capacity in the Adult Context

Mr K is a 91-year-old patient with dementia, heart disease, hypertension, osteoarthritis, diabetes and COVID-19 pneumonia who presents to the hospital in frail condition for the replacement of his nasogastric feeding tube. Nurse S approaches Mr K in the evening hours to replace the feeding tube but Mr K puts his hand up and says, 'Please don't', but cannot sustain conversation beyond this simple refusal. Mr K's son is his surrogate and is very clear that he wants his dad to get the feeding tube replaced because 'I'm not ready to lose him yet'.

REFLECTION POINT

While parents typically retain legal decision-making authority in cases like Iris' (because they are complying with recommended life-saving medical recommendations), an adolescent's refusal of medical treatment is distressing and invites further moral reflection (Case Study 16.3).

- How can clinicians elicit Iris' most pressing fears or worries about treatment and are there ways her clinical team and parents can help alleviate those?
- What 'smaller' choices can we give her (i.e. choices with lower stakes than refusing effective life-saving medical treatment) to help her feel a sense of control and autonomy?
- How should the medical team respond if the preferences of Iris and her parents were reversed with Iris wanting the treatment but her parents refusing?

COMPLEXITIES

In this section, we describe points of complexity that can arise when physicians apply the standard model of clinical ethics reasoning described previously. The complexities described here help to illustrate situations where involvement of a hospital's clinical ethics service can be useful.

One complexity of applying the standard model of moral reasoning involves determining how clinicians may ethically influence the outcome of a medical decision, that is, which model of the doctor-patient relationship is appropriate for a particular medial context.

CASE STUDY 16.3
Decision-Making Capacity in the Paediatric Context

Thirteen-year-old Iris is diagnosed with Hodgkin disease after experiencing months of unexplained weight loss and fever. Iris and her parents are told that with appropriate treatment, including chemotherapy, her chances of long-term survival are better than 90%. Without the treatment, Iris' chance of survival is extremely low, potentially zero. However, side effects of the treatment are significant and include severe fatigue, nausea, vomiting and hair loss. While her parents agree to begin the recommended treatment regimen immediately, Iris adamantly refuses, stating that 'Treatment sounds awful. I'd rather die.'

Three common models are medical paternalism, pure autonomy and shared decision-making. According to medical paternalism, the physician, not the patient or their surrogate, is the appropriate decision maker. Medical paternalism can be appropriate in the context of an emergency, when it can be impossible to follow the model of moral reasoning outlined earlier. On the pure autonomy model, the physician aims to describe only the clinical facts to the patient or surrogate (e.g. common risks and benefits of a treatment) without making a recommendation or attempting to influence their decision. The pure autonomy model can be appropriate in the context of ethically controversial decisions (e.g. whether to pursue an elective abortion) or when different medical goals tell in favour of different choices (e.g. whether to pursue continued aggressive treatment for longer life or comfort care with shorter life). According to the shared decision-making model, stakeholders are encouraged to exchange reasons in a deliberative process, but it is ultimately the patient (or their surrogate) who decides. In shared decision making, physicians may give recommendations in an attempt to influence stakeholders, but they may also use techniques of 'nudging' such as establishing 'default' positions (e.g. opt-in versus opt-out organ donation registries) or enlisting individuals with status and influence (e.g. an attending physician) to deliver key messages to stakeholders (Kostick et al., 2020). In some circumstances, clinicians may resort to stronger methods, such as triggering the investigation of a state agency (e.g. Child Protective Services) or replacing a surrogate decision maker (e.g. by pursuing a court-appointed guardian). The shared decision-making model should serve as the default approach in the context of most routine medical decisions in an established doctor-patient relationship (Emanuel and Emanuel, 1992; Quill and Brody, 1996; Siegler, 1981).

A second moral complexity that can arise is how to handle the strenuous refusals of medical treatment by patients who lack decision-making capacity. Mere ignorance or cognitive decline does not compromise a patient's personhood and one requirement of respecting persons is to take seriously their preferences about how they would like to be treated (Wasserman and Navin, 2018). There are several morally salient features that should be considered in these cases (American Society for Bioethics and Humanities, 2017). The first

is the patient's level of decision-making capacity. The refusal of a patient who almost meets the threshold of full decision-making capacity (even if they ultimately fall below it) weighs in favour of honouring the refusal. For example, a patient who has been determined to lack decision-making capacity because of only one compromised criterion of decision-making capacity (e.g. appreciation) is making a refusal that carries more weight than a patient who has three compromised criteria of decision-making capacity. Second, the potential of a treatment to restore the autonomy of the patient should be considered. A treatment that is not expected to restore a patient's decision-making capacity is a feature of these cases that weighs against providing that treatment over objection. Third, the nature of the refused medical intervention should be considered. Procedures that are highly invasive or require multiple iterations are features of a procedure's nature that weigh against providing them over strenuous patient objections. Interventions that would require physical or chemical restraints would also require special consideration. Fourth, the risk/benefit ratio of the medical intervention should be considered. An incapacitated patient refusing procedures with only moderate clinical benefits and comparable clinical risk would weigh in favour of honouring the refusal. Treatment refusals of child patients can be equally distressing and morally complex. While the choice of the child-patient typically carries less moral weight in these cases, because children are presumed to lack decision-making capacity and parents are presumed to have decisional authority, some treatment refusals of children will bear heeding, if not due to moral constraints (e.g. the informed preference of the child), then due to practical constraints (e.g. uncooperative patients can undermine the benefits of certain types of treatment).

A third moral complexity that can arise is clinician conscientious objection, which occurs when there is conflict between a clinician's moral integrity and providing medical goods or services that are legal and professionally permitted. These conflicts most commonly arise in the contexts of abortion, contraception, sterilization and physician-aid-in-dying. While there are extreme views for and against the permissibility of conscientious objection in healthcare, the conventional compromise asks that physicians disclose the availability of the relevant medical goods or services to the patient, refer them to a willing provider and not invoke conscientious objection in the context of a medical emergency (Brock, 2008). It is further stipulated that clinicians should constrain their conscientious objections to medical goods or services, not discriminatory refusals to treating certain types of patients (Wicclair, 2011). However, the antidiscrimination criterion is challenged by the fact that some medical procedures are only requested by certain types of patients (e.g. gender-affirming surgery for transgender persons) (Brummett and Campo-Engelstein, 2021). Clinical ethics services can assist in the parsing of morally permissible instances of conscientious objection and articulating the obligations of clinicians who object (e.g. disclosure and referral).

This section has described some of the many additional ethical complications that can arise when applying the standard model of clinical ethics reasoning outlined in this chapter. Consulting a hospital clinical ethics service is recommended when these complexities arise because trained consultants from a variety of disciplinary backgrounds can provide moral guidance to clinicians.

REFLECTION POINT

- Consider how the questions of clinical *ethical* reasoning (e.g. who should be the decision maker?) differ from other types of clinical questions (e.g. what treatment will best prevent the recurrence of breast cancer?).
- Although medical paternalism has been discredited as the appropriate *default* model of the doctor-patient relationship, in what situations might it still be ethically defensible?
- Is it ever ethically problematic for a clinician to recommend a specific course of care and if so, why?

SUMMARY

In this chapter we have outlined:

1. How the contemporary bioethics framework of principlism differs from the tradition of medical paternalism in moral reasoning.
2. How principlism is operationalized in a standard model of decision making for both adult and paediatric contexts.

3. Some ethical complexities that can arise when applying the standard model of moral decision making.

REFERENCES

American Society for Bioethics and Humanities, 2015. Improving competencies in clinical ethics consultation: An education guide (2nd ed.). American Society for Bioethics and Humanities.

American Society for Bioethics and Humanities, 2017. Addressing patient-centered ethical issues in health care: A case-based study guide. American Society of Bioethics and Humanities.

Appelbaum, P.S., 2007. Assessment of patients' competence to consent to treatment. New England Journal of Medicine 357 (18), 1834–1840. https://www.nejm.org/doi/full/10.1056/nejmcp074045

Belmont Commission, 1979. The Belmont Report (DHEW Publication Issue). http://ezp.slu.edu/login?url=http://search.ebscohost.com/login.aspx?direct=true&db=cat00825a&AN=slu.b1157558&site=eds-live

Berlinger, N., Jennings, B., Wolf, S.M., 2013. The Hastings Center Guidelines for decisions on life-sustaining treatment and care near the end of life: Revised and expanded, second edition. Oxford University Press.

Brock, D.W., 2008. Conscientious refusal by physicians and pharmacists: Who is obligated to do what, and why? Theoretical Medicine and Bioethics 29 (3), 187–200. https://doi.org/10.1007/s11017-008-9076-y

Brummett, A., Campo-Engelstein, L., 2021. Conscientious objection and LGBTQ discrimination in the United States. Journal of Public Health Policy 42 (2), 322–330. https://doi.org/10.1057/s41271-021-00281-2

Buchanan, A.E., Brock, D.W., 1989. Deciding for others: The ethics of surrogate decision making. Cambridge University Press.

Cantor, N.L., 2005. The bane of surrogate decision-making defining the best interests of never-competent persons. The Journal of Legal Medicine 26 (2), 155–205. https://doi.org/10.1080/01947640590949922

Danis, M., Fox, E., Tarzian, A., Duke, C.C., 2021. Health care ethics programs in US hospitals: Results from a national survey. BMC Medical Ethics 22 (1), 1–14. https://doi.org/10.1186/s12910-021-00673-9

DeMartino, E.S., Dudzinski, D.M., Doyle, C.K., Sperry, B.P., Gregory, S.E., Siegler, M., et al., 2017. Who decides when a patient can't? Statutes on alternate decision makers. The New England Journal of Medicine 376 (15), 1478. https://doi.org/10.1056/NEJMms1611497

Diekema, D., 2004. Parental refusals of medical treatment: The harm principle as threshold for state intervention. Theoretical Medicine and Bioethics 25 (4), 243–264. http://ezp.slu.edu/login?url=http://search.ebscohost.com/login.aspx?direct=true&db=cmedm&AN=15637945&site=eds-live

Emanuel, E.J., Emanuel, L.L., 1992. Four models of the physician-patient relationship. JAMA: Journal of the American Medical Association 267 (16), 2221. http://ezp.slu.edu/

login?url=http://search.ebscohost.com/login.aspx?direct=true&db=edb&AN=9205111328&site=eds-live

Fagerlin, A., Schneider, C.E., 2004. Enough: the failure of the living will. Hastings Center Report 34 (2), 30–42.

Goals of Medicine Project, 1996. The goals of medicine: Setting new priorities. Hastings Center Report 26 (Supplement), S1–S27.

Joint Commission on Accreditation of Healthcare Organizations, 1993. Patient rights. In Accreditation Manual for Hospitals, 1992.

Katz, A.L., Webb, S.A., Committee on Bioethics, 2016. Informed consent in decision-making in pediatric practice. Pediatrics 138 (2), e20161485. https://doi.org/10.1542/peds.2016-1485

Kostick, K.M., Trejo, M., Volk, R.J., Estep, J.D., Blumenthal-Barby, J.S., 2020. Using nudges to enhance clinicians' implementation of shared decision making with patient decision aids. MDM Policy & Practice 5 (1), 2381468320915906. https://doi.org/10.1177/2381468320915906

In Re Quinlan, 1976. 70 N.J. 10 https://law.justia.com/cases/new-jersey/supreme-court/1976/70-n-j-10-0.html

Lo, B., 2013. Resolving ethical dilemmas: A guide for clinicians, 5th ed. Wolters Kluwer Health/Lippincott Williams & Wilkins. http://www.loc.gov/catdir/enhancements/fy0838/2008034964-t.html

Navin, M., Wasserman, J.A., Stahl, D., Tomlinson, T., 2021. The capacity to designate a surrogate is distinct from decisional capacity: Normative and empirical considerations. Journal of Medical Ethics. https://doi.org/10.1136/medethics-2020-107078

Persad, G., Wertheimer, A., Emanuel, E.J., 2009. Principles for allocation of scarce medical interventions. The Lancet 373 (9661), 423–431. https://doi.org/10.1016/S0140-6736(09)60137-9

Quill, T.E., Brody, H., 1996. Physician recommendations and patient autonomy: Finding a balance between physician power and patient choice. Annals of Internal Medicine 125 (9), 763–769. https://doi.org/10.7326/0003-4819-125-9-199611010-00010

Salter, E.K., 2012. Deciding for a child: A comprehensive analysis of the best interest standard. Theoretical Medicine and Bioethics 33 (3), 179–198. https://doi.org/10.1007/s11017-012-9219-z

Siegler, M., 1981. Searching for moral certainty in medicine: A proposal for a new model of the doctor-patient encounter. Bulletin of the New York Academy of Medicine 57 (1), 56–69.

Veatch, R.M., 2009. Patient, heal thyself: How the new medicine puts the patient in charge. Oxford University Press.

Veatch, R.M., 2012. Hippocratic, religious, and secular medical ethics: The points of conflict. Georgetown University Press.

Veatch, R.M., Guidry-Grimes, L., 2020. The basics of bioethics, 4th ed. Routledge.

Wasserman, J.A., Navin, M.C., 2018. Capacity for preferences: Respecting patients with compromised decision-making. Hastings Center Report 48 (3), 31–39. https://doi.org/10.1002/hast.853

Wicclair, M.R., 2011. Conscientious objection in health care: An ethical analysis. Cambridge University Press.

17

CULTIVATING CLINICAL REASONING
The Need for the Health Humanities

INGRID BERG ■ NICOLE PIEMONTE

CHAPTER OUTLINE

CHAPTER AIMS

The aims of this chapter are:

- to explain the role of the health humanities in healthcare education and practice
- to explore ways of engaging with the health humanities that can cultivate clinical reasoning especially in the context of healthcare encounters that are inherently complex, ambiguous and interpersonal
- to demonstrate the importance of the patient's story when determining accurate diagnoses and appropriate treatment plans
- to invite readers to reflect on the ways they are personally affected by suffering and grief and how this can influence clinical reasoning.

'Study the humanities and the arts as part of your professional training only if you have to. You probably have to.'

Dr Mark Vonnegut, pediatrician (2014)

INTRODUCTION

Given that clinical reasoning encompasses both cognitive and noncognitive domains (Furze et al., 2022), somewhere between the application of biomedical knowledge and the interpretation of an individual patient's story lies an integrative exchange with the potential for therapeutic success or for serious treatment plan missteps. For trainees, the relative tidiness of a healthcare curriculum played out in lectures, read in textbooks and experienced through standardized patients gives way to the complexities of providing care within a system that often rewards efficiency rather than diagnostic precision and empathic connection. Thus, the work of the health humanities is to shape the internal cognitive and relational sensibilities of a clinician towards high-quality clinical reasoning – reasoning that is shaped by the ability to listen well, to foster connection and to navigate ambiguity.

While an education in the basic and clinical sciences provides a foundation for diagnostic and therapeutic interventions, the work of the health humanities is equally elemental in that its application not only contributes to the development of differential diagnoses and treatment plans, but also asks healthcare professionals to reflect on how to build trust with patients and support and accompany them through suffering and uncertainty. Interwoven, an education in traditional biomedicine and the humanities works synergistically to strengthen the clinical reasoning required each day by those in the health professions.

In this chapter, we propose that some of the most important cognitive and noncognitive domains of clinical reasoning can be developed and strengthened through an engagement with the health humanities. As described in Chapter 3 of this book, clinical reasoning is 'a multilayered and multicomponent capability' that allows clinicians to make 'difficult decisions in the conditions of complexity and uncertainty', which requires 'tolerance of ambiguity, reflexive understanding, practice artistry and collaboration'. As we will show, it is precisely the ability to engage in reflection and reflexive practice, to recognize the need for collaboration to address patients' complex needs and to tolerate – and even embrace – ambiguity that an engagement with the health humanities is intended to cultivate within current and future clinicians. We begin by offering a brief history of the development of the health humanities and what their place is in healthcare education before exploring the connection between the health humanities and clinical reasoning. Particular emphasis is placed on how engaging with the humanities can help trainees and practitioners better interpret and respond to the specific context(s) of patients' lives, an ability that is central to clinical reasoning (Ratcliffe and Durning, 2015).

THE HEALTH HUMANITIES: WHAT ARE THEY AND HOW DID THEY COME TO BE?

The health humanities have their roots in the 1960s and 1970s when technological advances in areas such as transplant medicine, genetics and the growth of critical care units with 'shifting standards of death' (Jones et al., 2017, p. 932–933) occurred alongside the women's rights, civil rights and patient rights movements. In 1965, an essay appeared in the *Journal of the*

American Medical Association lamenting that '... the laboratory test and the clinical experiment have to a large degree supplanted the consultation as the essential unit of medical practice'. The author warned that the elevation of science as an all-knowing entity would squelch '... the realization that sickness and death are inevitable sequelae of life, that science can never bring to an end human suffering' (Renner, 2015, p. 734, revisited from 1965).

During this time, philosophers, theologians, ethicists and clinicians joined the chorus in lamenting that medical care failed to address the lived experience of patients and also expressed concerns about 'the way medical students of the rising generation were being trained and, in particular, for what was lacking in their education' (Carson, 2003, p. 1). Medical educators who shared these concerns primarily focussed on three issues: depersonalization in medicine, the centrality of molecular biology in medical education and the teaching of 'mechanistic medicine' (Fox, 1985). Though it was not called 'medical humanities' at the time (the term would not become widely used until the 1980s and 1990s), prominent figures in medicine, such as renowned physician and bioethicist Edmund Pellegrino, advocated for the incorporation of the humanities into medical education (Carson et al., 2003). In 1967, The Penn State College of Medicine Department of Humanities became the first such department in a US medical school.

Welcoming scholars of literature, philosophy, history, anthropology, theology, sociology and disability studies (among many other areas), the medical humanities can be defined as '... an inter- and multidisciplinary field that explores contexts, experiences, and critical and conceptual issues in medicine and healthcare, while supporting professional identity formation' (Cole et al., 2015, p. 12). Champions of the medical humanities recognize that in order to help learners become the kind of clinicians who can fully address the complex needs of patients, they need a *way of knowing* beyond scientific knowledge – that is, they need a richer understanding of the complex human experience of health and illness that can come with an engagement with the humanities. The wisdom that the humanities offer can help clinicians navigate the realities that healthcare is laden with existential questions about the meaning of life and death, that clinical practice is inherently interpersonal, and that illness and suffering are about more than pathophysiology and the biological body.

In many ways, the humanities offer a new way of seeing, understanding and describing health and illness that helps to expand, nuance and enrich technical or scientific explanation. This is, in part, a result of the work of the early medical humanists – some of whom were theologians with an extensive background in hermeneutics – who were trained in interpretive philosophical frameworks that emphasized ethical listening, practical wisdom and attention to the particularities of the situation at hand (Carson, 2007). Given the moral ambiguity and relational complexity inherent to clinical decision making, the medical humanities encourage and embrace a tolerance for ambiguity and an ability to 'live in the question', while simultaneously attempting to uncover what is good and right for the situation at hand. Seeking 'not a philosophical answer, a truth, a good for all time, but a best judgement in this particular case', a clinician trained in the humanities might ask, for example, not only 'what do patients value the most?' but 'what does this particular patient, with this particular diagnosis, within this particular context value the most?' (Cole and Lagay, 2003, p. 165).

REFLECTION POINT

- What is your experience with the humanities?
- In what ways have the humanities – a book, film or song, for instance – helped you grapple with or better understand a difficult time in your own life?

THE MEDICAL HUMANITIES OR THE HEALTH HUMANITIES? DEFINING THE FIELD

The medical humanities should be distinguished from other philosophies that overlap, but yet retain their own discrete primary missions. Rita Charon, an internist, literary scholar and originator of Narrative Medicine (discussed later), warns that the medical humanities are not meant as a 'civilizing veneer' to edify or remediate the literary and artistic acumen of a healthcare professional schooled primarily in the biological sciences (Charon, 2017, p. 1668). To be sure,

appreciation for the arts is a likely – and perhaps even hoped for – byproduct of the medical humanities, but not its foremost goal. Rather than helping us become more 'cultured' or 'refined', the humanities intend to offer a deeper, broader and more critical understanding of healthcare education and practice. They offer us a new way of seeing and talking about the human elements of healthcare: the ways patients suffer beyond their physical bodies, the power dynamics inherent to clinical encounters, the way language influences how we understand health and illness, how social inequities exacerbate suffering, and so forth.

Likewise, the medical humanities are not synonymous with humanism in medicine, which also arose as a corrective to 'dehumanizing forces' in healthcare, specifically corporate and financial pressures, over-reliance on technology and decreased time with patients (Thibault, 2019, p. 1074). For Thibault (2019), humanizing medicine begins with centring patients in healthcare processes, appreciating patient and clinician stories, and applying rational, scientific processes to promote patient health. Empathy and exemplary bedside rapport are hallmarks of the humanistic clinician and several organizations, including the Gold Humanism Honor Society, have been championing and promoting these traits in healthcare professionals for many years. While engagement with the humanities hopefully does help to cultivate rapport and compassion, the medical humanities go further than this and help attune clinicians to the rich context of patients' lives through reflective practices. Cultivating a posture of openness and receptivity during a patient encounter and accompanying a patient throughout the trajectory of a chronic condition or challenging illness requires motivation to maintain that fortitude. Without that effort, clinical reasoning may crumple since a patient's clinical picture and needs change over time.

The growth of medical humanities has since evolved beyond explorations of medical education and the physician experience to encompass the delivery of healthcare through the intersection of all healthcare professionals, informal caregivers and patients. This expansiveness has prompted semantic debate within the field and support for a shift to the use of 'health humanities' to describe this work (Jones et al., 2017). The health humanities, according to Paul Crawford, afford an opportunity 'to generate diverse and even radical means of creating healthier and more compassionate societies'. He describes this creative scholarship as an amalgam of science, social science and the arts and humanities (Crawford, 2015). Interest in this field has grown exponentially in the 21st century with an increase from 12 to 140 baccalaureate programmes throughout the United States and Canada from 2000 to 2020 (Lamb et al., 2022). The health humanities bring together many stakeholders when it comes to the health and well-being of patients and communities. Given its impact on patient care, here, too, the inputs and development of sound clinical reasoning should have particular salience for health humanities scholars. We will continue to use the more expansive term of 'health humanities' for the remainder of this chapter.

THE INTERSECTION OF THE HEALTH HUMANITIES AND CLINICAL REASONING

An engagement with the arts and humanities can influence clinical reasoning in very real ways, although some are more obvious – or at least more obviously discussed in the literature – than others. We discuss some of the most profound ways that the humanities intersect with clinical reasoning, beginning with a discussion of some of the extant literature, which primarily highlights the influence of the humanities on improving clinical observation and grappling with ambiguity.

The Humanities, Clinical Reasoning and Ambiguity

As mentioned previously, clinical reasoning involves making difficult decisions when things are complex, uncertain and ambiguous. Interestingly, and importantly, much of the literature that explores the 'outcomes' of engaging with the humanities points to its ability to help clinicians and trainees tolerate, sit with or grapple with ambiguity (see, for instance, Bleakley, 2015; Ofri, 2017; Bentwich and Gilbey, 2017). While it is true that healthcare practitioners and educators acknowledge that uncertainty is inevitable and that there is a limit to our scientific and medical knowledge, we do not often encourage students and clinicians to sit with the discomfort of ambiguity or sort through the tangles of nuance for too long. Instead,

in healthcare education, we tend to emphasize knowledge that can be delivered, memorized, repeated and assessed – a tendency that is reinforced by high-stakes board exams within nearly every healthcare training programme that primarily assess scientific and technical knowledge. As a result, healthcare curricula tend to emphasize the acquisition of biomedical knowledge, often at the expense of developing qualities such as interpersonal connection, deep listening and communication, which are precisely the qualities that contribute to clinical acumen.

Because clinical care is rarely straightforward and because patients do not present in the clinic as multiple-choice questions, determining *what is the matter* and what to do for patients requires the ability to discern nuance and recognize the textures of patients' lives that affect health, illness, motivation and access to care. In other words, sound clinical reasoning involves recognizing and accounting for ambiguous information that is not readily discernible, measurable or fixable. This ability, however, is difficult to teach and will not be developed within students via lectures or passive didactic instruction. Rather, it is the kind of learning that the humanities offer that can help cultivate this ability in our future clinicians. As physician Danielle Ofri (2017) describes it: 'The humanities can offer doctors a paradigm for living with ambiguity and even for relishing it. Great works of literature, art, theater, and music specialize in ambiguity, confusion, and frailty. Unlike medicine, the humanities do not shy away from uncertainty. They revel in the depth and breadth that ambiguity affords' (p. 1657). Stories – whether novels, short stories, patient narratives or documentaries – take us through the twists and turns of human life and offer us truths about love, loss, sickness, beauty, death and suffering that are difficult to learn any other way. Stories, especially those with ambiguous, unsatisfactory or unfinished endings, show us that life can be uncertain and unpredictable and that patient care is not exempt from such contingencies.

In addition to the ability to embrace uncertainty, Charon (2001) argues that in order to engage in effective clinical care, clinicians must also have 'narrative competence', which is the 'ability to acknowledge, absorb, interpret, and act on the stories and plights of others' (p. 1897). For Charon, developing the skill of 'close reading' – the ability of a reader to pay attention to narrative features such as voice, mood, metaphor and temporality – can directly translate to patient care where clinicians must listen carefully to their patients' stories. Using the capacities one can learn through close reading, 'clinicians and their patients can face the unknown, tolerating the ambiguity that always surrounds illness' (Charon, 2016, p. 158). Becoming skilled at close reading allows a clinician to pay better attention to a patient's story, reflect on what is represented in that story and create a strong affiliation with the patient who tells it (Charon, 2007).

Like Narrative Medicine, Visual Thinking Strategies (VTS) in the context of healthcare training and practice have been shown to engage trainees and clinicians in thought processes analogous to clinical reasoning and to help them embrace uncertainty (Prince et al., 2022). VTS is a methodology for engaging participants in discussions about complex and ambiguous materials – such as works of art, literature or musical pieces – by encouraging learners to deconstruct and analyse the work via open-ended questions that focus on intentional and unhurried observation (Prince et al., 2022). Incorporating VTS into medical education was pioneered at Harvard Medical School in 2004 and the method is now used at more than 30 medical schools across the country (President and Fellows, 2023).

Peer-reviewed studies have demonstrated that VTS can help healthcare trainees and clinicians to hone observation, critical thinking, active listening and communication skills, as well as develop a tolerance for uncertainty (President and Fellows, 2023). For instance, Prince and colleagues (2022) piloted a study in which they incorporated VTS sessions into daily morning report sessions in an internal medicine residency training programme. Because the overall objective of morning report – which includes discussing a clinical case with attendees – is to 'challenge and refine participants' clinical reasoning abilities', the authors saw the morning report as a 'logical setting' for their pilot curriculum (Prince and colleagues, 2022, p. 1154). For four morning report sessions, the authors substituted a clinical case with a case from the humanities (a work of literature, music or visual art) that was not explicitly related to medicine or healthcare and a facilitator led them through a 30-minute analysis and discussion. Preliminary qualitative analysis of transcripts from the pilot curriculum revealed thought processes during group analyses of humanities cases analogous to that of clinical reasoning. Moreover, participant responses from each of the sessions alluded to a difficulty with synthesizing multiple meanings or confronting ambiguity, which may suggest that the humanities are 'a powerful tool for exploring and embracing ambiguity in clinical practice' (Prince et al., 2022, p. 1155).

While the extant literature, especially studies related to Narrative Medicine and VTS, highlights how engaging with the humanities may strengthen clinical thought processes, improve observation and help one tolerate uncertainty, we believe the health humanities can offer much more when it comes to clinical reasoning. We explore how the humanities can help reveal the power of language, the complexities of diagnostic errors and the nuances of shared decision making.

The Humanities, Clinical Reasoning and the Use of Language

Given that clinical reasoning is 'complex, contextual, and multifactorial' (Furze et al., 2022), there are many moments during a patient encounter when clinical reasoning can veer off course. One contributor to faulty clinical reasoning is a poor, insensitive or unreflective use of language. As one public health official in the UK observed in 2006, 'the way language is used in the health service is often opaque, alienating and disrespectful' (Cayton, 2006, p. 484). Indeed, stigmatizing language may be unleashed across the life cycle and particularly for members of marginalized communities. Pregnancy offers many examples of insensitive terminology such as the use of 'incompetent cervix' or 'habitual aborter' to describe women who have experienced frequent miscarriages. Denigrating mnemonics and other memory tricks are handed down throughout health science education such as the 'Fat, Female, Forty, Fertile and Feo' (feo means ugly in Spanish) to represent the common profile for a patient with gallstones (Zirulnik and Cartsonis, 2019). Such mnemonics and memory tricks, ostensibly designed to aid in clinical reasoning, undoubtedly shape the way trainees and clinicians view the people they care for. How we label patients, which is often thinly veiled as light-hearted or humorous, functions in a similar way. Cayton (2006), for instance, notes the insensitive labels placed on geriatric patients, specifically – crinklies, crumblies and frequent fliers – the latter term referring to the typically frail elderly who often require emergency room care and hospital admission. The perpetuation of such labels exacts a cost: 'Language both reflects and shapes our thinking and thus our behaviour' (Cayton, 2006). The glare of 'professional language that is pejorative, paternalistic, accusatory and aggressive' reflects a hierarchy and power dynamic that can rupture the relationship between clinician and patient (Zirulnik and Cartsonis, 2019).

Health humanities scholar Rebecca Garden (2019) observes that the health humanities can help illuminate how diagnostic determinations and labels can perpetuate the tendency to pathologize anyone who does not subscribe to heteronormative behaviours. She describes this work in the humanities as 'critical healing', which 'resists reductive medical narratives by excavating the possibilities of meaning and by restoring the potential for multiplicities of story, particularly the narratives of bodily and psychic difference generated by those who seek healthcare' (p. 1–2). If language is the conduit of narrative, then the clinician controls and perpetuates a patient story that might be read over and over again influencing care. To demonstrate this effect, Goddu et al. (2018) created two versions of a hypothetical patient with sickle cell disease utilizing language from actual medical records – one version using stigmatizing language and one with neutral language. Those resident physicians exposed to the stigmatizing chart had more negative attitudes towards the patient and managed the pain less aggressively. Language, then, has the potential to become a viral contagion on its own, creating a truncated version of truth and fallow soil for clinical reasoning to flourish. An inappropriate label such as 'drug seeker' that directly influences prescribing behaviours is a direct link to the role of language in clinical reasoning.

Goddu and colleagues (2018) were encouraged, however, to find that when participants reflected on the language used, they could identify how it had affected them. The authors note that 'this capacity for reflection may be a promising point of intervention' (Goddu and colleagues, 2018, p. 689). The health humanities offer that precise intervention. Through engagement with the humanities, arts and patient stories, new ways of knowing and seeing evolve and context more fully emerges: suddenly 'bad behaviour' or 'noncompliance' with medications or therapies may be due to cognitive decline or financial stressors, uncovered only through applying a clinical approach steeped in humane, compassionate and persistent questioning. Ultimately, inclusive and sensitive language that speaks to the human experience – and not simply to clinician frustrations – will propel patient care towards person-centred interventions rooted in nuance, relevance and a deeper understanding of the complexities of patients' lives.

The Humanities, Clinical Reasoning and Framing the Clinical Encounter

If a prerequisite to quality clinical reasoning is a sensitive and nonstigmatizing approach to language, the next building blocks might encompass further refinement in word choice, history gathering and attention to body language, countenance and attitude. All of these elements together have the potential to create a clinical context that welcomes a rich context of patient experience and compassionate rapport towards productive and therapeutic exchanges.

As discussed previously, stigmatizing language can be pervasive both within a patient encounter and throughout a patient's medical record. But what about when language is not inherently stigmatizing or controversial, but still significantly influences patient care? For example, Sinayev and colleagues (2015) found that when presented with a hypothetical situation about starting a new medication to treat newly diagnosed high cholesterol, research participants exhibited higher comprehension and willingness to try the medication when it was given as a percentage with a risk label, such as a '14% of patients experience dry mouth, a very common side effect'. Comprehension was reduced and medication initiation less likely when the same material about side effects was packaged in other less descriptive formats, such as percentage only, frequency only or frequency with a risk label. For health practitioners, counselling about medications, procedures, exercises and other interventions is a major feature of the clinical encounter. When it comes to whether and how a patient will proceed with a treatment plan, it is paramount that clinicians have a good sense of *how* to best counsel a patient, given their health literacy and numeracy, their worries and fears, and their attitudes about health, illness and treatment. Narrative medicine's focus on the close reading of patients and drawing from the humanities to prime that pump helps clinicians to *read the room* and assess a patient's understanding of decision points and instructions.

Likewise, history gathering is a basic and normative function for every healthcare professional and foundational in shaping the contours of a clinical encounter. Medical, surgical, mental health, medication, family and social histories represent the most commonly explored domains of patient health history. Most would agree that clinical reasoning is predicated on asking 'the right questions'. What is difficult to discern, however, is how often those relevant questions are missed. In an essay called 'The Unasked Question', Jeffrey L. Brown (2012), a paediatrician and Vietnam War veteran, recalled that decades after he had been deployed overseas and accumulated several health concerns, he realized that no healthcare professional had ever asked if he had served in the military. (The majority of veterans receive care outside the Veterans Administration system.) Nor had he ever been trained to routinely ask his patients or their family members that question. Wryly, he observes, 'Few of the veterans who visit their physician have the stereotyped appearance of young amputees, older men wearing gold-embroidered "I Am a Veteran" hats, or anxious patients taking tranquilizers' (p. 1870). Brown notes that his experience has left a *psychological imprint* and his exposure to Agent Orange means that he is at higher risk of neurological disease, leukaemia, diabetes and heart disease. Without that critical history, clinical reasoning, including differential diagnosis building, is stunted.

Similarly, obtaining a cursory family history or accepting at face value when a patient says they do not have, or do not know, their family history may unnecessarily restrict the clinical encounter, missing potential opportunities for screenings and unhelpfully narrowing the differential diagnosis (Andoh, 2023, p. E1). When it comes to family history, Joana Andoh, an ophthalmologist and daughter of Ghanaian immigrants, observes that 'unfortunately, discrimination, slavery, colonization, language barriers, physical separation and health literacy (or lack thereof) across generations are just some of the factors that affect how you might answer that question' (2023, p. E1). Andoh

reminds us that carrying a diagnosis – and knowing one's family history of other diagnoses – can be a sign of privilege, a marker of healthcare access and an opportunity to advocate for one's health. In short, patients without family health histories may indicate that they have been marked by war, forceful removal from family, refugee camp stays and forced migration. In the context of a clinical encounter, then, occupational and family history may be 'shadow histories' lost in the unasked and not-easily-spoken. An intentional integration of the arts and humanities in healthcare curricula can help cast light on these shadowy places, given the strong presence of crisis themes in many forms of art. Given that art, in all its varieties, often reflects humanity's struggles, the health humanities, especially within healthcare curricula, can help harness these themes to excavate these forgotten or ignored histories.

While the clinical encounter is shaped by the spoken – in the bundling of language when describing interventions and asking about history – it is also marked by the unspoken: nonverbal cues, body language and facial expressions. 'Microethics' is the term given to describe the interplay of all these factors within a clinical encounter and their effect on clinical reasoning (Komesaroff, 1995). Whether a clinician sits or stands, hides behind a laptop or maintains good eye contact, wears a white coat or casual dress, uses jargon or layperson's speak, breaks a silence or rests in that quiet space, nearly every microdecision leaves an interpersonal (ethical) imprint. As Sisk and Baker (2018) put it, 'The words, context, and framing of communication can all affect how patients and parents process information and make decisions' (p. E1).

The Humanities, Clinical Reasoning and Diagnostic Error

The reflective clinician will accept that their clinical reasoning, which encompasses differential diagnosis building and treatment plan design, is drawn from both personal and professional experience, as well as from didactic materials such as textbooks, lectures, journal articles and algorithms. Therapists and other clinicians know that hip pain might be related to a patient's golf swing, a penchant for high heels or always carrying a toddler on the same hip. Reasoning through these aetiologies may come from personal experience or from examples found in lectures or observed during clinical rotations. All of these various inputs coalesce, perhaps subconsciously, and underpin clinical reasoning. How or why they converge within a trainee to yield an accurate diagnosis and reasonable treatment strategy – or how or why a trainee might labour under diagnostic pitfalls and biases – can be difficult to predict, yet it is something healthcare practitioners and educators are called to discern.

Dumas and colleagues (2018) hypothesize that various *relational reasoning strategies* may help clinicians cross-check the cognitive processes that lead them, or their trainees, down the wrong rabbit holes. Relational reasoning includes a body of strategies that support a person's essential ability to identify meaningful patterns within a stream of information. In the context of healthcare, these relational reasoning strategies assist with clinical pattern recognition, assuming that 'prior medical knowledge, sufficient motivation, and accurate patient data' are in place (p. 711). These strategies include *analogy* (finding similarities), *anomaly* (recognizing discrepancies), *antimony* (noting incompatibilities) and *antithesis* (addressing oppositions). While Dumas and colleagues take care to note that using these strategies is not a fool-proof path towards consistent clinical excellence, they argue that the inherent metacognition these strategies support could be transformative in shaping clinical acumen.

In her essay 'Listening Lessons', physician Brittany Bettendorf (2023) recalls how she nearly ignored her patient's complaint of 'whooshing' in his ears, tempted to replace his concern with the common and typically benign complaint of 'ringing' in his ears. When a clinician changes the chief complaint, they risk barrelling down the wrong diagnostic pathway: 'The words were not interchangeable', she writes. 'I questioned how I could grant myself narrative permission to translate his choice of adjective' (p. 883). The patient was in need of urgent imaging and consultation with a neuro-interventionalist because the patient had abnormal connections between intracranial blood vessels, which could rupture and cause bleeding. Herein lies the danger of careless translation, of creating an approximation to a patient's stated concern.

Using a relational reasoning strategy, recognizing when a complaint is *not* similar to another, is just as important as noting when something rhymes. Indeed,

it may not be too far a stretch to draw a parallel between these relational reasoning strategies and the arts and humanities. Pattern recognition through the lens of metaphor, dialogue and lyrics, plot twists – all these elements of storytelling and narration – align with the relational aims of the strategies already described. In this sense, every word, every camera angle, every brushstroke has meaning and is a deliberate contextual piece of the clinical puzzle. What if we thought of the patient as the artist *and* co-consultant? It may take 7 years to become a licensed physician – the typical timeframe for most trainees to complete medical school and residency – and it took Lin-Manuel Miranda just as long to compose *Hamilton*, but most patients have been living in their bodies for far longer and are able to discern and express *what is the matter* better than anyone else.

Gabriel Swenson, for instance, knew something was very wrong with his body, as he recounted in his 2021 essay, 'Listening for Horses' (Swenson, 2021). Not long after suffering from a common cold, Swenson experienced 'paraesthesia' in both legs, stating that his legs felt weak. During his initial evaluation, his symptoms were attributed to the stress he was likely feeling after not getting into medical school. After a prescription for an anxiolytic, he asked incredulously, 'Was I even mentally stable enough to pursue medicine if my stress was causing me to go paralyzed?' Not convinced that his symptoms were simply stress related and because he knew his own body, Swenson returned to the emergency room and continued to advocate for himself. He eventually received the appropriate work-up, including a lumbar puncture, to confirm that he had developed Guillain–Barré syndrome – an inflammatory condition that can attack nerves, typically precipitated by a viral infection – and was admitted to the hospital.

In the aftermath of his near-complete recovery and eventual acceptance into medical school, Swenson ruminated on the old adage taught to clinicians: 'When you hear hoof beats, think horses, not zebras'. Although clinicians understand that 'common things are common', bilateral lower extremity weakness is not a sign of anxiety and was incompatible (antinomic) to the actual diagnosis. Here, one can only wonder how this patient's narrative was subsumed under the narratives created by his clinicians: *'Of course medical school rejection would be so terrible for him that he feels weak. I might feel the same way.'* Understanding the multiple narratives at work in this case, and how clinicians can get stuck in narrative loops, can reveal faulty clinical reasoning at work. An engagement with the humanities in the context of clinical reasoning can aid in strengthening the relational reasoning strategies used to reach appropriate diagnoses and treatment plans and may also help in postmortem analyses when patient care goes so wrong.

While antimonies were overlooked in this case, sometimes a failure to see anomalies (discrepancies between expectations and reality) can lead to faulty clinical reasoning. John Brown, the paediatrician and Vietnam veteran mentioned earlier, described years of medical encounters where no-one asked about his deployment or its possible relationship to his physical or mental health. As a result, no one explored possible pain or suffering caused by war experiences and instead pursued answers one might more typically expect to find. The exposures and characteristic injuries experienced during conflict can be conflict specific – burn pits in Afghanistan, for example – or ubiquitous across conflicts and eras, such as post-traumatic stress disorder or military sexual trauma. Therefore, for veterans, anomalies may become more common than expected. Recognizing this reality is essential for clinicians caring for veterans, because 'the ability and willingness to identify and resolve anomalies in data have been identified as critically important for success, both in clinical and scientific reasoning, and may represent a means to reduce diagnostic error' (Dumas et al., 2018, p. 710).

A similar parallel can be drawn to grief and loss in the aftermath of the COVID-19 pandemic and its relationship to patients' physical and mental health. De Leon Corona and colleagues (2022) warn that the grief unleashed by COVID-19 is a 'pandemic within the pandemic' and describe the phenomenon of 'bereavement overload', which refers to the accumulation of rapid-fire losses without time to process or adjust to any one of them. 'While losses are not necessarily destructive events', they say, 'multiple determinants can cause an imbalance and derangement of the grieving process' (p. 1244). Ongoing bereavement overload may very well manifest in somatic and psychic complaints with aetiologies that are difficult to pinpoint. Thus, a clinician may need even more creative strategies to help with diagnosis and treatment

when a clinical picture is befuddling. Corona and colleagues suggest that taking a 'loss history' – that is, asking open-ended and reflective questions to bereaved patients, family members and caregivers – may reveal an inventory of unexplored and unrecognized loss and grief. The treatment for otherwise fully explored and vetted somatic and mental health complaints might mean support groups, cognitive behavioural therapy or other forms of counselling. This process may also have other downstream effects, such as strengthening the rapport and trust between clinician and patient. Therapeutic listening as described earlier and bearing witness to grief and loss may be the most important treatment plan for a patient in the moment.

The health humanities, then, can unmoor our diagnostic biases and help us become more reflective about the language we use and the questions we ask in order to sharpen our clinical reasoning. The humanities remind us of the potential dangers of clinicians digging in their heels and anchoring too early on a particular diagnosis or treatment plan. Clinical reasoning requires ongoing reflective practice that helps clinicians untether from repetitive diagnostic wrong turns and let them drift away. Engaging in sound clinical reasoning may require multiple internal rough drafts before the copy is polished. It may mean opening new doors such as taking a loss history, even when the door has never been opened before.

REFLECTION POINT

- Can you think of a time when hearing your patient's story changed your initial assumptions about their diagnosis?
- What about a treatment plan? Did hearing more about your patient's past or current situation – perhaps who they live with, how they get to and from the clinic, what their greatest worries and fears are – change your ideas about the best treatment plan for them?

The Humanities, Clinical Reasoning and Shared Decision Making

The humanities remind us that clinical encounters are rarely certain, clear and succinct. Rather, they help us see that they are always an interpretive (hermeneutical) meeting of patient and clinician. Swedish philosopher and ethicist Fredrik Svenaeus has published a great deal of work concerning *medical hermeneutics*, which is grounded in the work of 20th century philosopher Hans Georg Gadamer (Gadamer, 1995; Svenaeus, 2003). Svenaeus, following Gadamer's philosophical hermeneutics, illuminates the 'interpretive structure' of the clinical encounter: the clinician listens for and discerns relevant information and determines what this information *means* for this particular patient in this particular circumstance. Svenaeus describes the clinical encounter as a 'coming together' of clinician and patient – of the two separate spheres of clinical knowledge and lived experience of illness – for the purpose of creating a mutual understanding that can benefit the health of the patient. Clinicians, therefore, are 'not first and foremost scientists who apply biological knowledge, but rather interpreters—hermeneuts of health and illness' (p. 416).

During the clinical encounter, the patient and clinician seek authentic understanding 'in and through language' with the aim of restoring health or finding healing (Svenaeus, 2003, p. 424). Central to both Gadamerian hermeneutics and medical hermeneutics is the idea that achieving a 'good' or 'authentic' understanding and determining what one ought to do within this understanding is always 'particularized' and dependent on the actual meeting of two different worlds. Thus, the clinician, through interpretation, must determine what is best for each unique patient within each unique situation. The clinician cannot simply apply abstract, universal principles to a decontextualized and dehistoricized patient. Interpreting the patient's story is necessary for the correct diagnosis and for creating treatment plans that are aligned with a patient's values, capabilities and resources. Thus, shared decision making is not simply developing a plan that a patient agrees with; rather, shared decision making involves authentically hearing, interpreting and responding to a patient's story – a story that helps the clinician discern the next best steps for *this particular patient* in *this particular situation*.

Knowing what to do for a patient depends on what an illness or injury *means* to a patient and their loved ones. In the context of end-of-life care, the complexity of decision making is intensified. Sometimes, the preferences a patient has previously voiced to a clinician can change (and maybe significantly so) once a family

member or friend enters the room. Most clinicians caring for patients with serious or terminal illnesses will experience the discomfort of suspecting their patient is suppressing their wishes in order to appease the wishes of their loved one(s). For instance, one of the authors of this chapter (I.B.) was recently caring for a patient with a terminal illness who expressed their desire not to undergo aggressive treatments at the end of life. A few family members, however, disagreed with the patient's wishes, eventually telling the nurse on the care team that they wanted their loved one to 'live longer' so that they had more time to share their religious beliefs with the patient so that they would be 'saved' before their death. When a family's goals are potentially in discordance with a patient's goals, it can start to feel, as the nurse who works with I.B. put it, as if one is *diffusing a bomb all day*. No matter how carefully a care team may try to elicit a patient's goals and wishes, complex family dynamics (intensified by feelings of grief, impending loss and religious beliefs) can create confusion and uncertainty about care decisions that have become, quite literally, life or death.

It may be difficult for a clinician to accept that concrete knowledge of the pathophysiology of disease or of the typical trajectory of recovery after a surgical procedure is not enough when it comes to understanding *what is the matter* and what to do for a patient who is suffering. An engagement with the arts and humanities – which underscore the complexities, confusion and existential pain of being human – can help clinicians make sense of the intricacies and ambiguity of patient care while also helping clinicians grapple with the internal conflicts and disappointments that come with caring for people who suffer in complex ways that cannot be *fixed* or *controlled*. The arts and humanities help give voice to the experience of both patients and clinicians as they bear witness to the remarkable achievements and inevitable failings of modern healthcare. As physician and health humanities scholar Arno Kumagai puts it:

> In addition to sharpening the powers of observation and analytical thinking, art also offers a way to explore the challenges and triumphs of providing care to those in need and to explore the meanings, feelings, and experiences of living and dying. It offers a way of understanding and expressing the moral dilemmas

of our time—the inequities of the healthcare system, the legacy of systemic racism, the crisis of climate change, the moral injuries of those working on the front lines of the pandemic—that goes beyond technical rationality and aspires toward the aesthetic, philosophical, and existential truths of a life in medicine.

(2022, p. 1116)

THE HEALTH HUMANITIES AS TREATMENT

While the humanities inform clinical reasoning by unpacking diagnostic biases, revealing the interpretive nature of clinical encounters and giving voice to the existential pain and beauty that comes with caring for others, it is sometimes the case that the humanities are a form of treatment themselves. The arts, such as music therapy (Warth et al., 2021), have been identified as essential nonpharmacological interventions in patient care. Strange as it may sound, literature may be equally therapeutic. The neurologist Harold Klawans (1990) describes in Newton's Madness how art, specifically literature, became an adjunctive treatment for one of his patients. In other words, the humanities and traditional biomedical approaches provided multimodal care.

HEALTH HUMANITIES AND SOFT SKILLS

Healthcare students are commonly taught that patient care requires a blend of 'hard skills' – the knowledge imparted by biomedicine – and 'soft skills', which help build compassion and bedside rapport. This oversimplified distillation of clinical work suggests these skills are cultivated on divergent roads rather than intersecting pathways. As discussed previously, it is the synergy between biomedicine and the humanities that helps clinicians get closer to *what is the matter and what to do about it*. The bifurcation of hard and soft skills is ultimately an unhelpful either/or construct that fails to account for the complexity of clinical reasoning that requires *both* the application of biomedicine and an attunement to a particular patient's context – a context that is best discerned through listening, interpreting a narrative and discerning what to do in collaboration with other people.

In many ways, the so-called soft skills of clinical reasoning *are* the hard skills; without the ability to listen, interpret and make collaborative decisions, it is impossible to discern what is troubling patients and how to help them. Referring to such abilities as soft skills implies that they are, as Lucinda Fickel (2015) puts it, 'easy', and, by extension, 'unworthy of effort or attention'. Such an implication is dangerous, given that these qualities might be the most important for a trainee or clinician to hone and given that they are not something one can simply memorize, cram or brush up on. Biomedical and technical knowledge, on the other hand, is studded with safety nets: an app, an online textbook or the colleague down the hall can help refresh the functional anatomy of the hip for the physical or occupational therapist, the procedure for performing an oral nerve block for the dental trainee, or the 'five rights' of medication administration for the nursing graduate. Wading through the uncertainty, clouding a patient story and sifting through ambiguity, however, are not skills gleaned from a textbook, a search engine or a quick scroll through social media.

Although one might argue that abilities to listen well, interpret difficult stories and make collaborative decisions can come with time and experience as a clinician, engaging with the humanities offers a buttress during the accumulation of that experience. More than this, the humanities can push clinicians with years of experience to go even deeper: to recognize the personal complexities, the social inequities and the economic and political injustices that contribute to illness, injury and suffering. Clinical reasoning calls upon healthcare professionals to trace the contours of a patient's life. It involves cognition *and* interpersonal skills, linking head and heart inextricably in an effort to care for patients and their families in all of their complexity.

REFLECTION POINT

- Think of some of the aspects of your training or practice that you've considered to be 'soft skills'.
- Given the fact that the clinical encounter is inherently complex, ambiguous and interpersonal, which of these humanities-inspired skills are actually *essential* to sound clinical reasoning?
- Which humanities-inspired skills – if absent – would make diagnosing a patient or developing a treatment plan extraordinarily difficult?

SUMMARY

Clinical reasoning requires the integration of biomedical knowledge with intra- and interpersonal wisdom to help patients who do not often present with clear, uncomplicated or strictly biomedical issues. Thus, diagnostic accuracy and sound therapeutic interventions require drawing on both cognitive and noncognitive domains. The health humanities can foster clinical reasoning and encourage a commitment to openness within a patient encounter that relentlessly seeks the patient's viewpoint and context alongside the application of biomedical know-how. As Dason (2022), a resident physician, observes, 'We cannot cage all human suffering into evidence-based medicine', highlighting the need for other ways of knowing when it comes to addressing the complex ways that patients and their families suffer (p. E1069). Practitioners who can accept the complexity of patient care and embrace the ways of knowing offered by both the humanities and biomedicine will ultimately have more to offer their patients. Supporting the collaboration between biomedicine and the humanities and recognizing the potential fruits of their intersection may 'spark their neural connections' (Bettendorf, 2023), setting up clinicians for greater diagnostic accuracy, and even pride and purpose within the art and science of clinical reasoning.

Physician and poet Shane Neilson reminds us that the 'real benefit of medicine [is] immersion in people's lives by choice' (as cited in Hanlon, 2012, p. 1818). Recognizing that clinical reasoning requires so much more than cognitive skill and technical know-how may help clinicians slow down enough to listen to their patients' rich and varied stories, rather than writing such things off as 'soft skills'. While future work is needed to explore how engaging with the humanities might improve patient outcomes or increase job satisfaction for healthcare professionals, our hope is that the literature explored throughout this chapter highlights how the health humanities can help students and practitioners more deeply interpret and respond to the specific contexts of patients' lives in order to strengthen their clinical reasoning.

REFERENCES

Andoh, J.E., 2023. The stories we don't know. JAMA, 329 (18), 1551. https://doi.org/10.1001/jama.2023.5891

Bentwich, M.E., Gilbey, P., 2017. More than visual literacy: Art and the enhancement of tolerance for ambiguity and empathy. BMC Medical Education 17 (1), 200. https://doi.org/10.1186/s12909-017-1028-7

Bettendorf, B.A., 2023. Listening lessons. JAMA 329 (11), 883. https://doi.org/10.1001/jama.2023.0521

Bleakley, A., 2015. Seven types of ambiguity in evaluating the impact of humanities provision in undergraduate medicine curricula. The Journal of Medical Humanities 36 (4), 337–357. https://doi.org/10.1007/s10912-015-9337-5

Brown, J.L., 2012. A piece of my mind: The unasked question. JAMA 308 (18), 1869–1870. https://doi.org/10.1001/jama.2012.14254

Carson, R.A., 2007. Engaged humanities: Moral work in the precincts of medicine. Perspectives in Biology and Medicine 50 (3), 321–333. https://doi.org/10.1353/pbm.2007.0025

Carson, R.A., 2003. Introduction. In: Carson, R.A., Burns, C.R., Cole, T.R. (Eds.), Practicing the medical humanities: Engaging physicians and patients. University Publishing Group, pp. 1–2.

Carson, R.A., Burns, C.R., Cole, T.R., 2003. Practicing the medical humanities: Engaging physicians and patients. University Publishing Group.

Cayton, H., 2006. The alienating language of health care. Journal of the Royal Society of Medicine 99 (10), 484. https://doi.org/10.1177/014107680609901002

Charon, R., 2001. The patient-physician relationship. Narrative medicine: A model for empathy, reflection, profession, and trust. JAMA 286 (15), 1897–1902. https://doi.org/10.1001/jama.286.15.1897

Charon, R., 2007. What to do with stories: The sciences of narrative medicine. Canadian Family Physician 53 (8), 1265–1267.

Charon, R., 2016. Close reading: The signature method of narrative medicine. In: Charon, R., DasGupta, S., Hermann, N., Irvine, C., Marcus, E.R., Rivera Colon, E., et al., (Eds.), The Principles and practice of narrative medicine. Oxford University Press, pp. 157–179.

Charon, R., 2017. To see the suffering. Academic Medicine: Journal of the Association of American Medical Colleges 92 (12), 1668–1670. https://doi.org/10.1097/ACM.0000000000001989

Cole, T.R., Carson, R.A., Carlin, N.S., 2015. Medical humanities: An introduction. Cambridge University Press.

Cole, T.R., Lagay, F.L., 2003. How the medical humanities can help revitalize humanism and how a reconfigured humanism can help nourish the medical humanities. In: Carson, R.A., Burns, C.R., Cole, T.R. (Eds.), Practicing the medical humanities: Engaging physicians and patients. University Publishing Group, pp. 157–177.

Crawford, P., 2015, March 30. Health humanities: We are here to collaborate, not to compete. The Guardian. http://www.theguardian.com/higher-education-network/2015/mar/30/health-humanities-here-to-collaborate-not-compete

Dason, E.S., 2022. Reflections of a chief resident. CMAJ: Canadian Medical Association Journal 194 (30), E1069. https://doi.org/10.1503/cmaj.220686

De Leon Corona, A.G., Chin, J., No, P., Tom, J., 2022. The virulence of grief in the pandemic: Bereavement overload during COVID. The American Journal of Hospice & Palliative Care 39 (10), 1244–1249. https://doi.org/10.1177/10499091211057094

Dumas, D., Torre, D.M., Durning, S.J., 2018. Using relational reasoning strategies to help improve clinical reasoning practice.

Academic Medicine: Journal of the Association of American Medical Colleges 93 (5), 709–714. https://doi.org/10.1097/ACM.0000000000002114

Fickel, L., 2015, May 1. What's in a terrible name? US News & World Report. https://www.usnews.com/opinion/knowledge-bank/2015/05/01/non-cognitive-skills-are-important-but-have-a-terrible-name

Fox, D.M., 1985. Who we are: The political origins of the medical humanities. Theoretical Medicine 6 (3), 327–341. https://doi.org/10.1007/BF00489733

Furze, J.A., Black, L., McDevitt, A.W., Kobal, K.L., Durning, S.J., Jensen, G.M., 2022. Clinical reasoning: The missing core competency in physical therapist education and practice. Physical Therapy 102 (9), 1–4. https://doi.org/10.1093/ptj/pzac093

Gadamer, H.G., 1995. Truth and method. Continuum.

Garden, R., 2019. Critical healing: Queering diagnosis and public health through the health humanities. The Journal of Medical Humanities 40 (1), 1–5. https://doi.org/10.1007/s10912-018-9533-1

Goddu, A.P., O'Conor, K.J., Lanzkron, S., Saheed, M.O., Saha, S., Peek, M.E., et al., 2018. Do words matter? Stigmatizing language and the transmission of bias in the medical record. Journal of General Internal Medicine 33 (5), 685–691. https://doi.org/10.1007/s11606-017-4289-2

Hanlon, V., 2012. "I am a doctor, and I write poems." CMAJ: Canadian Medical Association Journal 184 (16), 1818. https://doi.org/10.1503/cmaj.120299

Jones, T., Blackie, M., Garden, R., Wear, D., 2017. The almost right word: The move from medical to health humanities. Academic Medicine: Journal of the Association of American Medical Colleges 92 (7), 932–935. https://doi.org/10.1097/ACM.0000000000001518

Klawans, H.L., 1990. Newton's madness: Further tales of clinical neurology. HarperCollins.

Komesaroff, P.A., 1995. Troubled bodies: Critical perspectives on postmodernism, medical ethics, and the body. Duke University Press.

Kumagai, A.K., 2022. The powers of a fish: Clinical thinking, humanistic thinking, and different ways of knowing. Academic Medicine: Journal of the Association of American Medical Colleges 97 (8), 1114–1116. https://doi.org/10.1097/ACM.0000000000004684

Lamb, E.G., Berry, S.L., Jones, T., 2022. Baccalaureate programs in health humanities. HHC Curricular Toolkit. https://healthhumanitiesconsortium.com/publications/hhc-toolkit/

Ofri, D., 2017. Medical humanities: The Rx for uncertainty. Academic Medicine: Journal of the Association of American Medical Colleges 92 (12), 1657–1658. https://doi.org/10.1097/ACM.0000000000001983

President and Fellows of Harvard College, 2023. Training our eyes, minds and hearts: Visual thinking strategies for health care professionals—Overview. Retrieved May 1, 2023, from https://cmecatalog.hms.harvard.edu/training-our-eyes-minds-and-hearts-visual-thinking-strategies-health-care-professionals

Prince, G., Osipov, R., Mazzella, A.J., Chelminski, P.R., 2022. Linking the humanities with clinical reasoning: Proposing an integrative conceptual model for a graduate medical education humanities curriculum. Academic Medicine: Journal of the Association of American Medical Colleges 97 (8), 1151–1157. https://doi.org/10.1097/ACM.0000000000004683

Ratcliffe, T.A., Durning, S.J., 2015. Theoretical concepts to consider in providing clinical reasoning instruction. In: Trowbridge, R.L., Rencic, J.J., Durning, S.J. (Eds.), Teaching clinical reasoning. American College of Physicians, pp. 13–30.

Renner, W.F., 2015, revisited from 1965. Of science, humanism, and medicine. JAMA 314 (7), 734. https://doi.org/10.1001/jama.2014.11930

Sinayev, A., Peters, E., Tusler, M., Fraenkel, L., 2015. Presenting numeric information with percentages and descriptive risk labels: A randomized trial. Medical Decision Making. An International Journal of the Society for Medical Decision Making 35 (8), 937–947. https://doi.org/10.1177/0272989X15584922

Sisk, B.A., Baker, J.N., 2018. Microethics of communication—Hidden roles of bias and heuristics in the words we choose. JAMA Pediatrics 172 (12), 1115–1116. https://doi.org/10.1001/jamapediatrics.2018.3111

Svenaeus, F., 2003. Hermeneutics of medicine in the wake of Gadamer: The issue of phronesis. Theoretical Medicine and Bioethics 24 (5), 407–431. https://doi.org/10.1023/b:meta.0000006935.10835.b2

Swenson, G., 2021. Listening for horses. Academic Emergency Medicine: Official Journal of the Society for Academic Emergency Medicine 28 (6), 710–711. https://doi.org/10.1111/acem.14240

Thibault, G.E., 2019. Humanism in medicine: What does it mean and why is it more important than ever? Academic Medicine: Journal of the Association of American Medical Colleges 94 (8), 1074–1077. https://doi.org/10.1097/ACM.0000000000002796

Vonnegut, M., 2014. Foreword: Too long too short. In: Jones, T., Wear, D., Friedman, L.D. (Eds.), Health humanities reader. Rutgers University Press.

Warth, M., Koehler, F., Brehmen, M., Weber, M., Bardenheuer, H.J., Ditzen, B., et al., 2021. "Song of Life": Results of a multicenter randomized trial on the effects of biographical music therapy in palliative care. Palliative Medicine 35 (6), 1126–1136. https://doi.org/10.1177/02692163211010394

Zirulnik, M., Cartsonis, J., 2019, May 28. Opinion: Doctors privately use cruel words to describe their patients. Vice. https://www.vice.com/en/article/wjvpqy/opinion-doctors-use-cruel-words-to-privately-describe-their-patients

18

SHARED DECISION MAKING IN PRACTICE

JOY DOLL ▪ CINDY COSTANZO ▪ GAIL M. JENSEN

CHAPTER AIMS

The aims of this chapter are:

- to identify key attributes of shared decision making (SDM) in practice
- to recognize organizational characteristics that support and facilitate SDM
- to describe practice strategies that lead to successful outcomes when engaged in SDM.

INTRODUCTION

Health and well-being rely on the ability of a patient to make good decisions every day and over time. Healthcare providers often express frustration by the lack of engagement patients hold in the healthcare process and their own well-being. Yet healthcare systems and cultures clearly do not consistently support collaborative decision making of healthcare team members with patients. Additionally, systemic barriers create challenges for patients and clinicians in accessing health information to fully understand their care. Shared decision making (SDM) offers an avenue to address the disconnects in care by engaging patients in collaboration with healthcare professionals in making informed healthcare decisions. The chapter identi-

fies and describes the processes and good practices of SDM, as well as the importance of organizational culture in the influence of the adoption and sustainability of SDM. In addition, SDM models, measurement tools and decisional aids that augment SDM in practice will be shared. This chapter promotes the use of interprofessional, team-based practices and a patient-centred SDM model to ultimately improve clinical outcomes of care.

SHARED DECISION MAKING

Historically, decision making between healthcare professionals and patients has followed three definitive models: paternalism, consumerism and SDM (Fig. 18.1). A paternalistic model occurs when a provider or healthcare team makes the primary decisions and choices *for* the patient. A consumerist informative model occurs when the consumer decides *without* involvement of a provider or healthcare team (Charles et al., 1997). SDM occurs *with* the involvement of patients, providers and interprofessional team members in the decision-making process. SDM is defined as 'an approach where clinicians and patients share the best available evidence when faced with the task of making decisions, and where patients are supported

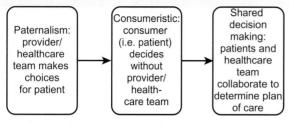

Fig. 18.1 ■ Patient decision-making approaches.

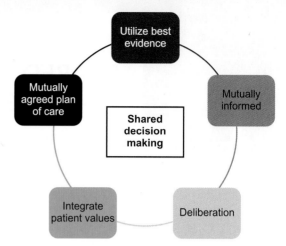

Fig. 18.2 ■ Components of shared decision making.

to consider options, to achieve informed preferences' (Barr et al., 2014).

SDM is the preferred practice and should be mainstreamed, but its implementation and execution continue to be challenging (Müller et al., 2016). Informed consent, informed choice, consumer rights, patient-centred care and chronic illnesses with a lifetime management approach have accelerated the shift from the once dominant paternalistic approach to SDM (Charles et al., 1997). Recently, interoperability, the sharing of data between systems and the importance of patient ownership of health data, has increased consumer awareness and access of their own health information. Health information technology infrastructure such as patient portals, wearables and remote patient monitoring systems are increasing patient access to health information. All of this infrastructure can support increased patient engagement promoting SDM (Martin et al., 2021).

SDM provides a forum for the healthcare team to involve the patient and family as part of the team. Today's complexity of care reinforces the need for SDM and requires that the interprofessional team become adept at utilizing this approach. As healthcare moves towards interprofessional collaborative practice, it is critical that patients and families are valued members of this team (Interprofessional Education Collaborative, 2016).

In SDM, the perspectives of the patient and/or family are valued as they collaborate with the healthcare team to make decisions about care (Interprofessional Education Collaborative, 2016). For SDM to be successful, several important actions are required. In SDM, interprofessional team members and patients must acknowledge that a decision should be made utilizing the best information both in data and patient experience, are mutually informed with an

understanding of the decision's risks and benefits, hold a period of deliberation and incorporate the patient's values and preferences as the team and patient arrive at a mutually agreed-upon care plan (Charles et al., 1997; Légaré et al., 2011a,b; Légaré and Witteman, 2013; Sepucha et al., 2016) (Fig. 18.2). Gravel et al. (2006) also acknowledge that SDM relies on provider motivation and a history of positive outcomes of SDM experienced by both the clinicians and patients involved. Although patients and healthcare team members often speak different languages, health literacy and the healthcare team's ability to provide health information in a manner that supports the patient's capacity to make an informed shared decision are vital (Edwards et al., 2009; Michaelson et al., 2019). Increased access to health information does not necessarily increase patient understanding. SDM can bridge the gap to ensure patients engage more effectively in their own care through engagement and translation of health information into a meaningful co-created care plan. In addition, SDM can ensure that access to data considers equity to ensure human dignity (Hedberg et al., 2022) (see Fig. 18.2).

SDM is not necessarily a natural process for the healthcare team. Légaré and Witteman (2013) identify three elements that are critical for SDM, including recognition that a decision needs to occur, knowledge of evidence-based practice and ensuring that the patients' values are part of the decision-making process.

Although SDM has been particularly addressed as a role for physicians, all members of the healthcare team can assist and be involved in SDM. Makoul and Clayman (2006) provide an integrative model that identifies essential elements of SDM. These attributes include the following:

- The problem is defined by patients and providers.
- Options are presented with supportive physician knowledge and recommendations.
- Benefits and risks are discussed.
- Patient values and preferences are included.
- The ability for the patient to follow through with the plan is discussed.
- There is an opportunity for any reclarification.
- The decision is made or deferred.
- Follow-up is organized.

Barriers to Shared Decision Making

Overcoming barriers to SDM can facilitate its adoption, implementation and use across healthcare settings. Historically, healthcare decisions were made utilizing a paternalistic approach, which continues across many healthcare settings today. Within the healthcare team, barriers can occur with or between individual practitioners and could include differences in healthcare knowledge, attitudes or beliefs that are not supportive of SDM and lack of agreement among team members when making a decision (Légaré et al., 2008; Légaré et al., 2014; Boland et al., 2019; Jones et al., 2022). Similar to the barriers seen in implementing interprofessional care, SDM faces challenges when healthcare team members do not dedicate or invest the time to discuss the processes of SDM (Pieterse et al., 2019). Lack of investment of time in identifying the processes of SDM leads to discrepancies in how decisions are made. Due to the nature of gathering diverse perspectives and knowledge on healthcare teams, conflict can occur among the team members and the patient. Although conflict is often identified in a negative light, SDM elicits conflict with the intent to co-create solutions and strategies for healthcare intervention and management. Healthcare team members must commit to SDM and not let issues such as individual practitioners' lack of motivation or self-confidence interfere with SDM (Légaré et al., 2008). SDM may also be a challenge when patients are not interested

in being part of the decision process. Depending on differences in culture and health beliefs, some patients may find the process of being asked to engage in SDM uncomfortable and countercultural. These beliefs can act as barriers to the successful implementation of SDM. Beyond providers and patients, systemic barriers exist for SDM, including time constraints, lack of resources to support SDM, reimbursement concerns and lack of organizational support. Some barriers may not actually exist but may be perceived to occur, such as lack of support for SDM by the healthcare system or healthcare team; such support and relevant infrastructure for implementation of SDM are necessary at team and organizational levels (Légaré et al., 2008).

REFLECTION POINT

- How do these barriers for SDM apply to your practice?

Shared Decision Making in Practice

SDM in practice environments calls upon healthcare teams to take on a healing- and wellness-oriented approach rather than a scientific approach based on cure and pathology. Such an approach recognizes not only *scientific* evidence but also human perspectives and aspirations in healthcare decisions. The first step in implementing SDM is ensuring that all healthcare team members are educated and understand how to engage in SDM (Muller et al., 2019; Boland et al., 2019). Team members must address their own professional socialization issues and enculturation, including attitudes of paternalism and power that often influence the patient, family and team. This is true for the clinical team as well as patients and family members engaged in SDM. Next, healthcare team members need to become comfortable with uncertainty, which will help them assist patients to recognize that much of healthcare includes varied levels of uncertainty that can be uncomfortable for all involved. Yet SDM offers an avenue for addressing uncertainty and further dialogue by all stakeholders, including patients, families and members of the healthcare team. Ultimately, addressing uncertainty and encouraging further dialogue in an open and honest forum can facilitate positive healthcare decisions (Braddock, 2013). The healthcare team should become aware of the access and understanding patients have of their own healthcare information. This requires the team to understand their own institution's health information technology infrastructure including patient portals and remote patient monitoring, along with where patients access both health education and their own health information. Patients vary in their engagement and savvy with these tools. Understanding patient engagement in these aspects can support improved SDM. Healthcare teams should also value and engage in health literacy strategies to ensure patients understand their health data to be fully engaged in the SDM.

Cultural Influences: Organizational on Shared Decision Making

Cultural beliefs and values have an influence on SDM. Healthcare providers' norms, language and practices are formed and framed within a cultural perspective that is unique to each individual and profession (Pecukonis et al., 2008). Both patients and healthcare professionals hold cultural beliefs and stereotypes about each other. Recognizing how beliefs and perceptions are formed about other people, professions and the roles that (healthcare) professionals play are important because all of these factors directly affect the development and implementation of SDM practices. Realizing the opportunities and challenges created by professionalism and intercultural interactions with the patient is important and helps identify opportunities and barriers to communication and collaboration. This, in turn, helps ensure that SDM promotes optimal health outcomes for both the patient and the healthcare organization (Légaré et al., 2008). Barriers between patients and providers can lead to medical errors, poor patient outcomes, decreased patient satisfaction and health disparities (Nelson, 2002).

Organizations are composed of individuals with beliefs, values and practices that are unique to each person but which unite and represent the overall organizational culture. Leadership, operational procedures and processes, policy, care practices and employee behaviours are influenced by the organizational culture. Shared decision-making processes are congruent with organizational cultures that demonstrate strong, mutually respectful relationships between the patient, family and interprofessional healthcare team. An organization that adopts and supports a shared

relationship model (i.e. relational coordination, relational coproduction and relational leadership) contributes to operational success and positive outcomes for the organization (Gittell et al., 2013; Moreau et al., 2012). SDM is a form of relational coordination and relational coproduction that not only addresses how to achieve the goals of treatment but most importantly allows patients to shape what those goals ought to be (Gittell, 2016). Adopting SDM principles can help interprofessional teams by supporting a shared mental model that has been identified as a strategy for success among interprofessional teams (Ginsburg and Tregunno, 2005). Fortunately, many of the SDM practice environment and organizational culture issues can be addressed simultaneously with interprofessional collaborative practice development.

REFLECTION POINT

- What attributes of SDM and key elements of organizational culture contributed to a collaborative team approach in Case Study 18.1?

Interprofessional Collaborative Practice and Shared Decision Making

The Core Competencies for Interprofessional Collaborative Practice (IPCP), released in 2011, provided a foundation for a wider discussion about interprofessional education and practice (Interprofessional Education Collaborative, 2011, 2016; 2023). Healthcare professions exhibit many differences, including their professional cultures, but they have one thing in common: their caring for the patient and family. Despite their differences, all healthcare professionals identify with 'a sense of shared purpose to support the common good in healthcare, and reflect a shared commitment to creating safer, more efficient and more effective systems of care' (Interprofessional Education Collaborative, 2011, p. 17). The common good is how health professionals are not only concerned about individual patient care but also how the communities in which we live can flourish (Doherty, 2020). The intent of interprofessional collaboration is that clinicians work 'deliberatively' together with the patient and family to provide optimal healthcare. Based on the principles and values of IPCP, healthcare professionals must learn to work in teams to collaborate 'with others

CASE STUDY 18.1

Shared Decision Making

Tom, a 45-year-old construction worker, has an appointment at a recently opened ambulatory care clinic in his neighbourhood. When making his appointment, Tom reported he experienced a fall a couple of days ago hurting his wrist and ankle. He also reviewed his patient portal and has some questions about items on his record. During the phone call for the appointment, the front desk staff asked Tom to begin thinking about options for his care and his priorities. The front desk scheduler explains to Tom that the clinic uses a healthcare team, and he may be seen by multiple professionals to address his issues and patients are a valued member of this team. She indicates Tom will have an active role in deciding his care.

After arriving for the appointment, the front desk receptionist reiterates to Tom that he will see a team and that at the clinic patients are encouraged to voice their desires for their care. Once Tom is checked in, the medical assistant brings him back to an examination room to get a brief history and also learns that he recently lost his job as a construction worker. The medical assistant encourages Tom to share this with the provider and also documents it in the electronic health record. During the patient interview, the medical assistant observes and notes that some cuts Tom received from the fall do not look well cleaned. The medical assistant mentions this to Tom and Tom asks what he could do to keep them clean. At this request, the medical assistant cleans the cuts and educates Tom how to properly keep the wounds clean. Before departing the examination room, the medical assistant encourages Tom to ask questions during his visit and share how he wants his care delivered. The medical assistant enters the ambulatory care pod, where clinicians can speak openly about patients, and shares information from the brief patient history.

As a result of previous physician visits, Tom believes that he will just be getting some medication and sent on his way. He does not realize that behind the doors of his room there is a large team of medical professionals collaborating to meet all of his needs. Tom is also viewed as a valued member of this team

who will be asked to help make decisions regarding his care. The healthcare team, including Tom, is committed to engaging patients in their healthcare and value-shared decision making as part of patient care. The team is composed of a medical assistant, medical resident, occupational therapist, pharmacist, physical therapist, psychologist, public health nurse, radiological technician and social worker. The team holds the value that all members of the team, including the patient, can speak up and advocate for the patient. Patients are informed about the opportunity to be engaged in their care and encouraged to engage in SDM as part of the team. The psychologist acts as the team coach supporting the team and its members, ensuring that the team works effectively. They ensure that the patient is included and is a facilitator for SDM among the team and the patient. The team engages in 'huddles' twice a day, where team members identify clinic issues for each session followed by a previsit planning session, where the healthcare team reviews the patient caseload for the session. When a patient's case is considered complex, any team member can identify the individual for case review at the weekly interprofessional care planning meeting.

The medical resident enters the room after being briefed by the medical assistant. She reviews with Tom the concerns the medical assistant reported. Tom also asks about some of the information in his patient portal which the resident pulls up and clarifies with him. She encourages him to use this tool and ask questions at every visit. Upon this review, the medical resident informs Tom that she wants him involved with deciding the next steps in his care. Tom tells her his priority is his wrist, but he is very concerned that if it is broken he will not have insurance for follow-up. The medical resident acknowledges this fear and tells Tom she would recommend a radiograph to determine whether it is broken. She would also like him to meet with the social worker to discuss options for job opportunities and insurance coverage. She would recommend a prescription of an antibiotic for his cuts because of risk of infection. Tom reports he would like to first determine whether

CASE STUDY 18.1

Shared Decision Making—cont'd

his wrist is broken with a radiograph. He feels this is a good first step.

Upon exiting the examination room, the medical resident with physician supervision identifies that she and Tom identified the following priorities:

- radiograph of wrist to determine potential fracture,
- prescription for antibiotic to address potential infection in his cuts and
- referral to social work to address recent job loss.

The resident knows he has access to many resources on the healthcare team but also recognizes that Tom is feeling overwhelmed from the fall and his job loss. The medical resident proceeds to review all the options with the patient including inviting him to attend the interprofessional team meeting later that week. Tom gets a little teary eyed, admitting to the resident that with his job loss, he will soon lose health insurance coverage. He is anxious about accessing other services because of cost. The resident recommends that because of the acuteness of his wrist injury, a radiograph is highly recommended at the appointment. He encourages Tom to take a moment to consider his options and leaves the examination room. The team recommends a social needs screening to identify his social needs.

Tom decides that he would like the radiograph and to visit the social worker. Due to transportation issues, he does not feel he can come back to the clinic for the interprofessional team meeting but is willing to have the team discuss options and have the social worker follow up with him. The social worker has access to a social care referral platform that can connect Tom with community-based organizations who can support his social needs.

When the healthcare team meets to discuss Tom's case, the medical resident reports concern for Tom, including the possibility of developing depression because of his recent job loss. The team decides that the social worker will contact Tom to discuss his options, especially related to his wrist fracture confirmed via the radiograph.

Through this collaboration of the interprofessional team and efforts to engage Tom in SDM, the healthcare team is able to work with his prioritized needs that include finding a new job, which is identified as a priority by both Tom and the healthcare team.

---

through shared problem-solving and SDM, especially in circumstances of uncertainty' (Interprofessional Education Collaborative, 2011, p. 24). Despite extensive literature supporting SDM as a valuable approach for the patient and single physician, emerging models for SDM with the interprofessional care team are increasingly supported as a means of helping the team engage in collaborative patient-centred care planning (Légaré et al., 2010).

Implementation of the Interprofessional Shared Decision-Making Model

Légaré et al. (2011a, 2014) implemented and tested an Interprofessional Shared Decision-Making (IP-SDM) model. They found the model useful and easy to understand for team members during the implementation phase of SDM. The authors report that the model served as an excellent guide, enhanced the team's understanding of the conceptual foundation of the SDM process and enhanced collaboration within the interprofessional team. Having a team member enact the role of a decisional coach has been found to be a successful strategy during the implementation process of IP-SDM (Shunk et al., 2014). Decision coaches can be any one of multiple team members who helps the patient, family and healthcare team members reach a decision based on the principles of SDM. Coaches help the team engage in effective SDM by overseeing the process and providing feedback to team members. Through this process, team members develop their abilities with SDM. Decision coaches can be members of the healthcare team who agree to take on this

TABLE 18.1	
Interprofessional Shared Decision-Making Model	
Steps	**Description**
1. Patient presents (at the healthcare centre) and a decision needs to be made	'Professionals share their knowledge and understanding of the options with the patient while recognizing equipoise[a] and the need for a decision' (Légaré et al., 2011b, p. 21).
2. Exchange of information	'The health professional(s) and the patient share information about the potential benefits and harms of the options, using educational material, patient decision aids and other evidence-based resources' (Légaré et al., 2011b, p. 22).
3. Value clarification	Clarifying values by all involved in the decision-making process.
4. Feasibility of options	The healthcare team has a good understanding of options available to the patient.
5. Decision	Team members agree upon a decision.
6. Support patient	Healthcare team members support the patient revisiting the decision as needed.

[a]Equipoise: a balance of forces or interests.

additional role to support the interprofessional healthcare team. The IP-SDM model with six process steps is outlined in Table 18.1.

Although there are limitations identified in using the IP-SDM model, Yu et al. (2014) identified that these limitations can be resolved by a deliberative interprofessional team that is engaged in respectful communication. The challenges with implementing interprofessional collaborative practice have been well documented and are no different from the support needed for SDM in the interprofessional team. Barriers to SDM for the interprofessional team include issues with knowledge and understanding of IP-SDM and patient-centred care among team members, team performance norms, individual team members' attitudes and perceptions towards IP-SDM, external factors such as reimbursement and organizational support by leadership (Chong et al., 2013). Clinicians may have differing opinions of how much patients should be involved in SDM. For example, a team member may value a patient engaged in rounds, whereas others may perceive this is not appropriate. Vetting the perspectives of the team and establishing clear team guidelines on patient involvement is critical to success. However, IP-SDM can be supported and facilitated through training of team members, establishing team commitments among team members and organizational support. The barriers and supports for both SDM and interprofessional care align. Overall, in order for SDM to be successful in the interprofessional care model, the healthcare team has to work through the basic principles of team development to

ensure that power dynamics are conducive to SDM and essentially work towards becoming a high-performing, *collaborative* team (Légaré et al., 2010). Teams have a shared professional responsibility for their individual and collective duty of care. Furthermore, there has to be support from the healthcare environment and the healthcare team in order for the SDM to be successful (Légaré et al., 2011a).

Important Influences for Successful Implementation and Sustainability of Shared Decision Making

Shared values, good communication, trust and supportive organizational culture are essential influences important for SDM to occur (Müller et al., 2016). SDM relies upon the healthcare team to ensure the patient perspective is valued. The development of this value occurs through building trust and relationships with patients through active listening and engaging in empathy. The process of SDM, which involves transparency and patient empowerment, can act as a venue to naturally facilitate trust building among the patient, family and healthcare team (Braddock, 2013). Epstein and Street called upon healthcare providers to promote SDM by developing a shared mind. A shared mind is characterized as a situation in which 'new ideas and perspectives emerge through the sharing of thoughts, feelings, perceptions, meanings and intentions among two or more people' (Epstein and Street, 2011, p. 455). Interprofessional teams need to see themselves working collaboratively with the patient as a 'shared mind' (Epstein and Street, 2011, p. 455).

Electronic Health Records for Successful Implementation and Sustainability of Shared Decision Making

Electronic health records (EHRs) can play an important part in the success of implementing and sustaining SDM. Essentially, EHRs can offer institutional support to the clinicians and the healthcare system to support SDM. Integrating processes to document SDM into EHRs has been identified as a strategy to accelerate the adoption of SDM into healthcare (Oshima Lee and Emanuel, 2013). Ideally, the EHR system can build a tailored SDM programme based on the patient's personal and clinical characteristics (Légaré et al., 2014). As part of this planning, access and availability is critical. For example, patients may access a portal, but may not understand it. For clinicians new to SDM, the EHR can include decisional aids and reminders to clinicians to engage in SDM with patients. Technology, such as EHRs, can help embed the tools and reminders needed to help SDM become a part of the healthcare team's daily processes. In a similar way to how patients use technology to manage and track health, EHRs can provide support to the healthcare team enacting SDM by providing reminders, decisional aids and tracking systems. Allowing patient access to these portions of the EHR also helps promote patient empowerment and SDM (Légaré et al., 2014). Electronic health records have been identified extensively in the literature as a tool to support the implementation of SDM (Archer et al., 2011; Tinetti et al., 2012). Although it is clear that EHRs can be a tool to implement SDM, clinicians must make a concerted effort to design processes to use the tools and document SDM in the EHR. In other words, simply building reminders and decisional aids into EHRs has not been proven to guarantee use. The opportunity exists to have EHRs support SDM but is commonly still underutilized (Davis et al., 2017). With the proliferation of artificial intelligence, remote patient monitoring, virtual care and other technological innovation along with the democratization of health data to patients, EHRs can be tools for data sharing and engagement (Abbasgholizadeh Rahimi et al., 2022). In addition, patient-reported outcomes are increasingly ripe for sharing into EHRs, which will provide direct opportunity for increased SDM using the EHR and other health information technology tools.

EHRs are not the only tools that can support SDM. Health information exchanges (HIEs) are repositories of EHR data aggregated and shared to promote patient safety. Depending on the national health system or region, HIEs can be statewide, regional or national. If accessible, the HIE provides the complete record of health information of all encounters a patient has experienced. This information can be helpful to clinicians to understand the comprehensive patient history.

Patient portals have also promoted access of patients to their health information. Recognizing and understanding how patients engage with these tools can help promote SDM.

Other health technology collects data and information on patients. Patients may engage with these tools, but these data may not be included as part of the EHR. It is important to ask patients which technology tools they use and explore how these tools can promote patient engagement and SDM.

Technology and access do not mean patients know or understand the information, even if they can access it, which can also be a barrier. Clinicians can be a bridge to building data literacy. It is also important to note that technology will continue to evolve and the tracking of health information may occur for many outside the healthcare ecosystem. For example, patients may track their exercise but this is never shared with their clinical team. With the democratization and access to health data, such as electrocardiograms (EKGs), some patients are more savvy and seeking more SDM from their clinical teams. Technology can drive patient desire for more collaboration with their healthcare team.

Decisional Aids for Successful Implementation and Sustainability of Shared Decision Making

Decisional aids have been instrumental in promoting SDM in encounters between interprofessional teams and the patient. Decisional aids provide patients with information on disease, describe complex health scenarios and treatment options for patients to improve the quality of the decision-making process (Sepucha et al., 2013) and reduce decisional conflict or uncertainty (Ruland and Bakken, 2002). The International Patient Decision Aids Standards Collaboration's focus is to increase the quality of decisional aids and they developed a criterion-based checklist involving 12 domains to evaluate the content and effective use of decision aids (McDonald et al., 2014). To date, there are over 1000 decisional aids that have been developed, used and studied within the healthcare system. The feasibility of continuing to produce these for every disease entity and treatment option has been brought into question. A universal decision support aid system has been proposed that allows clinicians and patients/families to input information specific to their situation and cultural context. This may be a promising solution that continues to be investigated (Légaré et al., 2018).

Outcomes of Shared Decision Making

SDM effectiveness with patient, provider, interprofessional team and organizational outcomes continues to be a focus of study. Establishing a consistent conceptual definition with methodologically sound measures must be a priority for continued research. Most outcome studies have focussed on disease-specific patient outcomes with variant results. Most of the literature focusses on contextual examples of SDM rather than themes or approaches that cross healthcare contexts. Although most models of SDM have been focussed on patient and physician, interprofessionalism naturally leans itself to SDM as teams include the patient and family as valued members. The ultimate outcome of SDM is to truly attain consensus on intervention. SDM is a complex experience recognizing the perspectives and values of multiple stakeholders. The success of SDM depends on the perspective of the player (Hsiao, et al., 2022). To accept that SDM is anything but nuanced and dynamic is critical to understand. For example, a patient and family will also change perspectives over time, based on diagnosis and experience with healthcare. The reality is that the values of SDM remain consistent in the interactions yet the outcomes of a SDM will be diverse to truly be considered a success.

SUMMARY

In this chapter, we have outlined:

- the attributes and barriers of SDM
- how interprofessional teams approach SDM in practice with consideration of the key, cultural and organizational factors that influence successful implementation of SDM, in particular shared values, good communication and trust

- other factors important for implementation and sustainability, including electronic health record and decisional aids
- a description of models, key outcomes and measurement of SDM.

REFERENCES

Abbasgholizadeh Rahimi, S., Cwintal, M., Huang, Y., Ghadiri, P., Grad, R., Poenaru, D., et al., 2022. Application of artificial intelligence in shared decision making: Scoping review. JMIR Medical Informatics 10 (8), e36199. https://doi.org/10.2196/36199

Archer, N., Fevrier-Thomas, U., Lokker, C., McKibbon, K.A., Straus, S.E., 2011. Personal health records: A scoping review. Journal of the American Medical Informatics Association 18 (4), 515–522. https://doi.org/10.1136/amiajnl-2011-000105

Barr, P.J., Thompson, R., Walsh, T., Grande, S.W., Ozanne, E.M., Elwyn, G., 2014. The psychometric properties of CollaboRATE: A fast and frugal patient-reported measure of the shared decision-making process. Journal of Medical Internet Research 16 (1), e3085. https://doi.org/10.2196/jmir.3085

Boland, L., Lawson, M.L., Graham, I.D., Légaré, F., Dorrance, K., Shephard, A., et al., 2019. Post-training shared decision making barriers and facilitators for pediatric healthcare providers: A mixed-methods study. Academic Pediatrics 19 (1), 118–129. https://doi.org/10.1016/j.acap.2018.05.010

Boland, L., Graham, I.D., Légaré, F., Lewis, K., Jull, J., Shephard, A., et al., 2019. Barriers and facilitators of pediatric shared decision-making: A systematic review. Implementation Science 14, 1–25. https://doi.org/10.1186/s13012-018-0851-5

Braddock, C.H., 2013. Supporting shared decision making when clinical evidence is low. Medical Care Research and Review 70 (1_suppl), 129S–140S. https://doi.org/10.1177/1077558712460280

Charles, C., Gafni, A., Whelan, T., 1997. Shared decision-making in the medical encounter: What does it mean? (or it takes at least two to tango). Social Science & Medicine 44 (5), 681–692. https://doi.org/10.1016/s0277-9536(96)00221-3

Chong, W.W., Aslani, P., Chen, T.F., 2013. Multiple perspectives on shared decision-making and interprofessional collaboration in mental healthcare. Journal of Interprofessional Care 27 (3), 223–230. https://doi.org/10.3109/13561820.2013.767225

Davis, S., Roudsari, A., Raworth, R., Courtney, K.L., MacKay, L., 2017. Shared decision-making using personal health record technology: A scoping review at the crossroads. Journal of the American Medical Informatics Association 24 (4), 857–866. https://doi.org/10.1093/jamia/ocw172

Doherty, R.F., 2020. Ethical dimensions in the health professions-e-book. Elsevier Health Sciences.

Edwards, M., Davies, M., Edwards, A., 2009. What are the external influences on information exchange and shared decision-making in healthcare consultations: A meta-synthesis of the literature. Patient Education and Counseling 75 (1), 37–52. https://doi.org/10.1016/j.pec.2008.09.025

Epstein, R.M., Street, R.L., 2011. Shared mind: Communication, decision making, and autonomy in serious illness. The Annals of Family Medicine 9 (5), 454–461. https://doi.org/10.1370/afm.1301

Ginsburg, L., Tregunno, D., 2005. New approaches to interprofessional education and collaborative practice: Lessons from the organizational change literature. J. Interprof. Care 19 (Suppl. 1), 177–187.

Gittell, J.H., Godfrey, M., Thistlethwaite, J., 2013. Interprofessional collaborative practice and relational coordination: Improving healthcare through relationships. Journal of Interprofessional Care 27 (3), 210–213. https://doi.org/10.3109/13561820.2012.730564

Gittell, J.H., 2016. Transforming relationships for high performance: The power of relational coordination. Stanford University Press.

Gravel, K., Légaré, F., Graham, I.D., 2006. Barriers and facilitators to implementing shared decision-making in clinical practice: A systematic review of health professionals' perceptions. Implementation Science 1, 1–12. https://doi.org/10.1186/1748-5908-1-16

Hedberg, B., Wijk, H., Gäre, B.A., Petersson, C., 2022. Shared decision-making and person-centred care in Sweden: Exploring coproduction of health and social care services. Zeitschrift für Evidenz, Fortbildung und Qualität im Gesundheitswesen 171, 129–134. https://doi.org/10.1016/j.zefq.2022.04.016

Hsiao, C.Y., Wu, J.C., Lin, P.C., Yang, P.Y., Liao, F., Guo, S.L., et al., 2022. Effectiveness of interprofessional shared decision-making training: A mixed-method study. Patient Education and Counseling 105 (11), 3287–3297.

Interprofessional Education Collaborative Expert Panel, 2011. Core competencies for interprofessional collaborative practice: Report of an expert panel. Interprofessional Education Collaborative.

Interprofessional Education Collaborative, 2016. Core competencies for interprofessional collaborative practice: 2016 update. Interprofessional Education Collaborative.

Interprofessional Education Collaborative, 2023. Core competencies for interprofessional collaborative practice: Preliminary draft revisions. Interprofessional Education Collaborative.

Jones, A., Knutsson, O., Schön, U.K., 2022. Coordinated individual care planning and shared decision making: Staff perspectives within the comorbidity field of practice. European Journal of Social Work 25 (2), 355–367. https://doi.org/10.1080/13691457.2021.2016649

Légaré, F., Kearing, S., Clay, K., Gagnon, S., D'Amours, D., Rousseau, M., et al., 2010. Are you SURE?: Assessing patient decisional conflict with a 4-item screening test. Canadian family physician, 56 (8), e308–e314.

Legare, F., Adekpedjou, R., Stacey, D., Turcotte, S., Kryworuchko, J., Graham, I., et al., 2018. Interventions for increasing the use of shared decision making by healthcare professionals. Cochrane Database Syst Rev, 7 (7), https://doi.org/10.1002/14651858.cd006732.pub4

Légaré, F., Witteman, H.O., 2013. Shared decision making: Examining key elements and barriers to adoption into routine clinical practice. Health Affairs 32 (2), 276–284. https://doi.org/10.1377/hlthaff.2012.1078

Légaré, F., Ratté, S., Gravel, K., Graham, I.D., 2008. Barriers and facilitators to implementing shared decision-making in clinical practice: Update of a systematic review of health professionals' perceptions. Patient Education and Counseling 73 (3), 526–535. https://doi.org/10.1016/j.pec.2008.07.018

Légaré, F., Stacey, D., Turcotte, S., Cossi, M.J., Kryworuchko, J., Graham, I.D., et al., 2014. Interventions for improving the adoption of shared decision making by healthcare professionals. Cochrane Database of Systematic Reviews 9, CD006732. https://doi.org/10.1002/14651858.CD006732.pub3

Légaré, F., Stacey, D., Brière, N., Desroches, S., Dumont, S., Fraser, K., et al., 2011a. A conceptual framework for interprofessional shared decision making in home care: Protocol for a feasibility study. BMC Health Services Research 11 (1), 1–7. https://doi.org/10.1186/1472-6963-11-23

Légaré, F., Stacey, D., Pouliot, S., Gauvin, F.P., Desroches, S., Kryworuchko, J., et al., 2011b. Interprofessionalism and shared decision-making in primary care: A stepwise approach towards a new model. Journal of Interprofessional Care 25 (1), 18–25. https://doi.org/10.3109/13561820.2010.490502

Makoul, G., Clayman, M.L., 2006. An integrative model of shared decision making in medical encounters. Patient Education and Counseling 60 (3), 301–312. https://doi.org/10.1016/j.pec.2005.06.010

McDonald, H., Charles, C., Gafni, A., 2014. Assessing the conceptual clarity and evidence base of quality criteria/standards developed for evaluating decision aids. Health Expectations 17 (2), 232–243. https://doi.org/10.1111/j.1369-7625.2011.00740.x

Martin, R.W., Brogård Andersen, S., O'Brien, M.A., Bravo, P., Hoffmann, T., Olling, K., et al., 2021. Providing balanced information about options in patient decision aids: An update from the International Patient Decision Aid Standards. Medical Decision Making 41 (7), 780–800. https://doi.org/10.1177/0272989X211021397

Michaelson, V., Pickett, W., Davison, C., 2019. The history and promise of holism in health promotion. *Health Promotion International* 34 (4), 824–832.

Moreau, A., Carol, L., Dedianne, M.C., Dupraz, C., Perdrix, C., Lainé, X., et al., 2012. What perceptions do patients have of decision making (DM)? Toward an integrative patient-centered care model. A qualitative study using focus-group interviews. Patient Education and Counseling 87 (2), 206–211. https://doi.org/10.1016/j.pec.2011.08.010

Müller, E., Hahlweg, P., Scholl, I., 2016. What do stakeholders need to implement shared decision making in routine cancer care? A qualitative needs assessment. Acta Oncologica 55 (12), 1484–1491. https://doi.org/10.1080/0284186X.2016.1227087

Müller, E., Strukava, A., Scholl, I., Härter, M., Diouf, N.T., Légaré, F., et al., 2019. Strategies to evaluate healthcare provider trainings in shared decision-making (SDM): A systematic review of evaluation studies. BMJ Open 9 (6), e026488. https://doi.org/10.1136/bmjopen-2018-026488

Nelson, A., 2002. Unequal treatment: confronting racial and ethnic disparities in health care. Journal of the National Medical Association 94 (8), 666.

Oshima Lee, E., Emanuel, E.J., 2013. Shared decision making to improve care and reduce costs. New England Journal of Medicine 368 (1), 6–8. https://doi.org/10.1056/NEJMp1209500

Pecukonis, E., Doyle, O., Bliss, D.L., 2008. Reducing barriers to interprofessional training: Promoting interprofessional cultural competence. Journal of Interprofessional Care 22 (4), 417–428. https://doi.org/10.1080/13561820802190442

Pieterse, A.H., Stiggelbout, A.M., Montori, V.M., 2019. Shared decision making and the importance of time. JAMA 322 (1), 25–26. https://doi.org/10.1001/jama.2019.3785

Ruland, C.M., Bakken, S., 2002. Developing, implementing, and evaluating decision support systems for shared decision making in patient care: A conceptual model and case illustration. Journal of Biomedical Informatics 35 (5-6), 313–321. https://doi.org/10.1016/S1532-0464(03)00037-6

Sepucha, K.R., Borkhoff, C.M., Lally, J., Levin, C.A., Matlock, D.D., Ng, C.J., Thomson, R., 2013. Establishing the effectiveness of patient decision aids: Key constructs and measurement instruments. BMC Medical Informatics and Decision Making 13 (2), 1–11. https://doi.org/10.1186/1472-6947-13-S2-S12

Sepucha, K.R., Breslin, M., Graffeo, C., Carpenter, C.R., Hess, E.P., 2016. State of the science: Tools and measurement for shared decision making. Academic Emergency Medicine 23 (12), 1325–1331. https://doi.org/10.1111/acem.13071

Shunk, R., Dulay, M., Chou, C.L., Janson, S., O'Brien, B.C., 2014. Huddle-coaching: A dynamic intervention for trainees and staff to support team-based care. Academic Medicine 89 (2), 244–250. https://doi.org/10.1097/ACM.0000000000000104

Tinetti, M.E., Fried, T.R., Boyd, C.M., 2012. Designing health care for the most common chronic condition—multimorbidity. JAMA 307 (23), 2493–2494. https://doi.org/10.1001/jama.2012.5265

Yu, C.H., Stacey, D., Sale, J., Hall, S., Kaplan, D.M., Ivers, N., et al., 2014. Designing and evaluating an interprofessional shared decision-making and goal-setting decision aid for patients with diabetes in clinical care-Systematic decision aid development and study protocol. Implementation Science 9 (1), 1–8. https://doi.org/10.1186/1748-5908-9-16

19

USING TELEHEALTH IN CLINICAL EDUCATION
Opportunities, Challenges and Considerations

REBECCA SUTHERLAND ▪ RACHEL BACON

CHAPTER AIMS

The aims of this chapter are:

- to provide an overview of the current use of tele-health in allied health
- to identify the challenges and strengths of tele-health for health service delivery
- to present key benefits, recommendations and considerations for using telehealth for student clinical placements experiences within accredited health programmes.

INTRODUCTION

Telehealth is an umbrella term that includes many different terms and types of services including tele-medicine, telepractice, telecare, tele-assessment, tele-audiology, telepsychiatry and telerehabilitation. In broad terms, telehealth describes healthcare services that are delivered remotely, using information technology services including phone calls and videoconferencing. Telehealth encompasses a range of health services, including assessment and treatment of a range of conditions (e.g. Sutherland et al., 2017; Burns, et al., 2019) along with health education and preventative activities (e.g. Vadheim et al., 2017). Digital health interventions more broadly include elements like mobile apps, such as those designed to provide speech sound interventions (e.g. Furlong et al., 2018) or to support therapeutic exercise for musculoskeletal pain (e.g. Thompson et al., 2022). However, in this chapter we will consider telehealth as the use of technology to connect clinicians to clients, either in real time or asynchronously. This chapter includes a specific focus on using telehealth for student clinical placements. Although the use of telehealth placements is recommended as part of an overall placement programme that includes face-to-face experiences, this chapter outlines some of the unique learning opportunities available to students and educators in this emerging area of clinical education. The chapter also provides recommendations and cautions to optimize telehealth student clinical placement experiences.

TELEHEALTH

What Is Telehealth?

The technology used for telehealth has ranged over time from cassette tapes, delivered via post and discussed over the telephone (e.g. Harrison et al., 1999), through to generic, low-cost Internet-based videoconferencing platforms (such as Zoom or Skype) and specially designed and built telehealth platforms, such as Coviu (e.g. Hodge et al., 2022), that allow for secure data and image sharing. While some early telehealth research and service delivery has involved custom-built videoconferencing equipment (e.g. Waite et al., 2010), most telehealth is now delivered over the phone or Internet using readily available equipment such as laptops and iPads, with or without additional webcams, speakers microphones and headsets (Keck and Doarn, 2014).

Telehealth service delivery models can be divided into three broad types: asynchronous and synchronous models and remote patient monitoring (Australian Digital Health Agency, 2022). Asynchronous types are also described as 'store and forward' systems (Deshpande et al., 2009) where images, data and video or audio recordings are collected from the remote site and transmitted to a healthcare professional at a distant site for later viewing and analysis (e.g. Haulman et al., 2020; O'Keefe et al., 2021). Synchronous telehealth models use information technologies, including video cameras, computers and Internet connection to allow patients and practitioners to communicate in real time. Videoconferencing, where clinician and patient communicate using over Internet connection, using computers, phones or specialized videoconferencing equipment are now a well-known type of synchronous telehealth. Hybrid models, which combine elements of store and forward technology with real-time communication, are also in use in many fields including dentistry (Thakkar et al., 2020), speech pathology and radiography. These hybrid models allow clinicians to combine face-to-face communication with prerecorded images and audio in assessment and intervention and to record patient responses for later analysis (Keck and Doarn, 2014). Finally, remote patient monitoring enables healthcare professionals to monitor patient health and clinical information at a distance (e.g. George and Cross, 2020).

Telehealth was seen as a service that was largely suitable to people with difficulties accessing services due to geographical barriers, particularly those in rural or remote areas. In Australia, for example, Medicare rebates for telehealth were limited to patients in particular geographic areas prior to COVID-19 (Fisk et al., 2020). However, due to social distancing regulations during the COVID-19 pandemic, telehealth was invaluable across disciplines and specialties, as a means of delivering healthcare much more broadly. Indeed, in Australia between the declaration of the pandemic in mid-March 2020 when changes were made to telehealth access (Fisk et al., 2020) and mid-February 2022 when many restrictions in Australia had eased, some 95.9 million telehealth services were delivered to 16.8 million patients (Australian Digital Health Agency, 2022). Small studies conducted during COVID-19 suggested that telehealth GP services, for example, have been well accepted by patients, with Javanparast et al. (2021) finding that high-risk patients felt that while their health had been managed differently because of the need to use telehealth, it had been managed quite well. It is also important to note that consumers reported that they valued flexibility and felt that not all issues (such as those requiring physical examination) are well suited to telehealth (Toll et al., 2022). Telehealth sessions were clearly important during stay-at-home orders and to prevent the spread of disease, but it has also become clear that telehealth has an important role to play in overcoming a range of barriers that may prevent clinicians and patients in coming together for healthcare services.

Telehealth in Allied Health Practice

Telehealth is in use across a wide range of medical and allied health professions, across Australia and internationally. Although there are conditions and treatments that are clearly not possible via telehealth, such as podiatrists performing wound care or physiotherapists providing hands-on care (e.g. Bennell et al., 2021), research, practice and professional statements from allied health organizations suggest that most professions have elements that are well suited to telehealth. These elements include observation, client and family meetings, interviewing, counselling, planning, monitoring, coaching and teaching. Some of these may need extra consideration or modification for telehealth use, such as a physiotherapist developing skills in describing or instructing a patient through a movement or exercise rather than relying on demonstration or a dietician guiding a patient through weight and other measurements as part of a nutrition assessment (Mauldin et al., 2021).

Some areas of practice may be enhanced or made easier by telehealth, such as scheduling family meetings with both parents of a child without physically requiring them to be present at an appointment. Telehealth may also allow greater engagement and insight into a patient's living situation, which may be useful across professions, for example, allowing an occupational therapist to observe a client moving around their own kitchen.

In contrast, some uses of telehealth are currently theoretically possible, or are being researched, but may not be within the realm of everyday practice yet, such as initial appointments regarding enteral feeding (e.g. Mundi et al., 2021) or physiotherapists accessing technology to measure range of movement. These tasks, as with all telehealth activities, should be approached within the framework of evidence-based practice that considers research findings, client perspectives and clinical expertise to guide decision making. The importance of patient-centred care and ensuring that clinicians attend to professional guidelines when considering telehealth is paramount.

Broadly, professional organizations state that telehealth services should meet the same standards of care as services that are delivered in person and that all services should consider the client's unique needs as well as the evidence base before undertaking telehealth services. For example:

- Speech Pathology Australia 'supports the use of telepractice as a service delivery model where it is based on current evidence-based practice and is at least equivalent to standard clinical care' (Speech Pathology Australia, 2022, p. 3).
- Occupational Therapy Australia 'supports the use of telehealth services that comply with WFOT principles and are client centred, evidence based, fit for purpose and within Occupational Therapy scope of practice' (OTA, 2020, p. 2.).
- The Australia Physiotherapists Association notes that 'Telehealth consultations should be conducted in accordance with existing best practice clinical standards and models of care for face-to-face consultations.' (Australian Physiotherapy Association, 2020, p. 4).
- For dieticians, 'It is the position of Dietitians Australia that clients can receive high-quality

and effective dietetic services … delivered via telehealth. Outcomes of telehealth-delivered dietetic consultations are comparable to those delivered in-person ...' (Kelly et al., 2020).
- The Australian Dental Association notes that 'In certain circumstances where a patient is seeking care from a dentist but is unable to attend a dental clinic in person, it may be necessary to conduct a consultation by audio or through a videoconferencing platform … It should be noted that a service may only be provided by teledentistry where it is safe and clinically appropriate to do so.' (Australian Dental Association, 2022).

In general, the use of telehealth is supported as long as safety, privacy and efficacy for each client are carefully considered. The use of telehealth does not change the need for the clinician to continue to follow all guidelines that would be part of face-to-face practice, particularly those around privacy and confidentiality (see later text).

STRENGTHS AND CHALLENGES OF TELEHEALTH

Challenges

Technology Factors

Technology barriers have long been a concern for both clinicians and clients in implementing telehealth (e.g. Dunkley et al., 2010). Early research on telehealth indicated that clinicians, such as speech pathologists, had very limited access to the types of equipment and Internet access they needed and believed that their clients would similarly struggle with technology (Dunkley et al., 2010). More recently, the community's familiarity with, and use of, a range of devices and services that allow telehealth has grown, but some barriers and challenges still remain. A 'digital divide' continues to exist (Thomas et al., 2022), with online access more restricted in rural and remote areas and to less socially and economically advantaged groups. Reliable, high-speed Internet coverage remains patchy (e.g. Svistova et al., 2022), even in some metropolitan areas, and those who rely solely on mobile (cell) phones for online access also experience lower levels of digital inclusion (Thomas et al., 2022). The cost of devices and accessing the Internet continue to exclude more disadvantaged groups and the difficulties in accessing, learning and mastering new skills mean that some groups, including older people and those with limited education, or majority language skills, may not be able to engage effectively with telehealth.

The infrastructure needed to use telehealth successfully can also prove a challenge to both clinicians and clients. In order to provide best practice, clinicians need to be able to access private areas in busy office or clinical spaces so that conversations are not overheard and so that clients are not seen on-screen by other members of staff or other patients. Similarly, clients need to be able to access appropriate spaces within their own homes to receive telehealth services: while it might suit a person living alone to engage in a telehealth session at their kitchen table, a young adult living in the family home may need privacy and a space where they cannot be overheard to participate comfortably in a telehealth psychology session (e.g. Pellicano et al., 2020).

Client Factors

There is no doubt that there are members of the community for whom telehealth is more challenging. There are concerns about using telehealth with older clients who may have limited experience and comfort with technology. Along with these factors, issues associated with ageing, including declining dexterity and sensory limitations, may hamper access to screen-based technology (Dykgraaf et al., 2022). Some research suggests that reliance on telehealth as the main service delivery option for older people appears to be 'far from optimal' (Svistova et al., 2022). It is possible that other forms of telehealth, such as simple telephone calls, may be a useful option for some people. Speech pathologists and others working in paediatrics also report challenges in engaging children with short attention spans and 'lack of video conferencing etiquette' (Sutherland et al., 2021, p. 6). Parents have been reported to prefer face to face over telehealth consultations for their children attending appointments for behavioural, mental health and developmental concerns (Hiscock et al., 2021) and the difficulties in working directly via telehealth with children and adults with significant disability are well established (Sutherland et al., 2018). It is important for clinicians to consider the way they provide services to these more vulnerable groups, recognizing that there

is unlikely to be a 'one size fits all' solution with telehealth. It is likely that engaging via telehealth with parents, carers and support people to coach them and support them to implement interventions may be the most useful and appropriate way to provide supports with some members of the community. The evidence for parent coaching via telehealth to support young autistic children, for example, is well established (Sutherland et al., 2018).

Privacy and Confidentiality

All health interactions, regardless of service delivery method, should be delivered in a way that upholds and maintains client privacy and in a manner that ensures that information about the client, and interactions with them, is kept confidential. Some of the challenges to this when delivering telehealth are novel and quite particular to this mode of interaction. Issues to consider include: ensuring that the clinician is in a private space where colleagues and others cannot see or hear the session; making sure that clients have access to private spaces for the sessions when needed; using appropriately secure Internet platforms for telehealth; managing risks around recording of sessions; and managing data when professionals are working outside a traditional setting (e.g. working from home).

Strengths

Access to Services

Obviously, one of the main strengths or benefits of telehealth is the ability to overcome barriers associated with the distance between clients and clinicians. While this has long been a known challenge in rural and regional areas, the COVID-19 pandemic has brought this into focus for metropolitan residents (see Caffery et al., 2022, for a useful discussion). Telehealth is proving to be useful not only in situations where patients need to travel vast distances to access medical services or allied health clinicians, it is also proving to be valuable in city settings, where barriers such as time, accessible or available transport, parking and its associated costs, child or elder care, and of course, the risks regarding disease transmission, all create barriers to accessing timely and high-quality healthcare (e.g. Ciccia et al., 2011). The use of telehealth has been shown to be well accepted by a range of groups, with time and cost savings the obvious benefits (e.g. Hiscock et al., 2021) although concerns exist regarding some types of telehealth treatments and for some people, including older patients with less familiarity with information technology.

Access to Speciality Services and Consultations

Both patients and clinicians may benefit from telehealth through the remote access to specialty services that may only be available in particular areas. In speech pathology, for example, patients with head and neck cancer may need specialist management to support their speech, eating and drinking (Collins et al., 2017). Not all speech pathologists have the knowledge, skills and experience to manage these complex cases and few are located in regional areas. For patients in these areas, access to such services in city areas can be costly and time consuming and even patients in metropolitan areas can find the travel and timing difficult. Hybrid models, where patients may be supported to access specialist services by local clinicians (who themselves receive mentoring), have been shown to be as effective as traditional face-to-face models (Ward et al., 2017). Similarly, telehealth has been used to support and monitor interdisciplinary teams engaging in swallowing assessments (videofluoroscopic swallow studies), making use of both synchronous (in real time) and asynchronous (by storing and forwarding video files) models to provide diagnostic information (Malandraki et al., 2013).

Telehealth Provides Access to Clients' Real-Life Needs

The ability to see clients and their families in situ provides clinicians with a rich opportunity to better understand their clients' context in a meaningful way. Telehealth provides occasions for clinicians to work directly with clients in their own homes, which can allow clinicians to develop a greater appreciation of aspects of clients' lives that may not be apparent in a face-to-face clinical setting and may lead to more functional, real-life problem solving with clients. For example, speech pathologists have commented on the usefulness in seeing and learning about family dynamics in telehealth sessions (Sutherland et al., 2021) and that children may be more relaxed in their own environment, compared with the clinic, leading to different observations of language and other communication skills. In published and unpublished comments from

our recent study (Bacon et al., 2022), the benefits of seeing clients in their own home were also articulated by exercise physiology and dietetics students. One student exercise physiologist noted that 'we can actually integrate an intervention within their current environment, so we find that it (telehealth) is actually working quite well' (p. 5), while another described the usefulness of being able to problem solve through seeing the environment their client was dealing with:

> We did a home assessment on somebody who was experiencing freezing (due to Parkinson's disease), … in the clinic we can give them all the strategies we want, but if they do not practice it or try it at home, it won't make a difference. Being able to use a video, and they show us exactly where they're freezing, and then give them a strategy to use, I think that was a huge thing that we'd never even really considered before.
> *(2022, p. 6)*

Similarly, a dietetics student commented on the usefulness of telehealth in getting accurate information from clients, saying '(when) they were in their own home, they could go to the fridge and they could grab stuff, or go, I don't know what brand I'm having, so they could check what it was, so it was a little bit easier for us to get the information that we needed' (Bacon et al., 2022).

REFLECTION POINT

- In your own experience, which clients or client groups have benefitted the most from telehealth? Which clients or groups have found it less useful?
- Have any clients or groups surprised you in their engagement with telehealth?
- What adaptations have you made or could you make to ensure that telehealth services are useful and accessible to your population?

TELEHEALTH CLINICAL PLACEMENT EXPERIENCES

This section of the chapter has been informed by work completed as part of a 2020–2021 Australian Collaborative Education Network (ACEN) Research Grant. The aims of the project were: (1) to conduct a systematic review to explore whether telehealth can support allied health students to develop competencies in interprofessional collaboration; (2) to compare the learning experiences provided by telehealth and face-to-face consultations during student clinical placements; and (3) to explore the perceived benefits, challenges and impacts of using telehealth for clinical placements for key stakeholders (students, supervising clinicians, patients and placement academics).

The project was conducted in an established urban allied health university clinic that provided discipline-specific services including nutrition and dietetics, physiotherapy, exercise physiology, optometry, counselling, psychology, occupational therapy, speech pathology and interprofessional services through a Parkinson's clinic, paediatric feeding clinic and a cancer wellness centre. Telehealth services were introduced from March 2020 because of the COVID-19 pandemic and included telephone calls and video conferencing with the students and clinical supervisors located on site.

In our systematic review (PROSEPRO registration number CRD42020189041) we searched seven data bases (CINAHL Plus (EBSCO interface), PsychINFO (EBSCO interface), Embase (EBSCO interface) MEDLINE (EBSCO and Web of Science interfaces) ERIC, Web of Science, and Scopus) up until 27 August 2020. We looked at both qualitative and quantitative studies written in English where there was one or more allied health university student (undergraduate/postgraduate) in interprofessional student teams and where at least one student in the interprofessional team provided care to a real or simulated patient through telehealth. We were interested in whether students were able to develop any of the Interprofessional Education Collaborative (IPEC) competencies (IPEC, 2016) from these experiences. For each paper, a quality appraisal was also conducted using the McGill Mixed Methods Appraisal Tool (MMAT) (Hong et al., 2018). We synthesized our data using a convergent, integrated approach to data synthesis according to the Joanna Briggs Institute (2022) methodology for mixed methods systematic reviews.

We also conducted a retrospective telephone survey with health students who had attended the university clinic between March 2020 and December 2020 and had participated in both face-to-face and telehealth consultations. The pilot-tested survey was informed by a validated student satisfaction questionnaire (Vivanti et al., 2014) and included three demographic items and ten items comparing their telehealth and face-to-face learning experiences. Students were required to rate each item in each setting using a five-point Likert scale with open-ended questions offered for clarification if required. We used either the Chi-squared test or the Fishers exact test to determine whether there was a difference in the students' learning experiences in the different consultation settings. Qualitative data were thematically analysed, using a descriptive approach, to support our understanding of these results.

In our final study, stakeholder experiences with telehealth student placements in the university clinic were explored in virtual focus groups held between November 2020 and March 2021. These discussions used semi-structured interview questions, were audiotaped and transcribed verbatim. They were thematically analysed independently by two researchers, then cross-checked for consistency with reflexivity applied. We were interested in finding out what the experiences of telehealth were like for students, their supervising clinicians, placement academics and the patients they saw, with a focus on the benefits and drawbacks, and what we could learn to inform future practice.

Fig. 19.1 (PRIMSA Diagram) and Table 19.1 (Data Extraction) show some of the results of our systematic review. Our results found that students perceived improvements in their practice across all four of the IPEC competencies:

1. Students reported greater understanding of patient's needs and the value of other team members (Bautista et al., 2020), worked co-operatively (Sweeney et al., 2018), improved their own clinical competency (Scott et al., 2020; O'Shea et al., 2019) and their patient's quality of care (Shortridge et al., 2018; Shortridge et al., 2016; Bautista et al., 2020) (IPEC Competency 1).
2. Students demonstrated an increased understanding of their own roles and scope of practice (Scott et al., 2020; O'Shea et al., 2019; Bautista et al., 2020; Shortridge et al., 2018) (IPEC Competency 2).

3. Students perceived their telehealth experiences to improve their communication skills, positively impacting on their ability to work with others (Scott et al., 2020; Sweeney et al., 2018; O'Shea et al., 2019) (IPEC Competency 3).

4. Students supported team skills development (Scott et al., 2020; Sweeney et al., 2018; Bautista et al., 2020; Shortridge et al., 2018) (IPEC Competency 4).

Overall, the studies in this review achieved low scores on the MMAT. As an emerging area of research, the included studies were predominantly pilot research (Scott et al., 2020; O'Shea et al., 2019; Bautista et al., 2020; Shortridge et al., 2018). As such, their contribution was in their descriptions of the development, implementation and evaluation of these teaching innovations. Learnings included: (1) the need for clear discipline-specific learning outcomes (O'Shea et al., 2019); (2) the need for experienced facilitators from all disciplines (O'Shea et al., 2019; Sweeney et al, 2018); and (3) the importance of adequate preparation and familiarity with the telehealth technology (Shortridge et al., 2016; Shortridge et al., 2018).

Our findings highlighted the potential of telehealth to support the development of interprofessional collaboration. Telehealth's functionality in bringing together expert clinicians and carers (even if geographically dispersed) facilitates interprofessional collaboration (Johnson and Robins, 2020), which is known to improve clinical performance, patient outcomes and patient satisfaction (Moffet et al., 2015; Wootton et al., 2007). However, our results need to be viewed with caution due to the small number of studies, low research quality and notable heterogeneity amongst the studies. In our review, technical challenges were reported in most studies devaluing the use of telehealth for interprofessional education. With recent technological developments, however, this may be less of a concern moving forward.

The results of our other two studies have been published elsewhere (Bacon et al., 2022; Bacon et al., 2023 under review). However, we have drawn on our research findings together with other published literature to inform the following discussion on the benefits, challenges and recommendations on using telehealth for clinical placement experiences.

Benefits of Using Telehealth Clinical Placement Experiences

Placement Capacity

Most accredited health courses require students to undertake clinical placements under the supervision of a clinical educator (Ahpra, 2021). Traditionally these placements have been completed face-to-face. During the COVID-19 pandemic, telehealth – which complied with government social distancing requirements – enabled students to continue their placement programmes (Pellegrini et al., 2021; Pelly et al., 2020; Pit et al., 2021). Telehealth offers new opportunities to increase clinical placement capacity, scope and efficiencies (Bacon et al., 2022; Liu and Miyazaki, 2000; Rutledge et al., 2020; Salter et al., 2020; Serwe et al., 2020). This includes:

1. Increasing the client base of student-led services, no longer constrained by geographic limitations;
2. Student placement opportunities in private and public health services with the option of attending placements remotely;
3. Virtual support for students and supervisors; and
4. Remote, peer and retrospective supervision models.

ILLUSTRATIVE EXAMPLE:

New Clinical Supervision Models Developed During Telehealth Placements

The rapid roll out of telehealth, due to the COVID-19 pandemic, forced some supervisors in our study to adopt a role more aligned to a team leader rather than student supervisor, changing the power dynamic (Bacon et al., 2022). Rather than students working under the directive of their supervisor, the students and supervisor worked together to deliver the new telehealth service most effectively. This approach worked well and is consistent with Wenger's (1998) Community of Practice theory, where student learning is enhanced through a sense of belonging and participation within the healthcare team.

Competency Development and Employability

The COVID-19 pandemic has given new impetus to including telehealth as a core competency for most health disciplines (Signal et al., 2020) and is now included in the competency standards for some disciplines (e.g. Accreditation Council for Occupational Therapy Education 2023). Importantly, there is emerging evidence suggesting that telehealth can provide high-quality clinical experiences for students within accredited health programmes (Bacon et al., 2022):

- Telehealth can provide a variety of different learning opportunities such as different client types and opportunities to use different telehealth technologies, for example, to deliver group therapy verses individual therapy (Bacon et al., 2022).
- Telehealth placement experiences can offer advantages over face-to-face placement experiences in developing communication capabilities including telephone etiquette, being more explicit when giving and receiving feedback, coaching, written exercise prescriptions, and resource development (Bacon et al., 2022; Pelly et al., 2020).
- Telehealth has some unique features that can support students in their development of person-centred care (Sutherland et al., 2021; Record et al., 2021). This includes:

  1. Allowing the health student to see the person they are treating in their usual home environment.
  2. Increasing efficiencies for service users by overcoming access barriers such as transport or child care.
  3. Allowing carers or family supports to be easily present.
  4. Providing the health student with more accurate assessment data, such as remote access to food items and medication.
  5. Supporting self-management by providing a pathway to greater motivation and accountability.
  6. Requiring clients to be more active participants in their healthcare delivery (doing *with* rather than *to*).

- Telehealth placement experiences can improve students' appreciation of and capability with telehealth (Bacon et al., 2022). With the rapid growth in telehealth technologies, funding and services resulting from the COVID-19 pandemic (Australian Digital Health Agency, 2022), telehealth is now becoming a mainstream health service and telehealth placement experiences can therefore improve students' employability (Thomas et al., 2022).
- Telehealth placement experiences can favour the development of capabilities in innovation and problem-solving skills and enhance the capacity for developing flexibility, adaptability, resourcefulness, reflective practice and risk assessment (Bacon et al., 2022).

ILLUSTRATIVE EXAMPLE:

Telehealth Extended Professional Boundaries
Telehealth clinical placements expanded traditional service boundaries and led to an increased use of 'hands-off' treatments, inclusion of other technologies such as exercise trackers, and new ways of assessing clients using video recordings (Bacon et al., 2022).

Recommendations for Telehealth Placement Experiences

Curriculum and Planning

Given the growing ubiquity of telehealth and the likelihood of hybrid services in the future, telehealth experiences are recommended as part of an overall placement programme that also includes face-to-face clinical placements. A number of steps may be taken at the curriculum level in order to prepare student clinicians for using telehealth as part of clinical placements. The first is to embed information about telehealth, including both current research and more practical knowledge and skills, into theoretical units within the health curricula prior to students commencing telehealth clinical placement experiences. Part of this may involve positioning telehealth in the context of a digitally connected world and providing a background to help students understand telehealth and its role in service provision including definitions and scope of telehealth (telephone, videoconferencing sessions and monitoring services).

Educators should highlight its role in: (1) expanding healthcare to underserviced areas (e.g. rural, remote, and vulnerable populations); and (2) offering more flexible services, including hybrid services. Further, academic units may provide specific instruction on how communication and clinical skills should be modified when using telehealth. Telehealth requires students, particularly students in 'hands-on' professions such as physiotherapy and exercise physiology, to learn to make verbal and non-verbal communication more overt and explicit with frequent clarification of the patient's understanding. Challenges associated with communicating via telehealth including changes in non-verbal communication, loss of touch, less natural turn-taking and more nuanced facial expressions and these concerns may be useful to address prior to engaging in telehealth in lecture and tutorial sessions.

As with all clinical placement programmes, telehealth clinical placement experiences should be positioned within the university's goals, policies, principles and values implement legal/risk management frameworks, compliance procedures and processes (Campbell et al., 2019). As previously discussed, privacy and confidentiality should be considered in all interactions, with particular emphasis on the unique issues that may arise when using telehealth.

Preparing, Supporting and Evaluating Telehealth Clinical Placements

The quality of a clinical placement is dependent on many factors independent of whether the placement is completed via telehealth or face-to-face, including the student supervisor relationship and factors related to the individual student. However, there are a number of practical steps that can be taken to prepare for, and enhance, telehealth learning experiences, as follows:

Preparing for telehealth learning experiences

- Develop an active community of practice for clinical educators providing telehealth clinical placement experiences to share learning and resources in this emerging area of clinical education.
- Make telehealth-focussed professional development regularly available to all academic and professional staff and industry and community partners who include telehealth clinical placements.

- Provide appropriate infrastructure and funding including technical support. To make telehealth clinical placements successful, the software and hardware need to be compatible.
- Provide students (and supervisors) with resources for learning about service provision in the telehealth context and how this differs from conventional placement experiences within their discipline.
- Train students in the telehealth technology to be used at each placement site prior to commencing any telehealth consultations (Cheng et al., 2021).
- Provide user guides for teleconsultation software and information on all the equipment that will be used.
- Give students time to become familiar with the telehealth technology used at their placement site, including troubleshooting problems that may arise during service provision.
- Co-locate students on-site with their educator. When students were also located off-site it is more difficult to develop trust with the students.

Supporting student learning using telehealth experiences

- Clearly identify the learning goals for telehealth placement experiences in the clinical placement course guides.
- Consider each individual student's capacity to engage with telehealth. Telehealth learning experiences can be challenging for some students. For example, students who are studying and providing services in their second or subsequent languages may find it more challenging to talk through the nuances of movements or exercises, compared with their ability to model this in a face-to-face setting. In other cases, students with hearing or vision disabilities may need to manage the complexity of making sure they are able to use accessibility features on telehealth platforms and other software. For some anxious students, starting with a telehealth consultation rather than a face-to-face consultation can scaffold their learning because it allows them to focus initially on fewer elements of delivery.
- Teaching resources such as mock clients/role plays, scripts and templates can be used to

scaffold students' development during telehealth placement experiences.

- The mute function can be used to support and guide students through the assessment phase of a telehealth consultation.
- Students completing telehealth placement experiences highly valued regular feedback being provided by their site supervisor against their usual competency assessment instruments. We found some competencies had to be assessed differently during telehealth clinical placements, e.g. practising 'hands-on' skills with other students and using 'think-alouds' to demonstrate clinical reasoning. Mechanisms should be put in place to ensure appropriate and supportive feedback is provided to students throughout their telehealth placement experiences that can be applied to meet their learning goals.
- Students need explicit communication and support to make connections between their face-to-face clinical placement experiences and telehealth placement experiences so that they can transform their learning across these two contexts. Such learning requires students to reflect on their experiences, recognize similarities and differences, seek new knowledge and create new understandings. This abstract analytical level of thinking is aligned with deep transformative learning.

Assessing and evaluating telehealth clinical placement experiences

- Assess student's development and demonstrated performance during telehealth placement experience against professional accreditation standards and unit learning outcomes as described for each discipline.
- Assessment tasks, such as an e-portfolio, that enable students to document evidence of the employability skills developed and demonstrated through their telehealth placement experiences is recommended.
- Assess telehealth learning experiences using standardized clinical placement assessments, as required by each discipline, enabling benchmarking and quality improvement.

- Regularly evaluate telehealth experiences and follow-up on evaluation outcomes to continually improve telehealth clinical placement experiences.

Final considerations

- Technical issues related to telehealth can be a barrier to positive clinical placement learning experiences. A solution-focussed approach is required to overcome medico-legal, connectivity and platform capacity barriers to optimize the opportunities with telehealth placement experiences. Appropriate infrastructure and funding, including technical support, are necessary for successful telehealth placement experiences.
- Developing the level of rapport required for some consultations (e.g. psychology) can be more challenging with telehealth.
- There is a need for greater access to assessment and intervention tools validated for use in telehealth.
- There are challenges with developing and accessing 'hands-on' skills such as assessments of strength or other body functions. For some 'hands-on' disciplines higher student supervision ratios may be required.
- There is a need for more research to extend the professional accreditation requirements to align better with this rapidly developing area of practice.

SUMMARY

Telehealth is a way of bringing healthcare to those who need it using information technologies. Telehealth is increasingly accepted and used across many areas of medicine and health and there is a need to integrate it in comprehensive healthcare especially when hands-on treatments are required. Telehealth does not change the need for the clinician to follow all legislation and guidelines associated with their professional responsibilities. Our research suggests that for accredited allied health courses, telehealth clinical placement experiences may offer some unique advantages including supporting students' development of person-centred care and employability skills.

REFLECTION POINT

- Consider your current role (educator/clinical supervisor/student) and identify the unique opportunities for telehealth in your own context?
- What are the challenges with using telehealth to support student learning? What can you do to optimize your telehealth clinical placement experiences?
- What resources, including human resources, might you need to ensure your telehealth clinical placement experiences are successful?

REFERENCES

Accreditation Council for Occupational Therapy Education (ACOTE), 2023. Standards and Interpretive Guide. https://acoteonline.org/download/5856/?tmstv=1706886053

AHPRA, 2021. Accreditation. AHPRA. http://www.ahpra.gov.au/Accreditation.aspx

Australian Dental Association, 2022. Guidelines for teledentistry. www.ada.org.au/Covid-19-Portal/Cards/Misc/Critical-Information-For-SA-Members/ADA-Guidelines-for-Teledentistry

Australian Digital Health Agency, 2022. Telehealth. https://www.digitalhealth.gov.au/initiatives-and-programs/telehealth

Australian Physiotherapy Association, 2020. Telehealth guidelines: Response to COVID-19. https://australian.physio/sites/default/files/APATelehealthGuidelinesCOVID190420FA.pdf

Bacon, R., Hopkins, S., Kellett, J., Millar, C., Smillie, L., Sutherland, R., 2022. The benefits, challenges and impacts of telehealth student clinical placements for accredited health programs during the COVID-19 pandemic. Frontiers in Medicine 9, 842685. https://doi.org/10.3389/fmed.2022.842685

Bacon, R., Hopkins, S., Georgousopoulou, G., Nahon, I., Hilly, C., Millar, C., et al., 2023. While allied health students prefer face-to-face clinical placement, telehealth can support competency development: Results from a mixed-methods study. Frontiers in Medicine, 10:1151980. https://doi.org/10.3389/fmed.2023.1151980.

Bautista, C.A., Huang, I., Stebbins, M., Floren, Lc, Wamsley, M., Youmans, S.I., 2020. Development of an interprofessional rotation for pharmacy and medical students to perform telehealth outreach to vulnerable patients in the COVID-19 pandemic. Journal of Interprofessional Care 34, 694–697. https://doi.org/10.1080/13561820.2020.1807920

Bennell, K.L., Lawford, B.J., Metcalf, B., Mackenzie, D., Russell, T., van den Berg, M., et al., 2021. Physiotherapists and patients report positive experiences overall with telehealth during the COVID-19 pandemic: A mixed-methods study. Journal of Physiotherapy 67 (3), 201–209. https://doi.org/10.1016/j.jphys.2021.06.009

Burns, C.L., Ward, E.C., Gray, A., Baker, L., Cowie, B., Winter, N., et al., 2019. Implementation of speech pathology telepractice services for clinical swallowing assessment: An evaluation of

service outcomes, costs and consumer satisfaction. Journal of Telemedicine and Telecare 25 (9), 545–551. https://doi.org/10.1177/1357633X19873248

Joanna Briggs Institute, 2022. JBI Reviewer's Manual: 8.4.1 MMSR questions that take a CONVERGENT INTEGRATED approach to synthesis and integration. Joanna Briggs Institute. https://jbi-global-wiki.refined.site/space/MANUAL/4689275/8.4.2+++MMSR+questions+that+take+a+CONVERGENT+SEGREGATED+approach+to+synthesis+and+integration

Campbell, M., McAllister, L., Smith, L., Tunny, R., Thomson, K., Barrett, M. (2019). Framework to support assurance of institution-wide quality in work integrated learning: Final Report. https://research.qut.edu.au/wilquality/wp-content/uploads/sites/261/2019/12/FINAL-FRAMEWORK-DEC-2019.pdf

Caffery, L.A., Muurlink, O.T., Taylor-Robinson, A.W., 2022. Survival of rural telehealth services post-pandemic in Australia: A call to retain the gains in the 'new normal'. Australian Journal of Rural Health 30 (4), 544–549. https://doi.org/10.1111/ajr.12877

Cheng, C., Humphreys, H., Kane, B., 2021. Transition to telehealth: Engaging medical students in telemedicine healthcare delivery. Irish Journal of Medical Science, 1–18. https://doi.org/10.1007/s11845-021-02720-1

Ciccia, A.H., Whitford, B., Krumm, M., McNeal, K., 2011. Improving the access of young urban children to speech, language and hearing screening via telehealth. Journal of Telemedicine and Telecare 17 (5), 240–244.

Collins, A., Burns, C.L., Ward, E.C., Comans, T., Blake, C., Kenny, L., et al., 2017. Home-based telehealth service for swallowing and nutrition management following head and neck cancer treatment. Journal of Telemedicine and Telecare 23 (10), 866–872. https://doi.org/10.1177/1357633X17733020

Dunkley, C., Pattie, L., Wilson, L., McAllister, L., 2010. A comparison of rural speech-language pathologists' and residents' access to and attitudes towards the use of technology for speech-language pathology service delivery. International Journal of Speech-Language Pathology 12 (4), 333–343.

Deshpande, A., Khoja, S., Lorca, J., McKibbon, A., Rizo, C., Husereau, D., et al., 2009. Asynchronous telehealth: A scoping review of analytic studies. Open Medicine 3, 39–61.

Dykgraaf, S.H., Desborough, J., Sturgiss, E., Parkinson, A., Dut, G.M., Kidd, M., 2022. Older people, the digital divide and use of telehealth during the COVID-19 pandemic. Australian Journal of General Practice 51 (9), 721–724. https://doi.org/10.3316/informit.616037628174926

Fisk, M., Livingstone, A., Pit, S.W., 2020. Telehealth in the context of COVID-19: Changing perspectives in Australia, the United Kingdom, and the United States. Journal of Medical Internet Research 22 (6), e19264.

Furlong, L., Morris, M., Serry, T., Erickson, S., 2018. Mobile apps for treatment of speech disorders in children: An evidence-based analysis of quality and efficacy. PloS One 13 (8), e0201513–e0201513. https://doi.org/10.1371/journal.pone.0201513

George, L.A., Cross, R.K., 2020. Remote monitoring and telemedicine in IBD: Are we there yet? Current Gastroenterology Reports 22 (3), 12. https://doi.org/10.1007/s11894-020-0751-0

Harrison, E., Wilson, L., Onslow, M., 1999. Distance intervention for early stuttering with the Lidcombe programme. International Journal of Speech-Language Pathology 1 (1), 31–36.

Haulman, A., Geronimo, A., Chahwala, A., Simmons, Z., 2020. The use of telehealth to enhance care in ALS and other neuromuscular disorders. Muscle and Nerve 61 (6), 682–691. https://doi.org/10.1002/mus.26838

Hiscock, H., Pelly, R., Hua, X., West, S., Tucker, D., Raymundo, C.-M., 2021. Survey of paediatric telehealth benefits from the caregiver perspective. Australian Health Review 46 (2), 197–203. https://doi.org/10.1071/AH21036

Hodge, M.A., Chan, E., Sutherland, R., Ong, N., Bale, G., Cramsie, J., et al., 2022. Tele-assessments in rural and remote schools – Perspectives of support teachers. Journal of Psychoeducational Assessment 40 (3), 360–380. https://doi.org/10.1177/07342829211059640

Interprofessional Education Collaborative, 2016. Core competencies for interprofessional collaborative practice. Interprofessional Education Collaborative.

Javanparast, S., Roeger, L., Kwok, Y., Reed, R.L., 2021. The experience of Australian general practice patients at high risk of poor health outcomes with telehealth during the COVID-19 pandemic: A qualitative study. BMC Family Practice 22 (1), 1–6. https://doi.org/10.1186/s12875-021-01408-w

Johnson, K., Robins, L., 2020. Interprofessional collaboration and telehealth: Useful strategies for family counsellors in rural and underserved areas. Interprofessional Collaboration and Telehealth 28, 1–10. https://doi.org/10.1177/1066480720934378

Keck, C.S., Doarn, C.R., 2014. Telehealth technology applications in speech-language pathology. Telemedicine Journal and e-Health 20 (7), 653–659. https://doi.org/10.1089/tmj.2013.0295

Kelly, J.T., Allman Farinelli, M., Chen, J., Partridge, S.R., Collins, C., Rollo, M., et al., 2020. Dietitians Australia position statement on telehealth. Nutrition and Dietetics 77 (4), 406–415.

Liu, L., Miyazaki, M., 2000. Telerehabilitation at the University of Alberta. Journal of Telemedicine and Telecare 6, 47–49. https://doi.org/10.1258/1357633001935554

Malandraki, G.A., Markaki, V., Georgopoulos, V.C., Bauer, J.L., Kalogeropoulos, I., Nanas, S., 2013. An international pilot study of asynchronous teleconsultation for oropharyngeal dysphagia. Journal of Telemedicine and Telecare 19 (2), 75–79. https://doi.org/10.1177/1357633x12474963

Mauldin, K., Gieng, J., Saarony, D., Hu, C., 2021. Performing nutrition assessment remotely via telehealth. Nutrition in Clinical Practice 36 (4), 751–768. https://doi.org/10.1002/ncp.10682

Hong, Q., Pluye, P., Fabregues, S., et al., (2018) Mixed Methods Appraisal Tool (MMAT) version 2018. Registration of Copyright (#1148552), Canadian Intellectual Property Office, Industry Canada.

Moffet, H., Tousignant, M., Nadeau, S., et al., 2015. In-home telerehabilitation compared with face-to-face rehabilitation after total knee arthroplasty: A noninferiority randomized controlled trial. Journal of Bone and Joint Surgery 97 (14), 1129–1141. https://doi.org/10.2106/jbjs.N.01066

Mundi, M.S., Mohamed Elfadil, O., Bonnes, S.L., Salonen, B.R., Hurt, R.T., 2021. Use of telehealth in home nutrition support:

Challenges and advantages. Nutrition in Clinical Practice 36 (4), 775–784. https://doi.org/10.1002/ncp.10736

Occupational Therapy Australia, 2020. Telehealth Guidelines 2020. http://ptaus.com.au/member-resources/covid-19/telehealth

O'Keefe, M., White, K., Jennings, J.C., 2021. Asynchronous telepsychiatry: A systematic review. Journal of Telemedicine and Telecare 27 (3), 137–145. https://doi.org/10.1177/1357633X19867189

O'Shea, M.C., Reeves, N.E., Bialocerkowski, A., Cardell, E., 2019. Using simulation-based learning to provide interprofessional education in diabetes to nutrition and dietetics and exercise physiology students through telehealth. Advances in Simulation 4 (S1), 28. https://doi.org/10.1186/s41077-019-0116-7

Pellegrini, W.R., DanisI, D.O., Levi, J.R., 2021. Medical student participation in otolaryngology telemedicine clinic during COVID-19: A hidden opportunity. Otolaryngology – Head and Neck Surgery, 164 (6), 1131–1133. https://doi.org/10.1177/0194599820970964

Pellicano, E., Brett, S., den Houting, J., Heyworth, M., Magiati, I., Steward, R., et al., (2020). "I want to see my friends": The everyday experiences of autistic people and their families during COVID-19. Sydney, Australia.

Pelly, F.E., Wiesmayr-Freeman, T., Tweedie, J., 2020. Student placement adaptability during COVID-19: Lessons learnt in 2020. Nutrition and Dietetics 77 (4), 481–483. https://doi.org/10.1111/1747-0080.12625

Pit, A.W., Velovski, S., Cockrell, K., Bailey, J., 2021. A qualitative exploration of medical student placement experiences with telehealth during COVID-19 and recommendations to prepare our future medical workforce. BMC Medical Education 21, 431. https://doi.org/10.1186/s12909-021-02719-3

Record, J.D., Ziegelstein, R.C., Christmas, C., Rand, C.S., Hanyok, L.A. 2021. Delivering personalized care at a distance: how telemedicine can foster getting to know the patient as a person. Journal of Personalized Medicine, 11 (2), 137. https://doi.org/10.3390/jpm11020137

Rutledge, C.M., Haney, T., Bordelon, M., Renaud, M., Fowler, C., 2020. Telehealth: Preparing advanced practice nurses to address healthcare needs in rural and underserved populations. International Journal of Nurse Education Scholarship 11, 61. https://doi.org/10.1515/ijnes-2013-0061

Salter, C., Oates, R.K., Swanson, C., Bourke, L., 2020. Working remotely: Innovative allied health placements in response to COVID-19. International Journal of Work Integrated Learning 21, 587–600. http://dhl.voced.edu.au/10707/572607

Scott Kruse, C., Karum, P., Shifflett, K., Vegi, L., Ravi, K., Brooks, M., 2020. Evaluating barriers to adopting telemedicine worldwide: A systematic review. Journal of Telemedicine and Telecare 24, 4–12. https://doi.org/10.1177/1357633X16674087

Serwe, K., Heindel, M., Keultjes, I., Silvers, H., Stovich, S., 2020. Telehealth student experiences and learning: A scoping review. Journal of Occupational Therapy Education 4, 1–16. https://doi.org/10.26681/jote.2020.040206

Shortridge, A., Steinheider, B., Ciro, C., Randall, K., Costner-lark, A., Loving, G., 2016. Simulating interprofessional geriatric patient care using telehealth: A team-based learning activity.

MedEdPORTAL 12, 10415. https://doi.org/10.15766/mep_2374-8265.10415

Shortridge, A., Ross, H., Randall, K., Ciro, C., Loving, G., 2018. Telehealth technology as e-learning: Learning and practicing interprofessional patient care. International Journal on E-Learning 17, 95–100.

Signal, N., Martin, T., Leys, A., Maloney, R., Bright, F., 2020. Implementation of telerehabilitation in response to COVID-19: Lessons learnt from neurorehabilitation clinical practice and education. New Zealand Journal of Physiotherapy 48, 117–126. https://doi.org/10.15619/NZJP/48.3.03

Speech Pathology Australia, 2022. *Telepractice in Speech Pathology.* Speech Pathology Australia: Melbourne, Australia

Sutherland, R., Trembath, D., Hodge, A., Drevensek, S., Lee, S., Roberts, J., et al., 2017. Telehealth language assessments using consumer grade equipment in rural and urban settings: Feasible, reliable and well tolerated. Journal of Telemedicine and Telecare 23 (1), 106–115. https://doi.org/10.1177/1357633X15623921

Sutherland, R., Trembath, D., Roberts, J., 2018. Telehealth and autism: A systematic search and review of the literature. International Journal of Speech and Language Pathology 20, 324–336. https://doi.org/10.1080/17549507.2018.1465123

Sutherland, R., Hodge, A., Chan, E., Silove, N., 2021. Barriers and facilitators: Clinicians' opinions and experiences of telehealth before and after their use of a telehealth platform for child language assessment. International Journal of Language Communication 56, 1263–1277. http://1460-6984.12666

Svistova, J., Harris, C., Fogarty, B., Kulp, C., Lee, A., 2022. Use of telehealth amid the COVID-19 pandemic: Experiences of mental health providers serving rural youth and elderly in Pennsylvania. Administration and Policy in Mental Health and Mental Health Services Research 49 (4), 530–538. https://doi.org/10.1007/s10488-021-01181-z

Sweeney, H.T., Knott, K., Rutledge, C.M., Britton, B., Fowler, C.N., Poston, R.D., 2018. How to prepare interprofessional teams in two weeks: An innovative education program nested in telehealth. International Journal of Nurse Education Scholarship 15, 1. https://doi.org/10.1515/ijnes-2017-0040

Thakkar, R., Kakkar, M., George, R., Singh, S., 2020. Telehealth and dental specialties during COVID-19 pandemic. SRM Journal of Research in Dental Sciences 11 (4), 199. https://doi.org/10.4103/srmjrds.srmjrds_83_20

Thomas, E.E., Haydon, H.M., Mehrotra, A., Caffery, L.J., Snoswell, C.L., Banbury, A., et al., 2022. Building on the momentum: Sustaining telehealth beyond COVID-19. Journal of Telemedicine and Telecare, 1–8. https://doi.org/10.1177/1357633X20960638

Thompson, D., Rattu, S., Tower, J., Egerton, T., Francis, J., Merolli, M., 2022. Mobile app use to support conditions may help improve pain intensity and self-reported physical function: A systematic review. Journal of Physiotherapy. 69, 23–24. https://doi.org/10.1016/j.jphys.2022.11.012

Toll, K., Spark, L., Neo, B., Norman, R., Elliott, S., Wells, L., et al., 2022. Consumer preferences, experiences, and attitudes towards telehealth: Qualitative evidence from Australia. PloS One 17 (8), e0273935. https://doi.org/10.1371/journal.pone.0273925 e0273935-e0273935

Vadheim, L.M., Patch, K., Brokaw, S.M., Carpenedo, D., Butcher, M.K., Helgerson, S.D., et al., 2017. Telehealth delivery of the diabetes prevention program to rural communities. Translational Behavioral Medicine 7 (2), 286–291.

Vivanti, A., Haron, N., Barners, R., 2014. Validation of a student satisfaction survey for clinical education placements in dietetics. Journal of Allied Health 43 (2), 65–71.

Waite, M.C., Theodoros, D.G., Russell, T.Gl, Cahill, L.M., 2010. Internet-based telehealth assessment of language using the CELF–4. Language, Speech, and Hearing Services in Schools 41, 445–458.

Ward, E.C., Wall, L.R., Burns, C.L., Cartmill, B., Hill, A.J., 2017. Application of telepractice for head and neck cancer management: A review of speech language pathology service models. Current Opinion in Otolaryngology and Head and Neck Surgery 25 (3), 169–174.

Wenger, E., 1998. Communities of practice: Learning, meaning, and identity. Cambridge University Press.

Wootton, R., Swinfen, P., Swinfen, R., Warren, M.A., Wilkinson, D., Brooks, P., 2007. Medical students represent a valuable resource for facilitating telehealth for the under-served. Journal of Telemedicine and Telecare 13, 92–97. https://doi.org/10.1258/1357633077832473

PART 4 Clinical Reasoning and the Professions

Clinical reasoning is at the heart of all health professions. There are many commonalities between the professions and there are significant differences. Clinical reasoning is also becoming more complex.

There are clearly many commonalities in clinical reasoning across the health professions. Most professions follow protocols for gathering information about patients that are very similar, if not identical. There are of course many differences in the clinical reasoning across the professions. Emergency physicians and paramedics will see new patients with acute conditions that need urgent attention, and they may never see these patients again. In contrast, other health professionals, such as dentists, optometrists and family practitioners, will see patients with whom they may have long-term professional relationships that can extend for decades as they provide routine care.

The proportion of long-term relationships in healthcare can be expected to grow as there is a steady increase in the proportion of the population with chronic conditions and disabilities. Because of the advances in science and healthcare practices, over many decades, we are getting better at treating many conditions. A problem is that while many acute conditions might be completely cured, many are not, and these become chronic conditions that need ongoing management for years. Many people, especially older people, have comorbidities (i.e. more than one chronic condition) and each comorbidity may complicate the management of the others. This makes the clinical reasoning involved far more complex than managing a surgical procedure in someone who is fit, young and otherwise healthy.

Newcomers to our health professions need to accept that there is going to be a rise in complexity and uncertainty that they will need to manage, often with others. To do this, they will need excellent clinical reasoning skills and a willingness to be comfortable working in a world of complexity and uncertainty. This will also require them to be comfortable working in interprofessional teams that can share and explain their clinical reasoning to each other. In Part 4, we take an in-depth look at how several health professions see their own clinical reasoning. We hope to raise awareness of the various issues around clinical reasoning within each health profession. Another hope is that this will open up the way for health professionals to understand the reasoning of their colleagues to improve the interprofessional healthcare that is going to be the future of healthcare for many practitioners.

20 METHODS IN THE STUDY OF CLINICAL REASONING

JOSE F. AROCHA ■ VIMLA L. PATEL

CHAPTER AIMS

This chapter aims:

- to provide a description of the most used methods for the investigation and assessment of clinical reasoning
- to classify such methods in terms of their nature and unit of analysis
- to show how the methods can be of utility for the study of clinical reasoning.

INTRODUCTION

Methods for the study of clinical reasoning are often selected based on the philosophical outlook considered by the researcher. Philosophically, quantitative methods are said to be characteristic of a positivist methodological approach to research, which posits the essentiality of quantifiable behaviour in the conduction of scientific research. In turn, qualitative methods are often based on a philosophy that proposes the constructive nature of human thought and action. Despite the difference in outlook, there has been a recent push to investigate thinking within a framework that forgoes, to some extent, the philosophical chasm between quantitative and qualitative research, while adopting a more pragmatic approach to research. From our view, this situation has positively affected the study of clinical reasoning. Indeed, its study in the fields of health has changed positively in recent years. Some of the major changes are the following:

First, some theories, notably dual-process theory (Croskerry, 2009), have become widely used to guide research studies and to explain cognitive processes, such as problem solving and reasoning. Second, new and not so new methodologies have been introduced and applied to the investigation of such processes, which promise to elucidate what goes on when a clinician interprets a patient problem. Third, the traditional and clearly delineated distinction between quantitative and qualitative research methods has become fuzzy (Haig, 2013) because new research increasingly makes use of both approaches in clinical reasoning investigations (e.g. Rice et al., 2014). Fourth, although in previous years the study of clinical reasoning was mostly focussed on medical tasks, there has been increasing research in other health fields, such as occupational therapy (Cramm et al., 2013), physiotherapy (Langridge et al., 2015) and nursing (Stec, 2016).

Methods of investigation of clinical reasoning can be grouped into those that look at outcomes to hypothesize the underlying cognitive processes and those that explore the processes of reasoning themselves. We found it useful to classify methodologies as quantitative or qualitative to the extent to which they generate numerical or verbal/gestural data. Also, some can be aggregated into statistics, while others are less suitable for aggregation. Specific studies can, of course, vary and use quantitative methods to identify average differences between groups together with qualitative methods to characterize individual performance (Patel et al., 2001). This chapter is devoted to the study of clinical reasoning as an individual process, leaving out methods designed to capture clinical reasoning as it occurs in teams or work groups (e.g. Patel et al., 2013).

QUANTITATIVE METHODS

Quantitative methodologies for investigating clinical reasoning have been used in various clinical problems. One of them is the study of diagnosis in perceptual tasks, such as X-ray or dermatological image interpretation (Jaarsma et al., 2015; Norman et al., 1992), where study participants are shown a series of slides after which they are asked to interpret or recall the information of the visual material. One goal of this research is to show how variations in the participants' performance (e.g. assessed through verbal recall) relate to variations on the experimental conditions (e.g. types of stimuli). These data are then quantified using descriptive statistics and subjected to standard statistical analysis (e.g. null-hypothesis testing). These methods have also been used to compare clinical performance by groups with different levels of expertise (Norman et al., 2007). The study of group differences serves to estimate population parameters. However, quantitative methods can also be used for investigating individuals (Runkel, 2007), although unfortunately little use has been made of such methods for this purpose. Next, we cover specific quantitative techniques recently applied to the study of clinical reasoning.

The Script Concordance Test

The Script Concordance (SC) test has gained considerable attention in recent years (Charlin et al., 2007).

The test, theoretically based on script theory (Schmidt and Rikers, 2007), assumes that clinicians develop increasingly coherent knowledge structures, called scripts, as their experience increases from students to seasoned practitioners. The test is also informed by dual-process theory. As clinicians' expertise increases in a given health field, they also develop two distinct thinking processes: 'analytical', which is slow, effortful and more characteristic of novices and 'nonanalytical', which is fast, subconscious and more characteristic of experts.

The SC test (Charlin et al., 2000; Lubarsky et al., 2013) is a psychometrically validated written instrument particularly designed to assess clinical reasoning. The test is normally developed with the help of a group of experts who generate vignettes describing clinical cases and provide interpretations of the cases. The vignettes should allow for different interpretations to reflect the various expert judgements and should not assume a single correct answer but alternative interpretations based on the response variations found among the experts who developed the vignettes. The interpretation selected by most experts is taken to be the 'best' answer, although other responses are also considered to be reasonable. After a case is introduced, a series of questions with several hypotheses below are presented. The questions are of the form 'If you were thinking of [e.g. diagnosis, investigation, treatment] and then you find a new [sign or symptom], your diagnosis becomes more or less likely [selected on a scale ranging from −2 to +2]?'. By presenting the case in partial form, adding new information over time and asking whether the selected hypothesis becomes more or less likely, the test can capture parts of the reasoning process. The SC test has been applied successfully in several health settings (e.g. Carriere et al., 2009; Kazour et al., 2017). Its relative ease makes the SC test an appealing way of studying clinical thinking. Computerized or online forms of the test are likely to make it even easier (Sibert et al., 2002). However, researchers should be aware of some validity and reliability concerns with the standard application and interpretation of SC test results (Lineberry et al., 2013).

The Repertory Grid Technique

The repertory grid technique was developed by Kelly (1991) to elicit and examine the personal constructs (e.g. personal beliefs) people use when interpreting a problem or situation. The theory posits that people interpret the world around them much like a scientist, generating hypotheses to understand and predict events. Kelly viewed personal constructs as existing along a bipolar dimension, where one construct was conceived in relation to its opposite, for instance, viewing a problem along the dimension of 'easy' versus 'difficult'. Thus, one assumption is that people's personal constructs can be elicited by placing them at some distance between two poles of the dimension. A benefit of the repertory grid is that it can be quantified and statistically analysed at the individual level.

The method has been applied to the study of clinical reasoning (Kuipers and Grice, 2009a, 2009b). Kuipers and Grice (2009a) illustrate the use of the technique by analysing an interview with an expert occupational therapist. The expert's constructs were elicited from a vignette describing a patient suffering from a neurological problem and a question, called an 'element', (e.g. 'what is the first thing you attend to when you see the client?'), which prompted the expert to generate a series of personalized questions regarding a therapy session. These 'elements' were then used to assist the expert in eliciting the polar constructs along which each element was situated within a numbered grid (Box 20.1). For instance, the expert in the study judged the element mentioned earlier to exist between 'assess functional issues' and its polar opposite 'reason and determine action' by numbering the element along a scale, e.g. with 5 if closest to the emerging construct and 1 if closest to the opposite construct (Kuipers and Grice, 2009a, pp. 280–281).

The method provided both qualitative data (from the interview) and quantitative data (from completing the grid). By applying a statistical method for finding clusters along dimensions in the data, called principal component analysis (PCA), it was possible to identify two components, labelled 'therapist role' and 'practice scope', which accounted for 83% of the variance in the expert's responses. Another study (Kuipers and Grice, 2009b) expanded the use of the repertory grid interview to explore differences between novice and expert occupational therapists before and after introducing a protocol designed to guide the process of clinical reasoning in cases of 'upper limb hypertonia'. The research showed differences between the groups: the novices significantly changed their reasoning so that they were more consistent with the protocol, while the experts did not. Although the repertory grid technique has not been extensively used, it is a promising theoretically based method for the study of clinical reasoning. A basic introduction to the use of repertory grid can be found in Pollock (1986).

Neuro-Imaging Methods

Recently researchers have looked at clinical reasoning processes using neuro-imaging methods (Chang et al., 2016; Durning et al., 2012; Durning, Costanzo, et al., 2013; Durning et al., 2016). The major aim of this kind of research is to uncover the brain structures that underlie the processes of reasoning and thinking. Basically, the method consists of carrying out one or more reasoning tasks while the study participant is in a functional magnetic resonance imaging (fMRI) scanner. The method has been applied to identify the neural structures involved in analytic and nonanalytic reasoning (Durning et al., 2015); memory structure and flexibility in thinking and the differences between experts and novices (Durning et al., 2016); the differences involved in answering questions versus thinking 'aloud' (Durning, Artino, et al., 2013); and clinical problem solving and recall by medical students (Chang et al., 2016).

REFLECTION POINT

Some scientists and philosophers maintain that the key to understanding human reasoning is by uncovering the neural processes underlying thinking and others maintain that many different approaches are needed to understand reasoning such as asking people what their thoughts are.
■ Which approaches do you think might be most suitable?

BOX 20.1
SCRIPT CONCORDANCE

Although the Script Concordance test is an outcome measure, the partial presentation of data allows a reasonable representation of the reasoning process. The repertory grid is based on the idea that people generate personal constructs as scientists generate hypotheses to interpret the world.

Multiple-choice questions (e.g. items from the US medical licensing examination) are often used during the scanning process, although concurrent and retrospective protocols have also been used (Durning et al., 2016). In a typical study, Durning et al. (2015) made use of dual-process theory as an explanatory framework and fMRI to investigate nonanalytic reasoning and thinking efficiency of internal medicine interns (novices) and board-certified internists (experts). The method used involved presenting a series of timed multiple-choice questions (e.g. 60 seconds for reading and 7 seconds for answering) to the participants, which they had to answer by pressing a button while they were in the scanner. After providing the responses, the participants were allowed some time to reflect on their answers, which was done to assess analytic reasoning. The results showed that although sharing a great deal of neural activation (e.g. in brain areas responsible for pattern recognition), novice and expert physicians also demonstrated some differences in the brain areas involved and in reasoning efficiency. Although the results of fMRI may be sometimes difficult to interpret, the method shows encouraging applicability to the study of clinical reasoning in controlled situations (Box 20.2).

Eye-Tracking Technology

Eye-tracking technology has become more available, less intrusive, smaller and simpler to use. A benefit of eye-tracking technology is that it precisely measures gaze behaviour (e.g. number, location and duration of eye fixations) providing evidence of the information that the clinician can focus attention on. Today's eye-tracking technology consists of non-intrusive small cameras that capture infrared light reflected on the cornea. Several eye-tracking studies have been recently conducted to investigate clinical reasoning (Blondon et al., 2015), where the method has been combined with

---

BOX 20.2
CLINICAL REASONING MEASURES

Clinical reasoning can be investigated with outcome and process measures. Using more than one kind of measure ensures a more complete description of clinical reasoning. Diverse measures using biological, behavioural and cognitive factors have been developed.

CASE STUDY 20.1
Investigation of Reasoning Strategies

A researcher is interested in assessing physiotherapy students' clinical reasoning skills. She knows that there are several methods of doing this because she is familiar with outcome-based performance measures, but she would like to understand the different strategies that students use to arrive at the solution of a patient problem. If the physiotherapist aims at capturing the actual process of reasoning, what quantitative methods might be the most useful to meeting their aims?

---

concurrent or retrospective verbal protocols. The vast majority of the studies to date have been conducted in visual domains, such as radiology (Krupinski, 2010), to identify the location of lesions or in the utilization of information technology (Tourassi et al., 2013). A review of the literature by Blondon et al. (2015) identified 10 studies that in various degrees can shed light on the process of clinical thinking. In one study, Tourassi et al. (2013) investigated the diagnostic accuracy in the processing of mammographies within a novice–expert paradigm. They showed that decision making in diagnostic accuracy could be predicted by the patterns of gaze behaviour, which suggests that eye-tracking may be a valid indicator of clinical reasoning (Case Study 20.1).

QUALITATIVE METHODS
Verbal Protocols

The methods described in this section vary widely in terms of their origins and applications and cover concurrent (Lundgren-Laine and Salantera, 2010) and retrospective (Elstein, 2009; Elstein et al., 1978) protocols. The more commonly used methods are the think-aloud and the explanation protocols. The first originates in the study of problem solving and computer simulation of thought (Elstein et al., 1978; Simon, 1993); the second originates in the analysis of text comprehension (Kintsch, 1998). In both cases, the researcher uses verbalizations as data, without involving introspection. That is, research participants are asked to verbalize their thoughts without 'theorizing' about their thinking. Examples of verbal report analyses can be found in Ericsson and Simon (1993) and Arocha et al. (2005).

Think-Aloud Protocol and Analysis

Think-aloud is still an extensively used technique for the study of clinical reasoning (Lee et al., 2016; Lundgren-Laine and Salantera, 2010). This is not surprising given the difficulties of investigating cognitive processes without making use of verbal data. As in many other methods, think-aloud protocols are based on a theory, in this case, the information processing model of Newell and Simon (1972). The method, to be applied successfully, needs a period of training before it can be used to collect data and requires study participants to follow some stringent criteria. The criteria pertain to the type of task that should be used, the kinds of instruction given to study participants and their familiarity with the task. Although criticisms have been raised against the method, e.g. the potential effect of the verbalization itself on the thought processes, it has been found to produce a reasonable description of the underlying thinking process (e.g. Durning, Costanzo et al., 2013).

In typical think-aloud research, clinicians are presented with a patient problem, frequently in written vignettes. A vignette may contain anything from a single sentence to a whole patient record including the clinical interview, the physical examination results and the laboratory results. The clinician is asked to read the information and verbalize whatever thoughts come to mind. If they pause for a few seconds, the experimenter intervenes with questions such as 'What are you thinking about?' or, more appropriately, with demands such as 'Please, continue', which encourages the clinician to carry on talking without introspecting. A detailed and lengthy description is provided by Ericsson and Simon (1993), although shorter introductions have been published (e.g. Lundgren-Laine and Salantera, 2010).

Once the protocol has been collected, it is subjected to an analysis aimed at uncovering the cognitive processes and the information that were used. The analysis of the protocol is then compared with a reference or domain model of the task to be solved. This model is frequently taken either from an expert collaborator in the study or from printed information about the topic, such as textbooks or scholarly expositions. For instance, in an earlier paper, Kuipers and Kassirer (1984) used a model of the Starling equilibrium mechanism, which was compared with the clinician's protocol. Patel et al. (Arocha et al., 2005; Patel et al., 1994) also used a reference model of the clinical problem generated by exceptional practitioners, which serves as a standard for comparison with the obtained protocol. More recently, researchers in fields other than medicine have proposed (Lundgren-Laine and Salantera, 2010) and used the think-aloud method (Lee et al., 2016). In one study (Lee et al., 2016), a group of nurses were given two scenarios describing patients with complex chronic diseases and were prompted to think aloud while interpreting the problem. The protocols were used to develop a detailed model of the nurses' reasoning process. Other researchers have used the think-aloud method in combination with other techniques. For instance, Power et al. (2017) used the method in tandem with the SC test. Also, Durning et al. (2013) combined its use with fMRI imaging and Balslev et al. (2012) had clinicians at different levels of expertise think aloud while solving diagnostic problems in paediatric neurology using eye-tracking technology.

Explanation Protocols

Explanation protocols are a form of retrospective protocol in which people are asked to explain a case to the researcher while the person is being audio-recorded. The explanation protocol is based on a number of assumptions (Arocha et al., 2005). First, information, such as a clinical case description, is processed serially. The information generated from a clinical problem passes through working memory first and is later linked to information in long-term memory, which provides context for interpretation. Second, the temporal sequence in an explanation protocol follows that of the underlying reasoning, in the sense that ideas that are verbalized first are processed first. Third, although the clinical problem may be the same, the reasoning strategies and the final response (e.g. final diagnosis) vary because people process clinical information at several levels of generality, from the very specific symptom level to the general diagnostic level. Research shows that the expertise of the clinician is the critical factor in determining the level of generality at which the clinical case is processed. Finally, both reasoning strategies and

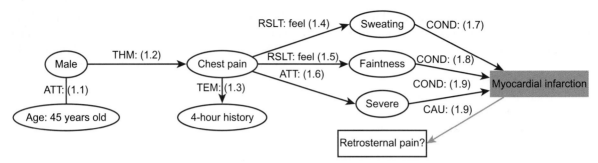

Fig. 20.1 ■ Network representation of propositional analysis generated from a clinician's verbal protocol.

inferences used during clinical reasoning are a function of the clinician's domain-specific prior knowledge.

In practice, the explanation protocol method involves asking research participants to explain the pathophysiology of a case. The transcription of the recorded session is analysed using propositional analysis, which represents the propositional structure of the explanation. Analysis consists of several steps: (1) segment the recorded protocol into clauses; (2) identify the propositions, or idea unit, in each clause; and (3) connect the propositions to reveal the overall semantics of the protocol. A semantic network can be developed from the list of propositions by representing concepts as nodes and relations as links between nodes. Fig. 20.1 shows a network representation of a propositional analysis generated from a clinician's verbal protocol. The oval nodes indicate patient-presented data, the pink box indicates suggested diagnosis and the white box indicates generated hypothetical symptom. The links indicate the direction of reasoning. The links from data to diagnosis refer to data-driven reasoning and the link (in pink) from diagnosis to hypothesis indicates hypothesis-driven reasoning. The text over the links designates semantic markers (e.g. ATT: attribute; CAU: cause; and COND: conditional). The resulting network is a connected conceptual map that represents the information used and the process of reasoning the clinician goes through. The method has been used to investigate patterns of explanations in novices and experts (Patel et al., 1994).

Video Data Collection and Analysis

Videotaping and video analysis can be very useful methodological tools for the study of behaviour

and cognition. There are various uses of video-based data collection. A video camera can be used to capture the stimulus material, such as patient simulation, and a video monitor can be used to present material to the study participants (Durning et al., 2012). Video can also be used as a data collection tool, where the video camera is positioned externally to the study participant, e.g. for analysing gestures, or can be used mounted on the participant's head (Pierce, 2005) to analyse the problem from the participant's point of view. It is especially the second use of video data collection that is more useful to the study of clinical reasoning (Unsworth, 2001b), especially when combined with concurrent or retrospective protocols (Box 20.3).

A benefit of video is that it can capture the context of reasoning. In fact, one may argue that videotaping and analysis allow a more complete characterization of cognitive processing, by providing extra non-verbal information, such as gestures, movements and gazes, which complements the information obtained from verbal protocols. Video data are helpful in analysing tasks designed to externalize someone's thought processes, for instance in physical therapy. In such tasks, both verbalizations and physical actions (e.g. pointing, gazing) can be analysed in a more complete fashion. Video recording has been used in several health disciplines, such as kinesiology, to conduct computer-based analysis of movements, or speech therapy, to analyse language production problems (Pierce, 2005), among others.

Several studies have been conducted in the health sciences using video recording and analysis (Bailliard, 2015). Roots et al. (2016) investigated osteopaths' clinical reasoning while assessing patients with low back pain. The session recorded the interaction between the health practitioner and the patient. After the session finished, the therapist was asked to watch the recording while commenting on the session. This part was audio-recorded for later analysis. Research from the point of view of the study participant has been conducted by Unsworth (2001b). In a study of expert and novice occupational therapists (Unsworth, 2001a), a small camera was strapped around the therapist's head and used to record a typical therapy session with a client. The therapists did not need any time for practice because the head-mounted camera did not disturb their normal work. After the session, the therapists were asked to think aloud while the recording of the session was being shown on a monitor to facilitate recall.

Video data analysis methods vary (Bailliard, 2015), ranging from qualitative to quantitative, the selection of which depends on the theoretical framework used, the objectives of the research and the nature of the data (Derry et al., 2010). Thematic or behavioural analyses exist, both top-down (i.e. categories are generated in advance) or bottom-up (i.e. coding is generated inductively from the data). These analyses can be carried out with the help of video software, which is commercially available (Case Study 20.2).

CASE STUDY 20.2
Choosing Methods

A nurse researcher wants to understand the knowledge that participants use during clinical reasoning in a particular study context. The researcher could not obtain think-aloud data because of the nature of the study context. Given these aims, what methods might be suitable to answer the nurse's question?

CONCLUSION

The panorama of current research methods for the study of clinical reasoning has changed a great deal. First, methodological pluralism is now a common occurrence in research studies. Although one may argue that a methodological fragmentation still exists, it is inspiring to see different methods used in single clinical reasoning studies. The distinction between quantitative and qualitative research methods is now less important as researchers make use of think-aloud in tandem with eye fixations, fMRI, video recording, repertory grids and the SC test. This way, mixed methods data can be collected and analysed that integrate numerical information with qualitative descriptions, which facilitates the comprehension of what goes on during clinical reasoning at several levels, from the purely behavioural, to the cognitive, to the neural. Although early research into clinical reasoning was somewhat characterized by methodological isolation, new methods and techniques have become increasingly used to capture different aspects of the same phenomenon. Approaching the study of clinical reasoning from different perspectives and integrating methods in single studies may facilitate a more complete understanding of the underlying processes and the settings where reasoning is deployed. Second, although not covered in this chapter, other major changes have occurred in the way clinical sciences are practised that may require methodological approaches that permit a fresh look at the processes of reasoning. Clinical reasoning can be considered, in the case of medicine for instance, as thinking through the various aspects of patient care to make a decision about the diagnosis or the therapeutic management of patient problems. This includes history-taking, physical examination, ordering laboratory and ancillary tests and making evidence-based patient management plans.

The increasing amount of research in allied health areas, such as nursing, occupational therapy, social work and physical therapy, has extended the scope of clinical reasoning to a variety of tasks not typically thought of being within its purview. Furthermore, given the considerable variety of these tasks, clinical reasoning can no longer be considered as a characteristic of the single individual because it is being increasingly carried out by teams and collaborative groups often through technological means, such as the electronic health record and decision support systems. The nature of clinical reasoning may need to be reconsidered and tackled with new eyes with the help of novel methods that can capture, holistically, the interactive processes generated by clinicians, patients and technology.

SUMMARY

In this chapter we have presented:

- a description of selected methods for the investigation of clinical reasoning in the health professions
- examples of their use in research on clinical decision making and thinking in medical and other healthcare settings
- comments about future methods and their potential integration to provide a more complete picture of the process of clinical reasoning.

REFLECTION POINT

- Consider what research questions you might pose if you were planning to research clinical reasoning.
- What methods would be useful for researching these questions?

Acknowledgement

The editors would like to thank Stephen Loftus for his valuable feedback on this chapter.

REFERENCES

Arocha, J.F., Wang, D., Patel, V.L., 2005. Identifying reasoning strategies in medical decision making: A methodological guide. J Biomed Inform 38 (2), 154–171. https://doi.org/10.1016/j.jbi.2005.02.001

Bailliard, A.L., 2015. Video methodologies in research: Unlocking the complexities of occupation. Can J Occup Ther 82 (1), 35–43. https://doi.org/10.1177/0008417414556883

Balslev, T., Jarodzka, H., Holmqvist, K., de Grave, W., Muijtjens, A.M., Eika, B., et al., 2012. Visual expertise in paediatric neurology. Eur J Paediatr Neurol 16 (2), 161–166. https://doi.org/10.1016/j.ejpn.2011.07.004

Blondon, K., Wipfli, R., Lovis, C., 2015. Use of eye-tracking technology in clinical reasoning: A systematic review. Stud Health Technol Inform 210, 90–94. https://www.ncbi.nlm.nih.gov/pubmed/25991108

Carriere, B., Gagnon, R., Charlin, B., Downing, S., Bordage, G., 2009. Assessing clinical reasoning in pediatric emergency medicine: Validity evidence for a Script Concordance Test. Ann Emerg Med 53 (5), 647–652. https://doi.org/10.1016/j.annemergmed.2008.07.024

Chang, H.J., Kang, J., Ham, B.J., Lee, Y.M., 2016. A functional neuroimaging study of the clinical reasoning of medical students. Adv Health Sci Educ Theory Pract 21 (5), 969–982. https://doi.org/10.1007/s10459-016-9685-6

Charlin, B., Boshuizen, H.P., Custers, E.J., Feltovich, P.J., 2007. Scripts and clinical reasoning. Med Educ 41 (12), 1178–1184. https://doi.org/10.1111/j.1365-2923.2007.02924.x

Charlin, B., Roy, L., Brailovsky, C., Goulet, F., van der Vleuten, C., 2000. The Script Concordance test: A tool to assess the reflective clinician. Teach Learn Med 12 (4), 189–195. https://doi.org/10.1207/S15328015TLM1204_5

Cramm, H., Krupa, T., Missiuna, C., Lysaght, R.M., Parker, K.C., 2013. Broadening the occupational therapy toolkit: An executive functioning lens for occupational therapy with children and youth. Am J Occup Ther 67 (6), e139–147. https://doi.org/10.5014/ajot.2013.008607

Croskerry, P., 2009. Clinical cognition and diagnostic error: Applications of a dual process model of reasoning. Adv Health Sci Educ Theory Pract 14 (Suppl. 1), 27–35. https://doi.org/10.1007/s10459-009-9182-2

Derry, S.J., Pea, R.D., Barron, B., Engle, R.A., Erickson, F., Goldman, R., et al., 2010. Conducting video research in the learning sciences: Guidance on selection, analysis, technology, and ethics. Journal of the Learning Sciences 19 (1), 3–53.

Durning, S.J., Artino, A.R., Boulet, J.R., Dorrance, K., van der Vleuten, C., Schuwirth, L., 2012. The impact of selected contextual factors on experts' clinical reasoning performance (does context impact clinical reasoning performance in experts?). Adv Health Sci Educ Theory Pract 17 (1), 65–79. https://doi.org/10.1007/s10459-011-9294-3

Durning, S.J., Artino Jr., A.R., Beckman, T.J., Graner, J., van der Vleuten, C., Holmboe, E., et al., 2013. Does the think-aloud protocol reflect thinking? Exploring functional neuroimaging differences with thinking (answering multiple choice questions) versus thinking aloud. Med Teach 35 (9), 720–726. https://doi.org/10.3109/0142159X.2013.801938

Durning, S.J., Costanzo, M., Artino Jr., A.R., Dyrbye, L.N., Beckman, T.J., Schuwirth, L., et al., 2013. Functional neuroimaging correlates of burnout among internal medicine residents and faculty members. Front Psychiatry 4, 131. https://doi.org/10.3389/fpsyt.2013.00131

Durning, S.J., Costanzo, M.E., Artino, A.R., Graner, J., van der Vleuten, C., Schuwirth, L., et al., 2015. Neural basis of nonanalytical reasoning expertise during clinical evaluation. Brain Behav 5 (3), e00309.https://doi.org/10.1002/brb3.309

Durning, S.J., Costanzo, M.E., Beckman, T.J., Artino Jr., A.R., Roy, M.J., van der Vleuten, C., et al., 2016. Functional neuroimaging correlates of thinking flexibility and knowledge structure in memory: Exploring the relationships between clinical reasoning and diagnostic thinking. Med Teach 38 (6), 570–577. https://doi.org/10.3109/0142159X.2015.1047755

Elstein, A.S., 2009. Thinking about diagnostic thinking: A 30-year perspective. Adv Health Sci Educ Theory Pract 14 (Suppl 1), 7–18. https://doi.org/10.1007/s10459-009-9184-0

Elstein, A.S., Shulman, L.S., Sprafka, S.A., 1978. Medical problem solving: An analysis of clinical reasoning. Harvard University Press.

Ericsson, A., Simon, H.A., 1993. Protocol analysis: Verbal reports as data, Rev. ed. MIT Press, Cambridge, Mass.

Haig, B.D., 2013. The philosophy of quantitative methods. In: Little, T.D. (Ed.), The Oxford handbook of quantitative methods, Vol. 1. Oxford University Press, pp. 7–31.

Jaarsma, T., Jarodzka, H., Nap, M., van Merrienboer, J.J., Boshuizen, H.P., 2015. Expertise in clinical pathology: Combining the visual and cognitive perspective. Adv Health Sci Educ Theory Pract 20 (4), 1089–1106. https://doi.org/10.1007/s10459-015-9589-x

Kazour, F., Richa, S., Zoghbi, M., El-Hage, W., Haddad, F.G., 2017. Using the Script Concordance test to evaluate clinical reasoning skills in psychiatry. Acad Psychiatry 41 (1), 86–90. https://doi.org/10.1007/s40596-016-0539-6

Kelly, G., 1991. The psychology of personal constructs: Clinical diagnosis and psychotherapy, Vol. 2. Routledge.

Kintsch, W., 1998. Comprehension: A paradigm for cognition. Cambridge University Press.

Krupinski, E.A., 2010. Current perspectives in medical image perception. Atten Percept Psychophys 72 (5), 1205–1217. https://doi.org/10.3758/APP.72.5.1205

Kuipers, B., Kassirer, J.P., 1984. Causal reasoning in medicine: Analysis of a protocol. Cognitive Science 8 (4), 363–385.

Kuipers, K., Grice, J.W., 2009a. Clinical reasoning in neurology: Use of the repertory grid technique to investigate the reasoning of an experienced occupational therapist. Aust Occup Ther J 56 (4), 275–284. https://doi.org/10.1111/j.1440-1630.2008.00737.x

Kuipers, K., Grice, J.W., 2009b. The structure of novice and expert occupational therapists' clinical reasoning before and after exposure to a domain-specific protocol. Aust Occup Ther J 56 (6), 418–427. https://doi.org/10.1111/j.1440-1630.2009.00793.x

Langridge, N., Roberts, L., Pope, C., 2015. The clinical reasoning processes of extended scope physiotherapists assessing patients with low back pain. Man Ther 20 (6), 745–750. https://doi.org/10.1016/j.math.2015.01.005

Lee, J., Lee, Y.J., Bae, J., Seo, M., 2016. Registered nurses' clinical reasoning skills and reasoning process: A think-aloud study. Nurse Educ Today 46, 75–80. https://doi.org/10.1016/j.nedt.2016.08.017

Lineberry, M., Kreiter, C.D., Bordage, G., 2013. Threats to validity in the use and interpretation of script concordance test scores. Med Educ 47 (12), 1175–1183. https://doi.org/10.1111/medu.12283

Lubarsky, S., Dory, V., Duggan, P., Gagnon, R., Charlin, B., 2013. Script concordance testing: From theory to practice: AMEE guide no. 75. Med Teach, 35(3), 184-193. https://doi.org/10.3109/0142159X.2013.760036

Lundgren-Laine, H., Salantera, S., 2010. Think-aloud technique and protocol analysis in clinical decision-making

research. Qual Health Res 20 (4), 565–575. https://doi.org/10.1177/1049732309354278

Newell, A., Simon, H.A., 1972. Human problem solving. Prentice-Hall.

Norman, G., Young, M., Brooks, L., 2007. Non-analytical models of clinical reasoning: The role of experience. Med Educ 41 (12), 1140–1145. https://doi.org/10.1111/j.1365-2923.2007.02914.x

Norman, G.R., Coblentz, C.L., Brooks, L.R., Babcook, C.J., 1992. Expertise in visual diagnosis: A review of the literature. Acad Med 67 (10 Suppl), S78–S83. https://doi.org/10.1097/00001888-199210000-00045

Patel, V.L., Arocha, J.F., Kaufman, D.R., 1994. Diagnostic reasoning and medical expertise. In: *Psychology of learning and motivation*, Vol. 31. Elsevier, pp. 187–252.

Patel, V.L., Arocha, J.F., Leccisi, M.S., 2001. Impact of undergraduate medical training on housestaff problem-solving performance: Implications for problem-based curricula. J Dent Educ 65 (11), 1199–1218. https://www.ncbi.nlm.nih.gov/pubmed/11765866

Patel, V.L., Kaufman, D.R., Kannampallil, T.G., 2013. Diagnostic reasoning and decision making in the context of health information technology. Reviews of Human Factors and Ergonomics 8 (1), 149–190.

Pierce, D., 2005. The usefulness of video methods for occupational therapy and occupational science research. Am J Occup Ther 59 (1), 9–19. https://doi.org/10.5014/ajot.59.1.9

Pollock, L.C., 1986. An introduction to the use of repertory grid technique as a research method and clinical tool for psychiatric nurses. J Adv Nurs 11 (4), 439–445. https://doi.org/10.1111/j.1365-2648.1986.tb01271.x

Power, A., Lemay, J.F., Cooke, S., 2017. Justify your answer: The role of written think aloud in script concordance testing. Teach Learn Med 29 (1), 59–67. https://doi.org/10.1080/10401334.2016.1217778

Rice, K.L., Bennett, M.J., Clesi, T., Linville, L., 2014. Mixed-methods approach to understanding nurses' clinical reasoning in recognizing delirium in hospitalized older adults. J Contin Educ Nurs 45 (3), 136–148. https://doi.org/10.3928/00220124-20140219-02

Roots, S.A., Niven, E., Moran, R.W., 2016. Osteopaths' clinical reasoning during consultation with patients experiencing acute low back pain: A qualitative case study approach. International Journal of Osteopathic Medicine 19, 20–34.

Runkel, P.J., 2007. Casting nets and testing specimens: Two grand methods of psychology, 2nd ed. revised and updated ed. Living Control Systems Publ.

Schmidt, H.G., Rikers, R.M., 2007. How expertise develops in medicine: Knowledge encapsulation and illness script formation. Med Educ 41 (12), 1133–1139. https://doi.org/10.1111/j.1365-2923.2007.02915.x

Sibert, L., Charlin, B., Corcos, J., Gagnon, R., Lechevallier, J., Grise, P., 2002. Assessment of clinical reasoning competence in urology with the script concordance test: An exploratory study across two sites from different countries. Eur Urol 41 (3), 227–233. https://doi.org/10.1016/s0302-2838(02)00053-2

Simon, H.A. (1993). The human mind: The symbolic level. *Proceedings of the American Philosophical Society*, 137(4), 638–647.

Stec, M.W., 2016. Health as expanding consciousness: Clinical reasoning in baccalaureate nursing students. Nurs Sci Q 29 (1), 54–61. https://doi.org/10.1177/0894318415614901

Tourassi, G., Voisin, S., Paquit, V., Krupinski, E., 2013. Investigating the link between radiologists' gaze, diagnostic decision, and image content. J Am Med Inform Assoc 20 (6), 1067–1075. https://doi.org/10.1136/amiajnl-2012-001503

Unsworth, C.A., 2001a. The clinical reasoning of novice and expert occupational therapists. Scandinavian Journal of Occupational Therapy 8 (4), 163–173.

Unsworth, C.A., 2001b. Using a head-mounted video camera to study clinical reasoning. Am J Occup Ther 55 (5), 582–588. https://doi.org/10.5014/ajot.55.5.582

21

CLINICAL REASONING AND BIOMEDICAL KNOWLEDGE IMPLICATIONS FOR TEACHING

DAVID R. KAUFMAN ■ NICOLE A. YOSKOWITZ ■ VIMLA L. PATEL

CHAPTER OUTLINE

CHAPTER AIMS

The aims of this chapter are:

- to discuss the relationship between basic science knowledge and clinical reasoning
- to identify the nature of biomedical knowledge and challenges integrating it in clinical contexts
- to review assumptions underlying different curricular models
- to present findings from cognitive research that address these matters.

INTRODUCTION

The landscape of healthcare is currently witnessing significant changes, with potential long-term impacts on clinical practice. There are competing views concerning the role of biomedical knowledge and its proper place in a health science curriculum. In this chapter, we consider some of these arguments in the context of empirical evidence from cognitive studies in medicine. Biomedical knowledge has undergone a dramatic transformation over the past 40 years, presenting formidable challenges to medical education

(Martin et al., 2004; Densen, 2011). The relationship between basic science conceptual knowledge and its application in clinical practice continues to be a matter of debate (Kulasegaram et al., 2015). In the past, medical schools have typically responded by adding new biomedical science content to existing courses, increasing the number of lectures and textbook readings (D'Eon and Crawford, 2005). This has changed as clinical courses have become more routine in the first 2 years of medical school (Martin et al., 2004) as has the format of teaching, which places a premium on active learning in clinically relevant contexts (Stott et al., 2016). In addition, basic science courses are increasingly competing with new curricular demands and objectives, for example, to improve professionalism and patient-centred care (Association of American Medical Colleges [AAMC], 2006, 2011).

In the past 25 years, information technology has had a profound effect on the practice of medicine, providing access to a wealth of information and decision support tools that have the potential to improve patient care substantially (Shortliffe and Chang, 2021; Hersh et al., 2014). Concerns have been raised about whether future health practitioners will continue to require the kinds of scientific training that their predecessors received. Although discoveries in science will continue to provide physicians with increasingly powerful investigative tools, it seems likely that the best clinical judgement will require a broader understanding of both biology and medicine than ever before (Prokop, 1992). For example, precision medicine is a groundbreaking approach that compiles and examines extensive data on a patient's history, lifestyle, genetics and environmental factors, aiming to customize the most effective treatment plan for the individual patient (Lamichhane and Agrawal, 2023). Clinicians who have a deeper understanding of basic science knowledge (BSK) will be better prepared to address more complex clinical situations and novel therapeutic strategies (Finnerty, 2010).

CURRICULAR AND EPISTEMOLOGICAL ISSUES

Clinical knowledge includes knowledge of disease entities and associated findings and BSK incorporates subject matter such as biochemistry, anatomy and physiology. It had been widely believed that biomedical and clinical knowledge can be seamlessly integrated into a coherent knowledge structure that supports clinical reasoning (Feinstein, 1973). Medical educators and researchers have argued over how best to promote clinical skill and foster robust conceptual change in students (Boshuizen and Schmidt, 1992; Clough et al., 2004; Patel and Groen, 1986).

Traditionally, the curricula of most medical schools during the first and second years involve preclinical courses that predominantly teach the basic sciences and clinical sciences in subsequent years. This began to change with problem-based learning (PBL), with instruction involving clinically meaningful problems being introduced at the beginning of the curriculum. This practice is guided by the assumption that scientific knowledge taught abstractly does not help students to integrate it in clinical practice (Norman and Schmidt, 2000). Many medical schools have embraced the idea of emphasizing a more clinically relevant basic science curriculum. The Association of American Medical Colleges (AAMC) (e.g. 2004, 2006, 2011) advocates reforming medical education to promote a more patient-centred approach and a more rigorous approach for ensuring that students and residents are acquiring the knowledge, skills, attitudes, values and teamwork orientation deemed necessary to provide high-quality patient care. The renewed focus on clinical skills and competencies introduces additional demands on an already crowded undergraduate curriculum. Similarly, the sheer amount of information in fundamental science disciplines is so enormous that expecting medical students to assimilate thoroughly a wide array of relevant biomedical concepts, related disease entities and findings within a limited time frame is not remotely tenable.

As expertise develops, the disease knowledge of a clinician becomes more dependent on clinical experience and clinical problem solving is increasingly guided by the use of exemplars, becoming less dependent on a functional understanding of the system in question (Patel and Kaufman, 2014). Biomedical knowledge, by comparison, is of a qualitatively different nature, embodying elements of causal mechanisms and characterizing patterns of perturbation in function and structure. Fig. 21.1 presents a knowledge organization reflected in the basic science disciplines with a deeper dive into cardiovascular physiology. Although it is a basic organizing scheme that focusses on the system level, it is helpful to think how certain concepts may inform clinical reasoning in adjacent areas.

REFLECTION POINT

- Reflect on how knowledge in medicine has changed and continues to change.
- How can the issues addressed in this section inform curricular change?

RESEARCH IN CLINICAL REASONING

In this section, we review some of the pertinent research in medical reasoning, particularly research that addresses the role of BSK in clinical medicine.

Clinical Reasoning Strategies and Expertise

Lesgold et al. (1988) investigated the abilities of radiologists at different levels of training and expertise to interpret chest X-ray images. Experts were initially able to detect a general pattern of disease with a gross anatomical localization, acting to constrain the possible interpretations. Novices had greater difficulty focussing

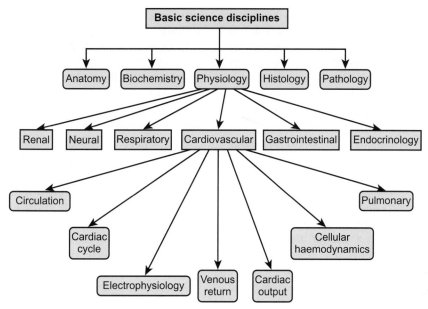

Fig. 21.1 ■ Classical organization scheme for biomedical knowledge.

on the important structures, being more likely to maintain inappropriate interpretations despite discrepant findings in the patient history. The authors concluded that the knowledge that underlies expertise in radiology includes the mental representation of anatomy, a theory of anatomical perturbation and the constructive capacity to transform the visual image into a three-dimensional representation. The less expert subjects had greater difficulty in building and maintaining a rich anatomical representation of the patient. Crowley et al. (2003) documented differences among subjects at varying levels of expertise in breast pathology corresponding to accuracy of diagnosis and aspects of task performance including feature detection, feature identification and data interpretation (Waite et al., 2019).

Norman et al. (1989) compared dermatologists' performance at various levels of expertise in tasks that required them to diagnose and sort dermatological slides according to the type of skin lesion. Expert dermatologists were more accurate in their diagnoses and took significantly less time to respond than novices. Experts grouped the slides into superordinate categories, such as viral infections, which reflected the underlying pathophysiological structure. Novices tended to classify lesions according to surface features such as scaly lesions. The

implication is that expert knowledge is organized around domain principles, which facilitate the rapid recognition of significant problem features. Experts use a qualitatively different kind of knowledge to solve problems based on a deeper understanding of domain principles.

Waite et al. (2019) conduct an extensive review on studies of radiological expertise. The review was motivated by the enduring high error rates in image analysis, which they estimate to be 33%. They argue that perceptual expertise peaks earlier than factual knowledge and begins very early in training but plateaus, leaving a persistent high level of error. The accuracy, error reduction and improvement of patient care in radiology can be enhanced through a more sophisticated understanding of perceptual expertise.

The picture that emerges from research on expertise across domains is that experts use a quite different pattern of reasoning from that used by novices or intermediates and organize their knowledge differently. Three important aspects are that experts (1) have a greater ability to organize information into semantically meaningful, interrelated chunks, (2) selectively focus on relevant information and (3) in routine situations, tend to use highly specific knowledge-based problem-solving strategies (Feltovich and Hoffman, 1997).

The use of knowledge-based strategies has given rise to an important distinction between a data-driven strategy (forward reasoning) in which hypotheses are generated from data and a hypothesis-driven strategy (backward reasoning) in which one reasons backwards from a hypothesis and attempts to find data that elucidate it. Forward reasoning is based on domain knowledge and is thus highly error-prone in the absence of adequate domain knowledge. Backward reasoning is slower and may make heavy demands on working memory and is most likely to be used when domain knowledge is inadequate. Backward reasoning is characteristic of nonexperts and experts solving nonroutine problems (Patel et al., 1989). In Fig. 21.2, forward reasoning is illustrated in a case of acute bacterial endocarditis. Clinical findings (e.g. fever and chills) coupled with clusters of other findings are suggestive of intermediate diagnostic constructs (often called 'facets') such as endocarditis. The cluster of facets led to the forward inference of acute bacterial endocarditis

with aortic insufficiency. Notice that there are no bidirectional or backward inferences.

In experiments with expert physicians in cardiology, endocrinology and respiratory medicine, clinicians showed little tendency to use basic science in explaining cases, whereas medical researchers showed preference for detailed, basic scientific explanations, without developing clinical descriptions (Patel et al., 1989). The pathophysiological explanation task requires subjects to explain the causal pattern underlying a set of clinical symptoms (Feltovich and Barrows, 1984). In one study (Patel and Groen, 1986), expert practitioners (cardiologists) were asked to solve problems within their domain of expertise. Their explanations of the underlying pathophysiology of the cases, whether correctly or incorrectly diagnosed, made virtually no use of BSK.

In a similar study (Patel et al., 1990), cardiologists and endocrinologists solved problems both within and outside their domains of expertise. The clinicians

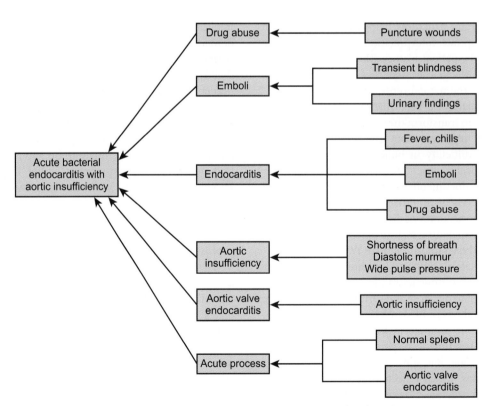

Fig. 21.2 ■ Forward reasoning in a case of acute bacterial endocarditis.

did not appeal to principles from basic biomedical science, even when they were working outside their own domain of expertise; rather, they relied on clinical associations and classifications to formulate solutions. The results suggest that basic science does not contribute directly to reasoning in clinical problem solving for experienced clinicians. However, biomedical information was used by practitioners when the task was difficult or when they were uncertain about their diagnosis. In these cases, biomedical information was used in a backward-directed manner, providing coherence to the explanation of clinical cues that could not be easily accounted for by their primary diagnostic hypothesis.

There have been many other studies highlighting the difficulty of integrating basic and clinical knowledge (e.g. Boshuizen and Schmidt, 1992; Patel et al., 1993; Kulasegaram et al., 2015; Woods, 2007). Pathophysiological information is used by physicians and senior medical students either when the problem-solving process breaks down or to explain findings that cannot be accounted for by the diagnostic hypotheses. In general, there is evidence to suggest that unprompted use of biomedical concepts in clinical reasoning decreases as a function of expertise. In addition, students have difficulty in applying basic science concepts in contexts that differ from the initial conditions of learning (Patel et al., 1990). On the other hand, the visual diagnosis studies suggest a more immediate role for BSK than does the work on expertise in the domains of cardiology and endocrinology. Certain domains necessitate a greater use of core biomedical concepts in understanding even basic problems.

We investigated subjects' mental models of cardiac output (Kaufman et al., 1996). The study characterized the development of understanding of the system as a function of expertise. The research also documented various conceptual flaws in the subjects' models and how these flaws affected subjects' predictions and explanations of physiological manifestations. Clinicians and medical students have variably robust representations of the structure and function of the system. We observed a progression of mental models as a function of expertise, as evidenced in predictive accuracy that increased with expertise and in the quality of explanations (Kaufman and Patel, 1998; Kaufman et al., 2009). Progression was also noted in the quality

of explanations in response to individual questions and problems and in terms of the overall coherence of subjects' representations of the cardiovascular and circulatory system (Patel et al., 2000).

The study documented a wide range of conceptual errors in subjects at different levels of expertise. There were particular misconceptions that, according to our analyses, were more likely to be a product of formal learning.

REFLECTION POINT

- Why do you think students have such difficulty assimilating basic science knowledge into clinical reasoning?
- What is different about visual diagnostic tasks?

Basic Science in Students' Explanations of Clinical Cases

A series of experiments were conducted to elucidate the role of basic science in clinical reasoning (Patel et al., 1990). In one study, medical students (who were either first-year students, second-year students who had completed all basic medical sciences but had not begun any clinical work or final-year students) were presented with three basic science tests (e.g. microcirculation) immediately before a clinical case of acute bacterial endocarditis (Patel et al., 1989). The subjects read basic science texts, recalled them in writing and then explained the clinical problem drawing on these texts. Subjects' recall of the basic science texts was poor, indicating a lack of well-developed knowledge structures in which to organize this information. Recall of the clinical text appeared to be a function of clinical experience, but there was no similar correlation between basic science and experience. In the explanation of the problem, second-year students made extensive use of BSK. Fourth-year students gave explanations that resembled those of expert physicians outside their domain of specialization, except that they used basic science information more liberally. The results indicate that BSK was used differently by the three groups of subjects.

In a second experiment (Patel et al., 1989), students recalled and explained cases when basic science information was provided after the clinical problem. Fourth-year students were able to use the basic science information in a highly effective manner. Second-year students were also able to use this information effectively, but diagnostic reasoning was not facilitated. First-year students were not able to use basic science information any more effectively when it was given after the clinical problem than when it was given before the clinical problem. These results suggest that reasoning towards a diagnosis from the facts of a case was frustrated by attempting to use BSK unless the student had already developed a strong diagnostic hypothesis. The addition of BSK seemed to improve the accuracy of diagnoses offered by final-year medical students but did not improve the accuracy of diagnoses by first- and second-year students. It is likely that final-year students, who had had some clinical experience, relied on clinically relevant features in a case to (broadly) classify the diagnosis and make selective predictions of features that could be explained by basic science concepts. This tendency of clinical solutions to subordinate basic scientific ones, and for basic science not to support the clinical organization of facts in a case, was evident among expert physicians, as discussed earlier. These results were also consistent with other findings, suggesting that unprompted use of biomedical concepts in clinical reasoning decreases as a function of expertise (Boshuizen and Schmidt, 1992).

Research evaluating the performance of PBL and conventional curricula (CC) programmes has found negligible differences in terms of clinical skills (Jolly, 2006). Nevertheless, the different curricula are predicated on different assumptions about how best to foster conceptual change. PBL programmes are based on the necessity of connecting scientific concepts to the conditions of application, whereas CC programmes emphasize the importance of fostering a foundation of general scientific knowledge that is broadly applicable. The CC runs the risk of imparting inert knowledge, much of which is not retained beyond medical school and is not readily applicable to clinical contexts. On the other hand, PBL curricula may promote knowledge that is so tightly coupled to specific contexts as to have minimum generality beyond the immediate problem set.

Patel et al. (1993) attempted to replicate the studies mentioned earlier in an established PBL medical school. Results showed that when basic science information was provided before the clinical problem, there was once again a lack of integration of basic science into the clinical context. This resulted in a lack of global coherence in knowledge structures, errors of scientific fact and disruption of the diagnostic reasoning process. When basic science was given after the clinical problem, there was integration of basic science into the clinical context. It was concluded that clinical problems cannot be easily embedded into a basic science context, but basic science can be more naturally embedded within a clinical context. It is our belief that when one is attempting to learn two unknown domains, it is better to learn one well so that it can be used as an 'anchor' for the new domain. BSK may act as a better anchor than clinical knowledge. It may be useful to introduce some core basic science at the beginning of the curriculum, followed by an early introduction of clinical problems that are thematically connected to the specific scientific concepts.

The findings of these studies suggest that, in conventional curricula, (1) basic science and clinical knowledge are generally separate, (2) clinical reasoning may not require BSK, (3) basic science is spontaneously used only when students have difficulty diagnosing the patient problem and (4) basic science acts to generate globally coherent explanations of the patient problem with connections among various components of the clinical problem. It is proposed that, in a conventional curriculum, the clinical aspect of the problem is viewed as separate from the biomedical science aspect, the two having different functions. In the PBL curriculum, basic science and clinical knowledge are spontaneously integrated. However, this integration results in students' inability to decontextualize the problem and draw on basic science concepts in other contexts. There are multiple competencies involved in the practice of medicine, some of which are best fostered in the context of real-world practice and others best acquired through a process of formal learning (Patel and Kaufman, 2021).

REFLECTION POINT

Consider this discussion of curricula.
- How did you experience these learning sequences in your own course?
- If you are a teacher, does the curriculum of your students differ from your own?
- Do you see a link between knowledge and clinical reasoning capacity development?

KNOWLEDGE ENCAPSULATION OR TWO WORLDS

We consider two theoretical hypotheses that differ on the role of biomedical knowledge in clinical reasoning. Patel and Groen (1991) proposed that clinical and BSK bases constitute 'two worlds' connected at discrete points. Schmidt and Boshuizen offered a more integrative theoretical perspective, built around a learning mechanism, *knowledge encapsulation*, which explains how biomedical knowledge becomes subsumed under clinical knowledge in the development of expertise (Schmidt and Boshuizen, 1993). The process of knowledge encapsulation involves the subsumption of biomedical propositions and associative relations under a small number of higher-level clinical propositions with the same explanatory power. These authors argued that through repeated application of knowledge in medical training and practice, networks of causal biomedical knowledge become incorporated into a comprehensive clinical concept (Van De Wiel et al., 2000).

The crux of the two-worlds hypothesis is that these two bodies of knowledge differ in important respects, including the nature of constituent knowledge elements and the kinds of reasoning they support. Clinical reasoning involves the coordination of diagnostic hypotheses with clinical evidence. Biomedical reasoning involves the use of causal models at varying levels of abstraction (e.g. organ and cellular levels). The evidence suggests that routine diagnostic reasoning is largely a classification process in which groups of findings become associated with hypotheses. BSK is not typically evident in expert think-aloud protocols in these circumstances.

Under conditions of uncertainty, physicians resort to scientific explanations that provide coherence, even when inaccurate. The role of basic science, aside from providing the concepts required to formulate clinical problems, is to create a basis for establishing coherence in the explanation of biomedical phenomena. Basic science does not provide the abstractions required to support clinical problem solving. Rather, it provides the principles that make it possible to organize observations that defy ready clinical classification and analysis. Biomedical knowledge also provides a means for explaining, justifying and communicating medical decisions. In the absence of basic science, the relationships between symptoms and diagnoses seem arbitrary.

The two-worlds hypothesis is consistent with a model of conceptual change in which clinical knowledge and BSK undergo both a joint and separate processes of reorganization. This is partly a function of the kinds of learning experience that students undergo. The premedical years are focussed primarily on the acquisition of biomedical knowledge. As students become increasingly involved in clinical activities, the prioritization of knowledge also shifts to concepts that support the process of clinical reasoning. Schmidt and Boshuizen (1993) proposed a developmental process in which students early in their training acquire 'rich elaborated causal networks explaining the causes and consequences of disease' in terms of biomedical knowledge (p. 207). Through repeated exposure to patient problems, the BSK becomes encapsulated into high-level simplified causal models explaining signs and symptoms. The knowledge structures remain available when clinical knowledge is not adequate to explain a clinical problem. Intermediates require additional processing time to accomplish a task compared with experts and, at times, even novices. For example, in pathophysiology explanations, intermediates generate lengthy lines of reasoning that use numerous biomedical concepts. On the other hand, experts use shortcuts in their line of reasoning, skipping intervening steps. A common finding is that intermediates recall more information from a clinical case than either novices or experts. Novices lack the knowledge to integrate the information, whereas experts selectively recall relevant information. Similarly, in pathophysiological explanation tasks, intermediates tend to use more biomedical knowledge and more elaborations than either novices or experts. The extra processing is caused by the fact that these subjects have accumulated a great deal of conceptual knowledge but have not fully tuned it to the performance of clinical tasks.

REFLECTION POINT

Reflect on the two proposed theories, namely, knowledge encapsulation and the two-worlds hypothesis. Can you think of different learning experiences that may be better explained by one theory or the other? The differences may be having an experience in which your knowledge appears to be seamless. On the other hand, sometimes you may have to do extra cognitive work to use basic science knowledge in addressing a clinical problem.

Schmidt and colleagues conducted several studies in which they varied the amount of time that an individual was exposed to stimulus materials (Van De Wiel et al., 2000; Schmidt and Boshuizen, 1993). They demonstrated that intermediates were negatively affected by having less time to process the stimulus material, whereas experts were largely unaffected by a reduction in time. The argument is that the immediate activation of a small number of highly relevant encapsulating concepts enables experts to rapidly formulate an adequate representation of a patient problem. On the other hand, students have yet to develop knowledge in an encapsulated form, relying more on biomedical knowledge and requiring more time to construct a coherent case representation. In other studies, Schmidt and Boshuizen (1993) demonstrated that expert clinicians could unfold their abbreviated lines of reasoning into longer chains of inferences that evoked more elaborate causal models when the situation warranted it.

The knowledge encapsulation theory may, on the one hand, overstate the capabilities of experts to activate elaborated biomedical models rapidly. On the other hand, by its focus on lines of reasoning, the theory may undermine the generative nature of expert knowledge. Lines of reasoning would suggest that experts have access to limited patterns of inference resulting from repeated exposure to similar cases. It is apparent that people learn to circumvent long chains of reasoning and chunk knowledge across intermediate states of inference as circumstances warrant this (Van De Wiel et al., 2000). This results in shorter, more direct inferences that are stored in long-term memory and are directly available to be retrieved in the appropriate contexts. We agree that repeated exposure to recurrent patterns of symptoms is likely to result in the chunking of causal inferences that will subsequently be available for reuse (Kaufman and Patel, 1998).

However, experts are also capable of solving novel and complex problems that necessitate the generation of new causal models based on a deep understanding of the system. This enables them to work out the consequences of a pathophysiological process that was never previously encountered (Kaufman and Patel, 1998). Mastery of biomedical knowledge may be characterized as a progression of mental models that reflect increasingly sophisticated and robust understandings of pathophysiological processes. Given the vast quantities of knowledge that need to be assimilated in 4-year medical curricula, it is not likely that one can develop robust understanding of the pathophysiology of disease. Clinical practice offers selective exposure to certain kinds of clinical cases. Even experts' mental models can be somewhat brittle when stretched to the limits of their understanding (Kaufman and Patel, 1998). Knowledge encapsulation may partially account for the process of conceptual change in biomedicine.

Boshuizen and colleagues (2020) introduced the 'Knowledge Restructuring through Case Processing' (KR-CP) theory, which represents an extension to knowledge encapsulation. The restructuring of medical knowledge is associated with the development of illness scripts. Illness scripts are knowledge frameworks that connect predisposing factors for a disease (such as genetic predisposition, lifestyle, previous illnesses and age) to the outcomes of that disease (the signs, symptoms and their progression). This information is unified through an understanding of the fault – the pathophysiological processes and pathoanatomical conditions that underpin the signs and symptoms. An extended discussion of KR-CP is beyond the scope of this chapter. Nevertheless, it is a theoretical framework that goes well beyond the knowledge restructuring that results in abbreviated lines of associated reasoning mechanism to one that may also explain the elaboration of causal models in understanding complex biomedical concepts as described in the two-worlds hypothesis.

Learning Mechanisms

Clearly, the diversity of biomedical knowledge and clinical reasoning tasks requires multiple mechanisms of learning. BSK plays a different role in different clinical domains (such as dermatology and radiology). This requires a relatively robust model of anatomical structures, which is the primary source of knowledge for diagnostic classification (Norman, 2000). In other domains, such as cardiology and endocrinology, BSK has a more distant relationship with clinical knowledge. Furthermore, the misconceptions evident in physicians' biomedical explanations would argue against well-developed encapsulated knowledge structures, where BSK can easily be retrieved and applied when necessary. Our contention is that neither conventional nor problem-based curricula can foster the kind of learning suggested by the encapsulation process. The challenge for medical schools is to strike the right balance between presenting information in applied contexts and allowing students to derive the appropriate abstractions and generalizations to further develop their models of conceptual understanding. The two-worlds hypothesis implies that each body of knowledge be given special status in the medical curriculum and that the correspondences between the two worlds need to be developed.

The design and reform of educational curricula in complex advanced knowledge domains, such as biomedicine, depend on the identification of those concepts and knowledge that are considered necessary to become an effective and skilled scientist-practitioner (Patel et al., 2009). Successful knowledge integration is predicated on presenting basic science information in a manner that creates explicit relationships between basic and clinical science (Kulasegaram et al., 2015). Diemers et al. (2015) similarly concluded that there is a need to provide students with varied patient experiences with the same underlying pathophysiological mechanism and to encourage students to link biomedical and clinical knowledge.

SUMMARY

There has been a long-standing concern that the amount of time devoted to basic science in medical curricula is decreasing. The concern is made more acute by the fact that new knowledge in the biological sciences is increasing rapidly and by the emergence of comparatively new scientific domains bioinformatics and personalized medicine 'that promise paradigm shifts in clinical thinking'. Advances in artificial intelligence promise to transform decision support and critically influence clinical reasoning processes. The downside is that these systems may induce complacency or automation bias. Enhancing biomedical understanding could act as a safeguard against complacency, equipping healthcare professionals with the resources needed to question and correct the

periodically incorrect assumptions of these systems. Although medical cognition research continues to flourish, less attention has been paid to the problem of integrating basic science knowledge into clinical reasoning. Given the enormous advances in basic medical science and the changing character of clinical practice, the time may be ripe to revisit old debates, invigorate new research efforts and determine how best to inform the biomedical curriculum for the coming decades.

REFLECTION POINT

- In what ways (if any) has your view of the place of BSK in clinical reasoning and the education of healthcare professionals changed as a result of reading this chapter?

REFERENCES

AAMC, 2004. Educating doctors to provide high quality medical care: A vision for medical education in the United States Report of the Ad Hoc Committee of Deans. AAMC, Washington, DC.

AAMC, 2006. Implementing the vision: Group on educational affairs responds to the IIME Dean's Committee report. AAMC, Washington, DC.

AAMC, 2011. Core competencies for interprofessional collaborative practice: Report on an expert panel. AAMC, Washington, DC.

Boshuizen, H.P., Schmidt, H.G., 1992. On the role of biomedical knowledge in clinical reasoning by experts, intermediates and novices. Cognitive Science 16 (2), 153–184.

Boshuizen, H. P., Gruber, H., & Strasser, J. (2020). Knowledge restructuring through case processing: The key to generalise expertise development theory across domains? Educational Research Review, 29, 100310.

Clough, R.W., Shea, S.L., Hamilton, W.R., Estavillo, J.A., Rupp, G., Browning, R.A., et al., 2004. Weaving basic and social sciences into a case-based, clinically oriented medical curriculum: One school's approach. Acad Med 79 (11), 1073–1083. https://doi.org/10.1097/00001888-200411000-00013

Crowley, R.S., Naus, G.J., Stewart J., 3rd, Friedman, C.P., 2003. Development of visual diagnostic expertise in pathology – An information-processing study. J Am Med Inform Assoc 10 (1), 39–51. https://doi.org/10.1197/jamia.m1123

D'Eon, M., Crawford, R., 2005. The elusive content of the medical-school curriculum: A method to the madness. Med Teach 27 (8), 699–703. https://doi.org/10.1080/01421590500237598

Densen, P., 2011. Challenges and opportunities facing medical education. Trans Am Clin Climatol Assoc 122, 48–58. https://www.ncbi.nlm.nih.gov/pubmed/21686208

Diemers, A.D., van de Wiel, M.W., Scherpbier, A.J., Baarveld, F., Dolmans, D.H., 2015. Diagnostic reasoning and underlying knowledge of students with preclinical patient contacts in PBL. Med Educ 49 (12), 1229–1238. https://doi.org/10.1111/medu.12886

Feinstein, A.R., 1973. An analysis of diagnostic reasoning. I. The domains and disorders of clinical macrobiology. Yale J Biol Med 46 (3), 212–232. https://www.ncbi.nlm.nih.gov/pubmed/4803623

Feltovich, P.J., Barrows, H.S., 1984. Issues of generality in medical problem solving. In: Schmidt, H., De Volder, M. (Eds.), Tutorials in problem-based learning: New Directions in training for the health professions. Van Gorcum, pp. 128–142.

Feltovich, P. J., & Hoffman, R. R. (Eds.), (1997). *Expertise in context.* Menlo Park, CA: AAAI Press.

Finnerty, E.P., 2010. The role and value of the basic sciences in medical education: An examination of Flexner's legacy. J Int Assoc Med Sci Educ 20 (3), 258–260.

Hersh, W.R., Gorman, P.N., Biagioli, F.E., Mohan, V., Gold, J.A., Mejicano, G.C., 2014. Beyond information retrieval and electronic health record use: Competencies in clinical informatics for medical education. Adv Med Educ Pract 5, 205–212. https://doi.org/10.2147/AMEP.S63903

Jolly, B., 2006. Problem-based learning, Vol. 40. Wiley Online Library, pp. 494–495.

Kaufman, D.R., Keselman, A., Patel, V.L., 2009. Changing conceptions in medicine and health. In: Vosniadou, S. (Ed.), International handbook of research on conceptual change. Routledge, pp. 323–355.

Kaufman, D.R., Patel, V.L., 1998. Progressions of mental models in understanding circulatory physiology. In: Singh, I., Parasuraman, R. (Eds.), Human cognition: A multidisciplinary perspective. Sage, pp. 300–326.

Kaufman, D.R., Patel, V.L., Magder, S.A., 1996. The explanatory role of spontaneously generated analogies in reasoning about physiological concepts. International Journal of Science Education 18 (3), 369–386.

Kulasegaram, K., Manzone, J.C., Ku, C., Skye, A., Wadey, V., Woods, N.N., 2015. Cause and effect: Testing a mechanism and method for the cognitive integration of basic science. Acad Med 90 (11 Suppl), S63–S69. https://doi.org/10.1097/ACM.0000000000000896

Lamichhane, P., Agrawal, A., 2023. Precision medicine and implications in medical education. Ann Med Surg (Lond) 85 (4), 1342–1345. https://doi.org/10.1097/MS9.0000000000000298

Lesgold, A., Rubinson, H., Feltovich, P., Glaser, R., Klopfer, D., Wang, Y., 1988. Expertise in a complex skill: Diagnosing x-ray pictures. In: Chi, M.T.H., Glaser, R.J., Farr, M.J. (Eds.), The nature of expertise. Lawrence Erlbaum, pp. 311–342.

Martin, J., Alpern, R., Betz, A., Deckers, P., Gabbe, S., Harris, E., et al., 2004. Educating doctors to provide high quality medical care: A vision for medical education in the United States. In: Washington, D.C.: Association of American Medical Colleges.

Norman, G., 2000. The essential role of basic science in medical education: The perspective from psychology. Clin Invest Med 23 (1), 47–51; discussion 52-44. https://www.ncbi.nlm.nih.gov/pubmed/10782317

Norman, G.R., Rosenthal, D., Brooks, L.R., Allen, S.W., Muzzin, L.J., 1989. The development of expertise in dermatology. Arch Dermatol 125 (8), 1063–1068. https://www.ncbi.nlm.nih.gov/pubmed/2757402

Norman, G.R., Schmidt, H.G., 2000. Effectiveness of problem-based learning curricula: Theory, practice and paper darts. Med Educ 34 (9), 721–728. https://doi.org/10.1046/j.1365-2923.2000.00749.x

Patel, V.L., Evans, D.A., Groen, G.J., 1989. Reconciling basic science and clinical reasoning. Teaching and Learning in Medicine: An International Journal 1 (3), 116–121.

Patel, V.L., Evans, D.A., Kaufman, D.R., 1990. Reasoning strategies and the use of biomedical knowledge by medical students. Med Educ 24 (2), 129–136. https://doi.org/10.1111/j.1365-2923.1990.tb02511.x

Patel, V.L., Groen, G.J., 1986. Knowledge based solution strategies in medical reasoning. Cognitive Science 10 (1), 91–116.

Patel, V.L., Groen, G.J., 1991. The general and specific nature of medical expertise: A critical look. In: Ericsson, K.A., Smith, J. (Eds.), Toward a general theory of expertise: Prospects and limits. Cambridge University Press, pp. 93–125.

Patel, V.L., Groen, G.J., Norman, G.R., 1993. Reasoning and instruction in medical curricula. Cognition and Instruction 10 (4), 335–378.

Patel, V.L., Kaufman, D., 2021. Cognitive informatics. In: Shortliffe, E.H., Cimino, J.J., Chang, M.F. (Eds.), Biomedical informatics: Computer applications in health care and biomedicine, 5th ed. Springer-Verlag, pp. 121–152.

Patel, V.L., Yoskowitz, N.A., Arocha, J.F., Shortliffe, E.H., 2009. Cognitive and learning sciences in biomedical and health instructional design: A review with lessons for biomedical informatics education. J Biomed Inform 42 (1), 176–197. https://doi.org/10.1016/j.jbi.2008.12.002

Prokop, D., 1992. Basic science and clinical practice: How much will a physician need to know. In: Marston, R., Jones, R. (Eds.), Medical education in transition. Princeton, NJ: The Robert Wood Johnson Foundation (pp. 51–57). Robert Wood Johnson Foundation.

Schmidt, H.G., Boshuizen, H.P., 1993. On acquiring expertise in medicine. Educational Psychology Review 5, 205–221.

Shortliffe, E.H., Chiang, M.F., 2021. Biomedical informatics: The science and the pragmatics. In: Shortliffe, E.H., Cimino, J.J. (Eds.), Biomedical informatics: Computer applications in health care and biomedicine, 5th ed. Springer, pp. 3–44. https://doi.org/10.1007/978-3-030-58721-5

Stott, M.C., Gooseman, M.R., Briffa, N.P., 2016. Improving medical students' application of knowledge and clinical decision-making through a porcine-based integrated cardiac basic science program. J Surg Educ 73 (4), 675–681. https://doi.org/10.1016/j.jsurg.2016.04.021

Van De Wiel, M.W., Boshuizen, H.P., Schmidt, H.G., 2000. Knowledge restructuring in expertise development: Evidence from pathophysiological representations of clinical cases by students and physicians. European Journal of Cognitive Psychology 12 (3), 323–356.

Waite, S., Grigorian, A., Alexander, R.G., Macknik, S.L., Carrasco, M., Heeger, D.J., et al., 2019. Analysis of perceptual expertise in radiology–Current knowledge and a new perspective. Frontiers in Human Neuroscience 13 (213), 323–356.

Woods, N.N., 2007. Science is fundamental: The role of biomedical knowledge in clinical reasoning. Med Educ 41 (12), 1173–1177. https://doi.org/10.1111/j.1365-2923.2007.02911.x

22 CLINICAL REASONING IN MEDICINE

OLGA KOSTOPOULOU ■ ALAN SCHWARTZ

CHAPTER AIMS

The aims of this chapter are:

- to describe the process of diagnostic reasoning in medicine
- to compare problem-solving and decision-making approaches to research on clinical reasoning and diagnostic error
- to introduce dual-process models of reasoning
- to explain educational implications of dual-process theory.

INTRODUCTION

How do physicians solve diagnostic problems? What is known about the process of diagnostic clinical reasoning? Why might a diagnosis be missed? In this chapter, we sketch our current understanding of answers to these questions by reviewing the cognitive processes and mental structures used in diagnostic reasoning in clinical medicine. We will not consider the parallel issue of developing a management plan. We draw upon two approaches that have been particularly influential in research in this field: problem solving and decision making.

Problem-solving research has usually focussed on how an ill-structured problem situation is defined and structured (normally by generating a set of diagnostic hypotheses). It is explored in the work of Elstein et al. (Elstein, 2009; Elstein et al., 1978), Bordage et al. (e.g. Bordage, 1994) and Norman (2005). Psychological decision research (also known as 'behavioural decision making') has typically looked at factors affecting diagnosis or treatment choice in well-defined, tightly controlled situations, as illustrated in the work of Kahneman et al. (Kahneman, 2003; Kahneman et al., 1982) and Schwartz and Bergus (2008). A common theme in both approaches is that human rationality is limited or 'bounded'. Nevertheless, researchers within the problem-solving paradigm have concentrated on identifying the strategies of experts, with the aim of facilitating the acquisition of these strategies by learners. Behavioural decision research, on the other hand, contrasts human performance with a normative statistical model of reasoning under uncertainty. It illuminates cognitive processes by examining people's inherent reasoning tendencies (cognitive heuristics) and the associated reasoning errors (cognitive biases) to which even experts are not immune. As a way of improving human reasoning, this literature concentrates on debiasing and decision aids.

A COMMON BASIS: DUAL-PROCESS THEORY

Both medical problem-solving and decision-making research have adopted dual-process or 'two systems' accounts of cognition described (with variations in details) by Kahnemann (Kahneman, 2002; Kahneman et al., 1982), Stanovich and West (2000) and, perhaps most accessibly, by Kahneman (2011). These accounts posit two distinct cognitive systems or types of processing. System 1 is a fast, automatic and intuitive mode of thinking that shares similarities with perception. Judgements made using System 1 take advantage of the power of pattern recognition, emotional cues and a set of cognitive heuristics and are susceptible to associated biases and the effect of the emotional state of the judge and emotional content of the judgement. System 1's accuracy is contingent on interactions between task features and the judge's prior experiences and memories. System 2 is a slow, effortful, analytic

mode that applies rules in an emotionally neutral manner (Fig. 22.1, from Kahnemann, 2003). When appropriate data are available, System 2 yields the most normatively rational response, but it is easily disrupted by high cognitive load. Therefore, both systems can lead to error under different conditions. Dual-process theory is broadly accepted among psychologists, with variations focussing on when and how the two systems activate and interact with one another (e.g. De Neys and Glumicic, 2008), differences in how experts and novices rely on each system, and conditions under which each system is expected to provide better performance (e.g. Rusou et al., 2013).

REFLECTION POINT

- Clinical reasoning operates through dual processes: a fast, intuitive process (System 1) and a slow, analytical process (System 2).

PROBLEM SOLVING: DIAGNOSIS AS HYPOTHESES GENERATION AND SELECTION

To solve a clinical diagnostic problem means first to recognize a 'malfunction' and then to set about identifying its causes. The diagnosis is thus an explanation of disordered function and, where possible, a causal explanation.

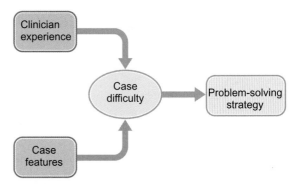

Fig. 22.1 ■ Effect on problem-solving strategy of case difficulty, clinician experience and case features. (With permission from The Noble Foundation; Kahneman, D., 2003. Maps of bounded rationality: A perspective on intuitive judgement and choice. In: Frangsmyr, T. (Ed.), Les Prix Nobel: The Nobel Prizes 2002. Stockholm, Sweden, Almqvist & Wiksell International, pp. 416–499.)

In most cases, not all the information needed to identify and explain the situation is available in the early stages of the clinical encounter. Physicians must outline potential diagnoses (a 'differential diagnosis'), consider their likelihood and severity and decide what information to collect, which aspects of the situation need attention and what can be safely set aside. Thus, data collection is both sequential and selective. Experienced physicians often go about this task almost automatically, sometimes very rapidly and in a confident manner; novices are slower and collect more information. There are several likely reasons for this. For example, novices may generate more diagnostic hypotheses on average than experts or they may generate less appropriate diagnostic hypotheses that do not help them reduce the 'problem space' quickly; they may experience greater uncertainty and think that more information may reduce this; or they may lack efficient strategies for information search. Behavioural decision research, on the other hand, contrasts human performance with a normative statistical model of reasoning under uncertainty. It illuminates cognitive processes by examining people's inherent reasoning tendencies (cognitive heuristics) and the associated reasoning errors (cognitive biases) to which even experts are not immune. As a way of improving human reasoning, this literature concentrates on debiasing and decision aids.

THE HYPOTHETICO-DEDUCTIVE METHOD

Early Hypothesis Generation and Selective Data Collection

In their pioneering studies on clinical reasoning, Elstein et al. (1978) found that diagnostic problems are solved by a process of generating a limited number of hypotheses, or problem formulations, early in the workup and using them to guide subsequent data collection and integration. Each hypothesis predicts which additional findings ought to be present if it were true. The workup is then a guided search for these findings; hence, the method is hypothetico-deductive and based on System 2 processes. Novices and experienced physicians alike attempt to generate hypotheses to explain clusters of findings, although the content of the experienced physicians' hypotheses is of higher quality.

Other clinical researchers have concurred with this view (Kuipers and Kassirer, 1984; Nendaz et al., 2005). It has also been favoured by medical educators (e.g. Kassirer and Kopelman, 1991), but the emergence of dual-process theory has redirected interest towards System 1 processes in hypothesis generation, with many authors and practitioners claiming that they lead to better diagnosis, at least in expert clinicians. Recent work has found that physicians' confidence about the first hypothesis that comes to mind can determine the appropriateness of the subsequent diagnostic process (Kourtidis et al., 2022).

Data Collection and Interpretation

Data obtained must be interpreted in the light of the hypotheses being considered. A clinician could collect data quite thoroughly but could nevertheless ignore, misunderstand or misinterpret a significant fraction. In contrast, a clinician might be overly economical in data collection but could interpret whatever is available quite accurately. Weiner and colleagues (Weiner et al., 2013; Weiner et al., 2010) used unannounced standardized patients (actors presenting as patients incognito to physicians) and real patients carrying concealed audio recorders and found that physicians often failed to probe for information and identify diagnoses based in patient context rather than physiology and paid greater attention to case features identified by physician inquiry than those revealed spontaneously by patients (Schwartz et al., 2016).

Although studies based on medical record reviews have often attributed diagnostic failures to inadequate data collection (e.g. Singh et al., 2007), experimental research has not found a strong association between thoroughness of data collection and diagnostic accuracy (Kostopoulou et al., 2017).

Consequently, some researchers switched to controlling the data presented to participants, to concentrate on data interpretation and problem formulation (e.g. Kuipers et al., 1988). Controlling the presentation of data facilitates analysis at the price of fidelity to clinical realities. This strategy is the most widely used in current research on clinical reasoning, the shift reflecting the influence of the paradigm of decision-making research. The analysis can focus on memory organization, knowledge utilization, data interpretation or problem representation (e.g. Bordage, 1994; Groves et al., 2003).

Kostopoulou and colleagues (2012) presented items of clinical information to participants sequentially – without the option of additional information search – to study 'predecisional information distortion', i.e. the tendency to change the value of incoming information to support a current belief (in this case, a leading diagnostic hypothesis) (see also Nurek et al., 2014). Sirota and colleagues (2017) gave the same block of initial information to all participants and asked them to think aloud before collecting further information. They found that if physicians did not explicitly mention cancer when they received the initial information, they were significantly less likely to give cancer as a possible diagnosis and refer the patient for further investigations at the end, irrespective of the information that they collected during the case.

Case Specificity

Problem-solving expertise varies greatly across cases and is highly dependent on the clinician's mastery of the particular domain (e.g. Kostopoulou et al., 2008). Differences among clinicians are to be found more in their understanding of the problem and their problem representations rather than in the reasoning strategies employed (Elstein et al., 1978). Thus, it makes more sense to talk about reasons for success and failure in a particular case than about generic traits or strategies of expert diagnosticians.

REFLECTION POINT

Reasoning depends on knowledge and the structure of knowledge in memory. General 'reasoning skills' may result in different outcomes depending on the experiences stored in the reasoner's memory.
- What experiences do physicians need to be exposed to?
- How might these experiences be organized in memory?

DIAGNOSIS AS PATTERN RECOGNITION

It has often been pointed out that the clinical reasoning of experts in familiar situations does not display explicit hypothesis testing; it is rapid, automatic and often nonverbal (e.g. Eva et al., 1998; Groen and Patel, 1985).

Expert reasoning in familiar situations looks more like a System 1 process of pattern recognition or direct automatic retrieval from a well-structured network of stored knowledge (Groen and Patel, 1985). Because experienced clinicians have a better sense of clinical realities and the likely diagnostic possibilities, they can more efficiently generate an early set of plausible hypotheses to avoid fruitless and expensive pursuit of unlikely diagnoses. The research emphasis thus shifted from the problem-solving process to the organization of knowledge in the long-term memory of experienced clinicians. Unlike hypothetico-deduction, pattern recognition and matching approaches neither require nor assume that causal reasoning takes place. Expert–novice differences are partly explicable in terms of the size of the knowledge store of prior instances available for pattern recognition. This theory of clinical reasoning has been developed with particular reference to pathology, dermatology and radiology, where the clinical data are predominantly visual. Additionally, better diagnosticians are thought to have more diversified and abstract links between clinical features or aspects of the problem (Bordage, 1994). Domain experts are better able to relate findings to each other and to potential diagnoses and to identify what additional findings are needed to complete a picture (Elstein et al., 1993). These capabilities suggest that more experienced physicians are working with more abstract representations and are not simply trying to match a new case to a specific previous instance. However, such a matching process may still occur with simple cases (where there is a larger store of specific memories) or with cases that are somehow memorable, because matching would be quicker than abstraction.

MULTIPLE REASONING STRATEGIES

The controversy about reasoning strategies in diagnosis can be resolved by positing that the strategy selected depends on the perceived characteristics of the problem. Norman et al. (1994) found that experienced physicians used a hypothetico-deductive strategy with difficult cases only. Easy cases are solved by pattern recognition and going directly from data to diagnostic classification – what Groen and Patel (1985) called *forward reasoning*. Difficult cases need systematic hypothesis generation and testing. Furthermore, there is an interaction between the clinician's level of skill and the perceived difficulty of the task (Elstein, 1994). Whether a problem is easy or difficult depends in part on the knowledge and experience of the clinician and the way the problem is conceptualized (Fig. 22.2). Mamede et al. (2008) found that when they suggested to participants that some clinical cases had been previously seen by experienced physicians who had failed to diagnose them, those cases took longer to diagnose and were diagnosed more accurately than when the same cases were presented as straightforward. Using a think-aloud methodology, they found more frequent mentions of findings, causal mechanisms and diagnoses for the supposedly difficult cases, suggesting that participants were using an analytical rather than intuitive approach for those cases.

DECISION MAKING: DIAGNOSIS AS OPINION REVISION

In the literature on medical decision making, reaching a diagnosis is conceptualized as a process of reasoning about uncertainty in a statistical manner and updating an opinion with imperfect information (the clinical evidence). As new information is obtained, the

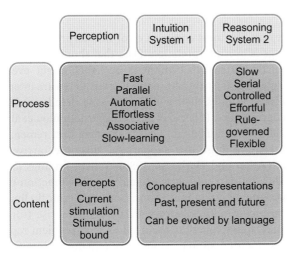

Fig. 22.2 ■ Characteristics of two cognitive systems for judgement. (With permission from The Noble Foundation; Kahneman, D., 2003. Maps of bounded rationality: A perspective on intuitive judgement and choice. In: Frangsmyr, T. (Ed.), Les Prix Nobel: The Nobel Prizes 2002. Stockholm, Sweden, Almqvist & Wiksell International, pp. 416–499.)

probability of each diagnostic possibility is continuously revised. Each posttest probability becomes the pretest probability for the next stage of the inference process. Bayes' theorem, the normative mathematical rule for this operation, states that the posttest probability is a function of two variables, pretest probability and the strength of the new diagnostic evidence. The pretest probability can be either the known prevalence of the disease or the clinician's belief about the probability of disease before new information is acquired. The strength of the evidence is measured by a *likelihood ratio*, the ratio of the probabilities of observing a particular finding in patients with and without the disease of interest.

This framework directs attention to two major classes of errors in clinical reasoning: errors in a clinician's beliefs about pretest probability, including either ignoring or over-relying on pretest probability and errors in assessing the strength of the evidence and revising the pretest probability. From the Bayesian viewpoint, the psychological study of diagnostic reasoning centres on errors in both components, which are discussed later in the chapter.

The revision of opinion, using Bayes' theorem, underlies teaching about diagnosis in evidence-based medicine (EBM) (Strauss et al., 2010). A variety of paper and online tools and spreadsheets have been developed to provide decision support or simplify EBM calculations. A typical example is the graphical Bayesian nomogram, which permits quick calculation of posterior probabilities from prior probability and likelihood ratio information. Fagan (1975) published the best-known nomogram, which is available on a pocket-sized card. Schwartz (2002) provides a widely used online version.

A COMMON CHALLENGE: DIAGNOSTIC ERROR

Singh et al. (2014) define diagnostic error as 'a missed opportunity to make a timely or correct diagnosis based on the available evidence'. The Committee of the National Academy of Medicine (Ball et al., 2015) proposed a more patient-centred definition: 'the failure to (a) establish an accurate and timely explanation of the patient's health problem(s) or (b) communicate that explanation to the patient' (p. 85).

Diagnostic error has attracted considerable interest in recent years due, in large part, to the patient safety movement. The US National Academy of Medicine (Ball et al., 2015) concluded that 'most people will experience at least one diagnostic error in their lifetime, sometimes with devastating consequences' (p. 1).

In acute care settings such as general practice, accident and emergency and after-hours care, diagnostic error accounts for most litigation cases (Gandhi et al., 2006; Silk, 2000). However, measuring the rate of diagnostic error is not an exact science, as all methods suffer from bias (Graber, 2013) (see Case Study 22.1).

ERRORS IN HYPOTHESIS GENERATION AND RESTRUCTURING

Neither pattern recognition nor hypothesis testing are error-proof strategies, consistent with statistical rules of inference from imperfect information. Kassirer and Kopelman (1991) illustrated and discussed errors that can occur in difficult cases in internal medicine and Graber et al. (2002) reviewed classes of error.

Because so much depends on the interaction between patient and clinician, prescriptive guidelines for the proper amount of hypothesis generation and testing are still unavailable for the student clinician and probably never will be. Perhaps the most useful advice is to emulate the hypothesis-testing strategy used by experienced clinicians when they are having difficulty.

Many diagnostic problems are so complex that the correct solution is not contained within the initial set of hypotheses. Restructuring and reformulating must occur through time as data are gradually obtained and the clinical picture evolves. Ideally, one would work purely inductively, reasoning only from the facts, but this strategy is never used because it is inefficient and produces high levels of cognitive strain (Elstein et al., 1978). It is much easier to solve a problem where some boundaries and hypotheses provide the needed framework. On the other hand, early problem formulation may also bias the clinician's thinking (Voytovich et al., 1985).

ERRORS IN DATA INTERPRETATION

Errors in interpreting the diagnostic value of clinical information have been found by several research

CASE STUDY 22.1
Screening Mammography

Screening mammography for breast cancer has an overall likelihood ratio of about 9 for a positive test: The odds of breast cancer are about nine times higher in a woman with a positive mammogram than a woman with a negative mammogram (Breast Cancer Surveillance Consortium, 2013). How likely is it that an average adult woman who gets a positive mammogram actually has breast cancer? What if she is younger than 40 years of age? A Bayesian reasoner, considering a breast cancer probability of 0.1% (1 breast cancer per 1000 women, or 1: 999 odds), should conclude that a woman with a positive mammogram will have about a 1% post-test probability of breast cancer. In a woman younger than 40 years of age, however, not only is the pretest probability lower than average (closer to 0.005%, or 5 breast cancers per 100,000 women), but the likelihood ratio of a positive test is lower (closer to 5). As a result, a positive test in a young woman suggests a 0.02% probability of breast cancer. How accurate was your estimate of the posttest probability, the pretest probability and the strength of the test?

teams. The most common error in interpreting findings is overinterpretation: Data that should not support a particular hypothesis and that might even suggest that a new alternative be considered are interpreted as consistent with hypotheses already under consideration (Elstein et al., 1978; Kostopoulou et al., 2009; Kourtidis et al., 2022). The data best remembered are those that support the diagnoses arrived at (Arkes and Harkness, 1980). Where findings are distorted in recall, it is generally in the direction of making the facts more consistent with typical clinical pictures. These errors are thought to arise from an adaptive function: the need to keep problem representations simple enough to remain within the capacity of working memory. Alternatively, decision makers need to find or create an alternative that is sufficiently superior to its competitors, so that it can be defended from postdecisional challenges that may occur to the decision maker or are posed by others

(Svenson et al., 2009). Finally, according to theories of cognitive consistency, data interpretation errors may arise from an inherent need to avoid cognitive tension by forming coherent representations, where perceptions, beliefs, attitudes and feelings are all consonant with each other (Simon et al., 2004).

Data interpretation errors occur not only postdiagnosis but also while clinical data are being evaluated and before a final diagnosis is given. This 'predecisional information distortion' is driven by certainty about the initial hypothesis and can lead to persistence with that hypothesis even in the absence of good evidence (Kostopoulou et al., 2012). In a series of online vignette-based experiments, Kourtidis et al. (2022) found that certainty about the initial diagnosis predicted the likelihood of diagnostic change and determined all aspects of the reasoning process. When confidence about the initial diagnosis was high, it was followed by less extensive information search, more biased evaluations of neutral information (i.e. they were perceived as supportive of the initial diagnosis), fewer diagnostic changes and fewer diagnostic alternatives offered. Suggesting diagnostic alternatives to physicians after they had given an initial diagnosis had no statistically significant impact on the process.

ERRORS IN PROBABILITY ESTIMATION

Many errors in probability revision result from reasoning tendencies, known as cognitive heuristics, which rely on the most salient and easily accessible information. These simple heuristics provide good estimates in most contexts but may yield systematic biases in others. For example, people are prone to overestimate the frequency of vivid or easily recalled events and to underestimate the frequency of events that are either very ordinary or difficult to recall (Tversky and Kahneman, 1981). As a result of this 'availability heuristic', clinicians may pursue investigations for rare but memorable diseases or injuries and may overlook more common explanations for the patient's symptoms. Memorability can be influenced by factors unrelated to probability, for example, high emotion (a missed diagnosis that led to patient death), novelty (an unusual presentation or disease), personal experience (it happened to me, to my family, to a friend, to

a colleague), recency (a patient I saw yesterday) or a good story (patient surviving against all odds).

People also overestimate the frequency of events that fit their ideas of a prototypical or representative case (Tversky and Kahneman, 1974). When this 'representativeness heuristic' comes into play, the probability of a disease, given a finding (also known as the 'positive predictive value' of a finding), can be confused with the probability of a finding, given the disease (i.e. the 'sensitivity' of the finding).

Small probabilities tend to be overestimated and large probabilities tend to be underestimated (Tversky and Kahneman, 1981). Cumulative prospect theory (Tversky and Kahneman, 1992) and similar theories provide formal descriptions of how people distort probabilities in risky decision making. The distortions are exacerbated when the probabilities are vague and not precisely known (Einhorn and Hogarth, 1986). Recent work in the science of emotion has also highlighted ways in which task-engendered emotions influence the estimation of probabilities and many other kinds of judgements (Lerner et al., 2015) (Box 22.1).

ERRORS IN PROBABILITY REVISION

Base-Rate Neglect

The basic principle of Bayesian inference is that a posterior probability is a function of two variables, the prior probability and the strength of the evidence. Some studies have found that, unless trained to use Bayes' theorem and to recognize when it is appropriate, physicians are just as prone as anyone else to misusing or neglecting base rates in diagnostic inference (Elstein, 1988). Other studies, however, have failed to find evidence of base-rate neglect (Gill et al., 2005). In

---

BOX 22.1
SOME COMMON BIASES IN ESTIMATING PROBABILITY

- Overestimating probability of easily recalled events
- Overestimating probability of events that fit a perceived pattern
- Overestimating small probabilities
- Underestimating large probabilities
- Overconfidence in probability estimates

fact, in some clinical disciplines, such as general practice (family medicine), physicians are particularly sensitive to base-rate information (Sirota et al., 2017).

Conservatism

In clinical case discussions, data are commonly presented sequentially. In this circumstance, people often fail to revise their diagnostic probabilities as much as they should, according to Bayes' theorem. This 'stickiness' has been called *conservatism* and was one of the earliest cognitive biases identified (Edwards, 1968). A heuristic explanation of conservatism is that people revise their diagnostic opinion up or down from an initial anchor, which is either given in the problem or subjectively formed. Final opinions are sensitive to the anchor and the adjustment up or down from this anchor is typically insufficient; therefore the final judgement is closer to the initial anchor than Bayes' theorem would require (Tversky and Kahneman, 1974).

The effect of conservatism is compounded when, in collecting data, there is a tendency to seek information that confirms the current hypothesis rather than data that facilitate efficient testing of competing hypotheses. This tendency has been called 'pseudodiagnosticity' (Kern and Doherty, 1982) or 'confirmation bias'. Information-processing approaches to studying decision making explain conservatism and confirmation bias in terms of how and in what order information is sampled from memory and the environment (Oppenheimer and Kelso, 2015).

CONFOUNDING PROBABILITY AND VALUE OF AN OUTCOME

Events deemed more serious may also be perceived as more likely, even when they are not, and may determine diagnosis and action. Probability revision errors that are systematically linked to the perceived cost of mistakes demonstrate the difficulties experienced in separating assessments of probability from preferences or values (Poses et al., 1985), a phenomenon also known as 'value-induced bias': events deemed more serious may also be perceived as more likely and determine diagnosis and action. Signal detection theory allows us to disentangle a decision maker's 'discrimination' (index d'), i.e. the ability to discriminate between positive and negative cases, such as cancer from no

cancer, from the decision maker's 'criterion' (index c), or threshold for action, which depends on trade-offs between the perceived costs and benefits of the different action outcomes, such as missing cancer versus diagnosing cancer in a healthy patient. Kostopoulou et al. (2019; 2020) used signal detection methodology to measure the discrimination and criterion of family physicians when dealing with patients who may need to be referred for cancer investigations. They found that, unlike discrimination, criterion seemed to be a stable characteristic of the physicians' referral decision making.

Order Effects

Given identical information, clinicians should reach the same diagnostic opinion, regardless of the order in which information is presented. Order effects mean that final opinions are also affected by the order of presentation of information. Some studies have found primacy effects in diagnostic judgements (e.g. Nurek et al., 2014) and others have found recency effects (Bergus et al., 1998). In other words, the information presented early in a case may be given more weight than information presented later (a primacy effect). A recency effect is said to occur when more weight is given to information presented later. Inconsistencies in the study results most likely stem from the different research methodologies and structure of the clinical cases used. This, nevertheless, does not invalidate the general finding that order of information matters (Box 22.2).

EDUCATIONAL IMPLICATIONS

What can be done to help learners acquire expertise in clinical reasoning? Particularly in light of the two-system theory of cognition, we endorse the multiple reasoning strategies position espoused by Norman and Eva (2010) and seek to identify educational implications from both intuitive and analytical models in problem solving and decision making.

PROBLEM SOLVING: EDUCATIONAL IMPLICATIONS

Even if experts in non problematic situations do not routinely generate and test hypotheses and instead retrieve a solution (diagnosis) directly from their structured knowledge, they clearly do generate and evaluate alternatives when confronted with problematic situations. For novices, most situations will initially be problematic and generating a small set of hypotheses is a useful procedural guideline. Because much expert hypothesis generation and testing are implicit, a model that calls it to the novice's attention will aid learning. The hypothetico-deductive model directs learners towards forming a conception of the problem and using this plan to guide the workup. This plan will include a set of competing diagnoses and the semantic relationships that facilitate separating between similar and different diagnostic candidates. This makes it possible to reduce unnecessary and expensive laboratory testing, a welcome emphasis in an era that stresses cost containment.

Clinical experience is needed in contexts closely related to future practice because transfer from one context to another is limited. In one way, this phenomenon reinforces a very traditional doctrine in medical education: Practical arts are learned by supervised practice and rehearsal supplemented by didactic instruction. In another way, it conflicts with traditional training, because the model implies that trainees will not generalize as much from one context (say, hospitalized patients) to another (say, ambulatory patients) as has traditionally been thought.

For reasoners to generalize from specific exemplars to more abstract patterns, clinical experience must be reviewed and analysed so that the correct general models and principles are abstracted from the experience. Given the emerging consensus about characteristics distinguishing experts from novices, an effective

route to the goal would be extensive, focussed practice and feedback with a variety of problems (Eshach and Bitterman, 2003).

DECISION MAKING: EDUCATIONAL IMPLICATIONS

Evidence-Based Medicine

EBM is particularly relevant for the diagnostic inference process discussed in this chapter because it is currently the most popular vehicle explicitly advocating a Bayesian approach to clinical evidence. Textbooks on EBM (e.g. Strauss et al., 2010) show how to use prevalence rates and likelihood ratios to calculate posterior probabilities of diagnostic alternatives (predictive value of a positive or negative test) and at least one recent study suggests that prevalence data may be readily available in the medical literature for inpatient adult medicine problems (Richardson et al., 2003). Formal statistical reasoning and decision analysis are likewise explained and advocated in an ever-growing number of works aimed at physicians (Kassirer and Kopelman, 1991; Lee, 2004; Mark, 2006; Sox et al., 1988). Decision theory, decision analysis and EBM seem to be on their way to becoming standard components of clinical education and training.

Decision Support Systems

Computer programs that run on microcomputers or in conjunction with electronic health records and can provide decision support have been developed. The role of these programs in medical education and in future clinical practice is still to be determined, but they hold out hope for addressing both cognitive and systemic sources of diagnostic error (Graber et al., 2002; Kostopoulou et al., 2017). Recent research finds that physicians are willing and able to adjust their risk estimates of cancer and subsequent referral decisions in response to a cancer risk algorithm when dealing with online patient vignettes even when their initial estimates are very different from the algorithm's (Palfi et al., 2022). Nevertheless, the evidence for the application and effectiveness of such electronic tools in clinical practice is discouraging (Medina-Lara et al., 2020; Price et al., 2019). A recent meta-review of systematic reviews of computer decision support systems found four significant challenges that remain for such systems to become more useful to physicians: improvement in knowledge representation, ability to update the system's knowledge to match advances in medicine, stronger interoperability with electronic health records, and better matching of decision support tools with clinicians' cognitive workflow (Nurek et al., 2015).

Debiasing

A number of researchers have proposed methods for debiasing judgements without resorting to formal methods of probability estimation and revision (Morewedge et al., 2015; Mumma and Wilson, 1995). General debiasing methods include educating decision makers about common biases, encouraging them to consider information that is likely to be underweighted or overlooked, e.g. consider alternative hypotheses, consider the opposite and so on, and making decision makers more accountable for their decisions. Evidence for the effectiveness of debiasing strategies for diagnostic reasoning is mixed (Graber, 2003). A recent systematic review by Lambe et al. (2016) found two interventions to be the most promising in reducing bias and improving diagnostic accuracy: (1) asking clinicians explicitly to consider alternative diagnoses and (2) guided reflection, i.e. using a structured process to reflect and reason. Guided reflection tended to improve diagnostic judgement relative to using intuition, particularly in complex cases. However, a more recent study by Lambe et al. (2018) found no evidence that guided reflection improves the diagnostic accuracy of advanced medical students, possibly because they already use some form of analytical reasoning.

REFLECTION POINT

To reduce the chances of missing a diagnosis, 'consider the opposite': Think actively of other diagnostic alternatives. Consider case findings that do not support your current hypothesis or that also support other hypotheses.

Embracing System 1

Not all educators and researchers agree that intuition must result in biased diagnosis or that it is inferior to analytical reasoning; some argue that intuition is an invaluable part of decision making, which should nei-

ther be ignored nor exclusively relied upon but tested by further analytical reasoning (Friedemann Smith and Nicholson, 2022). This 'gut feeling' is produced not by 'first impressions' but rather detection of conflict with the current hypothesis and irregularities in the way patients present (Woolley and Kostopoulou, 2013).

Some researchers have sought to demonstrate the conditions under which System 1 judgements can be better than System 2 judgements and under which conditions intuition can be further improved. In their review of heuristics in decision making, Gigerenzer and Gaissmaier (2011) identify fast-and-frugal trees as a valuable System 1 process that has received attention in diagnostic reasoning, both as a descriptive model of how physicians actually make diagnostic judgements and as a prescriptive approach to diagnosis that can outperform more complex, statistical clinical scoring rules, while being easier to apply. Research on fuzzy trace theory distinguishes between verbatim (System 2) and gist (System 1) encoding, retrieval and reasoning; research using the theory has demonstrated that reasoning from gist can lead to better decision making than reasoning from verbatim representations of the same problem. For a review, see Blalock and Reyna (2016).

Norman and Eva (2010) reviewed studies in diagnostic reasoning in which both experts and novices performed better and made fewer errors when explicitly instructed to use their experience (rather than analytical reasoning). The authors concluded that medical education should encourage both System 1 and System 2 judgement.

SUMMARY

- Research on the clinical reasoning of physicians has examined differences between expert and novice clinicians, psychological processes in judgement and decision making, factors associated with non-normative biases in judgement, improving instruction and training to enhance acquisition of good reasoning and the development, evaluation and implementation of decision support systems and guidelines.
- Concerns about diagnostic error have become a motivating force in the study of clinical reasoning

in medicine. Research in this area stands at the intersection of the interests of psychologists, medical sociologists, health policy planners, economists, patients and clinicians.

■ The prevailing view of two parallel and interacting cognitive systems, one fast and intuitive, the other slow and deliberative, has led to increased focus on how to study and improve each system and its interaction.

REFERENCES

Arkes, H.R., Harkness, A.R., 1980. Effect of making a diagnosis on subsequent recognition of symptoms. J Exp Psychol Hum Learn 6 (5), 568–575. https://www.ncbi.nlm.nih.gov/pubmed/6448908

Ball, J. R., Miller, B. T., Balogh, E. P., 2015. Improving Diagnosis in Health Care, 1st ed. National Academies Press. https://doi.org/10.17226/21794

Bergus, G. R., Chapman, G. B., Levy, B. T., Ely, J. W., Oppliger, R. A., 1998. Clinical diagnosis and the order of information. Medical Decision Making 18 (4), 412–417. https://doi.org/10.1177/02729 89X9801800409

Blalock, S.J., Reyna, V.F., 2016. Using fuzzy-trace theory to understand and improve health judgments, decisions, and behaviors: A literature review. Health Psychol 35 (8), 781–792. https://doi.org/10.1037/hea0000384

Bordage, G., 1994. Elaborated knowledge: A key to successful diagnostic thinking. Acad Med 69 (11), 883–885. https://doi.org/10.1097/00001888-199411000-00004

Breast Cancer Surveillance Consortium 2013. Performance measures for 1,838,372 screening mammography examinations from 2004 to 2008 by age—based on BCSC data through 2009. National Cancer Institute., USA.

De Neys, W., Glumicic, T., 2008, Mar. Conflict monitoring in dual process theories of thinking. Cognition 106 (3), 1248–1299. https://doi.org/10.1016/j.cognition.2007.06.002

Edwards, W., 1968. Conservatism in human information processing. In: Kleinmuntz, B. (Ed.), Formal representation of human judgement. Wiley, pp. 17–52.

Einhorn, H.J., Hogarth, R.M., 1986. Decision making under ambiguity. Journal of Business, S225–S250.

Elstein, Arthur S., 1988. Cognitive processes in clinical inference and decision making. In: Turk, D.C., Salovey, P. (Eds.), Reasoning, Inference and judgment in clinical psychology. New York, NY, Free Press, pp. 17–50.

Elstein, A.S., 1994. What goes around comes around: Return of the hypothetico-deductive strategy. Teaching and Learning in Medicine: An International Journal 6 (2), 121–123.

Elstein, A.S., 2009. Thinking about diagnostic thinking: A 30-year perspective. Adv Health Sci Educ Theory Pract 14 (Suppl 1), 7–18. https://doi.org/10.1007/s10459-009-9184-0

Elstein, A.S., Kleinmuntz, B., Rabinowitz, M., McAuley, R., Murakami, J., Heckerling, P.S., et al., 1993. Diagnostic reasoning of high- and low-domain-knowledge clinicians: A reanalysis.

Med Decis Making 13 (1), 21–29. https://doi.org/10.1177/02729 89X9301300104

Elstein, A.S., Shulman, L.S., Sprafka, S.A., 1978. Medical problem solving: An analysis of clinical reasoning. Harvard University Press.

Eshach, H., Bitterman, H., 2003. From case-based reasoning to problem-based learning. Acad Med 78 (5), 491–496. https://doi.org/10.1097/00001888-200305000-00011

Eva, K.W., Neville, A.J., Norman, G.R., 1998. Exploring the etiology of content specificity: Factors influencing analogic transfer and problem solving. Acad Med 73 (10 Suppl), S1–5. https://doi.org/10.1097/00001888-199810000-00028

Fagan, T.J., 1975. Letter: Nomogram for Bayes theorem. N Engl J Med 293 (5), 257. https://doi.org/10.1056/NEJM197507312930513

Friedemann Smith, C., Nicholson, B.D., 2022. Creating space for gut feelings in the diagnosis of cancer in primary care. Br J Gen Pract 72 (718), 210–211. https://doi.org/10.3399/bjgp22X719249

Gandhi, T.K., Kachalia, A., Thomas, E.J., Puopolo, A.L., Yoon, C., Brennan, T.A., et al., 2006. Missed and delayed diagnoses in the ambulatory setting: A study of closed malpractice claims. Ann Intern Med 145 (7), 488–496. https://doi.org/10.7326/0003-4819-145-7-200610030-00006

Gigerenzer, G., Gaissmaier, W., 2011. Heuristic decision making. Annu Rev Psychol 62, 451–482. https://doi.org/10.1146/annurev-psych-120709-145346

Gill, C.J., Sabin, L., Schmid, C.H., 2005. Why clinicians are natural Bayesians. BMJ 330 (7499), 1080–1083. https://doi.org/10.1136/bmj.330.7499.1080

Graber, M., 2003. Metacognitive training to reduce diagnostic errors: Ready for prime time? Acad Med 78 (8), 781. https://doi.org/10.1097/00001888-200308000-00004

Graber, M., Gordon, R., Franklin, N., 2002. Reducing diagnostic errors in medicine: What's the goal? Acad Med 77 (10), 981–992. https://doi.org/10.1097/00001888-200210000-00009

Graber, M.L., 2013. The incidence of diagnostic error in medicine. BMJ Qual Saf 22 (Suppl 2), ii21–ii27. https://doi.org/10.1136/bmjqs-2012-001615

Groen, G.J., Patel, V.L., 1985. Medical problem-solving: Some questionable assumptions. Med Educ 19 (2), 95–100. https://doi.org/10.1111/j.1365-2923.1985.tb01148.x

Groves, M., O'Rourke, P., Alexander, H., 2003. The clinical reasoning characteristics of diagnostic experts. Med Teach 25 (3), 308–313. https://doi.org/10.1080/0142159031000100427

Kahneman, Daniel, 2011. Thinking, fast and slow. Farrar, Strauss and Giroux. New York.

Kahneman, D., 2002. Maps of bounded rationality: A perspective on intuitive judgement and choice. In: Frangsmyr, Y. (Ed.), Les Prix Nobel: The Nobel Prizes 2002. Almqvist & Wiksell International, pp. 416–499.

Kahneman, D., 2003. Maps of bounded rationality: A perspective on intuitive judgement and choice. In: Frangsmyr, T. (Ed.), Les Prix Nobel: The Nobel Prizes 2002. Almqvist & Wiksell International.

Kahneman, D., Slovic, P., Tversky, A., 1982. Judgement under uncertainty: Heuristics and biases. Cambridge University Press.

Kassirer, J.P., Kopelman, R.I., 1991. Learning clinical reasoning. Williams & Wilkins.

Kern, L., Doherty, M.E., 1982. Pseudodiagnosticity' in an idealized medical problem-solving environment. J Med Educ 57 (2), 100–104. https://doi.org/10.1097/00001888-198202000-00004

Kostopoulou, O., Mousoulis, C., Delaney, B., 2009. Information search and information distortion in the diagnosis of an ambiguous presentation. Judgment and Decision Making 4 (5), 408–419.

Kostopoulou, O., Oudhoff, J., Nath, R., Delaney, B.C., Munro, C.W., Harries, C., et al., 2008. Predictors of diagnostic accuracy and safe management in difficult diagnostic problems in family medicine. Med Decis Making 28 (5), 668–680. https://doi.org/10.1177/0272989X08319958

Kostopoulou, O., Porat, T., Corrigan, D., Mahmoud, S., Delaney, B.C., 2017. Diagnostic accuracy of GPs when using an early-intervention decision support system: A high-fidelity simulation. Br J Gen Pract 67 (656), e201–e208. https://doi.org/10.3399/bjgp16X688417

Kostopoulou, O., Russo, J.E., Keenan, G., Delaney, B.C., Douiri, A., 2012. Information distortion in physicians' diagnostic judgments. Med Decis Making 32 (6), 831–839. https://doi.org/10.1177/0272989X12447241

Kourtidis, P., Nurek, M., Delaney, B., Kostopoulou, O., 2022. Influences of early diagnostic suggestions on clinical reasoning. Cogn Res Princ Implic 7 (1), 103. https://doi.org/10.1186/s41235-022-00453-y

Kuipers, B., Kassirer, J.P., 1984. Causal reasoning in medicine: Analysis of a protocol. Cognitive Science 8 (4), 363–385.

Kuipers, B., Moskowitz, A.J., Kassirer, J.P., 1988. Critical decisions under uncertainty: Representation and structure. Cognitive Science 12 (2), 177–210.

Lambe, K.A., Hevey, D., Kelly, B.D., 2018. Guided reflection interventions show no effect on diagnostic accuracy in medical students. Front Psychol 9, 2297. https://doi.org/10.3389/fpsyg.2018.02297

Lambe, K.A., O'Reilly, G., Kelly, B.D., Curristan, S., 2016. Dual-process cognitive interventions to enhance diagnostic reasoning: A systematic review. BMJ Qual Saf 25 (10), 808–820. https://doi.org/10.1136/bmjqs-2015-004417

Lee, T.H., 2004. Interpretation of data for clinical decisions. In: Goldman, L., Ausiello, D. (Eds.), Cecil textbook of medicine, 22nd ed. Saunders, pp. 23–28.

Lerner, J.S., Li, Y., Valdesolo, P., Kassam, K.S., 2015. Emotion and decision making. Annu Rev Psychol 66, 799–823. https://doi.org/10.1146/annurev-psych-010213-115043

Mamede, S., Schmidt, H.G., Rikers, R.M., Penaforte, J.C., Coelho-Filho, J.M., 2008. Influence of perceived difficulty of cases on physicians' diagnostic reasoning. Acad Med 83 (12), 1210–1216. https://doi.org/10.1097/ACM.0b013e31818c71d7

Mark, D.B., 2006. Decision-making in clinical medicine. In: Fauci, A.S., Braunwald, E., Kasper, D.L., Hauser, S.L., Longo, D.L., Jameson, J.L., Loscalzo, J. (Eds.), Harrison's principles of internal medicine, 17th ed. McGraw-Hill, pp. 16–23.

Medina-Lara, A., Grigore, B., Lewis, R., Peters, J., Price, S., Landa, P., et al., 2020. Cancer diagnostic tools to aid decision-making in primary care: Mixed-methods systematic reviews and cost-effectiveness analysis. Health Technol Assess 24 (66), 1–332. https://doi.org/10.3310/hta24660

Morewedge, C.K., Yoon, H., Scopelliti, I., Symborski, C.W., Korris, J.H., Kassam, K.S., 2015. Debiasing decisions. Policy Insights From the Behavioral and Brain Sciences 2 (1), 129–140. https://doi.org/10.1177/2372732215600886

Mumma, G.H., Wilson, S.B., 1995. Procedural debiasing of primacy/anchoring effects in clinical-like judgments. J Clin Psychol, 51 (6), 841–853. https://doi.org/10.1002/1097-4679(199511)51:6<841::aid-jclp2270510617>3.0.co;2-k

Nendaz, M.R., Gut, A.M., Perrier, A., Louis-Simonet, M., Reuille, O., Junod, A.F., et al., 2005. Common strategies in clinical data collection displayed by experienced clinician-teachers in internal medicine. Med Teach 27 (5), 415–421. https://doi.org/10.1080/01421590500084818

Norman, G., 2005. Research in clinical reasoning: Past history and current trends. Med Educ 39 (4), 418–427. https://doi.org/10.1111/j.1365-2929.2005.02127.x

Norman, G.R., Eva, K.W., 2010. Diagnostic error and clinical reasoning. Med Educ 44 (1), 94–100. https://doi.org/10.1111/j.1365-2923.2009.03507.x

Norman, G.R., Trott, A.D., Brooks, L.R., Smith, E.K.M., 1994. Cognitive differences in clinical reasoning related to postgraduate training. Teaching and Learning in Medicine: An International Journal 6 (2), 114–120.

Nurek, M., Kostopoulou, O., Delaney, B.C., Esmail, A., 2015. Reducing diagnostic errors in primary care. A systematic meta-review of computerized diagnostic decision support systems by the LINNEAUS collaboration on patient safety in primary care. Eur J Gen Pract 21 Suppl (sup1), 8–13. https://doi.org/10.3109/13814788.2015.1043123

Nurek, M., Kostopoulou, O., Hagmayer, Y., 2014. Predecisional information distortion in physicians' diagnostic judgments: Strengthening a leading hypothesis or weakening its competitor? Judgment and Decision Making 9 (6), 572–585.

Oppenheimer, D.M., Kelso, E., 2015. Information processing as a paradigm for decision making. Annu Rev Psychol 66, 277–294. https://doi.org/10.1146/annurev-psych-010814-015148

Palfi, B., Arora, K., Kostopoulou, O., 2022. Algorithm-based advice taking and clinical judgement: Impact of advice distance and algorithm information. Cogn Res Princ Implic 7 (1), 70. https://doi.org/10.1186/s41235-022-00421-6

Poses, R.M., Cebul, R.D., Collins, M., Fager, S.S., 1985. The accuracy of experienced physicians' probability estimates for patients with sore throats. Implications for decision making. JAMA 254 (7), 925–929. https://www.ncbi.nlm.nih.gov/pubmed/3894705

Price, S., Spencer, A., Medina-Lara, A., Hamilton, W., 2019. Availability and use of cancer decision-support tools: A cross-sectional survey of UK primary care. Br J Gen Pract 69 (684), e437–e443. https://doi.org/10.3399/bjgp19X703745

Richardson, W.S., Polashenski, W.A., Robbins, B.W., 2003. Could our pretest probabilities become evidence based? A prospective survey of hospital practice. J Gen Intern Med 18 (3), 203–208. https://doi.org/10.1046/j.1525-1497.2003.20215.x

Rusou, Z., Zakay, D., Usher, M., 2013. Pitting intuitive and analytical thinking against each other: The case of transitivity. Psychon Bull Rev 20 (3), 608–614. https://doi.org/10.3758/s13423-013-0382-7

Schwartz, A. (2002). *Nomogram for Bayes' theorem*. Retrieved 27 July 2023 from http://araw.mede.uic.edu/cgi-bin/testcalc.pl

Schwartz, A., Bergus, G.R., 2008. Medical decision making: A physician's guide. University Press, Cambridge.

Schwartz, A., Weiner, S.J., Binns-Calvey, A., Weaver, F.M., 2016. Providers contextualise care more often when they discover patient context by asking: Meta-analysis of three primary data sets. BMJ Qual Saf 25 (3), 159–163. https://doi.org/10.1136/bmjqs-2015-004283

Silk, N., 2000. What went wrong in 1,000 negligence claims. Health Care Risk Report 7, 13–15.

Simon, D., Snow, C.J., Read, S.J., 2004. The redux of cognitive consistency theories: Evidence judgments by constraint satisfaction. J Pers Soc Psychol 86 (6), 814–837. https://doi.org/10.1037/0022-3514.86.6.814

Singh, H., Meyer, A.N., Thomas, E.J., 2014. The frequency of diagnostic errors in outpatient care: Estimations from three large observational studies involving US adult populations. BMJ Qual Saf 23 (9), 727–731. https://doi.org/10.1136/bmjqs-2013-002627

Singh, H., Thomas, E.J., Khan, M.M., Petersen, L.A., 2007. Identifying diagnostic errors in primary care using an electronic screening algorithm. Arch Intern Med 167 (3), 302–308. https://doi.org/10.1001/archinte.167.3.302

Sirota, M., Kostopoulou, O., Round, T., Samaranayaka, S., 2017. Prevalence and alternative explanations influence cancer diagnosis: An experimental study with physicians. Health Psychol 36 (5), 477–485. https://doi.org/10.1037/hea0000461

Sox, H.C., Blatt, M.A., Higgins, M.C., 1988. Medical decision making. Butterworth-Heinemann.

Stanovich, K.E., West, R.F., 2000. Individual differences in reasoning: Implications for the rationality debate? Behav Brain Sci 23 (5), 645–665; discussion 665–726. https://doi.org/10.1017/s0140525x00003435

Strauss, S.E., Glasziou, P., Richardson, W.S., 2010. *Evidence-based medicine: How to practice and teach it*, 4th ed. Churchill Livingstone.

Svenson, O., Salo, I., Lindholm, T., 2009. Post-decision consolidation and distortion of facts. Judgment and Decision Making 4 (5), 397–407.

Tversky, A., Kahneman, D., 1974. Judgment under uncertainty: Heuristics and biases. Science 185 (4157), 1124–1131. https://doi.org/10.1126/science.185.4157.1124

Tversky, A., Kahneman, D., 1981. The framing of decisions and the psychology of choice. Science 211 (4481), 453–458. https://doi.org/10.1126/science.7455683

Tversky, A., Kahneman, D., 1992. Advances in prospect theory: Cumulative representation of uncertainty. Journal of Risk and Uncertainty 5, 297–323.

Voytovich, A.E., Rippey, R.M., Suffredini, A., 1985. Premature conclusions in diagnostic reasoning. J Med Educ 60 (4), 302–307. https://doi.org/10.1097/00001888-198504000-00004

Weiner, S.J., Schwartz, A., Sharma, G., Binns-Calvey, A., Ashley, N., Kelly, B., et al., 2013. Patient-centered decision making and health care outcomes: An observational study. Ann Intern Med 158 (8), 573–579. https://doi.org/10.7326/0003-4819-158-8-201304160-00001

Weiner, S.J., Schwartz, A., Weaver, F., Goldberg, J., Yudkowsky, R., Sharma, G., et al., 2010. Contextual errors and failures in individualizing patient care: A multicenter study. Ann Intern Med 153 (2), 69–75. https://doi.org/10.7326/0003-4819-153-2-201007200-00002

Woolley, A., Kostopoulou, O., 2013. Clinical intuition in family medicine: More than first impressions. Ann Fam Med 11 (1), 60–66. https://doi.org/10.1370/afm.1433

23 CLINICAL REASONING IN NURSING

BARBARA J. RITTER ■ MICHAEL J. WITTE

CHAPTER OUTLINE

CHAPTER AIMS

This chapter aims:

- to discuss theoretical perspectives pertaining to clinical reasoning
- to review studies relevant to understanding nurses' clinical reasoning
- to explore errors in diagnostic reasoning, implications and recommendations
- to highlight educational strategies to promote clinical reasoning.

INTRODUCTION

Clinical reasoning represents the essence of nursing practice. It is intrinsic to all aspects of care provision and is critical to all forms of nursing education, research and practice. An understanding of nurses' clinical reasoning is important to nursing research because of the need for a rigorous basis to evaluate nursing practice and education and a need to develop and test theories of nurses' cognitive processes and reasoning skills. Research is also needed to describe and explain the relationship between nurses' reason-ing and patient outcomes in order to demonstrate the essential role that nursing plays in the healthcare delivery system.

Knowledge about clinical reasoning is important to nursing education because education and teaching that is based on inappropriate or irrelevant models of reasoning can not only lead to waste but also result in graduates who are ill prepared to reason well in practice. Clinical reasoning is important to nursing practice because patient care provision is becoming increasingly more complex and difficult, requiring sound reasoning skills to maintain patient stability, provide high-quality care with positive outcomes and avoid the costly, even deadly, mistakes that can occur from faulty reasoning and errors in decision making.

DEFINITION OF CLINICAL REASONING

The literature provides several definitions of nurses' clinical reasoning. Gordon (2019) saw nurses' reasoning as a form of clinical judgement that occurs in a series of stages: encountering the patient; gathering clinical information; formulating possible diagnostic hypotheses; searching for more information to confirm or reject these hypotheses; reaching a diagnostic decision; and determining actions. Ritter (1998) viewed clinical reasoning as a process involving inclusion of evidence to facilitate optimum patient outcomes. Therefore, nurses' clinical reasoning can be defined as the cognitive processes and strategies that nurses use to understand the significance of patient data, to identify and diagnose actual or potential patient problems, to make clinical decisions to assist in problem resolution, and to achieve positive patient outcomes. According to O'Neill et al. (2005), clinical decision making is a complex task geared towards the identification and management of patients' health needs that requires a knowledgeable practitioner combined with reliable information and a supportive environment. Using this rubric, with experience, nurses develop a method of reasoning that provides them with an 'intuitive grasp' of the whole clinical situation, without having to always rely on the step-by-step analytical approach of the nursing process. These authors advocated a nursing curriculum that would include activities that would foster students' skills in intuitive judgement.

THEORETICAL PERSPECTIVES

Several different theoretical perspectives have helped provide an understanding of clinical reasoning. In this chapter we focus on three perspectives that have proved to be particularly useful in nursing: information processing, decision analysis and hermeneutics.

Information Processing Theory

Information processing theory (IPT) was first described by Newell and Simon (1972) in their seminal work examining how individuals with a great deal of experience in a specific area (domain expertise) reasoned during a problem-solving task. A fundamental premise of IPT is that human reasoning consists of a relationship between an information processing system (the human problem solver) and a task environment (the context in which problem solving occurs). A postulate of this theory is that there are limits to the amount of information that one can process at any given time and that effective problem solving is the result of being able to adapt to these limitations.

Miller's (1956) earlier classic work had demonstrated that an individual's working, short-term memory (STM) can hold only 7 ± 2 symbols at a time. Newell and Simon (1972) showed that the capacity of STM could be greatly increased, however, by 'chunking' simple units into familiar patterns. Individuals with a great deal of knowledge and experience in a particular domain can more easily chunk information pertaining to that domain and can therefore make more efficient use of their STM during reasoning.

Another memory bank identified by Newell and Simon (1972) is long-term memory (LTM), which has a vast capacity for information storage. The theory proposes that information gained from knowledge and experience is stored throughout life in LTM and that it takes longer to access LTM information than the small amount of information temporarily stored in STM. According to this theory, the information stored in LTM may need to be accessed by associating it with related information, which helps explain why experts reason so well within their domain. Indeed, cognitive research has demonstrated that experts possess an organized body of domain-specific conceptual and procedural knowledge that can be easily accessed using reasoning strategies (heuristics) and specific reasoning processes that are gradually learned through academic learning and through clinical experience (Glaser and Chi, 1988; Joseph and Patel, 1990).

Decision Analysis Theory

Decision analysis theory (DAT) was introduced in medicine in the latter half of the 20th century as a method of solving difficult clinical problems. DAT methods include use of Bayes' theorem, decision trees, sensitivity analysis and utility analysis. Bayes' theorem involves the use of mathematical formulas, tabular techniques, nomograms and computer programs to determine the likelihood of meaning of given clinical data.

Several nursing studies have demonstrated the applicability of decision theory to nurses' decision making. In her classic study examining the relationship between the expected value (anticipated outcome) that nurses assign to each of their outcomes and their ranking of nursing actions, Grier (1976) demonstrated that nurses select actions that are consistent with their expected values, which seems to support the use of decision trees in some instances of nurses' reasoning and decision making. Lipman and Deatrick (1997) found that nurse practitioner students who used a decision tree made better decisions about diagnosis and treatment choices for both acute and chronic conditions. Lauri and Salantera (1995) studied decision-making models and the variables related to them. Findings were that the nature of nursing tasks and the context yielded the greatest difference in decision-making approach. Conflict and ambiguity significantly increase task complexity. Therefore, recommendations should consider task complexity during model design when developing decision models for use in nursing. Narayan et al. (2003) examined decision analysis as a tool to support an analytical pattern of reasoning; they found that decision analysis is especially valuable in difficult and complex situations where there are mutually exclusive options and there is time for deliberation. Simulated cases provide a way to weave clinical experiences into memory. In this way, the thought process of working through a simulated case becomes an episodic memory in the same way that a true patient encounter does, utilizing the steps of information gathering, information processing, data analysis and formulation of diagnoses. This involves using the various heuristics while promoting critical thinking, clinical reasoning, diagnostic reasoning, performance and outcomes and is inherently valuable in clinical situations, where timely decision-making is critical.

Hermeneutics

Hermeneutics is the art and study of interpretation. In nursing studies, hermeneutics, combined with phenomenology, has been used as a rigorous research approach for some years (e.g. Benner, 1994). The intention of studies into nurses' reasoning guided by this approach is to understand the clinical world of nurses and its meanings from their subjective perspective, in particular, their reasoning as they make decisions about patient care. Benner et al. (1992) used a hermeneutic phenomenological approach to study the development of expertise in critical care nursing practice. Their findings indicated that nurses at different levels of expertise 'live in different clinical worlds, noticing and responding to different directives for action' (Benner et al., 1992, p. 13). Findings from a later study by the same authors (Benner et al., 1996) indicate that this clinical world is shaped by experience that teaches nurses to make qualitative distinctions in practice. They also found that beginner nurses were more task oriented, while those with more experience focussed on understanding their patients and their illness states.

Studies of nurses' clinical judgement, intuition, problem solving and decision making, and diagnostic reasoning have contributed to the understanding of nurses' clinical reasoning.

Clinical Judgement Studies

Nurses' clinical judgement represents a composite of traits that assists them in reasoning (Tanner, 1987). Benner et al. (1992), in their hermeneutic phenomenological study, described characteristics of clinical judgement exhibited by critical care nurses with varying levels of practice experience when they reasoned about patient care. Characteristics of clinical judgement that were identified in the most experienced subjects included:

1. The ability to recognize patterns in clinical situations that fit with patterns they had seen in other similar clinical cases;
2. A sense of urgency related to predicting what lies ahead;
3. The ability to concentrate simultaneously on multiple, complex patient cues and patient management therapies; and
4. An aptitude for realistically assessing patient priorities and nursing responsibilities.

The characteristics of clinical judgement identified by Benner et al. (1996) assist in our understanding of nurses' clinical reasoning by identifying and describing some of the cognitive traits or skills that nurses use during reasoning. These insights help further the theoretical understanding of nurses' judgement that can be used by educators to teach their students to reason better. These insights also provide nurses in practice with knowledge that will help them to make better decisions about patient care.

Problem Solving and Decision-Making Studies

One of the primary objectives of clinical reasoning is to make decisions to resolve problems. Thus, research into nurses' problem solving and decision making should provide understanding about the processes involved in their clinical reasoning.

A number of researchers have investigated the complexity of nurses' decision-making tasks and situations and have identified a range of reasoning strategies, including hypothetico-deduction, intuition and pattern recognition. These studies have emphasized the importance of consultation with experienced colleagues in this learning process.

Intuition Studies

Several investigators have proposed that intuition is an important part of nurses' reasoning processes. A classic study that continues to guide nursing research on intuition was conducted by Pyles and Stern (1983) to explore the reasoning of a group of critical care nurses with varying levels of expertise. The investigators identified a 'gut feeling' experienced by the more seasoned nurse subjects, which they believed was as important to nurses' reasoning as their formal knowledge about patient cases. Subjects said they used these gut feelings to temper information from specific clinical cues; they also emphasized the importance of previous clinical experience in developing intuitive skills. Rew (1990) also demonstrated the important role that intuition played in nurses' reasoning and decision making. Subjects described their intuitive experiences as strong feelings or perceptions about their patients, as well as about themselves and how they responded to their patients. These perceptions also involved anticipated outcomes that they sensed without having to go through an analytical reasoning process.

Diagnostic Reasoning Studies

Ritter (2000) studied the combination of two models, information processing and hermeneutics (Fig. 23.1 and Box 23.1), to explain diagnostic reasoning. Although previous research related to clinical reasoning used either information processing or hermeneutical models, neither model alone fully describes all components of diagnostic reasoning. This study systematically examined nurse practitioners' (NPs) diagnostic reasoning using both models.

Findings suggest that both models operated among the 10 NPs who participated in this study. Furthermore, there is a relative blend of both models in practice. The NPs in this study used the information processing model 55% of the time and the hermeneutical model 45% of the time. Two categories, one information processing (gathering data) and one hermeneutical (skilled know-how), account for 57% of the themes.

Gathering data, by NPs, involves using their senses to purposefully collect specific meaningful information about a patient so that diagnostic meaning can be assigned to the information. The variables of gathering facts and generating the hypothesis (Fig. 23.1) were used most often. These findings are in alignment with previous research in that some aspects of information processing were used more than others. This study also emphasizes that the process of gathering data is important when generating a hypothesis. It is also important to guard against prematurely closing the diagnostic reasoning process before considering any viable alternative diagnosis.

Skilled know-how is independent of reliance on analytical thinking but rather involves processing numerous complex variables, simultaneously, in an unconscious, automatic, efficient manner. In the study, expert NPs demonstrated skilled know-how when they meticulously gathered, and skilfully acquired, the appropriate data to formulate a diagnosis. The NPs also had a very good sense of which data were appropriate.

The fact that NPs use a combination of both models is the most significant finding of this study. Expert nurse practitioners' diagnostic reasoning behaviours demonstrate how the individual components of the models overlap and blend into each other (Fig. 23.2).

Pirret (2016) compared nurse practitioners and physicians reasoning using DPT. Dual processing identifies diagnostic reasoning via intuitive (System I) and analytical (System II) processes. The degree to which each is used is dependent on the clinical situation.

System I processes rely on pattern recognition, are fast, intuitive, and are used when clinicians are involved in familiar case presentations. Intuition relies on past experiences, needs little mental effort and is sometimes described as a gut feeling. Pattern recognition can rely on a few pieces of critical information

Information processing model

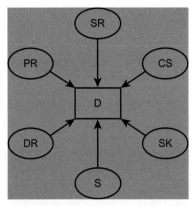

Gather facts Generate hypothesis Gather data Evaluate hypothesis   Diagnosis

Hermeneutical model

PR = pattern recognition; SR = similarity recognition; CS = common-sense understanding;
SK = skilled know-how; S = sense of salience; DR = deliberative rationality; D = diagnosis

Fig. 23.1 ■ Representation of the information processing and hermeneutical model components.

BOX 23.1

HERMENEUTICAL MODEL DEFINITION OF TERMS

- Commonsense understanding is a common understanding of diverse situations of life in general.
- Deliberative rationality is the ability to change one's interpretation of a situation by considering other alternatives.
- Pattern recognition is the ability to recognize relationships among cues.
- Sense of salience is understanding certain events to be more important than others.
- Skilled know-how is already having the knowledge and ability to do something well. It implies some independence from analytical thinking.
- Similarity recognition is the ability to recognize similarities with past experiences even if the current experience differs from the previous.

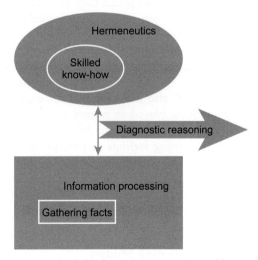

Fig. 23.2 ■ Blended information processing and hermeneutical model.

---

gained from the clinical context. There is often a rapid recognition that the patient's presentation resembles previous cases.

System I processes include cognitive shortcuts or rules of thumb, commonly termed heuristics, to reduce the cognitive load and to simplify the diagnostic reasoning process. These heuristics are based on experience, patient characteristics and the context in which the patient presents. Heuristics enable clinicians to reach a diagnosis quickly without resorting to the intensive System II processes of exploring all the possibilities, a so-called differential diagnosis.

If the patient presentation is not familiar or if the clinician is uncertain, the slower, logical and deliberate System II processes are used. System II thinking makes use of the hypothetico-deductive model. The hypothetico-deductive model is an approach which uses a combination of inductive and deductive reasoning to guide clinicians to the correct diagnoses. Novices can be helped in System II thinking by using Clinical Practice Guidelines as these can remind the novices of what needs to be considered.

Pirret (2016) used an intuitive/analytical reasoning instrument and maxims questionnaire to compare: (1) the diagnostic reasoning style of NPs and resident doctors and (2) the influence of diagnostic reasoning style on their abilities to deal with a complex case. The results showed NPs incorporated more System I (intuitive) processes when compared with residents; however, both groups made use of certain maxims. The use of System I or System II thinking was related to the diagnostic reasoning style of each individual. However, all participants used System II thinking when required.

Conclusions were that both NPs and resident doctors used intuition and hypothetico-deductive reasoning to aid in diagnosis. The NPs tended to use more System I nonanalytical reasoning than the residents. However, both NPs and resident doctors resort to analytical reasoning when dealing with a complex case. Both System I and II processes are prone to diagnostic error.

Errors in Clinical Reasoning

The Institute of Medicine (IOM) published a series of reports on quality and safety in healthcare. The reports, with their evidence-based focus, have increasingly been used to guide informed decisions for changes in professional practice that will improve the quality of healthcare and clinical outcomes. The first report in the series, 'To Err is Human: Building a Safer Health System' (2000), provided the groundwork for reform by drawing attention to the estimated 98,000 preventable deaths per year attributable to quality and safety deficits in the healthcare industry in the United States. This report was followed by 'Crossing the Quality Chasm: A New Health System for the 21st Century'

(2001), which concluded that 'care should be safe, effective, patient-centered, timely, efficient and equitable' (p. 39). A subsequent report, 'Health Professions Education: A Bridge to Quality' (2003), operationalized those characteristics by identifying specific competencies (see the immediate, following Reflection Point) that are essential to increasing safety and quality regardless of the healthcare discipline.

REFLECTION POINT

The IOM (2003) proposed core competencies that all health professionals, regardless of discipline, should demonstrate:

- the provision of patient-centred care,
- working in interprofessional teams,
- using evidence-based practice,
- applying quality improvement approaches and
- utilizing informatics.

To what extent does your local institution actively pursue and promote these competencies?

More than 12 years later, the IOM published another landmark study entitled 'Improving Diagnosis in Health Care' (2015). The report noted that most patients will eventually experience one or more diagnostic errors, such as delayed or simply inaccurate diagnoses. The report emphasized that far too little attention has been paid to diagnostic errors – an issue that will 'likely worsen' if it is not addressed. The IOM made a number of recommendations (see the following Reflection Point).

REFLECTION POINT

IOM recommendations:
1. Promote effective collaboration in the diagnostic process among clinicians.
2. Improve training for healthcare professionals so that it emphasizes communication, clinical reasoning and teamwork.
3. Place more emphasis on learning from diagnosis errors and close calls in clinical practice.

The IOM report (2015) also suggests that all electronic health records (EHRs) should align with clinical workflows, demonstrate usability, facilitate the flow of information among patients and providers, and provide clinical decision support (CDS). The IOM found that although getting the right diagnosis is a key quality indicator in healthcare, efforts to find ways to improve diagnosis and reduce diagnostic errors have been quite limited. Improving diagnosis is a complex challenge, partly because making a diagnosis is often a collaborative and inherently inexact process that may unfold over time and across different healthcare settings. To improve diagnosis and reduce errors, the IOM called for a payment and care delivery environment that supports the diagnostic process: more effective teamwork among healthcare professionals, patients and families; enhanced training for healthcare professionals; more emphasis on identifying and learning from diagnostic errors and near misses in clinical practice; and a dedicated focus on new research.

The committee also recommended that healthcare professional education and training emphasize clinical reasoning and teamwork. It urged better alignment of health information technology (IT) with the diagnostic process and said US federal agencies should develop a coordinated research approach. It is clearly critical that there is support for the development of sound data tools as a baseline for evaluating current practices in the diagnostic process and then to use these data to measure and compare outcomes accurately.

Decision Support

Diagnostic decision support tools can provide support to clinicians and patients throughout each stage of the diagnostic process. This would include information acquisition, information integration and interpretation, as well as the formation of a working diagnosis, and making a diagnosis (Del Fiol et al., 2008; Zakim et al., 2008). Tools such as info-buttons can be integrated into EHRs and provide direct links to relevant online information resources, such as medical textbooks, clinical practice guidelines and appropriateness criteria at the point of care (Del Fiol et al., 2008).

An important challenge is the development of an electronic workflow to standardize and improve communication. Making clinical and patient information available via computerized clinical decision support (CDS) puts important information in providers' hands at critical points in the diagnosis and treatment process. Information technology has improved clinicians'

ability to follow up on diagnostic tests in a timely fashion, which should reduce the incidence of delayed diagnoses and human error. CDS encompasses a variety of tools that enhance decision making in the clinical workflow. Clinicians can now access and use the scientific evidence base at the point of care into their decision-making processes.

Population and Clinical Reasoning

Clinical reasoning is a key component of efforts to improve healthcare that also emphasize population health. For example, in the United States, the Institute of Healthcare Improvement (IHI) has been promoting the triple aim (Berwick et al., 2008). These aims are:

- improving the patient experience of care (including quality and satisfaction)
- improving the health of populations
- reducing the per capita cost of healthcare.

Clinical reasoning clearly plays a role in the first aim of improving the patient experience of care. However, the other aims also affect clinical reasoning and are affected in turn by clinical reasoning. If healthcare professionals are aware of the characteristics of their local population, they can focus attention on these issues. For example, Shazhzad et al. (2019) discussed a study where primary care practices made the effort to identify low vitamin D levels in an immigrant community and designed health promotion activities together with screen-and-treat programmes that targeted these groups. Initiatives like this require collaboration between many stakeholders, government, providers, insurers, academia, employers and unions, the media, philanthropy, political leaders, community organizations and others. These initiatives can then also reduce the cost of delivering healthcare. Other initiatives related to decision-making include Healthy People 2030 (https://health.gov/healthypeople).

These initiatives emphasize the importance of shared decision making between patients and their healthcare providers. The new technology becoming available, such as the telehealth movement, helps this shared decision making and fundamentally changes the relationship between patients and providers towards interactions that support informed, directional conversations to improve health. Other Healthy People 2030 objectives that support telehealth include goals to deliver reliable and actionable health information, goals to connect with culturally diverse and hard-to-reach populations, and a goal to provide sound principles in the design of programmes and interventions that result in healthier behaviours.

The IOM reports point to improved communication, teamwork and collaboration as the best ways to improve our healthcare delivery system and outcomes (Fig. 23.3). For nearly a decade, Grumbach and Bodenheimer (2002) have acknowledged that these changes can promote patient-centred care with the *patient-centred medical home* and, using collaborative teams in promoting evidenced-based performance outcome, improving diagnostic reasoning and health outcomes. The *patient-centred medical home* is a model for the organization of primary care that delivers the core functions of primary healthcare: comprehensive care, patient-centred care, shared decision making, coordinated care, accessible services, quality and safety (AHRQ, 2017).

The AHRQ also recognizes the central role of health IT in successfully operationalizing and implementing the key features of the medical home. Health IT includes electronic medical records (EMR) with meaningful use outcome measures. Meaningful use outcomes of an EHR are defined as evolving through three stages. These are: data capture and sharing, advanced clinical process and improved outcomes. Additionally, AHRQ notes that creating accessible, affordable and high-quality primary care delivery platforms will require significant workforce development and fundamental payment reform inclusive of value-based pay-for-performance measures (AHRQ, 2017).

Educational Focus on Clinical Reasoning

Nurses increasingly need well-developed reasoning skills to assist them in understanding and resolving the complex patient problems encountered in practice.

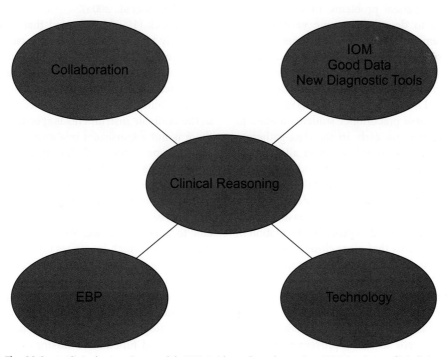

Fig. 23.3 ■ Clinical reasoning model. *EBP,* Evidence-based practice; *IOM,* Institute of Medicine.

Barrows and Pickell (1991, p. 3) remind us that 'ambiguities and conflicting or inadequate information are the rule in medicine'. This is equally true in nursing, where dealing with complex patient problems with uncertain and unpredictable outcomes requires continuous astute reasoning and accurate and efficient decision making. Thus, the ability to think critically is essential. Lee et al. (2006) emphasize the importance of both cognitive and metacognitive skills (thinking about one's thinking) in clinical reasoning to promote the use of self-regulated learning and facilitate the development of critical thinking and reflective practice abilities.

The cognitive skills that today's nursing students need to learn in order to reason accurately and make decisions effectively in practice have caused nurse educators to adjust their teaching methods. More creative teaching methods have been adopted that are designed to improve students' reasoning skills and furnish them with a repertoire of creative approaches to care. Much of the nursing education literature has begun to focus on ways to teach critical thinking (CT). Fonteyn and Cooper (1994) proposed using case studies to improve nursing students' reasoning skills by teaching them to identify potential patient problems, to suggest nursing actions and to describe outcome variables that would allow them to evaluate the effectiveness of their actions. Case studies provide the advantage of allowing nurse educators to give continuous feedback in the safe environment of simulation and to provide reality-based learning. Lipman and Deatrick (1997) found that beginning nurse practitioner students tended to formulate diagnoses too early in the data-gathering phase, thus precluding consideration of all diagnostic options. When they used a case study approach, incorporating algorithms to guide the decision-making process, students developed a broader focus and diagnostic accuracy improved. To increase realism, case studies can be designed to provide information in chronological segments that more closely reflect real-life cases, in which clinical events and outcomes evolve over time (Fonteyn, 1991). One well-known form of case study is problem-based learning (PBL).

PBL develops students' ability to reflect continuously on their reasoning and decision making during patient care and leads to self-improvement through practice. PBL significantly increases CT, clinical reasoning, problem solving and transfer of knowledge gained (Evenson and Hmelo, 2000). Once students have developed their reasoning skills in this manner, they can apply them while caring for real patients in the clinical setting. In practice, nurses first identify (from data initially obtained in report form and confirmed by patient assessment) the most important patient problems on which to focus during their nursing shift. Information from the patient, the family and other members of the healthcare team should be included in a plan of care that will assist in resolving the problems identified. As the shift progresses, nurses continuously evaluate and refine their plan of care based on additional data obtained from further patient assessment, additional clinical data and information from all individuals involved in carrying out the plan of care. PBL can simulate all of this.

Other methods that have been suggested by nurse educators to improve students' CT skills include clinical experience, conferences, computer simulations, clinical logs, collaboration, decision analysis, discussion, e-mail dialogue, patient simulations, portfolios, reflection, role modelling, role playing and writing position papers (Baker, 1996; Fonteyn and Cahill, 1998; O'Neill et al., 2005).

Videbeck (1997b) indicated that as well as being effectively taught, CT must be assessed in an appropriate manner. She pointed out that standardized paper-and-pencil tests are often selected as an evaluation measure because normative data are available and reliability has been established. However, none of the available instruments is specific to nursing and there is not a consistent relationship between scores on this type of test and clinical judgement. The use of faculty-developed instruments to assess student outcomes is strongly recommended. Course-specific measures, such as clinical performance criteria or written assignments, have the advantage of being specific to nursing practice. Videbeck (1997a) suggested that a model which integrates CT in all aspects of the programme (definition, course objectives and evaluation) be used.

In the future, educators must strive to devise additional methods to develop and improve nurses' clinical reasoning. Further changes will be required in the structure and function of nursing curricula. Students need to learn to improve the ways in which they identify significant clinical data and determine the meaning of data in regard to patient problems. They also need to learn how to reason about patient problems in ways that facilitate decisions about problem resolution.

Teaching strategies which promote clinical reasoning are those in which the educator designs classroom activities to engage the students. Students frequently need to reason their way critically through nursing principles, concepts and theories, so that accurate application and transfer of knowledge occurs in an integrated and intuitive way. Computer-assisted instruction can provide high-quality instruction that is intellectually challenging (Luge and Assal, 1992). Access to online videoconferencing, journals, websites, interactive programmes and distance learning hold rich promise for promoting creative and effective teaching environments (Fetterman, 1996). Many of the initiatives discussed come under the label of Health Systems Science, which is gaining a great deal of attention in healthcare and the education of health professionals. There is a need for research to explore how Health Systems Science and clinical reasoning affect each other (Gordon et al., 2022).

Practice

The ultimate goal of both research and educational endeavours related to clinical reasoning in nursing is to improve nurses' reasoning in practice and, ultimately, to achieve more positive patient outcomes. Nursing literature suggests that nurses' reasoning and interventions have a significant effect on patient outcome (Fowler, 1994). The relationship between nurses' reasoning and patient outcomes requires identification of the specific patient outcome indicators associated with nurses' reasoning and explication of the measurements of these indicators. If nursing is to continue to play a proactive role in healthcare provision, it is essential to identify the role that nurses' reasoning and decision making play in overall patient outcomes.

A major difficulty in demonstrating the influence of nurses' reasoning on patient outcomes is the complex nature of the outcomes. These outcomes span a broad range of effects or presumed effects that are influenced not only by nursing and other healthcare providers but by many other variables. These include time, environmental conditions, support systems and

patient history. Decision support systems and expert systems are currently being developed to assist nurses in practice to reason more efficiently and to make better clinical decisions. Expert system development began in research laboratories in the mid-1970s and was first implemented in commercial and practical endeavours in the early 1980s (Frenzel, 1987). Fonteyn and Grobe (1994) suggested that an 'expert system' could be designed to represent the knowledge and reasoning processes of experienced nurses and could then be used to assist less experienced nurses to improve their reasoning skills and strategies. Iliad is one such expert system case-based teaching programme, which was effective in improving nurse practitioner students' diagnostic abilities (Lange et al., 1997). Expert system shells (a computer system that emulates the decision-making ability of a human expert), coupled with a focus on the concise nursing problems encountered within a specific area of nursing practice and a common taxonomy, provide a means to expedite and facilitate the growth and development of such expert systems for use in nursing practice (Bowles, 1997). However, in more recent times, there has been a surge in the development of artificial intelligence (AI) systems. These AI systems are based on machine learning and have the potential to supersede the more traditional expert systems that are rule-based. This is because of increases in computer power and access to large volumes of data. These developments have provided modern AI systems the opportunities to learn on vast amounts of data and seek out correlations not obvious to human observers of that same data. There are major implications arising from using such AI systems in nursing that have yet to be explored. For example, it may be possible for such AI systems to assist nurses in their clinical reasoning. Göcke and Rosenthal-von der Putten (2020) discuss the implications of AI in more detail.

FUTURE DIRECTIONS IN PRACTICE RELATED TO NURSES' CLINICAL REASONING

The relationship between nurses' reasoning and patient outcomes should receive greater attention in future research to demonstrate the important role that nurses play in healthcare delivery. There will be an increasing need to develop meaningful data sets related to patient outcomes. These data sets should contain the actions that nurses commonly choose after reasoning about specific patient problems and intervention outcomes. Prior to the development of these data sets, the indicators of patient outcome that are related to nurses' reasoning and decision making need to be identified and described in a manner that facilitates their measurement. Computerized support systems, including AI, will play an ever-increasing role in assisting nurses to reason, to make decisions about appropriate nursing actions and to evaluate their impact on patient outcome. Recommendations proposed emphasize collaboration, communication, teamwork and decision support modalities as well as teaching strategies which promote critical thinking and clinical reasoning. Further studies are needed to evaluate the effect of these interventions on diagnostic error rates as well as improved population and individual health outcomes.

SUMMARY

Nurses increasingly need well-developed reasoning skills to assist them in understanding and resolving the complex patient problems encountered in practice. Barrows and Pickell (1991) remind us that 'ambiguities and conflicting or inadequate information are the rule in medicine' (p. 3). This is equally true in nursing, where dealing with complex patient problems with uncertain and unpredictable outcomes requires continuous astute reasoning and accurate and efficient decision making. Thus, the ability to think critically is essential. Lee et al. (2006) emphasize the importance of both cognitive and metacognitive skills in clinical reasoning and promote the use of self-regulated learning, learning that is guided by metacognition (thinking about one's thinking), to facilitate the development of critical thinking and reflective practice abilities.

REFERENCES

AHRQ, 2017, September 2020. The SHARE approach—achieving patient-centered care with shared decisionmaking: A brief for administrators and practice leaders. The Agency for Healthcare Research and Quality. https://www.ahrq.gov/health-literacy/professional-training/shared-decision/tool/resource-9.html

Baker, C.R., 1996. Reflective learning: A teaching strategy for critical thinking. J Nurs Educ 35 (1), 19–22. https://doi.org/10.3928/0148-4834-19960101-06

Barrows, H., Pickell, G. 1991. Developing clinical problem-solving skills: A guide to more effective diagnosis and treatment. Norton Medical Books.

Benner, P., 1994. Sage publications. Interpretive phenomenology: Embodiment, caring, and ethics in health and illness.

Benner, P., Tanner, C., Chesla, C., 1992. From beginner to expert: Gaining a differentiated clinical world in critical care nursing. ANS Adv Nurs Sci 14 (3), 13–28. https://doi.org/10.1097/00012272-199203000-00005

Benner, P., Tanner, C., Chesla, C. (Eds.), 1996. Expertise in nursing practice: Caring, clinical judgment, and ethics. Springer.

Berwick, D.M., Nolan, T.W., Whittington, J., 2008. The triple aim: Care, health, and cost. Health Aff (Millwood) 27 (3), 759–769. https://doi.org/10.1377/hlthaff.27.3.759

Bowles, K.H., 1997. The barriers and benefits of nursing information systems. Comput Nurs 15, 197–198.

Del Fiol, G., Haug, P.J., Cimino, J.C., Narus, SP., Norlin, C., Mitchell, JA., 2008. Effectiveness of topic-specific infobuttons: A randomized controlled trial. J Am Med Inform Assoc 15 (6), 752–759.

Evenson, D.H., Hmelo, C.E. (Eds.), 2000. Problem-based learning: A research perspective on learning interactions. Lawrence Erlbaum Associates.

Fetterman, D.M., 1996. Videoconferencing on-line: Enhancing communication over the Internet. Educational Researcher 25 (4), 23–27.

Fonteyn, M.E., 1991. A descriptive analysis of expert critical care nurses' clinical reasoning. Unpublished PhD thesis, The University of Texas, Austin.

Fonteyn, M.E., Cahill, M., 1998. The use of clinical logs to improve nursing students' metacognition: A pilot study. J Adv Nurs 28 (1), 149–154. https://doi.org/10.1046/j.1365-2648.1998.00777.x

Fonteyn, M.E., Cooper, L.F., 1994. The written nursing process: Is it still useful to nursing education? J Adv Nurs 19 (2), 315–319. https://doi.org/10.1111/j.1365-2648.1994.tb01086.x

Fonteyn, M.E., Grobe, S.J., 1994. Expert system development in nursing: Implications for critical care nursing practice. Heart Lung 23 (1), 80–87.

Fowler, L.P., 1994. Clinical reasoning of home health nurses: A verbal protocol analysis. Unpublished PhD thesis. University of South Carolina.

Frenzel, L.E., 1987. Understanding expert systems. Longman Higher Education.

Glaser, R., Chi, M.T.H., 1988. Overview. In: Chi M.T.H., Glaser R., Farr M.J. (Eds.), The nature of expertise. Lawrence Erlbaum, Hillsdale, NJ, xv–xxviii.

Göcke, B.P., Rosenthal-von der Pütten, A. (Eds.), 2020. Artificial intelligence: Reflections in philosophy, theology, and the social sciences. Brill Mentis, Boston MA.

Gordon, J., Ghilardi, M.F., Cooper, S.E., 2019. Accuracy of planar reaching movements. Exp Brain Res 99, 112–130. https://doi.org/10.1007/BF00241416

Gordon, D., Rencic, J.J., Lang, V.J., Thomas, A., Young, M., Durning, S.J., 2022. Advancing the assessment of clinical reasoning across the health professions: Definitional and methodologic recommendations. Perspect Med Educ 11 (2), 108–114. https://doi.org/10.1007/s40037-022-00701-3

Grier, M.R., 1976. Decision making about patient care. Nurs Res 25 (2), 105–110.

Grumbach, K., Bodenheimer, T., 2002. A primary care home for Americans: Putting the house in order. JAMA 288 (7), 889–893. https://doi.org/10.1001/jama.288.7.889

Institute of Medicine, 2000. To err is human: Building a safer health system. National Academies Press (US). https://doi.org/10.17226/9728

Institute of Medicine, 2001. Crossing the quality chasm: A new health system for the 21st century. National Academies Press (US). https://doi.org/10.17226/10027

Institute of Medicine, 2003. Health professions education: A bridge to quality. National Academies Press (US). https://doi.org/10.17226/10681

Institute of Medicine, 2015. Improving diagnosis in health care. National Academies Press (US). https://doi.org/10.17226/21794

Joseph, G.M., Patel, V.L., 1990. Domain knowledge and hypothesis generation in diagnostic reasoning. Med Decis Making 10 (1), 31–46

Lange, L.L., Haak, S.W., Lincoln, M.J., Thompson, C.B., Turner, C.W., Weir, C. et al., 1997. Use of Iliad to improve diagnostic performance of nurse practitioner students. J Nurs Educ 36 (1), 36–45.

Lauri, S., Salanterä, S., 1995. Decision-making models of Finnish nurses and public health nurses. J Adv Nurs 21 (3), 520–527. https://doi.org/10.1111/j.1365-2648.1995.tb02736.x

Lee, J., Chan, A.C., Phillips, D.R., 2006. Diagnostic practise in nursing: A critical review of the literature. Nurs Health Sci 8 (1), 57–65. https://doi.org/10.1111/j.1442-2018.2006.00267.x

Lipman, T.H., Deatrick, J.A., 1997. Preparing advanced practice nurses for clinical decision making in specialty practice. Nurse Educ 22 (2), 47–50. https://doi.org/10.1097/00006223-199703000-00018

Luge, C.F., Assal, J.P., 1992. Designing computer assisted instruction programs for diabetic patients: How can we make them really useful? Proc Annu Symp Comput Appl Med Care, 215–219.

Miller, G.A., 1956. The magical number seven, plus or minus two: Some limits on our capacity for processing information. Psychol Rev 101 (2), 343–352. https://doi.org/10.1037/0033-295x.101.2.343

Narayan, S.M., Corcoran-Perry, S., Drew, D., Hoyman, K., Lewis, M., 2003. Decision analysis as a tool to support an analytical pattern-of-reasoning. Nurs Health Sci 5 (3), 229–243. https://doi.org/10.1046/j.1442-2018.2003.00157.x

Newell, A., Simon, H.A., 1972. Human problem solving. Prentice-Hall.

O'Neill, E., Dluhy, N.M., Chin, E., 2005. Modelling novice clinical reasoning for a computerized decision support system. J Adv Nurs 49 (1), 68–77. https://doi.org/10.1111/j.1365-2648.2004.03265.x

Pirret, A.M., 2016. Nurse practitioners' versus physicians' diagnostic reasoning style and use of maxims: A comparative study. The Journal for Nurse Practitioners 12 (6), 381–389.

Pyles, S.H., Stern, P.N., 1983. Discovery of Nursing Gestalt in critical care nursing: The importance of the Gray Gorilla syndrome. Image J Nurs Sch 15 (2), 51–57. https://doi.org/10.1111/j.1547-5069.1983.tb01356.x

Rew, L., 1990. Intuition in critical care nursing practice. Dimens Crit Care Nurs 9 (1), 30–37. https://doi.org/10.1097/00003465-199001000-00011

Ritter, B., 1998. Why evidence-based practice? CCNP Connection 11 (5), 1–8.

Ritter, B., 2000. An analysis of expert nurse practitioners' diagnostic reasoning [University of San Francisco].

Shahzad, M., Upshur, R., Donnelly, P., Bharmal, A., Wei, X., Feng, P., et al., 2019. A population-based approach to integrated healthcare delivery: A scoping review of clinical care and public health collaboration. BMC Public Health 19 (1), 708. https://doi.org/10.1186/s12889-019-7002-z

Tanner, C.A., 1987. Teaching clinical judgement. Annu Rev Nurs Res 5, 153–173.

Videbeck, S.L., 1997a. Critical thinking: A model. J Nurs Educ 36 (1), 23–28. https://doi.org/10.3928/0148-4834-19970101-07

Videbeck, S.L., 1997b. Critical thinking: Prevailing practice in baccalaureate schools of nursing. J Nurs Educ 36 (1), 5–10. https://doi.org/10.3928/0148-4834-19970101-04

Zakim, D., Braun, N., Fritz, P., Alscher M.D., 2008. Underutilization of information and knowledge in everyday medical practice: Evaluation of a computer-based solution. http://www.biomedcentral.com/1472-6947/8/50

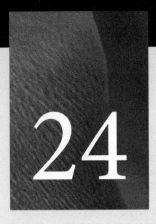

24

CLINICAL REASONING IN PHYSIOTHERAPY

MARK JONES ■ GAIL M. JENSEN ■ GINA MARIA MUSOLINO

CHAPTER AIMS

The aims of this chapter are:

- to introduce the concept of 'Noise' in human judgement as it relates to clinical reasoning
- to discuss the importance of clinical reasoning as a component of clinical practice excellence
- to appraise CR frameworks providing context and focus to the learning and teaching continuum *from novice to expert*
- to examine strategies for translation of CR theory to practice
- to value the importance of patient narrative for efficacious CR and virtuous clinical judgements
- to interpret factors influencing CR quality.

INTRODUCTION

Clinical reasoning (CR) may be defined as a reflective process of inquiry and analysis carried out by a health professional in collaboration with the patient with the aim of understanding the patient, their context and their clinical problem(s) in order to guide evidence-based practice. CR reflects a biopsychosocial practice philosophy requiring a broad scope, including understanding:

- the individual's health problem(s) or clinical presentation,
- the individual,
- their physical and social environment and
- their unique, lived experiences with their health problem(s).

Precise analysis of each element guides health education and best management, promoting understanding, shared decision making and active participation/self-efficacy. CR requires a broad scope of focus including diagnostic, psychosocial, interactive, collaborative, ethical, procedural and prognostic reasoning. CR is impacted by timing, sequencing and opportunities for reflection and self-assessment. Whilst striving for excellence in clinical practice, one must be aware of potential biases and common errors in CR processes and judgements.

To assist in understanding CR, three core frameworks are updated herein: CR in a biopsychosocial framework, CR focus and hypothesis categories to promote excellence in clinical judgement and practice. The concept of 'noise' as unwarranted variability in human judgement is highlighted. We consider quality aspects of CR and clinical judgements, including application of critical thinking standards with suggestions for evaluating and addressing noise in analytical judgements.

WHY DO PHYSIOTHERAPISTS NEED TO STUDY AND PRACTICE CLINICAL REASONING?

Research Evidence Only Provides a Guide, Not a Prescription, to Practice

Despite exponential growth over recent decades, our current body of research is far from conclusive to sufficiently inform the full scope of clinical decisions required in practice (Jones et al., 2006; Kerry et al., 2013; Moseley et al., 2014; Villas Boas et al., 2013). Studies of physiotherapy effectiveness have limitations that include high dropout rates or follow-up losses, lack of masking (patient, therapist, measurer), lack of adequate identification of population subgroups, artificial isolation of treatment interventions in determining effectiveness and lack of sustainable outcomes evidence. Hence, clinicians face the daunting challenge of maintaining best practice based on best evidence when the evidence is still largely unavailable or incomplete. Even when research testing therapeutic interventions for the condition of interest is available, numerous issues must be considered for the clinician to have confidence in the applicability of the findings, including whether their patient matches the population studied (often made difficult by lack of homogeneity of subjects and insufficient consideration of psychosocial variables) and whether the intervention tested can be replicated. Very few studies provide sufficient detail and justification of the assessments and treatments to enable clinicians to fully replicate the assessments and management (educatively, behaviourally and humanistically) with confidence. More recently, Clinical Practice Guidelines (CPGs) have begun to consider the numerous internal and external variables that impact healthcare, e.g. patients' values and beliefs; information technologies to facilitate guideline adherence, both bedside decision-support software for clinicians and mobile apps for patients; considerations of patient multimorbidities; cost-effectiveness from both system and patient perspectives; inclusion of psychological and general health questionnaires with activity level scales; recognition that CPGs are considered outdated after 3 years due to healthcare progressions and should be reassessed. These variables can assist in clinical decision making when expert insights are combined with ratings of evidence, experience and guided appraisal. However, CPGs do not replace the inherent need for sound CR judgements. CPGs assist in avoiding unwarranted variations in practice, such as 'Noise' and can improve quality and safety (Atkins et al., 2004; Horvath, 2004; Panteli et al., 2019; Woolf et al., 2012).

Human Judgement Is 'Noisy'

Kahneman et al. (2021) define 'Noise' in human judgement as objective variability in professional judgements that should not vary, often due to cognitive bias and emotional reactions. They provide extensive examples of both nonhealth and health-related findings demonstrating noise across and within individuals' judgements. For example, within the judicial system, judges were tougher the hungrier they were!

Examples of studies illustrating inconsistency in medical judgements cited by Kahneman and colleagues include:

- Physicians having only fair agreement assessing MRI scans for the degree of spinal stenosis;
- Physicians being significantly more likely to prescribe opioids at the end of a long day and more likely to order cancer investigations early in the day.

So how do physiotherapists do? When considering diagnostic judgements, variability occurs when therapists are using different classification systems. However, research looking at therapists using the same classification system shows there is still considerable judgement variability. For example:

- Therapists' agreement using a pathoanatomical classification for low back pain has been reported as varying from 39% to 72% (Karayannis et al., 2012)

- Examples of judgement variability within different systems of classification include:
  - Mechanical diagnosis and therapy classification of derangement, dysfunction and postural patterns has been shown to have 93% to 100% agreement across credentialed therapists, but poor agreement in others, and conflicting neck pain classification agreement (Garcia et al., 2018);
  - Treatment-based low back pain classification (acute, subacute, return to participation – manipulation, stabilization, specific exercise, traction) based on specific initial assessment findings has been reported as having 31% to 83% agreement (Karayannis et al., 2012);
  - Movement system impairment classification has been reported to have 75% to 83% agreement (Karayannis et al., 2012; Sahrmann et al., 2017) and
  - Cognitive functional therapy classification (of pain as specific, nonspecific, peripheral, central, low back pain/pelvic girdle, control impairment, movement impairment with fear avoidance) has been shown to have between 73% and 97% agreement (Vibe Fersum et al., 2009; Karayannis et al., 2012).

Diagnosis of the precise source of symptoms, i.e. specific symptomatic structure or tissue, is limited by the challenge of pathology being common in the asymptomatic population and poor diagnostic validity of many, if not most, tests. This has resulted in the ubiquitous use of 'nonspecific' classifications where a symptomatic pathology cannot be established. However, in the absence of confirmed symptomatic pathology there is still significant specificity in therapists' diagnostic judgements, for example deciding whether pain symptoms are local somatic nociception or somatic referral, visceral referral, vascular or neuropathic. Even with the classification of spinal pain from local somatic nociception, skilled therapists have between 91% and 98% agreement identifying the symptomatic cervical segment in patients presenting with neck pain disorders (Schneider et al., 2013).

Noise also exists in physiotherapists' judgements regarding precautions/contraindications to examination and treatment, for example:

- Barakatt et al. (2009) demonstrated 77% agreement between two physiotherapists' judgements regarding low back pain irritability over 48 patients;
- 73 final-year undergraduate students from 15 European countries correctly recognized potential red flag pathological process in 53% of cases (Lackenbauer et al., 2018);
- 969 American physical therapists' judgements on six cases of potential lower extremity deep vein thrombosis in outpatient practice underestimated the two high probability cases 87% and 64% respectively and 32% and 27% reported they would not have contacted the referring physician in those cases (Riddle et al., 2004).

Contrastingly, however, in a review of 78 case reports where physical therapists referred patients to physicians, 78.8% were referred upon initial encounter with resulting diagnoses of medical conditions. Most of the patients being referred presented with unknown causes of recent worsening of symptoms, inconsistent presentation with primary medical diagnoses, unusual symptoms including fatigue and unexplained weakness and insufficient treatment responses. Following referral, additional diagnostics led to the following diagnoses: fractures, tumours, visceral manifestations which were predominantly cardiovascular in nature and medication-disorders (Boissonnault and Ross, 2012). Direct access to physiotherapy without the need for practitioner referral allows the patient more control for care choices. The focus today on population health and the need to reason and to make judgements based upon numerous screens and standardized measures is even more important when dealing with the elderly and safe ageing in place (Wilson et al., 2022, p. 9). 'Physiotherapists can leverage their integration within the medical community by providing referrals to other healthcare team members for any identified evolving health or cognitive issues'. (Wilson et al., 2022)

Other essential physiotherapy CR judgements have *not* been investigated. What is the noise in our:

- Psychosocial judgements?
- Judgements regarding the underlying cause(s) or contributing factor(s) to the onset and maintenance of patients' health problems?

- Procedural reasoning judgements regarding what to address in management, what to address first, what to reassess and judgement regarding progression of management?
- Prognostic judgements?

Judgements from one patient to the next, even with the same general health problem, can be expected to vary according to the unique patient presentation. There should, however, arguably be consistency in broad judgements such as problem classification, recognition of potentially relevant psychosocial factors, broad management, safety considerations and prognosis. Kahneman et al. (2021) highlight that noise, or unwanted variability in professional judgement, can be traced to the tendency for human bias.

Bias is systematic predictable error of judgement when an accurate judgement can be confirmed (e.g. weight scale consistently 2 lb off). Subjective judgements that are randomly different such as subjective assessment of strength or range of movement is noise and hence the need for objective measurement where possible. When truth cannot be confirmed (i.e. non-verifiable judgements) as is the case with most physiotherapy judgements, we need to look for bias in the judgement process (examples in Box 24.1).

Bias does not just influence analysis, it also affects what we perceive and screen. Noise occurs in individual biases that create judgement variability (e.g. Do we always find psychosocial factors in chronic presentations? Do we judge all physical impairments as necessarily relevant?). We should also recognize environmental influences can lead to bias with busy clinical environments, sleep deprivation and fatigue often impairing clinical decision making (Walston et al., 2022).

What Can We Do About 'Noise'?

Kahneman and colleagues (2021) advocate the use of a 'noise audit' for assessment of judgement variability in a group of professionals. Extrapolating this to a physiotherapy noise audit any aspect of the CR process or judgements could be examined. Analysis of audit findings would provide a deeper understanding of the variability found, for example:

- Exploring therapists' personal concepts regarding the purpose of physiotherapy in different areas of practice;
- Examining the different focus or categories of clinical judgements therapists' consciously considered;
- Exploring what information therapists seek or use to inform each category of judgement;
- Exploring criteria therapists use for making specific judgements, for example:
  - Diagnostic categorizations
  - Relevance and significance of potential psychosocial factors or physical findings
  - Dominant pain mechanism(s)
  - Need for caution in physical examination and treatment versus referral for further investigation(s)
  - Prognosis

Kahneman and colleagues (2021) also report on the success of two strategies of 'decision hygiene' to preemptively reduce bias and unwanted variability in judgements, 'nudges' and 'boosting'. Nudges are strategies targeting behaviours to reduce the effects of bias, such as:

- Using a structured examination protocol or using explicit CR frameworks;
- Analysing complex judgements (e.g. physical diagnosis(es) broken down into hypotheses

---

BOX 24.1
EXAMPLES OF BIAS IN THE PHYSIOTHERAPY JUDGEMENT PROCESS

- Priming influence of prior information such as a referral or imaging
- Overemphasis on first impression or intuition, commonly characterized as 'fast-thinking'
- Ascertainment bias, i.e. when thinking is shaped by prior expectation (e.g. stereotyping based on someone's appearance, socioeconomic status, etc.)
- Confirmation bias, i.e. tendency to seek confirmatory evidence and ignore negating evidence (ongoing analysis biased by first impression)
- Excessive coherence, i.e. ignoring what does not make sense. This relates well to what Maitland taught about how to 'make the features fit' or avoid ignoring something that does not make sense, instead keep exploring until you can make sense of it.

regarding dominant pain mechanism, source of symptoms, potential pathology and key physical impairments); and

■ Using CPGs and clinical decision aids.

Boosting involves teaching decision makers about common biases (see Box 25.1) and providing practice to recognize bias. This has been shown to improve judgement performance and decrease noise. Other boosting strategies include:

■ Delaying intuition: The fast versus slow thinking distinction implies we should avoid intuition and rely totally on our slower analytical reasoning. However, there is evidence that intuition combined with analytical thinking is better than analytical alone (Kahneman et al., 2021). Rather than ignoring intuition, delay it to avoid the bias it often creates.
■ Promote intellectual humility to recognize what we do not know.
■ Continually revise and develop knowledge, reasoning and skill. Interestingly, Kahneman and colleagues (2021) reported variation in skill accounted for 44% of variation in medical diagnostic decisions and policies that improve skill are better than providing uniform decision guidelines. Of course, we need to use clinical guidelines and decision tools but proficient skill with interviewing, physical assessment, shared decision making, management and CR matters more.

Fast and Slow Reasoning in Physiotherapy Practice

In addition to being holistic and collaborative in their reasoning, expert physiotherapists use a combination of fast and slow reasoning as required by the complexity and familiarity of the patient's unique clinical presentation and context. Kahneman (2011) describes fast thinking as automatic, effortless first impressions and intuition (e.g. pattern recognition) and slow thinking as analytical deliberations requiring more attention, time and effort. Although shortcuts in thinking such as pattern recognition can be effective when working with very familiar presentations where little problem solving is required, errors are likely to occur if relied on in less familiar, more complex presentations.

Humans are prone to find and accept coherence based on limited information, especially in fast thinking. Kahneman (2011, p. 86) has characterized this trait, associated with many of our biases, such as 'What You See Is All There Is' – the assumption, or acceptance, that the information at hand is all that is available. We build a story (explanation) from the information we have and if it is a good, coherent story, we believe it. Paradoxically, coherent stories are easier to construct when there is less information for sense-making. Although overreliance on fast reasoning can clearly lead to errors, experts working with familiar problems function largely on pattern recognition (Boshuizen and Schmidt, 2008; Jensen et al., 2007; Kaufman et al., 2008; Schwartz and Elstein, 2008).

While there is risk of error in relying on fast thinking, overanalysis can also lead to errors in judgement (Lehrer, 2010; Schwartz and Elstein, 2008). Decision support systems can assist clinical judgement. However, the uniqueness of individual patient presentations suggests that these will be insufficient on their own for most categories of clinical judgement.

When one considers the large number of first-impression, fast-thinking judgements that inform our understanding of the patient and their problems, this dimension of CR should not be dismissed. Kahneman et al. (2021) also acknowledge the value of fast reasoning (e.g. intuition). However, they advise basing initial judgements on the slower analytical process and only then factoring insights from intuition. Utilizing input and perspectives from more experienced colleagues and mentors also helps to reduce bias (Walston et al., 2022).

Examples of fast reasoning in clinical practice include quick recognition of:

■ the need to clarify patients' responses,
■ discerning patients' discomfort, needs and emotions,
■ observing postural, movement and control impairments,
■ adjusting a hands-on intervention midtreatment.

When an existing approach is inadequate, there is an inherent need for a reflective openness that has been described as 'adaptive expertise' (Cutrer et al., 2017). There is a need to reframe problems and combine this with an ability to adapt, to explore and to invent creative solutions.

This includes integrating fast and slow thinking as well as managing uncertainty (Cooke and Lemay, 2017).

REFLECTION POINTS

- Can you identify any 'Noise' in your own clinical judgements?
- Can you spot any of the common human biases that may have crept into your CR?
- Why is it important to be cognizant of noise influencing CR?

THREE FRAMEWORKS TO SITUATE CR IN PHYSIOTHERAPY

CR is increasingly acknowledged as important in clinically focussed publications, conference presentations and practice competencies. However, outside scholarly works that focus on CR (e.g. Edwards et al., 2004a; Jensen et al., 2007; Musolino and Jensen, 2020), CR is often referred to as a broad construct without reference to the scope of clinical judgements that should be considered or the dynamics of the reasoning process. Three frameworks that can provide context and focus to the learning and practice of CR in physiotherapy are the biopsychosocial framework, CR strategies and hypothesis categories.

CR in a Biopsychosocial Framework

Physiotherapists must consider all factors potentially contributing to a person's health. The biopsychosocial perspective (Engel, 1977) recognizes that disability is the result of the cumulative effects of the biological health condition (disease, illness, pathology, disorder), external environmental influences (e.g. physical, social, economic, political) and internal personal influences (e.g. age, gender, education, beliefs, culture, coping style, self-efficacy) (Borrell-Carrió et al., 2004; Epstein and Borrell-Carrió, 2005; Imrie, 2004). The biopsychosocial model of health contrasts with the biomedical model that previously dominated medicine and physiotherapy practice where disease and illness were primarily attributed only to pathogens, genetic or developmental abnormalities or injury.

The World Health Organization International Classification of Functioning, Disability and Health (ICF) model (Fig. 24.1) provides a biopsychosocial framework illustrating the scope of knowledge and CR required for physiotherapists to holistically understand and competently manage patient healthcare.

The boxes across the middle of the diagram depict the relationship between a patient's body function and impairments, their capabilities to do activities and participate in life situations (e.g. work, family, sport, leisure). Bidirectional arrows reflect the reciprocal relationships whereby different factors have the potential to influence each other. Formerly, functional restrictions, physical impairments and pain would have been conceptualized as the end result of a specific injury/pathology or syndrome, but the reciprocal arrows highlight that these can also be associated with, and even maintained by, environmental and personal influences. A holistic understanding of a patient's clinical presentation therefore necessitates attention and analysis of their physical health, environmental and personal factors. The ICF model provides focussed contextualization of the scope of knowledge and CR required in physiotherapy practice. A framework of CR strategies provides further assistance to understanding and learning CR.

Focus of Our CR: CR Strategies

It is common for CR presentations and discussions to focus on diagnosis alone, with diagnosis often limited to categorizing the problem, injury or pathology. Understanding the associated pathogenesis of a confirmed health problem is important so that we can understand the rationale and mechanisms of medical and physiotherapy therapeutic interventions and the expected progression and prognosis. Some suspected pathologies require further investigation and possibly medical management. Other known or suspected pathologies may not require further medical investigation yet do require more caution in physical examination and treatment, for example an inflammatory presentation, suspected neuropathic pain or a possible structural instability. However, CR that overfocusses on pathology at the expense of other factors, such as the psychosocial, physical impairment and environmental influences, is risking an incomplete understanding of a patient's issues. Pathology can be asymptomatic and symptoms can exist without detectable pathology. Symptomatic pathology exhibits a continuum of presentations, relating to stage and severity of pathol-

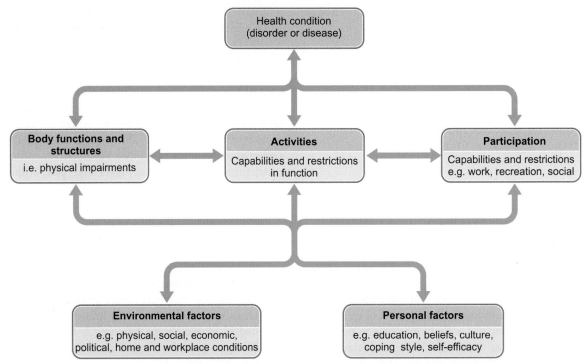

Fig. 24.1 ■ An adaptation of World Health Organization International Classification of functioning, ssdisability and health framework. (Adapted with permission from World Health Organization (2001). International classification of functioning, disability, and health. World Health Organization, Geneva.)

ogy and interactions from other health comorbidities and psychosocial and environmental influences. Reasoning about diagnosis/pathology represents only a portion of the reasoning that occurs in clinical practice. Treating the root cause is often critical for success rather than just focussing on the treatment of symptoms. Across the health professions, CR research and theory elucidates a range of CR foci. We suggest the following CR strategies capture the scope of reasoning necessary to apply the ICF biopsychosocial model to physiotherapy practice (Box 24.2).

Expert physiotherapists attend to these various reasoning strategies and move dialectically in their reasoning between a biological and psychosocial focus, in a fluid and seemingly effortless manner (Edwards et al., 2004a). For example, a diagnostic test may elicit a patient response that is more reflective of their fear of movement rather than any underlying pathology. Even though the diagnostic test may

have good validity, the expert clinician will recognize the need to switch dialectically from biological to biopsychosocial thinking. Although CR strategies provide a framework to assist clinicians in recognizing the different foci of reasoning required in biopsychosocial practice, it is also helpful to recognize that different and varying categories of clinical judgements are required across these different reasoning strategies.

REFLECTION POINTS

- Do you explicitly assess patients' psychosocial status? If so, what do you assess, how do you assess it and how do you judge a psychosocial feature as contributing to a patient's presentation?
- Why is full consideration of the patient's narrative so vital to CR and clinical judgements?

BOX 24.2
APPLYING THE INTERNATIONAL CLASSIFICATION OF FUNCTIONING, DISABILITY AND HEALTH BIOPSYCHOSOCIAL MODEL TO PHYSIOTHERAPY

Diagnostic reasoning: Depending on the health problem this may encompass pathology or pathophysiological process, clinical syndrome, source of symptoms or functional limitation(s). There is also the identification of associated cognitive, physical, physiological and anatomical impairments with consideration of pain mechanism, if appropriate, and the broad scope of potential contributing factors to the development and maintenance of the health problem.

Psychosocially focussed reasoning: The assessment here is associated with understanding individuals' (and at times family's, carers') illness and/or disability experiences. This requires getting the person's story, or narrative, and how it incorporates their understanding (including the personal meaning of their understanding) of their problem(s). It includes their perceptions regarding its effects on their life, their expectations for management, any associated emotions and their ability to cope. It also includes assessment of the effects these personal perspectives have on their clinical presentation, particularly whether these perspectives are facilitating or obstructing their recovery.

Reasoning about procedure: Analyses need to consider the selection, implementation and progression of treatment procedures. Although clinical guidelines provide broad direction, typically focussing only on diagnostic categorization, practising therapists need to reason adaptively about how best to apply guidelines to patients' individual presentations and goals. Progression of treatment is then guided by judicious outcome reassessment that attends to both impairment and function/disability-related outcomes.

Interactive reasoning: This is the thinking and behaviour involved in the purposeful establishment of rapport and the ongoing management of the patient/client–therapist therapeutic alliance. The nature and manner (e.g. communication, confidence, nonverbal behaviours, time allowed) of the examination and therapy influences the level of trust and the success of the therapeutic relationship in general.

Collaborative reasoning: Shared decision making is a healthcare partnership between the therapist and the individual (and sometimes other relevant individuals) in making choices about goals and care. This is based on explanation and understanding of the therapist's analysis and the patient's preferences (Jones et al., 2022). Shared decision making also applies to the healthcare team.

Reasoning about teaching: This concerns how the therapist goes about helping patients to understand what is happening and helping them to comply with treatment (e.g. rehabilitative exercises) and bring about behavioural change.

Prognostic reasoning: This is the clinical judgement about whether a person's health problem(s) can be resolved, improved or deterioration lessened. Although prognostic judgements are not precise, there needs to be a thorough consideration of biological, environmental and personal factors that can and cannot be changed.

Ethical reasoning: The CR of physiotherapists has an ethical component. For example, the effect of power dynamics can influence who has the right to make and accept decisions. The personal and professional values of therapists and patients can all have an effect on the decisions taken.

Categories of Clinical Judgements Required: Hypothesis Categories

CR is a hypothesis-oriented, iterative thinking process comprised of key elements (Elder and Paul, 2019). Hawkins et al. (2019, p. 5) relate this thinking to CR stating:

Whenever we think, we think for a purpose within a point of view based on assumptions leading to implications and consequences. We use concepts, ideas, and theories to interpret data, facts, and experiences in order to answer questions, solve problems, and resolve issues.

That is, rather than simply teaching and learning a prescribed patient examination and analysis, clinicians, students and educators should:

- Consider the purpose of each area of clinical practice.
- Identify the questions that need to be answered to achieve that purpose.
- Reflect on the information important to answering those questions.
- Foster patient–practitioner interaction that assures we are gaining full insight into the patient's narrative and understanding the lived experiences

that impact their health. This includes the patient's perceptions, support systems and their home/work environments. These may need to be revisited with subsequent encounters.

- Consider the inferences or categories of clinical judgement that need to be formulated and what information specifically informs each category.
- Identify, review and critique the theory and conceptual knowledge underpinning the examination, analysis and evidence-based management.
- Identify assumptions inherent in assessment and management approaches and adopt strategies to minimize unjustified assumptions.
- Ensure the reasoning is truly hypothesis-oriented and iterative.
- Reflect on the breadth of our reasoning by recognizing the point of view we are taking and ponder whether other perspectives should also be considered.

It is not appropriate to stipulate a definitive list of clinical judgements all physiotherapists must consider. It is more important to understand and to learn how to think critically. This is because these skills will help us cope with changes in knowledge and practice. Nevertheless, awareness of different categories of clinical judgement can help to critique and to optimize those judgements. Examples of categories of judgements that might be formulated are highlighted in Box 24.3.

As physiotherapists follow their structured examination appropriate for each area of practice, they should recognize patient cues that in turn should elicit hypotheses in one or more categories. That is, CR across the different hypothesis categories occurs simultaneously and with varying emphasis depending on the context and nature of the clinical situation and problems encountered. There are many different types of clinical patterns, including patterns within all hypothesis categories (Box 24.4).

REFLECTION POINT

Which of the different types of clinical patterns (Box 24.4) do you use in your clinical judgements? If there are some you agree are important but are not well developed in your working knowledge, you might consider building your knowledge of these through further study and peer discussions.

As specific hypotheses are considered, informed by knowledge of clinical patterns, tentative judgements should be 'tested' for the remaining features of the pattern through further patient inquiry, physical tests and ultimately with the physiotherapy intervention. Thinking of interpretations of patient information as hypotheses discourages premature conclusions and promotes synthesis of the full clinical story and physical assessment. Patient information typically has implications for several different hypothesis categories. The reasoning regarding each of these hypothesis categories would then continue to evolve throughout the ongoing initial assessment and ongoing management. Utilizing the biopsychosocial framework, CR strategies and hypothesis categories framework collectively highlight core areas of knowledge essential to holistic CR, assisting students and practising physiotherapists to better understand and improve their own CR.

Quality of CR and Clinical Judgements

Critical Thinking Standards

So how can we judge the quality of CR thought processes that underpin our clinical judgements and reasoning? Elder and Paul (2019) promote standards of judging the quality of analytical thinking with clear application to CR. The following standards are proposed for students, clinicians and educators when considering the quality of CR:

- **Depth and breadth:** Is the depth and breadth of assessment sufficient for a thorough, holistic analysis? Kahneman (2011) highlights the common cognitive error of assuming 'What You See Is All There Is', that is, assuming if the patient does not volunteer the information, it is not there or it is not significant. Avoiding this error of assumption in CR requires screening for other symptoms, psychological factors, physical and social environmental factors, features that signal the need for precaution in the physical examination and treatment and need for further medical investigation.
- **Relevance and significance:** Is the relevance and significance attributed to assessment findings justified? For example: What is the relationship

BOX 24.3
HYPOTHESIS CATEGORIES FRAMEWORK

ACTIVITY AND PARTICIPATION CAPABILITY AND RESTRICTION

- Activity: functional abilities and restrictions (e.g. walking, lifting, sitting) that are volunteered and further screened for. To gain a complete picture, it is important that the clinician identifies those activities the patient is capable of alongside those that are restricted.
- Participation: abilities and restrictions to participate in life situations (e.g. work, recreation/sport, family), including modified participation (e.g. modified work duties).

PSYCHOSOCIAL

Incorporating personal life circumstances (e.g. culture, home, work and life generally) and the individual's perspectives on their experiences and social influences, such as:

- Understandings, for example of their health problem, its cause or factors they believe contribute to it.
- Beliefs, for example regarding management and its likely effect.
- Self-concept or how their health problem may have affected how they feel about themselves.
- Openness to new ideas because this can influence their receptiveness to recommended management.
- Motivation to change because participation in physiotherapy requires effort and commitment.
- Confidence to help themselves or their self-efficacy: if this is low, strategies to reinforce and facilitate self-efficacy will be required.
- Expectations, for example regarding recovery and goals they want to pursue.
- Distress (e.g. anxiety, grieving, anger, fear, self-worth, depression, etc.) and how the distress relates to their problem(s) or symptom(s).
- Behaviour and coping strategies (e.g. adaptive or unhelpful?).
- Social factors, including education and health literacy, culture, social and living situation, work status and influence of health problem on their work, perceived level of support at home, in their social groups and at work as support is a well-recognized factor influencing health outcomes.

PHYSIOTHERAPY DIAGNOSIS OR PROBLEM CLASSIFICATION

Examples of common problem classifications used in physiotherapy include:
- Pathology or pathophysiological process
- Clinical syndrome or disorder
- Pain mechanisms if pain is a symptom
- Source of symptom(s) or functional limitation(s), i.e. hypotheses regarding specific structures or tissues that are involved without specific reference to pathology.

IMPAIRMENTS IN BODY FUNCTION OR STRUCTURE

Any loss or abnormality of cognitive, psychological, physiological, structure, movement system or function.

CONTRIBUTING FACTORS TO THE DEVELOPMENT AND MAINTENANCE OF THE PROBLEM

Predisposing or associated factors involved in the development or maintenance of the patient's problem(s). Both intrinsic and extrinsic factors should be considered, including environmental, psychosocial, behavioural, physical/biomechanical and hereditary.

PRECAUTIONS AND CONTRAINDICATIONS TO PHYSICAL EXAMINATION AND TREATMENT

Medical (e.g. comorbidities), environmental, psychosocial, behavioural and physical factors and red flags (signs and symptoms that may indicate the presence of more serious pathology and systemic or viscerogenic pathology/disease) identified that inform:

- Whether a physical examination should be carried out at all (versus immediate referral for further medical consultation or investigation) and, if so, the extent of examination that can be safely performed that will minimize the risk of aggravating the patient's symptoms/condition
- Whether specific safety tests are indicated (e.g. cervical arterial dysfunction testing, neurological examination, blood pressure/heart rate, balance assessment, instability tests)
- Whether any treatment should be undertaken (versus referral for further consultation/investigation)
- The appropriate dose/strength of any physical interventions planned

MANAGEMENT/TREATMENT SELECTION AND PROGRESSION

1. Overall health management of the patient, including consultation and referral to other healthcare professionals, health promotion interventions (e.g. fitness assessment and management) and patient advocacy as required (e.g. with insurers or employers).
2. Specific therapeutic interventions (educational and physical) and underlying reasoning required to determine which impairments to address, prioritizations, the strategy/procedure and dosage, outcome measures to reassess and the self-management appropriate for optimizing change (in understanding, impairment, activity and participation); progression of treatment informed by outcome reassessment has the same considerations.

PROGNOSIS

The therapist's informed hypotheses regarding the natural course of the health problem(s), the efficacy of therapeutic

---

BOX 24.3
HYPOTHESIS CATEGORIES FRAMEWORK—CONT'D

interventions addressing the person's unique presentation, and an estimate of time required. Whether an individual's problem(s) can be resolved or improved, or whether assistance can be given to live with the problem depends in part on whether the factors underpinning the problem are modifiable or not. Broadly an individual's prognosis is determined by:

- The nature of the health problem(s), for example whether it is a permanent and sometimes progressive disorder

or whether it is an injury that will heal through natural recovery and be assisted by physiotherapy intervention.
- The extent of the health problem(s).
- The natural course of the problem(s).
- The efficacy of therapeutic interventions.
- The person's ability and willingness to make the necessary changes (e.g. in lifestyle, psychosocial and physical contributing factors) to facilitate recovery or improved quality of life.

---

between a patient's understanding of their problem and the meaning their understanding has to them with respect to their threat perception, expectations for recovery, expectations for management and their coping strategies?

- **Clarity, accuracy and precision:** To what extent is patient information clear, accurate and precise? To what extent is the clinician's analysis and reporting clear, accurate and precise? For example:
  - recognizing the need to clarify patient answers for precision to ensure accuracy of information;
  - using the appropriate diagnostic classification supported by the findings;
  - being able to report/explain the analysis with clear, accurate and precise reference to patient findings, supporting research and personal experience.

Metacognition

In addition to physiotherapists' critical thinking and analytical skills, their metacognitive skills also influence the quality of their CR. Metacognition is a form of reflective self-awareness that incorporates monitoring of ourselves (e.g. our performance, our thinking, our knowledge) as though we are outside ourselves observing and critiquing our own practice. There is an integral link between cognition (i.e. perception, interpretation, synthesis, planning), metacognition and learning from clinical practice experience (Higgs et al., 2008a; 2008b). Although, all therapists think, not all therapists think about their thinking. It is this self-awareness and self-critique that prompt the

---

BOX 24.4
DIFFERENT TYPES OF CLINICAL PATTERNS

- Epidemiology of different health conditions
- Diagnostic or problem classification clinical syndromes (e.g. pathology or physiological processes, clinical syndrome, source of symptoms or functional limitations, associated cognitive, physical, physiological and anatomical impairments, pain mechanisms, contributing factors to development and maintenance of health problem and disability)
- Patterns of pathology, clinical syndrome, physiological processes (e.g. degenerative, inflammatory, ischaemic, tissue strain), source of symptoms or functional limitations, pain/symptom mechanisms
- Patterns of activity and participation restrictions, symptoms
- Patterns of impairments (e.g. cognitive, physical, physiological, anatomical, movement systems) common to problem classification (e.g. spinal stenosis, functional instability, chronic obstructive pulmonary disease, multiple sclerosis, etc.)
- Patterns of environmental, personal and physical predisposing or contributing factors to the development and maintenance of the health problem and disability
- Patterns of medical conditions, medications, symptoms and signs that signal the need for precautions to physical examination and treatment and/or referral for further medical consultation
- Patterns of management strategies for different diagnostic and clinical health conditions
- Patterns of factors suggesting poor to good prognosis (e.g. pathology/illness, impairments, environmental and personal factors)

---

metacognitive therapists to reconsider their hypotheses, plans and management.

Metacognition should also include reflection and critique of assumptions embedded in current knowledge, reasoning and practice; open-mindedness to other perspectives; critique of information regarding its accuracy, precision, completeness and relevance; and imagination to look beyond one's own perspective, including contemplation of possibilities beyond what is empirically known at the present time (Brookfield, 2008; Paul and Elder, 2007). Everyone has assumptions that underpin what they believe, feel, know and do. These assumptions manifest in different forms, including professional beliefs, values and stereotypical views about human nature and social organization that underpin our attitudes and actions. Becoming aware of our own perspectives and habitual ways of thinking and acting in practice, along with the assumptions that form the basis for those perspectives and actions, is an essential element of critical thinking and skilled CR. That is, transforming habits of thinking requires critical reflection of the premises or assumptions underpinning our thinking. The need for this is not always obvious as people often acquire their beliefs/ perspectives, points of views and habits of thinking unconsciously through their professional and personal experiences. As such, there is a tendency to fall back on what is available and familiar rather than critically appraising what we know or believe. Unjustified assumptions in clinical practice can be minimized through a range of safeguards, including those listed in Box 24.5.

This self-awareness is not limited to testing formal hypotheses and thinking about treatments. Metacognitive awareness of performance is also important; underpinning the experienced therapist's immediate recognition that a particular phrasing of a question or explanation is not clear or a procedure needs to be adjusted or perhaps should be abandoned.

Lastly, metacognition is important to recognizing limitations in knowledge and ability. Health professionals who lack metacognitive awareness will learn less. Experts not only know a lot in their area of practice, but they also know what they do not know. That is, the expert is typically very quick to recognize a limitation in their knowledge (e.g. a patient's medication they are unfamiliar with, a medical condition, the distribution of a peripheral sensory or motor nerve) and act on this by consulting a colleague or appropriate resource. In short, metacognition and critical

---

BOX 24.5
SOME SAFEGUARDS AGAINST UNJUSTIFIED ASSUMPTIONS

- Qualifying patients' meanings
- Screening to ensure information is not missed
- Testing for competing hypotheses
- Attending to 'negatives' or features of a presentation that do not fit favoured hypotheses and explanations
- Verifying our assessment of the patient's story with the patient
- Openly subjecting and comparing our own reasoning to others

---

reflection are important means to continue professional formation and career-long learning.

Data Collection and Procedural Skills

CR is only as good as the information on which it is based. Incomplete and inaccurate information obtained through the patient interview, physical examination and monitoring of outcomes (during and after treatments) can lead to inaccurate analyses that compromise specific treatment and overall management. The breadth of this information will then be complemented by the depth needed to understand individual patients in their uniqueness and clarify what is meaningful for them.

There are many situations in which skilled listening identifies patient responses that require clarification to understand their meaning accurately. For example, patients' perceptions of their problems may be based on superficial understandings of what their health professionals, doctors, or others, have advised. Our assessments need to find out what these perceptions actually mean to the patient with respect to the cause, management and the future. Clarifying relationships between beliefs, cognitions, emotions and behaviours with the history of the patient's symptoms and disability helps identify the key factors contributing to a patient's pain/disability experience. Explicit screening questions that assess beyond what the patient spontaneously offers as already discussed contribute to this completeness.

As with the patient interview, the quality of information obtained from the physical examination is influenced by the physiotherapist's procedural skills.

Errors in assessments of physical tests and measures along with analysis of function underpin the importance of using reliable objective tests, measures and diagnostic procedures with the strongest psychometric properties wherever possible. When objective measurement is not available, findings should be rechecked for consistency, related to other findings (e.g. impairments in joint mobility compared with functional analysis findings) and cautiously integrated with more objective findings to guide reasoning judgements.

Knowledge Organization

The importance of knowledge to physiotherapists' CR is highlighted in Jensen's expertise research. Expert physiotherapists were seen to possess a broad, multidimensional knowledge base acquired through professional education and reflective practice where both patients and other health professionals were valued as sources for learning (Jensen et al., 2007). Well-structured knowledge is essential to domain competence. Well-structured knowledge is not simply how much an individual knows but how that knowledge is organized. For knowledge to be accessible in practice, it needs to be linked to practice.

All forms of knowledge are important, including clinicians' broader worldviews, their philosophy of practice and their medical and profession specific knowledge. The ICF biopsychosocial model, CR strategies, hypothesis categories and frameworks presented earlier provide means for physiotherapy knowledge organization that directly links theory to practice. Equally important is our professional craft knowledge (Higgs et al., 2008b). Craft knowledge comprises professional knowledge such as procedural, communication and teaching knowledge and skills. It is underpinned by theory that has been contextualized through clinical experience.

Although clinical trials, CPGs, clinical prediction rules and theory extrapolated from basic science all provide helpful direction for management of different problems, these should not be taken as unchallenged prescriptions (Greenhalgh et al., 2014). Instead, physiotherapists must judge how their patient matches the population in reported evidence and then tailor their management to the individual patient's unique lifestyle, goals, activity and participation restrictions, perspectives, pain type, potential pathology and physical impairments. Because fully research-supported management efficacy is still lacking for most clinical problems, advanced theoretical and craft knowledge, combined with metacognitive, trained reasoning, is the physiotherapist's preeminent tool to optimize management effectiveness for individual patients. Optimizing care usually involves a therapeutic alliance.

Therapeutic Alliance

Ferreira et al. (2013, p. 471) define the therapeutic alliance as 'the sense of collaboration, warmth, and support between the client and therapist'. Collaboration requires understanding, not just of the health problem but also the person behind the problem – their purpose(s) for seeking care, their goals, their perspectives on their experiences. As therapists, we do not have absolute control of health outcomes, but there needs to be an explicit focus on understanding the person, not just the problem. There also needs to be collaborative engagement that addresses the perspectives of a patient so that we can enhance their participation and promote outcomes that are meaningful to the person. Physical therapy is a relational practice where the CR process requires contextual collaboration (Jensen et al., 2007; Jensen et al., 2019; Weiner, 2022).

The way an examination and therapy are provided is important, especially with respect to patient rapport. If the physiotherapist shows interest, empathy and confidence, patients are likely to respond positively. Patients are more willing to volunteer relevant information and to participate in self-management, more motivated to change and likely to be satisfied with their care (Ferreira et al., 2013; Hall et al., 2010; Klaber Moffett and Richardson, 2009; Matthias et al., 2013). Building rapport is an ongoing process that commences with initial introductions and continues through the examination and subsequent management. There are numerous ways rapport is enhanced but central is demonstrating interest in the person, not just their problem. This requires empathy and validation of a patient's concerns. Although the patient interview and physical examination are largely about gaining information to understand the patient and their problems, the nature and way this is done are also important. The tone of voice, the nonverbal behaviours, the time allowed and the responses to patients all affect how a patient perceives the therapist. These factors are a strong influence on the confidence of the patient and the success of the therapeutic relationship (Ferreira et al., 2013; Hall et al., 2010). The patient–therapist relationship is founded on the perceptions each has about the other and by how each person perceives and understands themselves (and their roles) as a 'self'. Merleau-Ponty offered a concept of the 'self' as embodied (1962, p. 137), meaning that a person's sense of self (and their consciousness) is expressed in the physical and social world of that person via such things as their gestures, movements and actions. The idea of embodiment helps us understand that illness or disability 'is not simply a biological dysfunction of a body part but a pervasive disturbance of our being in the world' (Carel, 2012, p. 326). In other words, health problem symptoms and disability can profoundly affect a person's sense of self and how they experience their place in the world. Our questions and responses (verbal and nonverbal) are interpreted by patients with symptoms and disability from this position of a changed sense of self (Greenfield and Jensen, 2010). If we forget this, then in our CR conclusions we can reduce the experiences of a person's health problems to a merely prescriptive label, such as 'chronic pain or chronic obstructive pulmonary disease', and we can also reduce patients' capacity to act for change (Edwards et al., 2014; Ricoeur, 2006). Sensitivity to embodiment requires empathy.

Empathy in a clinical context refers to therapists' cognitive abilities to understand what their patients are experiencing and therapists' affective abilities to project themselves imaginatively into their patients' situations (Braude, 2012). Having, and conveying, empathy are probably personal skills acquired throughout life. When empathy is applied in practice, patients are more likely to feel they have been given a voice, have been heard and have been believed, all of which strengthen the therapeutic alliance. Many patients report negative experiences with medical and other healthcare professionals whom they felt did not listen or believe them (e.g. Edwards et al., 2014; Epstein and Borrell-Carrió, 2005; Johnson, 1993; Payton et al., 1998). Without good rapport and empathy, the patient is less likely to collaborate, potentially compromising CR and jeopardizing the eventual outcome. The importance of empathic collaboration (as in collaborative reasoning), not simply cooperation, is underscored by the evidence that patients who have been given an opportunity to share in the decision making and take greater responsibility for their own management are more satisfied with their healthcare and have a greater likelihood of achieving better outcomes (Arnetz et al., 2004; Edwards et al., 2004b; Trede and Higgs, 2008).

SUMMARY

In this chapter, we have outlined:

- The critical need for physiotherapists to understand the components of CR given the limitations of research evidence and CPGs and the biases in human judgement that leads to unwanted variability or noise
- Fast and slow reasoning processes and the critical role of adaptive expertise
- How CR fits within a biopsychosocial framework and is aligned with the ICF model
- A framework of CR strategies that aids understanding, learning and transforming CR theory to practice
- A framework of hypothesis categories, or clinical judgements, required across the different CR strategies
- Factors that influence the quality of CR and clinical judgements, including critical thinking standards, metacognition, data collection and procedural skills, knowledge organization and therapeutic alliance.

REFLECTION POINT

- How can you synthesize the ideas, frameworks and strategies presented in this chapter into a coherent model to guide your own CR?

REFERENCES

Arnetz, J.E., Almin, I., Bergström, K., Franzen, Y., Nilsson, H., 2004. Active patient involvement in the establishment of physical therapy goals: Effects on treatment outcome and quality of care. Advances in Physiotherapy 6 (2), 50–69.

Atkins, D., Best, D., Briss, P.A., Eccles, M., Falck-Ytter, Y., Flottorp, S., et al.; GRADE Working Group, 2004. Grading quality of evidence and strength of recommendations. BMJ 328 (7454), 1490. https://doi.org/10.1136/bmj.328.7454.1490

Barakatt, E.T., Romano, P.S., Riddle, D.L., Beckett, L.A., 2009. The reliability of Maitland's Irritability Judgments in patients with low back pain. J Man Manip Ther 17 (3), 135–140. https://doi.org/10.1179/jmt.2009.17.3.135

Boissonnault, W.G., Ross, M.D., 2012. Physical therapists referring patients to physicians: A review of case reports and series. J Orthop Sports Phys Ther 42 (5), 446–454. https://doi.org/10.2519/jospt.2012.3890

Borrell-Carrió, F., Suchman, A.L., Epstein, R.M., 2004. The biopsychosocial model 25 years later: Principles, practice, and scientific inquiry. Ann Fam Med 2 (6), 576–582. https://doi.org/10.1370/afm.245

Boshuizen, H.P., Schmidt, H.G., 2008. The development of clinical reasoning expertise. In: Higgs, J., Jones, M.A., Loftus, S., Christensen, N. (Eds.), Clinical reasoning in the health professions, 3rd ed. Elsevier, pp. 113–121.

Braude, H.D., 2012. Conciliating cognition and consciousness: The perceptual foundations of clinical reasoning. J Eval Clin Pract 18 (5), 945–950. https://doi.org/10.1111/j.1365-2753.2012.01898.x

Brookfield, S., 2008. Clinical reasoning and generic thinking skills. In: Higgs, J., Jones, M., Loftus, S., Christensen, N. (Eds.), Clinical reasoning in the health professions, 3rd ed. Elsevier, pp. 65–75.

Carel, H., 2012. Nursing and medicine. In: Luft, S., Overgaard, S. (Eds.), The Routledge companion to phenomenology. Routledge, Taylor & Francis Group, pp. 623–632.

Cooke, S., Lemay, J.F., 2017. Transforming medical assessment: Integrating uncertainty into the evaluation of clinical reasoning in medical education. Acad Med 92 (6), 746–751. https://doi.org/10.1097/ACM.0000000000001559

Cutrer, W.B., Miller, B., Pusic, M.V., Mejicano, G., Mangrulkar, R.S., Gruppen, L.D., et al., 2017. Fostering the development of master adaptive learners: A conceptual model to guide skill acquisition in medical education. Acad Med 92 (1), 70–75. https://doi.org/10.1097/ACM.0000000000001323

Edwards, I., Jones, M., Carr, J., Braunack-Mayer, A., Jensen, G.M., 2004a. Clinical reasoning strategies in physical therapy. Phys Ther 84 (4), 312–330; discussion 331-315: https://www.ncbi.nlm.nih.gov/pubmed/15049726

Edwards, I., Jones, M., Higgs, J., Trede, F., Jensen, G., 2004b. What is collaborative reasoning? Advances in Physiotherapy 6 (2), 70–83.

Edwards, I., Jones, M., Thacker, M., Swisher, L.L., 2014. The moral experience of the patient with chronic pain: Bridging the gap between first and third person ethics. Pain Med 15 (3), 364–378. https://doi.org/10.1111/pme.12306

Elder, L., Paul, R., 2019. The thinker's guide to intellectual standards: The words that name them and the criteria that define them. Rowman & Littlefield.

Engel, G.L., 1977. The need for a new medical model: A challenge for biomedicine. Science 196 (4286), 129–136. https://doi.org/10.1126/science.847460

Epstein, R.M., Borrell-Carrió, F., 2005. The biopsychosocial model: Exploring six impossible things. Families, Systems, & Health 23 (4), 426.

Ferreira, P.H., Ferreira, M.L., Maher, C.G., Refshauge, K.M., Latimer, J., Adams, R.D., 2013. The therapeutic alliance between clinicians and patients predicts outcome in chronic low back pain. Phys Ther 93 (4), 470–478. https://doi.org/10.2522/ptj.20120137

Garcia, A.N., Costa, L., de Souza, F.S., de Almeida, M.O., Araujo, A.C., Hancock, M., et al., 2018. Reliability of the mechanical diagnosis and therapy system in patients with spinal pain: A systematic review. J Orthop Sports Phys Ther 48 (12), 923–933. https://doi.org/10.2519/jospt.2018.7876

Greenfield, B.H., Jensen, G.M., 2010. Understanding the lived experiences of patients: Application of a phenomenological approach to ethics. Phys Ther 90 (8), 1185–1197. https://doi.org/10.2522/ptj.20090348

Greenhalgh, T., Howick, J., Maskrey, N., 2014. Evidence based medicine: A movement in crisis? BMJ 348, g3725. https://doi.org/10.1136/bmj.g3725

Hall, A.M., Ferreira, P.H., Maher, C.G., Latimer, J., Ferreira, M.L., 2010. The influence of the therapist-patient relationship on treatment outcome in physical rehabilitation: A systematic review. Phys Ther 90 (8), 1099–1110. https://doi.org/10.2522/ptj.20090245

Hawkins, D., Elder,, L., Paul, R., 2019. The thinker's guide to clinical reasoning: Based on critical thinking concepts and tools. Rowman & Littlefield.

Higgs, J., Fish, D., Rothwell, R., 2008a. Knowledge generation and clinical reasoning in practice. In: Higgs, J., Jones, M.A., Loftus, S., Christensen, N. (Eds.), Clinical reasoning in the health professions, 3rd ed. Elsevier, pp. 163–172.

Higgs, J., Jones, M.A., Titchen, A., 2008b. Knowledge, reasoning and evidence for practice. In: Higgs, J., Jones, M.A., Loftus, S., Christensen, N. (Eds.), Clinical reasoning in the health professions, 3rd ed. Elsevier, pp. 151–161.

Horvath, B., 2004. A new process for writing clinical guidelines. Virtual Mentor 6 (12), 547–549. https://doi.org/10.1001/virtualmentor.2004.6.12.jdsc1-0412

Imrie, R., 2004. Demystifying disability: A review of the International Classification of Functioning, Disability and Health. Sociol Health Illn 26 (3), 287–305. https://doi.org/10.1111/j.1467-9566.2004.00391.x

Jensen, G., Gwyer, J., Hack, L., Mostrom, E., Nordstrom, T. (Eds.), 2019. Educating physical therapists. Slack.

Jensen, G., Gwyer, J.M., Hack, L.M., Shepard, K.F., 2007. Expertise in physical therapy practice, 2nd ed. Saunders-Elsevier.

Johnson, R., 1993. Attitudes don't just hang in the air …': Disabled people's perceptions of physiotherapists. Physiotherapy 79 (9), 619–627.

Jones, M., Grimmer, K., Edwards, I., Higgs, J., Trede, F., 2006. Challenges in applying best evidence to physiotherapy. Internet Journal of Allied Health Sciences and Practice 4 (3), 11.

Jones, M.A., Lewis, J.M., Hall, K., 2022. Clinical reasoning and shared decision making. In: Lewis, J., Fernandez-de-las-Penas, C. (Eds.), The shoulder: Theory & practice. Handspring Publishing, pp. 188–198.

Kahneman, D., 2011. Thinking, fast and slow. Farrar, Straus and Giroux.

Kahneman, D., Sibony, O., Sunstein, C.R. (2021). Noise: A flaw in human judgment. Hachette UK.

Karayannis, N.V., Jull, G.A., Hodges, P.W., 2012. Physiotherapy movement based classification approaches to low back pain:

Comparison of subgroups through review and developer/expert survey. BMC Musculoskelet Disord 13, 24. https://doi.org/10.1186/1471-2474-13-24

Kaufman, D.R., Yoskowitz, N.A., Patel, V.L., 2008. Clinical reasoning and biomedical knowledge: Implications for teaching. In: Higgs, J., Jones, M.A., Loftus, S., Christensen, N. (Eds.), Clinical reasoning in the health professions, 3rd ed. Elsevier, pp. 137–149.

Kerry, R., Madouasse, A., Arthur, A., Mumford, S.D., 2013. Analysis of scientific truth status in controlled rehabilitation trials. J Eval Clin Pract 19 (4), 617–625. https://doi.org/10.1111/j.1365-2753.2012.01855.x

Klaber Moffett, J.A., Richardson, P.H., 2009. The influence of the physiotherapist-patient relationship on pain and disability. Physiotherapy Theory and Practice 13 (1), 89–96. https://doi.org/10.3109/09593989709036451

Lackenbauer, W., Janssen, J., Roddam, H., Selfe, J., 2018. Keep/refer decision making abilities of European final year undergraduate physiotherapy students: A cross-sectional survey using clinical vignettes. European Journal of Physiotherapy 20 (3), 128–134.

Lehrer, J., 2010. How we decide. Houghton Mifflin Harcourt.

Matthias, M.S., Salyers, M.P., Frankel, R.M., 2013. Re-thinking shared decision-making: Context matters. Patient Educ Couns 91 (2), 176–179. https://doi.org/10.1016/j.pec.2013.01.006

Merleau-Ponty, M., 1962. Phenomenology of perception C. Smith, trans. Routledge & Kegan Paul, London.

Moseley, A.M., Elkins, M.R., Janer-Duncan, L., Hush, J.M., 2014. The quality of reports of randomized controlled trials varies between subdisciplines of physiotherapy. Physiother Can 66 (1), 36–43. https://doi.org/10.3138/ptc.2012-68

Musolino, G.M., Jensen, G.M., 2020. Clinical reasoning and decision making in physical therapy: Facilitation, assessment, and implementation. Slack Publications.

Panteli, D., Legido-Quigley, H., Reichebner, C., Ollenschläger, G., Schäfer, C., Busse, R., 2019. Clinical practice guidelines as a quality strategy. In: Busse, R., Klazinga, N., Panteli, D., Quentin, W. (Eds.), Improving healthcare quality in Europe: Characteristics, effectiveness and implementation of different strategies. European Observatory on Health Systems and Policies, pp. 233–264. https://www.ncbi.nlm.nih.gov/books/NBK549283/

Paul, R., Elder, L., 2007. A guide for educators to critical thinking competency standards. Foundation for Critical Thinking.

Payton, O.D., Nelson, C.E., Hobbs, M.S.C., 1998. Physical therapy patients' perceptions of their relationships with health care professionals. Physiotherapy Theory and Practice 14 (4), 211–221.

Ricoeur, P., 2006. In: Deneulin, S., Nebel, M., Sagovsky, N. (Eds.), Transforming unjust structures: The capability approach. Springer, pp. 17–26.

Riddle, D.L., Hillner, B.E., Wells, P.S., Johnson, R.E., Hoffman, H.J., Zuelzer, W.A., 2004. Diagnosis of lower-extremity deep vein thrombosis in outpatients with musculoskeletal disorders: A national survey study of physical therapists. Phys Ther 84 (8), 717–728. https://doi.org/10.1093/ptj/84.8.717

Sahrmann, S., Azevedo, D.C., Dillen, L.V., 2017. Diagnosis and treatment of movement system impairment syndromes. Braz J Phys Ther 21 (6), 391–399. https://doi.org/10.1016/j.bjpt.2017.08.001

Schneider, G.M., Jull, G., Thomas, K., Smith, A., Emery, C., Faris, P., et al., 2013. Intrarater and interrater reliability of select clinical tests in patients referred for diagnostic facet joint blocks in the cervical spine. Arch Phys Med Rehabil 94 (8), 1628–1634. https://doi.org/10.1016/j.apmr.2013.02.015

Schwartz, A., Elstein, A.S., 2008. Clinical reasoning in medicine. In: Higgs, J., Jones, M.A., Loftus, S., Christensen, N. (Eds.), Clinical reasoning in the health professions, 3rd ed. Elsevier, pp. 223–234.

Trede, F., Higgs, J., 2008. Collaborative decision making. In: Higgs, J., Jones, M.A., Loftus, S., Christensen, N. (Eds.), Clinical reasoning in the health professions, 3rd ed. Elsevier, pp. 31–41.

Vibe Fersum, K., O'Sullivan, P.B., Kvale, A., Skouen, J.S., 2009. Inter-examiner reliability of a classification system for patients with non-specific low back pain. Man Ther 14 (5), 555–561. https://doi.org/10.1016/j.math.2008.08.003

Villas Boas, P.J., Spagnuolo, R.S., Kamegasawa, A., Braz, L.G., Polachini do Valle, A., Jorge, E.C., et al., 2013. Systematic reviews showed insufficient evidence for clinical practice in 2004: What about in 2011? The next appeal for the evidence-based medicine age. J Eval Clin Pract 19 (4), 633–637. https://doi.org/10.1111/j.1365-2753.2012.01877.x

Walston, Z., Whelehan, D.F., O'Shea, N., 2022. Clinical decision making in physical therapy - Exploring the 'heuristic' in clinical practice. Musculoskelet Sci Pract 62, 102674. https://doi.org/10.1016/j.msksp.2022.102674

Weiner, S.J., 2022. Contextualizing care: An essential and measurable clinical competency. Patient Educ Couns 105 (3), 594–598. https://doi.org/10.1016/j.pec.2021.06.016

Wilson, C.M., Arena, S.K., Boright, L.E., 2022. State of the art physiotherapist-led approaches to safe aging in place. Arch Physiother 12 (1), 17. https://doi.org/10.1186/s40945-022-00142-5

Woolf, S., Schunemann, H.J., Eccles, M.P., Grimshaw, J.M., Shekelle, P., 2012. Developing clinical practice guidelines: Types of evidence and outcomes; values and economics, synthesis, grading, and presentation and deriving recommendations. Implement Sci 7, 61. https://doi.org/10.1186/1748-5908-7-61

25

CLINICAL REASONING IN DENTISTRY

SHIVA KHATAMI ■ MICHAEL MACENTEE ■
STEPHEN LOFTUS ■ HSINGCHI VON BERGMANN

CHAPTER OUTLINE

CHAPTER AIMS

The aims of this chapter are:

- to present a conceptual framework for clinical reasoning in dentistry
- to identify sources of uncertainty in clinical reasoning in dentistry
- to provide direction for future research and education of clinical reasoning in dentistry.

INTRODUCTION

Clinical reasoning is a core component of healthcare in which clinical problems are identified, explored, analysed and managed (Khatami et al., 2012). It involves a process of interacting with 'problem spaces' within a multilayered context of the clinician, the patient, the clinical problem and a larger social, cultural and global environment (see Chapter 11, 'The context of emerging clinical reasoning'); Higgs and Jones, 2008; Schuwirth et al., 2020). Clinical reasoning is the interactive and interpretive process to understand clinical situations, frame problems and make diagnostic and therapeutic decisions to solve those problems (Khatami et al., 2012).

A CONCEPTUAL FRAMEWORK

Evolution of Clinical Reasoning in Dentistry

The biomedical model dominated how health professions perceive and respond to health and disease (Parsons, 1951; Foucault, 1994; Adams, 1999) until clinicians became more sensitive to the psychosocial determinants of health (Engel, 1977; Frank et al., 2020; MacEntee, 2006; Marmot et al., 2008). Emphasis on the centrality of the patient supports the concept of health as a general feeling of physical, psychological and social well-being. This understanding of health includes culture and history and takes into account health and healthcare inequality (Pérez-Wilson et al., 2021).

Dentistry has seen a parallel evolution from treating only disease to treating the whole person within specific sociocultural contexts (Al-Sahan et al., 2020a; Baelum and Lopez, 2004; Khatami and MacEntee, 2011). A growing focus on prevention has highlighted the individual, social and behavioural context of diseases together with a need for equitable access to oral healthcare services (Watt et al., 2019). Indeed, data on oral health are difficult to interpret meaningfully because of uncertainty about the relevance of clinical measurements of oral conditions and how people feel about them (MacEntee and Mathu-Muju, 2014; Winkelmann et al., 2022). This uncertainty significantly influences how we perceive inequity in the global burden of oral diseases and access to care (Watt et al., 2019). The focus now on equity has broadened dental practice from mostly private dental clinics to include hospitals, schools, community-based clinics and long-term care facilities, along with an interprofessional approach to care (Field, 1995; Formicola et al., 2006). The advent of telemedicine and teledentistry extends even further the context of dental practice from physical to virtual interactions with patients and peers (Howell and Fukuoka, 2022). All these changes have had implications for dental education and how we teach clinical reasoning.

Following the Institute of Medicine report (Field, 1995), dental educators were also challenged to accommodate a broader awareness of environmental and psychosocial determinants of health in an already crowded professional curriculum focussed narrowly on science and psychomotor skills (MacEntee, 2010; Polverini, 2017). Alternative curricular models emerged promoting problem-solving skills, developing competencies and community-service learning, although their effectiveness in developing and assessing how dentists make decisions is unclear, probably because of our limited understanding of the process of clinical reasoning (Khatami and MacEntee, 2011; Yazdani and Abardeh, 2019).

Exploring Clinical Reasoning

Clinical reasoning in dentistry, as in other healthcare disciplines, has a broad focus encompassing prevention, biological diagnosis and treatment of diseases from the perspectives of society and individual patients (Khatami and MacEntee, 2011). Inconsistencies in diagnosis and treatment planning emphasize the need for better diagnostic tests with more sensitivity and specificity, better practice guidance and improved decision-support systems for dentists (Kay et al., 1992; Kawahata and MacEntee, 2002). Decision-support systems are now being influenced by artificial intelligence (AI). AI is having impacts across many disciplines and professions. There are many unanswered questions about AI that will need to be explored in coming years. To what extent do we allow AI to make decisions for

us or do we restrict AI to providing suggestions for us to consider? How do AI systems shape our communications with them and with others? Brand (2020), for example, makes the controversial claim that although AI systems cannot think the way that humans do, they can answer moral problems. It is clear that the moral and ethical implications of using AI are yet to be worked out in detail. We maintain, however, that clinicians should continue to be the principal custodians of the moral and ethical implications of those decisions (Schwendicke et al., 2020; Mörch et al., 2021; Pereira, 2021). Many AI systems build on existing efforts to support clinical reasoning from the field of medical decision theory.

Medical Decision Theory

Decision analysis, preference-based measurement, rating scales, standard gamble techniques, time trade-offs, quality-adjusted life (tooth) years, game theory and Bayesian-based utility measures have all been applied as theoretical foundations for exploring decision making within the general context of medical decision theory (Matthews et al., 1999).

Decision analysis applies a sequential process of developing and revising diagnostic and treatment decisions by constructing and proceeding along the trunk and branches of decision trees (Kawahata and MacEntee, 2002). Bayesian-like rules are applied to weigh all possible decisions by identifying the expected outcomes, estimating their probability, evaluating their risks and benefits and assigning a utility value to each. The probability and utility values are then evaluated to reach the most reasonable decision within the clinical context of the decision. However, Chambers et al. (2010) found that applications of Bayesian formulas to epidemiological data were not a typical part of how dental students or experienced dentists made decisions about the presence or prognosis of disease. The absence or uncertainty of sufficient available evidence frequently compromises confidence in the diagnosis (MacEntee and Mathu-Muju, 2014). Moreover, rational treatment decisions based on the rules of decision analysis can conflict with a patient's preferences and a clinician's ethical principles (Weir et al., 2017). Decision trees also require a certain degree of artistry in their design and the creativity for constructing and interpreting them can contradict the conceptual framework of decision theory which is based on logic. Even so, medical decision theory has been used as the basis for computer-based decision support systems.

Decision Support Systems

Bayes' theorem informed the development of earlier computer-based decision support systems for diagnosis and treatment planning in dentistry (e.g. Sims-Williams et al., 1987), followed by neural networks (e.g. Brickley and Shepherd, 1996) and fuzzy logic (e.g. Wang et al., 2016). There has also been an emphasis on language, symbols and semantics within the context of dentistry even in the presence of uncertainty (Kawahata and MacEntee, 2002). Symbolic computations, such as fuzzy logic, for example, offer the possibility of managing uncertainty in rule-based clinical decisions (Zadeh, 2008; Amirkhani et al., 2017). However, decision support systems are essentially reductionist methods for solving problems and pose ethical and legal concerns without empirical evidence to support the decision recommended (Mörch et al., 2021). Computerized systems cannot always manage the multilayered meanings within the clinical interactions between patient and dentist (Loftus, 2015), although they offer educational opportunities for simulating diagnostic and treatment decisions on virtual patients (Cook et al., 2010). In response to the challenge of managing complexity in clinical reasoning in dentistry we offer a conceptual framework that integrates many of the factors involved (Fig. 25.1).

A Framework for Dentists

The multilayered context of clinical reasoning can be viewed as a group of overlapping ovals integrating oral problems within the perspectives of the dentist, the patient and the larger healthcare environment, supplemented by scientific, conditional, collaborative, narrative, ethical, pragmatic and part-whole reasoning strategies (Fig. 25.1).

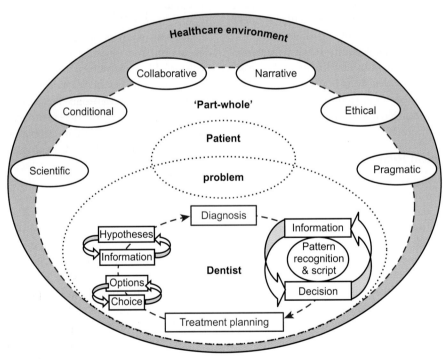

Fig. 25.1 ■ A conceptual framework of strategies for clinical reasoning in dentistry. (With permission from Khatami, S., MacEntee, M. I., Pratt, D. D., Collins, J. B., 2012. Clinical reasoning in dentistry: A conceptual framework for dental education. J. Dent. Educ. 76(9), 1116–1128.)

Reasoning Strategies

Scientific

The hypothetico-deductive (HD) process of reasoning follows a scientific method of systematically observing, measuring and collecting information, followed by the formation, testing and modification of a list of tentative diagnoses. An experienced clinician uses their experience, together with methodical reasoning, to evaluate the findings and reach a definitive diagnosis (Khatami et al., 2012; Schuwirth et al., 2020). Most dentists take a systematic approach with appropriate diagnostic aids to explore and interpret a patient's psychosocial history and clinical status. They plan the content and sequence of treatment by dealing with any acute disorder before rehabilitating and stabilizing long-term function. Familiarity with the routines (and rituals) of this approach in many instances achieves the goal of a diagnosis through a mixture of conscious and subconscious decisions. Indeed, experienced dentists have mental routines that enable rapid and efficient gathering and processing of all relevant information (Benner et al., 2011).

Conditional

Using a conditional approach means that provisional measures may be taken before every effort is made to reduce uncertainty to an acceptable level before any irreversible decision is made.

Collaborative

Communications between patient and clinician mean that responsibility can be shared when deciding treatment, especially when treatment options may challenge a patient's original beliefs and expectations (Al-Sahan et al., 2020b).

Narrative

This strategy assumes that the general experience and multilayered meaning of disease and health of patients is organized into a story, perhaps an illness narrative. Dentists need to work with patients' stories as these stories influence health-related behaviours and expected treatment outcomes. This might include stories of previous encounters with similar problems that help make sense of the current situation (Al-Sahan et al., 2020a).

Ethical

Principle-based ethics have tended to dominate how many dentists resolve ethical problems. There are alternatives such as the ethics of virtue and narrative. These may provide greater scope for dealing with the difficulties of clinical uncertainty (Charon et al., 2016). The ethics of virtue relies on the development of moral character. This approach encourages personal reflections on strengths, weaknesses and the nuances encountered in particular cases, rather than the broad generalities of the principle-based approach (Geisler, 2006; Oakley, 2016).

Pragmatic

The pragmatic approach to the social, economic and political environment of healthcare permeates all clinical practice. Clinicians must temper their idealism with realistic and practical offerings of care and confront challenges to resources, risks and benefits, and cost-effectiveness of treatment. All this must occur within the context of the dentist's own cognitive and technical skills (Schell, 2008).

Part-Whole Approach

Several reasoning strategies are used to focus in and out of different conceptual spaces, refocus on different aspects of a clinical problem, move from one problem to another, and relate it all to the patient as a whole (Rama Fiorini et al., 2014). The clinical encounter can be seen in hermeneutic terms because the dentist must carefully interpret many parts, such as clinical findings, clinical ability and patient expectations to create a whole, a diagnosis and treatment plan that is acceptable to all (Svenaeus, 2000).

Backward-Deductive and Forward-Inductive Approach

It has been shown that experienced professionals can reason both forwards or backwards as they analyse and diagnose problems (Laufer and Glick, 1996). When they reason forward, experienced practitioners select a small number of tentative or preliminary diagnoses that they are willing to change as more information emerges. Novices, in contrast, often prefer a backward process of reasoning where they quickly form one diagnosis to which they may remain steadfastly attached despite emerging information that this might be wrong (McKendry, 2015).

Pattern-Recognition and Scripts

Visual and descriptive cues often help dentists quickly and easily recognize the pattern of specific diseases, such as dental caries, periodontal disease and other abnormalities. This recognition allows them to bypass the more laborious processes of making and testing hypotheses (Weir et al., 2017). Demineralized lesions on teeth, for example, present in a range of colours and textures from which dentists can identify a pattern recognized from previous clinical experiences (Maupomé et al., 2010). Nonetheless, assessing the aetiology and risk of dental caries and tooth loss can require a more elaborate exploration that extends from physical to psychosocial considerations (Baelum, 2010). The 'caries scripts' often consist of information about the composition of saliva and oral bacteria and details of a patient's diet, hygiene and socioeconomic status leading to an assessment of caries risk and therapeutic options. Similarly, visual cues about the normal versus abnormal appearance of gingiva and periodontium trigger the scripts for gingivitis and periodontal disease (Baelum and López, 2004). However, to classify the severity of each disease and appropriate treatment, additional historical, behavioural, social, economic, clinical and possibly radiographic information is required (Watt et al., 2019).

Decision Analysis

As mentioned earlier, most dentists do not quantify the probability or utility value associated with Bayes theorem. Medical Decision Theory claims to be normative (how practitioners should act). However, descriptive studies show that practitioners integrate their knowledge and practical experience to interpret the problem, deal with uncertainty and select treatment options (Chambers et al., 2010; Khatami et al., 2012). Examples are the descriptive studies that show how hermeneutics and narrative play a central role in integrating knowledge into decisions, even though many practitioners are not familiar with these concepts (Svenaeus, 2000; Loftus and Greenhalgh, 2010).

REFLECTION POINT

A Clinical Challenge

Angela is a 74-year-old retired teacher who consults you with Wendy, her daughter, who explains that her mother does not speak English. They have consulted three dentists recently about the sensitivity to cold drinks from an incisor tooth. They are anxious because of the cost of dental treatment.

Angela is hypertensive, which is under control, and has early signs of Parkinson's disease.

Her upper left central incisor, with a ceramic crown, is very sensitive to cold. She has no posterior teeth and her lower incisors are very abraded, but this does not bother her.

To minimize the cost of treatment for this and future dental problems, Wendy asks if her mother should have complete dentures.

How might your social background and professional experience influence your care for Angela?

UNCERTAINTY IN CLINICAL REASONING

The uncertainties of clinical practice challenge all clinicians, whether novice or mature practitioners. Many students struggle with three domains of uncertainty. The first domain is the boundaries of available knowledge. The second domain is their incomplete mastery of the knowledge and skills they have acquired. The third domain arises from the first two and is the difficulty in distinguishing between personal ignorance and the limitations of present knowledge (Beresford, 1991; Khatami, 2010; Lukšaitė et al., 2022). Han et al. (2011) claimed that it is not necessary to eliminate uncertainty but to accept and acknowledge it. They proposed a three-dimensional taxonomy of uncertainty that they state can help us to clarify the many sources of uncertainty so that we can deal with them more effectively. Katz (1984) suggested that being honest with patients about our uncertainty can, in fact, be reassuring for patients about our sincerity. Katz goes on to say that being honest and sincere about uncertainty with patients is one way of taking advantage of the placebo effect because honesty builds trust.

However, it is claimed that many clinicians still deceive themselves and their patients to create an illusion of certainty that can be subject to risks from flawed or deceptive reasoning (Katz, 1984; Knafl and Burkett, 1975; MacEntee and Mathu-Muju, 2014). More experienced clinicians, however, are more likely to accept uncertainty and develop a 'professional rhetoric' to manage uncertainty when communicating with colleagues (Lingard et al., 2003). This need to master a professional rhetoric shows that dealing with uncertainty in clinical reasoning is both an art and a science (MacEntee, 2007; MacEntee and Mathu-Muju, 2014).

Other sources of uncertainty range from different philosophies of care to rapid scientific advances (Knafl and Burkett, 1975; MacEntee and Mathu-Muju, 2014; Nadanovsky and Sheiham, 1995; Watt et al., 2019). There are many examples of how advances in biomaterials, computer-aided design and computer-aided manufacturing (CAD/CAM) add more to the uncertainty of treatment (Marinello, 2016; Mörch et al., 2021). In addition, the validity of diagnostic indicators for caries, periodontal disease and other mouth disorders are all subject to serious interpretive challenges (Baelum, 2010; Baelum and López, 2004; Fuller et al., 2015; Buenahora et al., 2021; Nadanovsky and Sheiham, 1995).

The clinical reasoning of dentists is under pressure from other sources. Commercial interests may also influence the demand for specific dental treatments and approaches to care even if untested or lacking robust evidence (Jerrold and Karkhanehchi, 2000; Kearns et al., 2015; MacEntee, 2005; Mialon, 2020; Newsome and Langley, 2014). Discrepancies in priorities of treatment objectives by clinicians, patients and third-party payers compounded by commercial interests can create ethical conflicts. The cost of treatment is also a strong influence on how patients and clinicians rationalize and make treatment choices (Spinler et al., 2021; Vernazza et al., 2015). Furthermore, unclear definitions for standards of care can cause moral and ethical dilemmas, fear of litigation and clinical decisions to provide less than appropriate care (Bryant et al., 1995; Smith and Thomson, 2017). However, growing sensitivity to the social determinants of health and the benefits of intersectional or transdisciplinary care challenge dental professionals to extend their clinical reasoning beyond traditional limits (MacEntee, 2011; Muirhead et al., 2020; Wallace et al., 2015). Unfortunately, dental education does not always acknowledge that uncertainty is an integral and substantially unavoidable aspect of clinical reasoning (von Bergmann and Shuler, 2019).

REFLECTION POINT

- How do you keep up-to-date with changing knowledge in the profession?
- What ethical issues do you confront in your practice and how do you deal with them?

ASSESSING AND TEACHING CLINICAL REASONING

Dentists develop a professional identity that shapes how they approach clinical challenges. Professional identity is shaped by factors of the learning environment, such as the pressure to be technically proficient, role modelling and mentoring, and the development of reflective skills as part of their clinical reasoning skills that should continue developing throughout their careers (Kwon et al., 2022). However, teaching and assessing these skills poses challenges for dental educators (Khatami and MacEntee, 2011). There is limited evidence that problem-based learning (PBL) methods and the HD model of problem solving enhance the critical reasoning of dental students unless presented in a clinical context that is relevant and familiar to students (von Bergmann et al., 2007; Whitney et al., 2016). Similarly, assessment of competency should acknowledge the practical context and complexity of the clinical setting (Kelleher et al., 2021; MacEntee, 1996; Paley, 2004; Thorne and Sawatzky, 2014).

The HD model has been the dominant theory explaining how experienced dentists should search for, identify and organize key points of information and generate a diagnosis (Crespo et al., 2004). Dental students are taught to start by generating a list of hypotheses and working backwards to confirm or reject each hypothesis. Experts are usually more rapid and rely on experience to recognize patterns or illness scripts from previous clinical encounters (Charlin et al., 2000). Experienced dentists typically recognize dental caries, for example, from a mental script that relates to the colour and size of demineralized dental lesions

(Bader and Shugars, 1997). Rapid pattern recognition has been called System 1 thinking and the more deliberative and analytical thinking, System 2 (Kahnemann, 2011). According to Maupomé et al. (2010), dental students often use a more laborious dual processing model with HD reasoning and pattern recognition together. However, the accuracy of one system over the other is unclear (Norman et al., 2017; Weir et al., 2017). There are other approaches to understanding and teaching clinical reasoning such as the use of narrative.

A narrative approach allows the subjective experience, beliefs and expectations of patients to be integrated into the biomedical story (Loftus, 2015). Allowing patients to tell their stories and validating their experience can be therapeutic in itself. Health professionals, such as dentists, need to develop a narrative sensitivity towards patients. A narrative sensitivity can develop into practical wisdom or phronesis. Phronesis is the ability to customize care for this particular patient, in this particular time and place, under these particular circumstances. The development of phronesis is helped by reflection on the challenges of practice ideally with an experienced mentor and becomes an important part of the professional identity of the dentist (Kinsella and Pitman, 2012).

SUMMARY

The clinical reasoning of dentists can be complex and can be viewed from a number of perspectives. The conceptual framework model (Fig. 25.1) shows many of the perspectives that can be considered in clinical reasoning. We now accept that the wider context of clinical practice, such as sociocultural influences, and access to resources can shape the clinical reasoning that needs to occur. Clinical reasoning can be viewed as thinking backwards or forwards or a mixture of the two. Clinical reasoning can also be seen in terms of rapid pattern recognition or more careful analytical deliberation or a mixture of the two. We can view clinical reasoning from the perspective of logic and medical decision analysis or from the perspective of narrative interpretation. A major concern is how we manage uncertainty. Related to this is the challenge of working with change in many formats such as the need to work with AI. All these influences help to shape the professional identity of a dentist who is ethical,

constantly working to improve and humble enough to accept the limits of their own abilities. Clinical reasoning is at the heart of all this.

REFERENCES

Adams, T., 1999. Dentistry and medical dominance. Social Science & Medicine 48 (3), 407–420. https://doi.org/10.1016/s0277-9536(98)00316-5

Al-Sahan, M.M., MacEntee, M.I., Bryant, S.R., 2020a. A metatheory explaining how patients manage tooth loss. Gerodontology 37 (3), 258–270. https://doi.org/10.1111/ger.12457

Al-Sahan, M.M., MacEntee, M.I., Thorne, S., Bryant, S.R., 2020b. A qualitative synthesis of theories on psychosocial response to loss of breasts, limbs or teeth. Journal of Dentistry 103S, 100014. https://doi.org/10.1016/j.jjodo.2020.100014

Amirkhani, A., Papageorgiou, E.I., Mohseni, A., Mosavi, M.R., 2017. A review of fuzzy cognitive maps in medicine: Taxonomy, methods, and applications. Computer Methods and Programs in Biomedicine 142, 129–145. https://doi.org/10.1016/j.cmpb.2017.02.021

Bader, J.D., Shugars, D.A., 1997. What do we know about how dentists make caries-related treatment decisions? Community Dentistry and Oral Epidemiology 25 (1), 97–103. https://doi.org/10.1111/j.1600-0528.1997.tb00905.x

Baelum, V., Lopez, R., 2004. Periodontal epidemiology: Towards social science or molecular biology? Community Dentistry and Oral Epidemiology 32 (4), 239–249. https://doi.org/10.1111/j.1600-0528.2004.00159.x

Baelum, V., 2010. What is an appropriate caries diagnosis? Acta Odontologica Scandinavica 68 (2), 65–79. https://doi.org/10.3109/00016350903530786

Benner, P.E., Hooper-Kyriakidis, P.L., Stannard, D., 2011. Clinical wisdom and interventions in acute and critical care: A thinking-in-action approach. Springer Publishing Company.

Beresford, E.B., 1991. Uncertainty and the shaping of medical decisions. Hastings Center Report 21 (4), 6–11.

Brand, L., 2020. Why machines that talk still do not think, and why they might nevertheless be able to solve moral problems. In: Göcke, B.P., Rosenthal-von der Pütten, A. (Eds.), Artificial intelligence: Reflections in philosophy, theology and the social sciences. Brill Mentis, pp. 203–217.

Brickley, M.R., Shepherd, J.P., 1996. Performance of a neural network trained to make third-molar treatment-planning decisions. Medical Decision Making: An International Journal of the Society for Medical Decision Making 16 (2), 153–160. https://doi.org/10.1177/0272989X9601600207

Bryant, S.R., MacEntee, M.I., Browne, A., 1995. Ethical issues encountered by dentists in the care of institutionalized elders. Special Care in Dentistry: Official Publication of the American Association of Hospital Dentists, the Academy of Dentistry for the Handicapped, and the American Society for Geriatric Dentistry 15 (2), 79–82. https://doi.org/10.1111/j.1754-4505.1995.tb00482.x

Buenahora, M.R., Peraza-L, A., Díaz-Báez, D., Bustillo, J., Santacruz, I., Trujillo, T.G., et al., 2021. Diagnostic accuracy of clinical visualization and light-based tests in precancerous and cancerous lesions of the oral cavity and oropharynx: A systematic review and meta-analysis. Clinical Oral Investigations 25 (6), 4145–4159. https://doi.org/10.1007/s00784-020-03746-y

Chambers, D.W., Mirchel, R., Lundergan, W., 2010. An investigation of dentists' and dental students' estimates of diagnostic probabilities. Journal of the American Dental Association 141 (6), 656–666. https://doi.org/10.14219/jada.archive.2010.0253

Charlin, B., Tardif, J., Boshuizen, H.P., 2000. Scripts and medical diagnostic knowledge: Theory and applications for clinical reasoning instruction and research. Academic Medicine: Journal of the Association of American Medical Colleges 75 (2), 182–190. https://doi.org/10.1097/00001888-200002000-00020

Charon, R., DasGupta, S., Hermann, N., Irvine, C., Marcus, E.R., Colsn, E.R., et al., 2016. The principles and practice of narrative medicine. Oxford University Press.

Cook, D.A., Erwin, P.J., Triola, M.M., 2010. Computerized virtual patients in health professions education: A systematic review and meta-analysis. Academic Medicine: Journal of the Association of American Medical Colleges 85 (10), 1589–1602. https://doi.org/10.1097/ACM.0b013e3181edfe13

Crespo, K.E., Torres, J.E., Recio, M.E., 2004. Reasoning process characteristics in the diagnostic skills of beginner, competent, and expert dentists. Journal of Dental Education 68 (12), 1235–1244.

Engel, G.L., 1977. The need for a new medical model: A challenge for biomedicine. Science 196 (4286), 129–136. https://doi.org/10.1126/science.847460

Field, M.J. (Ed.), 1995. Dental education at the crossroads: Challenges and change. National Academies Press.

Foucault, M., 1994. The birth of the clinic: An archaeology of medical perception. Pantheon Books.

Formicola, A.J., Myers, R., Hasler, J.F., Peterson, M., Dodge, W., Bailit, H.L., et al., 2006. Evolution of dental school clinics as patient care delivery centers. Journal of Dental Education 70 (12), 1271–1288.

Frank, J., Abel, T., Campostrini, S., Cook, S., Lin, V.K., McQueen, D.V., 2020. The social determinants of health: Time to re-think? International Journal of Environmental Research and Public Health 17 (16), 5856. https://doi.org/10.3390/ijerph17165856

Fuller, C., Camilon, R., Nguyen, S., Jennings, J., Day, T., Gillespie, M.B., 2015. Adjunctive diagnostic techniques for oral lesions of unknown malignant potential: Systematic review with meta-analysis. Head & Neck 37 (5), 755–762. https://doi.org/10.1002/hed.23667

Geisler, S.L., 2006. The value of narrative ethics to medicine. The Journal of Physician Assistant Education 17 (2), 54–57.

Han, P.K., Klein, W.M., Arora, N.K., 2011. Varieties of uncertainty in health care: A conceptual taxonomy. Medical Decision Making: An International Journal of the Society for Medical Decision Making 31 (6), 828–838. https://doi.org/10.1177/0272989x11393976

Higgs, J., Jones, N., 2008. Clinical decision making and multiple problem spaces. In: Higgs, J., Jones, M.A., Loftus, S., Christensen, N. (Eds.), Clinical reasoning in the health professions. Butterworth-Heinemann, pp. 3–18.

Howell, S.E., & Fukuoka, B., 2022. Teledentistry for patient-centered screening and assessment. Dental Clinics 66 (2), 195–208.

Jerrold, L., Karkhanehchi, H., 2000. Advertising, commercialism, and professionalism: A history of the ethics of advertising in dentistry. The Journal of the American College of Dentists 67 (4), 39–44.

Kahnemann, D., 2011. Thinking fast and slow. Farrar, Straus and Giroux.

Katz, J., 1984. Why doctors don't disclose uncertainty. Hastings Center Report 14 (1), 35–44.

Kawahata, N., MacEntee, M.I., 2002. A measure of agreement between clinicians and a computer-based decision support system for planning dental treatment. Journal of Dental Education 66 (9), 1031–1037.

Kay, E.J., Nuttall, N.M., Knill-Jones, R., 1992. Restorative treatment thresholds and agreement in treatment decision-making. Community Dentistry and Oral Epidemiology 20 (5), 265–268. https://doi.org/10.1111/j.1600-0528.1992.tb01696.x

Kearns, C.E., Glantz, S.A., Schmidt, L.A., 2015. Sugar industry influence on the scientific agenda of the National Institute of Dental Research's 1971 National Caries Program: A historical analysis of internal documents. PLoS Medicine 12 (3), e1001798. https://doi.org/10.1371/journal.pmed.1001798

Kelleher, M., Kinnear, B., Sall, D.R., Weber, D.E., DeCoursey, B., Nelson, J., et al., 2021. Warnings in early narrative assessment that might predict performance in residency: Signal from an internal medicine residency program. Perspectives on Medical Education 10 (6), 334–340. https://doi.org/10.1007/s40037-021-00681-w

Khatami, S. (2010). Clinical reasoning in dentistry (Doctoral dissertation, University of British Columbia). https://open.library.ubc.ca/soa/cIRcle/collections/ubctheses/24/items/1.0071103 (accessed 02.02.23).

Khatami, S., MacEntee, M.I., 2011. Evolution of clinical reasoning in dental education. Journal of Dental Education 75 (3), 321–328.

Khatami, S., MacEntee, M.I., Pratt, D.D., Collins, J.B., 2012. Clinical reasoning in dentistry: A conceptual framework for dental education. Journal of Dental Education 76 (9), 1116–1128.

Kinsella, E.A., Pitman, A. (Eds.), 2012. Phronesis as professional knowledge: Practical wisdom in the professions, vol. 1. Springer Science & Business Media.

Knafl, K., Burkett, G., 1975. Professional socialization in a surgical specialty: Acquiring medical judgment. Social Science & Medicine 9 (7), 397–404. https://doi.org/10.1016/0037-7856(75)90140-7

Kwon, J.H., Shuler, C.F., von Bergmann, H., 2022. Professional identity formation: The key contributors and dental students' concerns. Journal of Dental Education 86 (3), 288–297. https://doi.org/10.1002/jdd.12810

Laufer, E.A., Glick, J., 1996. Expert and novice differences in cognition and activity: A practical work activity. In: Engeström, Y., Middleton, D. (Eds.), Cognition and communication at work. Cambridge University Press, pp. 177–198.

Lingard, L., Garwood, K., Schryer, C.F., Spafford, M.M., 2003. A certain art of uncertainty: Case presentation and the development of professional identity. Social Science & Medicine 56 (3), 603–616. https://doi.org/10.1016/s0277-9536(02)00057-6

Loftus, S., 2015. Embodiment in the practice and education of health professionals. In: Green, B., Hopwood, N. (Eds.), Body/Practice:

The body in professional practice, learning and education. Springer, pp. 139–156.

Loftus, S., Greenhalgh, T., 2010. Towards a narrative mode of practice. In: Higgs, J., Fish, D., Goulter, I., Loftus, S., Reid, J., Trede, F. (Eds.), Education for future practice. Sense, pp. 85–94.

Lukšaitė, E., Fricker, R.A., McKinley, R.K., Dikomitis, L., 2022. Conceptualising and teaching biomedical uncertainty to medical students: An exploratory qualitative study. Medical Science Educator 32 (2), 371–378. https://doi.org/10.1007/s40670-021-01481-x

MacEntee, M.I., 1996. Measuring the impact of oral health in old age: A qualitative reaction to some quantitative views. Gerodontology 13 (2), 76–81. https://doi.org/10.1111/j.1741-2358.1996.tb00158.x

MacEntee, M., 2005. Prosthodontics: Have we misjudged the cause and lost direction? The International Journal of Prosthodontics 18 (3), 185–187.

MacEntee, M.I., 2006. An existential model of oral health from evolving views on health, function and disability. Community Dental Health 23 (1), 5–14.

MacEntee, M.I., 2007. Where science fails prosthodontics. The International Journal of Prosthodontics 20 (4), 377.

MacEntee, M.I., 2010. The educational challenge of dental geriatrics. Journal of Dental Education 74 (1), 13–19.

MacEntee, M.I., 2011. Muted dental voices on interprofessional healthcare teams. Journal of Dentistry 39 (Suppl 2), S34–S40. https://doi.org/10.1016/j.jdent.2011.10.017

MacEntee, M.I., Mathu-Muju, K.R., 2014. Confronting dental uncertainty in old age. Gerodontology 31 (Suppl 1), 37–43. https://doi.org/10.1111/ger.12109

Marinello, C., 2016. The digital revolution in prosthodontics: Can it benefit older people? Gerodontology 33 (2), 145–146. https://doi.org/10.1111/ger.12228

Marmot, M., Friel, S., Bell, R., Houweling, T.A., Taylor, S., Commission on Social Determinants of Health, 2008. Closing the gap in a generation: Health equity through action on the social determinants of health. Lancet 372 (9650), 1661–1669. https://doi.org/10.1016/S0140-6736(08)61690-6

Matthews, D.C., Gafni, A., Birch, S., 1999. Preference based measurements in dentistry: A review of the literature and recommendations for research. Community Dental Health 16 (1), 5–11.

Maupomé, G., Schrader, S., Mannan, S., Garetto, L., Eggertsson, H., 2010. Diagnostic thinking and information used in clinical decision-making: A qualitative study of expert and student dental clinicians. BMC Oral Health 10, 11. https://doi.org/10.1186/1472-6831-10-11

McKendry, S., 2015. Critical thinking skills for healthcare. Routledge.

Mialon, M., 2020. An overview of the commercial determinants of health. Global Health 16 (1), 74. https://doi.org/10.1186/s12992-020-00607-x

Mörch, C.M., Atsu, S., Cai, W., Li, X., Madathil, S.A., Liu, X., et al., 2021. Artificial intelligence and ethics in dentistry: A scoping review. Journal of Dental Research 100, 1452–1460. https://doi.org/10.1177/00220345211013808

Muirhead, V.E., Milner, A., Freeman, R., Doughty, J., Macdonald, M.E., 2020. What is intersectionality and why is it important in oral health research? Community Dentistry and Oral Epidemiology 48 (6), 464–470. https://doi.org/10.1111/cdoe.12573

Nadanovsky, P., Sheiham, A., 1995. Relative contribution of dental services to the changes in caries levels of 12-year-old children in 18 industrialized countries in the 1970s and early 1980s. Community Dentistry and Oral Epidemiology 23 (6), 331–339. https://doi.org/10.1111/j.1600-0528.1995.tb00258.x

Newsome, P.R., Langley, P.P., 2014. Professionalism, then and now. British Dental Journal 216 (9), 497–502. https://doi.org/10.1038/sj.bdj.2014.355

Norman, G.R., Monteiro, S.D., Sherbino, J., Ilgen, J.S., Schmidt, H.G., Mamede, S., 2017. The causes of errors in clinical reasoning: Cognitive biases, knowledge deficits, and dual process thinking. Academic Medicine: Journal of the Association of American Medical Colleges 92 (1), 23–30. https://doi.org/10.1097/ACM.0000000000001421

Oakley, J., 2016. Virtue ethics and public policy: Upholding medical virtue in therapeutic relationships as a case study. The Journal of Value Inquiry 50, 769–779.

Paley, J., 2004. Clinical cognition and embodiment. International Journal of Nursing Studies 41 (1), 1–13. https://doi.org/10.1016/s0020-7489(03)00081-6

Parsons, T., 1951. The social system. The Free Press.

Pereira, L.M., 2021. The carousel of ethical machinery. AI & Society 36, 185–196. https://doi.org/10.1007/s00146-020-00994-0

Pérez-Wilson, P., Marcos-Marcos, J., Morgan, A., Eriksson, M., Lindström, B., Álvarez-Dardet, C., 2021. 'A synergy model of health': An integration of salutogenesis and the health assets model. Health Promotion International 36 (3), 884–894. https://doi.org/10.1093/heapro/daaa084 PMID: 32968813

Polverini, P.J., 2017. Oral health research and scholarship in 2040: Executive summary. Journal of Dental Education 81 (9), 1137–1143. https://doi.org/10.21815/JDE.017.070

Rama Fiorini, S., Gärdenfors, P., Abel, M., 2014. Representing part-whole relations in conceptual spaces. Cognitive Processing 15 (2), 127–142. https://doi.org/10.1007/s10339-013-0585-x

Schell, B.A.B., 2008. Pragmatic reasoning. In: Schell, B.A.B., Schell, J.W. (Eds.), Clinical and professional reasoning in occupational therapy. Lippincott Williams & Wilkins, pp. 169–187.

Schuwirth, L.W.T., Durning, S.J., King, S.M., 2020. Assessment of clinical reasoning: Three evolutions of thought. Diagnosis 7 (3), 191–196. https://doi.org/10.1515/dx-2019-0096

Schwendicke, F., Samek, W., Krois, J., 2020. Artificial intelligence in dentistry: Chances and challenges. Journal of Dental Research 99 (7), 769–774. https://doi.org/10.1177/0022034520915714

Sims-Williams, J.H., Brown, I.D., Matthewman, A., Stephens, C.D., 1987. A computer-controlled expert system for orthodontic advice. British Dental Journal 163 (5), 161–166. https://doi.org/10.1038/sj.bdj.4806228

Spinler, K., Aarabi, G., Walther, C., Valdez, R., Heydecke, G., Buczak-Stec, E., et al., 2021. Determinants of dental treatment avoidance: Findings from a nationally representative study. Aging Clinical and Experimental Research 33 (5), 1337–1343. https://doi.org/10.1007/s40520-020-01652-7

Smith, M.B., Thomson, W.M., 2017. 'Not on the radar': Dentists' perspectives on the oral health care of dependent older people. Gerodontology 34 (1), 90–100. https://doi.org/10.1111/ger.12227

Svenaeus, F., 2000. The hermeneutics of medicine and the phenomenology of health: Steps towards a philosophy of medical practice. Kluwer Academic Publishers.

Thorne, S., Sawatzky, R., 2014. Particularizing the general: Sustaining theoretical integrity in the context of an evidence-based practice agenda. Advances in Nursing Science 37 (1), 5–18. https://doi.org/10.1097/ANS.0000000000000011

Vernazza, C.R., Rousseau, N., Steele, J.G., Ellis, J.S., Thomason, J.M., Eastham, J., et al., 2015. Introducing high-cost health care to patients: Dentists' accounts of offering dental implant treatment. Community Dentistry and Oral Epidemiology 43 (1), 75–85. https://doi.org/10.1111/cdoe.12129

von Bergmann, H., Dalrymple, K.R., Wong, S., Shuler, C.F., 2007. Investigating the relationship between PBL process grades and content acquisition performance in a PBL dental program. Journal of Dental Education 71 (9), 1160–1170.

von Bergmann, H., Shuler, C.F., 2019. The culture of certainty in dentistry and its impact on dental education and Practice. Journal of Dental Education 83 (6), 609–613. https://doi.org/10.21815/JDE.019.075

Wallace, B.B., MacEntee, M.I., Pauly, B., 2015. Community dental clinics in British Columbia, Canada: Examining the potential as health equity interventions. Health & Social Care in the Community 23 (4), 371–379. https://doi.org/10.1111/hsc.12151

Wang, K.J., Chen, K.H., Huang, S.H., Teng, N.C., 2016. A prognosis tool based on fuzzy anthropometric and questionnaire data for obstructive sleep apnea severity. Journal of Medical Systems 40 (4), 110. https://doi.org/10.1007/s10916-016-0464-y

Wasserman, J., Loftus, S., 2023. Changing demographic and cultural dimensions of populations: Implications for healthcare and decision-making. In: Higgs, J., Jensen, G., Loftus, S., Christensen, N. (Eds.), Clinical reasoning in the health professions, 5th ed. Elsevier, Edinburgh, pp. XX.

Watt, R.G., Daly, B., Allison, P., Macpherson, L., Venturelli, R., Listl, S., et al., 2019. Ending the neglect of global oral health: Time for radical action. Lancet 394 (10194), 261–272. https://doi.org/10.1016/S0140-6736(19)31133-X

Weir, C.R., Rubin, M.A., Nebeker, J., Samore, M., 2017. Modeling the mind: How do we design effective decision-support? Journal of Biomedical Informatics 71S, S1–S5. https://doi.org/10.1016/j.jbi.2017.06.008

Whitney, E.M., Aleksejuniene, J., Walton, J.N., 2016. Critical thinking disposition and skills in dental students: Development and relationship to academic outcomes. Journal of Dental Education 80 (8), 948–958.

Winkelmann, J., Gómez Rossi, J., van Ginneken, E., 2022. Oral health care in Europe: Financing, access and provision. Health Systems in Transition 24 (2), 1–169. https://apps.who.int/iris/bitstream/handle/10665/355605/HiT-24-2-2022-eng.pdf?sequence=1

Yazdani, S., Abardeh, M.H., 2019. Five decades of research and theorization on clinical reasoning: A critical review. Advances in Medical Education and Practice 10, 703–716. https://doi.org/10.2147/AMEP.S213492

Zadeh, L.A., 2008. Is there a need for fuzzy logic? Information Sciences 178 (13), 2751–2779.

26

CLINICAL REASONING IN OCCUPATIONAL THERAPY

CHRIS CHAPPARO ■ JUDY RANKA

CHAPTER AIMS

The aim of this chapter is to examine clinical reasoning in occupational therapy from five perspectives:

- a brief history of clinical reasoning in occupational therapy
- the content of therapist thinking that has been found to influence occupational therapy action
- the conceptual notions about the thinking processes that underpin clinical decision making in occupational therapy
- how occupational therapists may use a hermeneutical approach to synthesize multiple sources of information, thoughts, beliefs into a coherent understandable whole
- how occupational therapists may use cognitive strategies during the process of reasoning.

INTRODUCTION

Answers to six questions lie at the heart of occupational therapy (OT) assessment and intervention, which is a complex, dynamic process, based on observation of the interaction between people and their environments as they perform relevant and valued everyday activity.

- What is the situation?
- What is wanted/needed/possible in this situation?
- What will I do?
- How will I do it?
- Is it 'right'?
- Why am I doing it?
- Did it work?

People access OT when they, family members or others, call for help because of reduced participation in daily occupations or activities. Disruptions to participation in occupational performance are inherently complex, severe and enduring, impacting all ages and sociocultural backgrounds. The professional practice of therapists is impacted by a configuration of client demographic, social, cultural, political, technological or epidemiological sources, contributing to the complexity of therapy. Under conditions of such complexity, uncertainty and change, occupational therapists (OTs) aim to develop and implement therapy programmes which enable people and their families to engage in desired life activities and ensure their quality of life.

For decades, clinical reasoning, or 'thinking like a therapist', has been targeted as critical to selecting the 'best' therapeutic intervention for the moment and delivering it in the interests of each individual situation (Mattingly and Fleming, 1994; Rogers and Masagatani, 1982; Scanlan et al., 2021; Schell and Schell, 2018). It is a nonlinear, circular style of thinking which involves gathering and analysing information about people, and their situation, who are referred to OT, as well as deciding on therapeutic actions which 'fit' their specific circumstances and needs. It combines cognitive and metacognitive strategies such as analysis, planning, problem solving and evaluation together with precognitive intuition. It involves a dynamic process of analysing the client situation in the present and imagined future contexts (Durning and Artino, 2011). Finally, it is a tacit, highly imagistic and deeply phenomenological mode of thinking (Schell and Schell, 2018), which is informed in part by an overarching metacognitive frame comprised of salient beliefs, attitudes and expectancies held by the therapist (Chapparo, 1999; Shafaroodi et al., 2014; Unsworth, 2017).

Although the importance of reasoning in OT has been clearly established in previous decades, it remains a hypothetical construct, the understanding of which continues to evolve (Márquez-Álvarez et al., 2019). Several questions remain unanswered about the thinking processes used in clinical reasoning. What personal and contextual elements are involved in the reasoning process? How do therapists combine science, experience and their personal commitments to make decisions about their actions? Why do therapists make decisions the way they do?

CLINICAL REASONING IN OCCUPATIONAL THERAPY: HISTORICAL PERSPECTIVE

Clinical reasoning has been studied by occupational therapy researchers since the mid-1970s with the first formal publication in 1982 (Rogers and Masagatani, 1982). Throughout the development of the OT profession, elements of what is termed clinical reasoning have been referred to as: treatment planning (Day, 1973; Pelland, 1987); the evaluative process (Hemphill-Pearson, 1982); clinical thinking (Line, 1969); a subset of the OT process (Christiansen and Baum, 1997); and problem solving (Hopkins and Tiffany, 1988). More recently, there has been a move away from use of the term 'clinical reasoning' in preference to 'professional reasoning' (Unsworth and Baker, 2016), 'occupational reasoning' (Rogers and Holm, 1991) and 'therapist thinking', as many therapists are employed outside of clinical settings and provide interventions for 'consumers', 'clients' and 'people' rather than 'patients'. The development of the profession has influenced various reasoning strategies used in current practice as well as the methods that have been used for studying them.

OT was founded on humanistic values (Myers, 2019). The view of occupation early in the profession's development centred on the relationship between health and the ability to organize the temporal, physical and social elements of daily living (Breines, 1990). Influential in the creation of treatment principles was a thinking mode described by pragmatic theorist, John Dewey (1910), who claimed that actions of professionals depended upon *a unique mental analysis to obtain an understanding of the significance and meaning in a person's everyday life*. From this evolved a client-centred philosophy which emphasized the rights of all people to access opportunities to establish a balanced, wholesome life. These original humanistic values remain in current therapist thinking which focuses not only on maintaining clients' well-being through occupation, but also on scaffolding occupational and social support for all people and communities and advocating for politically supported and socially valued occupational opportunities (Braveman and Suarez-Balcazar, 2009). Understanding of the 'lived experience' of people's occupational performance is a goal of the reasoning process.

In the middle of the 20th century, growing pressure from medicine called for a more scientific rationale for OT practice (Licht, 1947), which approximated medical explanations of human function (Kielhofner and Burke, 1983). Clinical decision making became reductionist, with linear decision-making processes for intervention aimed at improving isolated units of function, such as particular physical or psychological attributes (e.g. Day, 1973; Molineux and Baptiste, 2011). Central to this process was a procedural reasoning style that continues to be recognized as one element of current therapist thinking (Schell and Schell, 2018).

The last three decades have seen a resurgence of scientific and reductionist thinking in the evidence-based practice movement which promotes a systematic approach to therapist thinking (Jeffery et al., 2021; Thomas and Law, 2013). Several terms have been generated which emphasize the use of knowledge from research and other types of formal inquiry to interpret client situations and make intervention plans. These include evidence-based practice (EBP) (Krueger et al., 2020; Nott and Chapparo, 2020), research utilization (RU) (Myers, 2019) and knowledge translation (KT) (Miciak et al., 2021) Although the original intention was that evidence-based decisions should be based on 'knowledge of *individual client characteristics and preferences* in the formulation of clinical decisions' (Dubouloz et al., 1999, p. 445), clinical experience, clinical research (Sackett et al., 1996, p. 71) and current interpretations of evidence constitute a narrow form of reasoning that adheres to knowledge generated by controlled trials and statistical measurement (National Health and Medical Research Council, 2009; Hoffmann et al., 2013). Clinical reasoning that is solely based on this view of evidence and which does not consider testimonial evidence of lived experiences (Watson, 2021) has been described as 'self-referential, closed on itself, and not shaped by the logic of priorities established within the field of the social rights to health' (Di Costanzo, 2012) and therefore distant from the original focus of OT.

REFLECTION POINT

OT practice in the 21st century continues to be characterized by theoretical conflict, as the profession reexamines its direction and place in the changing landscape of culturally relevant social health practice. The original belief in clients' rights to choice and autonomy is reflected in the phenomenological and hermeneutic approaches that have largely been used to study OT clinical reasoning and the influence of medicine on clinical reasoning is illustrated by the analytic EBM (evidence-based medicine) approach.

SOURCES OF KNOWLEDGE USED DURING OCCUPATIONAL THERAPY CLINICAL REASONING

There are both internal and external influences on the decisions therapists make about their actions. One way to describe these influences is to consider them as *sources of knowledge that act as motivators for decision making*, which address the questions:

- 'what do therapists think about' when they reason and
- 'how' do they obtain and use knowledge.

The Client/Therapy Context

The context contains powerful factors which establish knowledge about the conditions (e.g. organizational, cultural and societal values) and constraints (e.g. human and financial resources, policies) that contribute to a *practical knowledge schemata* used by therapists to determine potential outcomes of therapy (Schell and Schell, 2018). Therapy experiences are remembered by therapists as total contextual patterns of what is possible and include people, actions, contexts and objects, rather than as decontextualized elements or general rules (McBee et al., 2017). Contextual patterns contribute to therapists' perceptions of the amount of control they have over their ability to carry out planned actions (Shafaroodi et al., 2014). Therapists reason according to their internalized values and theoretical perspectives, which may be either consistent with, or at odds with, the client or therapy context. If practice beliefs and values of therapists fail to account for prevailing therapy/client contexts, the resulting dilemma for clinical reasoning is one of conflict between what therapists perceive should be done, what the client wants done and what the context will allow (Carrier et al., 2015).

Clients and Their Life Contexts

Fundamental to the OT clinical reasoning process is a core ethical tenet that the intervention be in concert with clients' needs, goals, lifestyles and personal and cultural values (American Occupational Therapy Association, 2020; Chapparo et al., 2017a). To this end, Mattingly and Fleming (1994) originally described one of the primary goals of OT clinical reasoning as determining the *meaning of reduced participation* in occupational performance from the client's perspective. Knowledge from multiple sources of information is used during the process of assessment and intervention to build a conceptual model of the client situation (Mattingly and Fleming, 1994; Schell and Schell, 2018). Therapists constantly update their understanding of how clients view themselves, how clients view therapy and the therapist, and what clients think should be done. Knowledge is used by therapists in the reasoning process to build a conceptual model of the client situation (Schell and Schell, 2018) (Box 26.1).

Theory and Science

One contribution to clinical decision making is therapists' scientific knowledge about disease, human function and human occupation, gleaned largely from theory and evidence (Schell and Gillen, 2018). Termed *professional knowledge*, it is conceptualized as applied theory whereby a process of 'naming' and 'framing' the problem occurs (Márquez-Álvarez et al., 2019). The process requires identifying and classifying abstract constructs according to some theory base (such as function, depression, sensory processing, motor control, occupational role, cognitive ability or social justice) and 'fitting' them with the client situation. The identified construct becomes a cognitive mechanism which can facilitate the selection of strategies for assessment and treatment (Schell and Gillen, 2018).

Theoretical knowledge alone, however, is an insufficient basis for effective clinical reasoning in occupational therapy for many reasons. First, occupational therapy has a theory base that is incomplete. Second,

---

BOX 26.1

TYPES OF KNOWLEDGE CONTRIBUTING TO UNDERSTANDING OF THE CLIENT'S OCCUPATIONAL NEED

- Knowledge of the client's motivations, desires and tolerances
- Knowledge of the context within which occupational performance occurs
- Knowledge of the client's abilities and deficits
- Insight into the existing relationship with the client, its tacit rules and boundaries
- Predictive knowledge of the client's potential in the long term

---

therapists are required to make decisions in situations of uncertainty. Under these conditions, *practical knowledge* (a personal theory derived from experience) is also required (Mattingly and Fleming, 1994). Practical knowledge is integrated with theoretical knowledge to form a reasoning strategy that has been termed 'deliberative rationality' (Pena, 2010) and/or 'intuition' (McKenna et al., 2020).

Personal Beliefs of the Therapist

Clinical reasoning is not a linear process but is an ongoing series of linked personal encounters. The fourth source of knowledge is *personal knowledge*, comprising the beliefs, values and attitudes of the therapist, which provides a thinking 'disposition' (bias) (Scheffer and Rubenfeld, 2000). These are the fundamental assumptions about what we 'know to be true' about ourselves, others and occupational therapy. They can range from tentatively held beliefs to strong convictions and differ from person to person as well as from situation to situation. The place of personal beliefs in clinical reasoning contributes to defining the limits of 'acceptability' in any given clinical situation (Chapparo, 1999).

Attitude–Behaviour Expectancy

Although 'therapeutic use of self' is a widely supported part of intervention (Cave et al., 2019), the impact of *attitude* on occupational therapist thinking during reasoning has received little attention (Solman and Clouston, 2016). After defining clinical reasoning as a purposive social interaction, Chapparo (1999) used elements of attitude–behaviour theory (Ajzen, 2002) to demonstrate the impact of attitude on therapist thinking. In this model, therapy is found to be mediated through intention (what therapists choose to do) and expectancies (the perceived expectations of self and others). This refers to the extent to which therapists believe that their therapy will meet the expectations of other people whose opinions they value. These other people may be clients or family members or other professionals. Attitude (what therapists expect as outcomes of therapy) develops from sets of beliefs derived from the personal, theoretical and contextual knowledge outlined earlier. This conceptual model of reasoning is not an explanation of the effects of *general* beliefs and attitudes on clinical reasoning, but of the effects of a *particular attitude towards a particular personal behaviour*, in this instance, occupational therapy for a *particular* client. Attitudes of therapists about their actions may be the primary motivators in decision making and are derived from salient beliefs triggered by specific and changing events in therapy. Although these propositions have long found support in attitude–behaviour research (Ajzen, 2002; Bandura, 1997), further research in occupational therapy is required (Shafaroodi et al., 2014).

Internal Frame of Reference

Clearly, clinical reasoning in occupational therapy is a phenomenon involving balancing personal, client-related, theoretical and organizational sets of knowledge. How therapists orchestrate their knowledge to determine which element receives precedence in reasoning is not yet clear. One emerging hypothesis is that the knowledge used for clinical reasoning is housed within a highly individualized *personal internal frame of reference*, which has precognitive and cognitive elements that comprise knowledge in the form of beliefs and attitudes representing the therapist's personal view of any clinical event (Creek and Lawson-Porter, 2007; Shafaroodi et al., 2014). This knowledge is organized into facts about the therapist's everyday practice world (external elements), perceptions of what is real in everyday practice (internal elements), and judgements about the everyday practice world which are verified through action (attitude). It is used during the clinical reasoning process to order, categorize and simplify complex data for planning therapist action (or nonaction). In it resides the sum of the cultural and personal biases of the therapist which colour and interpret clinical reality and, ultimately, clinical reasoning (Fig. 26.1).

USING KNOWLEDGE IN LINES OF REASONING

Considering the diverse content of the knowledge platform that guides thinking, it is not surprising to find researchers proposing that multiple lines of reasoning are used by occupational therapists. In the third section of this chapter, we explore how therapists use their knowledge to form pictures of client problems, client potential, therapy action and outcome and address the question 'how are these knowledge categories interrelated in therapist thinking?' Much of this information

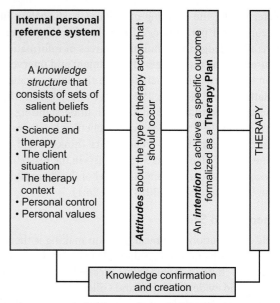

Fig. 26.1 ▪ The therapist internal personal reference system. A personal knowledge structure that is shaped by beliefs, attitudes and expectations. Therapy (action) is preceded by an intention to act in a particular way (therapy plan). Intentions are shaped by attitudes towards the salient therapy situation. Attitudes are shaped by a constellation of beliefs about aspects of the therapy situation.

has been derived from what is considered the keystone study into clinical reasoning in occupational therapy, commissioned by the American Occupational Therapy Association (AOTA) (Mattingly and Fleming, 1994). Although it was a relatively small, culturally and geographically localized study with inherent biases, it still exerts disproportional influence on how clinical reasoning in OT internationally is described and taught today.

Diagnostic, Procedural and Abductive Reasoning: 'What Is *the Problem* of Occupation?'

OTs are thought to use a logical line of thinking which parallels deductive inquiry when they try to understand the impact of health and contextual barriers to occupational participation experienced by people. Two forms of scientific reasoning identified by early OT researchers are *diagnostic reasoning* (Rogers and Holm, 1991) and *procedural reasoning* (Mattingly and Fleming, 1994). These processes involve a progression from problem sensing to problem definition and problem resolution. The focus is on the problem and therapists draw on their knowledge of occupations, therapy procedures, health and disability to address it. Diagnostic reasoning may start before the therapist approaches a client and results in early ideas about which information is required to form an occupational perspective of 'the problem'. This has been termed *abductive reasoning* (Råholm, 2010). It is the process of generating early hypotheses, personal theories or explanations and precedes deductive and inductive procedural reasoning processes when knowledge about the situation is incomplete (Thompson, 2012).

At this stage of reasoning, therapists are thought to generate two to four hypotheses regarding the cause and nature of functional problems and several more concerning possible directions for treatment (Mattingly and Fleming, 1994; Unsworth and Baker, 2016). Hypotheses generated are then subjected to a process of critical reflection and consideration of evidence which involves *critical thinking* to differentiate between fact, judgement and opinion (Alfaro-Lefevre, 2013). Without critical reflection, therapists cut short the act of inquiry, resulting in ineffective scientific reasoning (Lau et al., 2020). Questions which may prompt hypothesis generation in this line of reasoning may include those in Box 26.2 (Cooper and Deshaies, 2013).

Narrative and Interactive Reasoning: 'What Does Occupational Participation *Mean* to the Person?'

In implementing a therapy programme that will potentially change life roles and functions for people, OTs are faced with profound problems of understanding.

'Therapeutic use of self', a highly valued OT skill, is used in this type of reasoning (Taylor, 2020). Often done through facilitating story telling of a person's life experience (Haines and Wright, 2023), this involves coming to an understanding of the meaning of illness, life participation, disability and therapy outcome from the person's perspective, a process incorporating *narrative* and *interactive* reasoning. Such understanding involves making an interpretation of the story.

Two dimensions of meaning making are involved in narrative reasoning. *Meaning schemes* are habitual, implicit rules for interpreting and are strongly linked to scientific knowledge. For example, a therapist with experience in stroke rehabilitation expects to see signs of left hemiplegia when examining a client with a diagnosis of right cerebrovascular accident. *Meaning perspectives* refer to assumptions and beliefs within which new experiences are interpreted. For example, OTs make interpretations about clients based on values espoused by the notion of a 'helping profession' and their judgements are focussed on client performance and satisfaction with occupational participation. Both meaning schemes and meaning perspectives selectively order and delimit narrative reasoning by implicitly determining therapists' expectations and therefore their intentions in therapy and how they communicate this with clients (Hartog et al., 2020). Questions that may prompt these lines of reasoning are given in Box 26.3.

BOX 26.2
QUESTIONS RELATING TO PROCEDURAL REASONING IN OT

- What is the problem of occupation?
- What are all the factors associated with this problem?
- Are there assessment and intervention protocols for this problem?
- What interventions have/might be used?
- What evidence (fact: experience: opinion) supports the use of these assessments/interventions?
- What are the expected outcomes?

BOX 26.3
QUESTIONS RELATING TO NARRATIVE AND INTERACTIVE REASONING IN OT

- Who is the client and others in this situation?
- What are their concerns and goals?
- How do the client and others perceive the current status of occupational participation?
- What impact has (problem) had on the occupational participation of client (and others)?
- How does the client (and others) experience the problem and its impact?
- What is the best way for me to engage this client (and others) in an assessment and intervention process?
- What is the best future I can see for this client (and others) over time?
- What needs to happen to achieve this?

Ethical Reasoning: 'What *Should* Happen?'

Interactions with clients and others, navigation of service delivery systems and the way law and political policy are put in place may prompt ethical uncertainty, ethical distress or ethical dilemmas. In the process of choosing a therapeutic action using the reasoning processes outlined above, OTs are often forced to balance one personal value against another. Ethical uncertainty occurs when a therapist is uncertain about which personal values to apply to decide whether a situation is a moral problem. Ethical distress occurs when a therapist knows the 'right' course of action (e.g. type of intervention; time offered for intervention; the law) but feels constrained to act otherwise by broader imperatives of the service delivery system (e.g. overly large caseloads). Ethical dilemmas occur when a therapist must deal with ethical problems where there is no defensible alternative guiding an outcome (Bushby et al., 2015; VanderKaay et al., 2020; Watson, 2021). Box 26.4 lists some questions which arise during the process of ethical reasoning.

Conditional Reasoning: 'What Will Be the Outcome?'

Conditional reasoning involves projecting an imagined future for the client and draws on therapist experience (Mattingly and Fleming, 1994). The term 'conditional' is used in three different ways. First, problems are identified and solutions are devised. Second, therapists imagine how the present client situation could be changed. Third, potential success is determined by a line of thinking whereby therapists reconcile the actual (problem/therapy) and the possible (intention/planned therapy) in terms of therapy outcome (change). This involves reflection, whereby the therapist's action turns in on itself; conflict, whereby therapists seek to reconcile choices made; and judgement, whereby therapists weigh soundness of decisions. Box 26.5 contains questions which prompt this line of reasoning.

Pragmatic Reasoning: 'What *Can Be Done* Now?'

Pragmatic reasoning focusses on what is achievable within the client's world (Schell and Schell, 2018). As outlined earlier, this includes organizational constraints, values and resources, practice trends and reimbursement issues, and the skills of the therapist. Studies confirm that therapists' thinking is increasingly influenced by social influences from their practice world. Research highlights the place of conformity to the expectations of colleagues (Shafaroodi et al., 2014), organizational issues, access to resources and lack of skills and knowledge as being barriers to reasoning (da Silva Araujo et al., 2022). Questions which prompt this line of reasoning may include those in Box 26.6.

BOX 26.5
QUESTIONS RELATING TO CONDITIONAL REASONING IN OT

- Where will participation in occupation happen?
- What context has the client (others) identified as most important?
- What future(s) can be imagined for the client (others)?
- What critical skills/supports might shape the future of occupational performance?
- How can I support the client (others) to see a picture of a positive future and work towards it?
- Will it work?

BOX 26.4
QUESTIONS PROMPTING ETHICAL REASONING

- Is what I have decided to do/am doing/told to do, 'right'?
- Do I agree with the team's/other professional's decision about this client situation?
- Is this decision safe for me, client and others?
- Does my thinking uphold expected professional standards?
- Am I thinking 'within the law'?

BOX 26.6
QUESTIONS RELATING TO PRAGMATIC REASONING

- What organizational supports and constraints should I consider (for me and for the client) in developing a plan of action?
- What knowledge and skill level do I need to carry out what needs to be done?
- What knowledge and skill level do others in the client situation require to carry out what needs to be done?

REFLECTION POINT

It is unclear whether therapists use exclusive forms of thinking or whether the different styles of reasoning that have been identified in each piece of research were constructed through the research process of attempting to describe in words a largely internal, tacit phenomenon (Robertson, 2012). Descriptions of the various clinical reasoning processes that exist may reflect the epistemology of the researchers at the time (Robertson, 2012), such as anthropology (Mattingly and Fleming, 1994), medicine (Dutton, 1995; Rogers and Holm, 1991), cognitive psychology (Chapparo et al., 2017b) and social psychology (Merkebu et al., 2020).

CONSTRUCTING THE WHOLE STORY FROM ITS PARTS: USING HERMENEUTICS

Clearly, the lines of thinking used at any time during therapy relate to the salient goal and form of therapy (for example, occupational diagnosis, exploring alternatives with others, setting short-term goals, evaluating intervention, discharge planning). What is not clear is how therapists 'fuse' these lines of thinking to create a coherent whole. This part of the chapter proposes that a type of hermeneutical thinking strategy is used by OTs to consolidate disparate lines of knowledge and reasoning.

TABLE 26.1	
Characteristics of a hermeneutical approach as they apply to interpreting information used in the OT clinical reasoning process	
Hermeneutic Characteristic	**Application to Therapist Thinking**
Interpretation from one source of information is *partial*	■ Multiple perspectives of the 'problem' of occupation and its resolution are considered most effective in the reasoning process (client, others, therapist) ■ Every person's perspective is unique ■ There is no single interpretation that presents the complete picture ■ Any one interpretation of another person's lived experience can only ever be partial
Interpretation is *situated*	■ Therapist thinking is *situated in a time/place reality* constructed by the subjective contextual experiences of the client(s), therapist and others
Reasoning is a form of *dialogue*	■ Information obtained during the reasoning process is viewed as *external dialogue* between the client, others and therapist, as well as text reports (evidence, assessment results, professional reports) and behavioural observations ■ The reasoning process also happens through *internal dialogue* within the therapist's own thinking
Acceptance of *ambiguity*	■ Information obtained is not considered an exact representation of the experience of occupational performance itself, but rather the perception of it ■ Information used is *polyvocal* and may contain conflicting perceptions ■ Experiences change over time and context ■ Various reasoning processes are used to understand the various meanings that clients, other people, therapists attribute to 'the problem'
Interpretation of *parts* and the *whole* experience	■ The reasoning process attempts to understand the relationship between *parts* of client's (and others') experience of occupational performance (e.g. specific tasks, such as eating or dressing) and the way in which those parts relate to each other as a *whole* (overall occupational role performance as a self-maintainer and 'fit' in context) ■ Parts are *fused* into a cohesive whole which contains all lines of reasoning

From Chapparo, C., 2023. Hermeneutik. In: Ritchl, C., Weigl, R., Stamm, T. (Eds.), Wissenschaftliches arbeiten und schreiben: Verstehen, anwenden, nutzen für die praxis, 2nd ed. Springer.

There is increasing interest in examining how hermeneutic methods are used in OT clinical reasoning and other health professions (MacLeod et al., 2023). *Hermeneutics* has been described as an information gathering and interpretation method which focusses on discovering the meanings contained in descriptions of people's life experience (Santiago et al., 2020). Hermeneutic approaches have been used in OT primarily as research methodologies and rarely reported as a method of inquiry that is part of everyday clinical reasoning. Terms such as exploration, interpretation, investigation, revealing and unmasking have been associated with this approach. Clinical reasoning can be described as a specific example of hermeneutic inquiry. It goes beyond factual description of experience in order *to understand meanings* which may not be immediately apparent (Koch, 1996). It requires a receptive disposition towards things beyond our understanding. Understanding is constructed through therapist thinking by synthesis or *fusion* of a number of information sources (Gadamer, 1996). It uses polyvocal input through dialogue, text (medical charts, therapy notes, images, emails, patient care guidelines, published evidence), observation of actions, perceptions, imagination, thoughts, emotions, desires and intentions. The final interpretation is an understanding which is attributable to a *fusion* of all pertinent perspectives to the reasoning problem (Chapparo, 2023). This process addresses aspects of reasoning which other linear approaches are unable to accommodate. It imposes coherence on the multiple tracks of thought outlined earlier and allows further thinking to generate therapy plans and actions (Robertson, 2012). Some aspects of hermeneutical inquiry and their proposed alignment with therapist thinking in OT clinical reasoning are outlined in Table 26.1.

INFORMATION PROCESSING, COGNITIVE STRATEGY USE AND CLINICAL REASONING

Clinical reasoning in OT requires therapists to extend or abstract their knowledge beyond what they know and beyond the context in which they do therapy, implicating the role of cognition in this process (Lam Wai Shun et al., 2022). Cognitive deficiencies

in decision making have been shown to be associated with poor outcomes (Merkebu et al., 2020). This part of the chapter addresses the question 'what *thinking strategies* do therapists use to obtain, manipulate and generate knowledge of clients, self, situations and therapy?'

Cognition has been defined in many ways. In this chapter it is defined as an interaction of thinking processes which involve all forms of awareness and knowing such as sensing, perceiving, conceiving, remembering, questioning, evaluating, problem solving and decision making (VandenBos, 2007). Cognition subsumes metacognition (thinking about one's own thinking) enabling us to orchestrate multiple tasks and parts of tasks into a seamless whole. The role of cognition in clinical reasoning is not related to the structure of cognition per se, but how therapists use their lines of thinking strategically to suit a specific therapy situation, termed *cognitive strategy use* (Siegler, 2007).

Cognitive strategies are mental thinking tactics (Siegler, 2007). They are used daily when we need to: identify important, unfamiliar or difficult information; understand and retain information; retrieve information from memory stores; manipulate and apply information; plan and modify responses using information; and simultaneously cope with internal and external distractions during task performance (Ramsden, 2013).

Cognitive strategy use is dependent on information processing which is conceptualized as a flexible self-organizing system (Dajani and Uddin, 2015). Models of information processing trace the staged flow of information from registering sensory input, processing it and responding to it. This processing system is controlled by an executive system, which is generally considered to have two main functions: awareness of the skills, strategies and resources needed to perform each task; and self-regulatory strategies to monitor thinking processes and engage in corrective strategies when processing is not going smoothly (Huitt, 2003). Central to applying the theory to occupational therapy clinical reasoning is the assumption that successful reasoning requires both automatic (precognitive) and deliberate (cognitive) use of information (Kahneman, 2011). In many instances, occupational therapy requires therapists to use high-level thinking strategies to 'know the unknown' (e.g. conditional reasoning). At the same time, therapists access and use other knowledge so automatically that they can 'do without thinking' (e.g. in procedural and pragmatic reasoning), for example be able to think ahead to the next sequence of a therapy session while automatically positioning a client or themselves safely for a wheelchair transfer.

During clinical reasoning, therapists gather information from people, things and events in their environment (using attending and sensory gathering strategies). They match the sensory information with what they have learned and experienced, noting similarities and differences, and store the information for future use (recall strategies). These representations of therapy become deeper and more powerful with repetition over time. Therapists' understanding of client problems, worldviews and therapy outcomes becomes more precise as they apply their knowledge using a range of cognitive strategies across a wide range of clients and therapeutic tasks (generalizing, planning, decision making and self-evaluating strategies). They become strategic thinkers, which presupposes that therapists simultaneously know what must be accomplished (goal) and can make plans (planning), initiate strategic behaviour (initiation), pay attention to their own and the client's performance (monitor), and evaluate their thinking and resulting actions in relation to the goals (reflection, self and situation evaluation).

Each therapy situation demands particular client information to be chosen, constructed, processed, stored, recalled, organized and used for a particular therapy purpose. Such cognitive strategy use implies salient use of a general set of cognitive strategies required in a particular moment. Chapparo et al. (2017b) constructed a conceptual model of how people use cognitive strategies during task performance. Termed the Perceive, Recall, Plan and Perform (PRPP) System (Fig. 26.2) it is centred on four processing 'quadrants' connected by multidirectional arrows that mirror the four-staged flow of information in theoretical models of information processing. These quadrants include attention and sensory perception (Perceive), memory (Recall), response planning and evaluation (Plan) and performance monitoring (Perform). Built on earlier notions from instructional psychology (Romiszowski, 1984) as well as applied cognitive task analysis, it has been used to explain people's ability to use cognitive strategies to think through routine and complex work tasks effectively (Challita et al., 2019; Lewis et al., 2016; Nott and Chapparo, 2020).

Perceive: Attention and Sensory Perception Strategies (Cognitive Strategies for Attending to and Sensing Information)

Once sensory input from a client or therapy context captures our attention and we focus on it, details of the information are registered and we create sensory pictures of clients, ourselves and therapy events. Initial interpretation of sensory data is thought to precede conscious thinking, implying that client and contextual information is always interpreted preconsciously in the first instance (Hogarth, 2014). The more attention we pay to a given bit of sensory information (for example, a wrist joint or listening to a client narrative), the more elaborately the information will be retained. The top left-hand quadrant (Perceive) in Fig. 26.2 outlines some specific strategies from the PRPP System associated with this first stage of information processing. These strategies are observable behaviours that signal whether therapists are attending to and dealing with sensory input that is needed for therapy (Chapparo et al., 2017b).

Recall Strategies (Cognitive Strategies Used to 'Know' and Use What Is Known)

Sensory images of people, things and contexts are transferred to a working memory, which is what we are thinking about at any given time. Memories of our personal, client and therapy experiences are then configured efficiently into long-term memory structures called schemas. Schemas serve as filters for ongoing experience, allowing us to come to conclusions about what we see, hear or do automatically (Hattie and Yates, 2014) without having to 'think too hard' and is often referred to as 'automaticity' (Chapparo et al., 2017b). This line of thinking is depicted by arrows from Perceive (sensory) to Recall (memory) to Perform (action) in the central part of Fig. 26.2. This is similar in concept to Kahneman's (2011) view of System 1 automatic reasoning. In clinical reasoning this enables us to interpret the present based on experience from the past and answer the question 'Do I know…?' (Chapparo et al., 2017b).

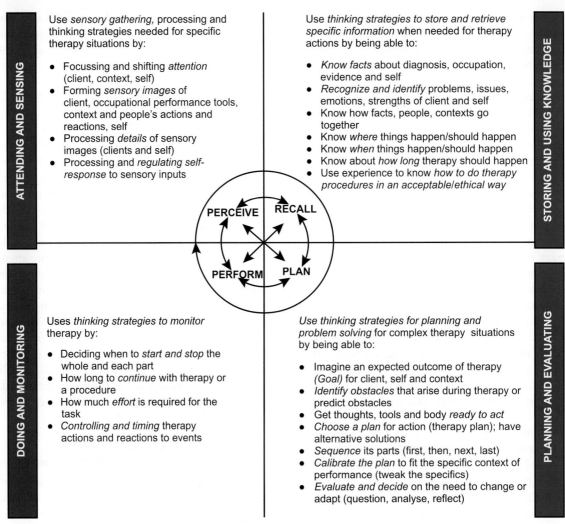

Fig. 26.2 ■ The Perceive, Recall, Plan and Perform (PRPP) System of Task Analysis Conceptual Model. Hypothesized cognitive strategies that are used in clinical reasoning during every therapy situation. (From Chapparo, C., Ranka, J. L., Nott, M. T., 2017b. Perceive, Recall, Plan and Perform (PRPP) system of task analysis. In: Curtin, M., Egan, M., Adams, J. (Eds.), Occupational therapy for people experiencing illness, injury or impairment (7th ed.). Elsevier, pp. 236–250).

Three broad categories of knowledge are stored and retrieved for use during clinical reasoning. These are:

Factual knowledge (Facts): 'Do I know WHAT…?' The storing and recalling of facts enable therapists to store information from formal evidence, recognize sensory data from clients and situations and the meaning that is attached to them. It makes a major contribution to practical knowledge and is the basis for diagnostic and procedural reasoning. Sensory images

from therapy situations are assigned categorical and language codes which assist with fast, efficient storage and retrieval. Labels such as pain, activities of daily living and so on become fused with our own personal understanding of these terms and are used to assign meaning to client and therapy events.

Schematic knowledge (Schemes): 'Do I know WHERE…?';'Do I know WHEN…?'; 'Do I know HOW LONG…?' Schematic memory represents what we have learned about where, when and how long something happens. This type of knowledge is based on experiences located in personal time and space and probably contributes to pragmatic reasoning. Schematic information provides us with a personally constructed 'map' or a model for how, when and where to act as a therapist.

Procedural knowledge: 'Do I know HOW…?' Procedural memory enables us to perform therapeutic procedures based on experience. It has been shown to be the most resistant to forgetting and foremost in the natural inclination for therapists to 'do what they know' in the first instance. Experienced therapists often seem to 'do therapy' without thinking because they have highly developed procedural knowledge.

The top righthand quadrant (Recall) in Fig. 26.2 outlines some specific cognitive strategies from the PRPP System associated with this second stage of information processing.

Planning Strategies (Cognitive Strategies Used to Map Out, Programme and Evaluate Future Action)

Planning strategies are executive functions (organizing, planning, evaluating, goal setting) that are applied to all information for use in a particular way or when what we know is not enough. When reasoning through complex therapy events, we process information with reference to a particular goal, an idea, an understanding of an outcome (what will happen?). With an outcome in mind, efficient strategic thinkers use cognitive strategies that prepare them to put a therapy plan into action. Knowledge is used as a platform for this aspect of reasoning (arrow from Recall to Plan Fig. 26.2). Planning strategies are then used to modify habitual responses that may be demanded by the client situation or therapy context. Rapid searches for additional information are used throughout the problem-solving process (arrow from Plan to Perceive, Fig. 26.2). Problem solving before, during and upon review is paramount during this stage of clinical reasoning and includes the problem-solving questioning in the immediately following Reflection Point.

REFLECTION POINT

Problem solving is paramount when planning around complexity or novelty and is stimulated by the following self-generated questions:

- What obstacles might/did get in the way?
- How can I get myself and the client ready for therapy?
- What is the best choice of therapy approach, place and tool to use for this specific therapy task?
- How do I have to sequence therapy?
- What do I have to do to make my responses fit the client expectation/therapy context/my abilities?
- What personal reactions to client and therapy events do I have to consciously inhibit?

Effective clinical reasoning happens when therapists reflect on their own plans and performance and make considered decisions (Fox and Christoff, 2014). Some of the cognitive strategies involved in the planning aspect of information processing during clinical reasoning are listed in the lower-right quadrant in Fig. 26.2 (Plan).

Perform Strategies (Cognitive Strategies Used to Time, Control and Monitor Therapy)

After planning, the last stage of information processing focusses on using thinking strategies to initiate and control therapy action (arrow from Plan to Perform, Fig. 26.2). Actively responding to information that is processed requires being able to initiate both starting and stopping of responses (verbal, motor, gestural, affective), timing responses 'in the moment', controlling actions and monitoring effort. Therapist actions and client/contextual reactions to them are fed back into the system as further sensory input and result in not only remembering what has been done and how (arrows from Perform to Perceive, Perform to Recall), but also the thinking that preceded it (arrow from Perform to Plan). For this attending, sensing, knowing, thinking, doing system to be effective, therapists must have a firm outcome (goal) in mind and be able to bring the goal back into focus for review as they 'do' therapy.

SUMMARY

Clinical reasoning in OT is based on the complex interaction between people and their environments as they perform relevant and valued everyday activity in unique ways and contexts. As contemporary therapy becomes increasingly aligned with community service delivery systems in public health, social welfare and education, there are suggestions for 'clinical' reasoning to be termed 'professional' reasoning. There is general agreement that:

- There are multiple lines of reasoning in OT, providing a multifaceted view of clients' problems, capacities, futures and therapy outcomes. Ethics and pragmatics further frame our views of clinical reasoning.
- Each therapist constructs a personal internal frame of reference, in which information about clients and the client situation are thought to be 'fused' with the therapist's personal beliefs about such things as perceived level of skill, ethics and perceived level of control. Such images make clinical reasoning an intensely personal process.
- Using methods similar to hermeneutic inquiry, discrete lines of reasoning are fused by means of therapist thinking into a coherent whole, allowing therapists to view the whole situation in context and discover the meaning of occupation and associated problems for clients and others.
- Finally, from a cognitive perspective, clinical reasoning is thought to be served by an attending, sensing, knowing, thinking, doing, dual processing cognitive system which is part automatic and part deliberate thinking. It operates strategically within the frame of the occupational therapy profession to apply multiple thinking strategies 'in the moment' to suit therapy.

REFLECTION POINT

Current explanations of clinical reasoning in OT are continually evolving. It is a highly individualistic mode of social interaction which is informed by scientific knowledge and method, cultural competence, creative imagination, intuition and interpersonal skill and operates within the frame of the OT profession.

REFERENCES

Ajzen, I., 2002. Perceived behavioral control, self-efficacy, locus of control, and the theory of planned behavior. Journal of Applied Social Psychology 32, 665–683.
Alfaro-Lefevre, R., 2013. Critical thinking and clinical judgment: A practical approach to outcome-focused thinking, 5th ed. Elsevier.
American Occupational Therapy Association, 2020. Occupational therapy practice framework. The American Journal of Occupational Therapy, 74 (Suppl. 2), 74124100101–741241001087 https://doi.org/10.5014/ajot.2020.74S2001
Bandura, A., 1997. Self efficacy: The exercise of control. WH Freeman.
Braveman, B., Suarez-Balcazar, Y., 2009. Social justice and resource utilization in a community-based organization: A case illustration of the role of the occupational therapist. Am J Occup Ther 63 (1), 13–23. https://doi.org/10.5014/ajot.63.1.13
Breines, E., 1990. Genesis of occupation: A philosophical model for therapy and theory. Australian Occupational Therapy Journal 37 (1), 45–49.
Bushby, K., Chan, J., Druif, S., Ho, K., Kinsella, E.A., 2015. Ethical tensions in occupational therapy practice: A scoping review. British Journal of Occupational Therapy 78 (4), 212–221.
Carrier, A., Levasseur, M., Bédard, D., Desrosiers, J., 2015. Clinical reasoning process: Cornerstone of effective occupational therapy practice. In: Söderback, I. (Ed.), International handbook of occupational therapy interventions. Springer International, pp. 73–82.
Cave, B., Wegner, L., Katie, C., 2019. Therapeutic use of self: Essential stuff not 'fluff'. Australian Occupational Therapy Journal 66 (S1), 57.
Challita, J., Chapparo, C., Hinitt, J., Heard, R., 2019. Patterns of cognitive strategy use common in children with reduced social competence derived from parent perceptions. Aust Occup Ther J 66 (4), 500–510. https://doi.org/10.1111/1440-1630.12574
Chapparo, C., 1999. Working out: Working with Angelica- Interpreting practice. In: Ryan, S.E., McKay, E.A. (Eds.), Thinking and reasoning in therapy: Narratives from practice. Stanley Thornes, pp. 31–50.
Chapparo, C., 2023. Hermeneutik. In: Ritchl, C., Weigl, R., Stamm, T. (Eds.), Wissenschaftliches arbeiten und schreiben: Verstehen, anwenden, nutzen für die praxis, 2nd ed. Springer.
Chapparo, C., Ranka, J.L., Nott, M.T., 2017a. Occupational performance model (Australia): A description of constructs, structure and propositions. In: Curtin, M., Egan, M., Adams, J. (Eds.), Occupational therapy for people experiencing illness, injury or impairment E-book. Elsevier, pp. 134–147.
Chapparo, C., Ranka, J.L., Nott, M.T., 2017b. Perceive, Recall, Plan and Perform (PRPP) system of task analysis. In: Curtin, M., Egan, M., Adams, J. (Eds.), Occupational therapy for people experiencing illness, injury or impairment, 7th ed. Elsevier, pp. 236–250.
Christiansen, C., Baum, C. (Eds.), 1997. Occupational therapy: Enabling function and well-being. Slack.
Cooper, C., Deshaies, L., 2013. Mosby's field guide to occupational therapy for physical dysfunction: Overview and occupational therapy process. Elsevier.
Creek, J., Lawson-Porter, A., 2007. Contemporary issues in occupational therapy: Reasoning and reflection. John Wiley & Sons.
da Silva Araujo, A., Anne Kinsella, E., Thomas, A., Demonari Gomes, L., Quevedo Marcolino, T., 2022. Clinical reasoning in occupational therapy practice: A scoping review of qualitative and conceptual peer-reviewed literature. Am J Occup Ther 76 (3), 7603205070. https://doi.org/10.5014/ajot.2022.048074

Dajani, D.R., Uddin, L.Q., 2015. Demystifying cognitive flexibility: Implications for clinical and developmental neuroscience. Trends Neurosci 38 (9), 571–578. https://doi.org/10.1016/j.tins.2015.07.003

Day, D.J., 1973. A systems diagram for teaching treatment planning. Am J Occup Ther 27 (5), 239–243. https://www.ncbi.nlm.nih.gov/pubmed/4716361

Dewey, J., 1910. How we think. University of Chicago Press.

Di Costanzo, C., 2012. Science and rights: The 'clinical reasoning' within health needs assessment. GSTF Journal of Law and Social Sciences (JLSS) 1 (2), 84.

Dubouloz, C.J., Egan, M., Vallerand, J., von Zweck, C., 1999. Occupational therapists' perceptions of evidence-based practice. Am J Occup Ther 53 (5), 445–453. https://doi.org/10.5014/ajot.53.5.445

Durning, S.J., Artino, A.R., 2011. Situativity theory: A perspective on how participants and the environment can interact: AMEE Guide no. 52. Med Teach 33 (3), 188–199. https://doi.org/10.3109/0142159X.2011.550965

Dutton, R., 1995. Clinical reasoning in physical disabilities. Williams & Wilkins.

Fox, K.C., Christoff, K., 2014. Metacognitive facilitation of spontaneous thought processes: When metacognition helps the wandering mind find its way. In: Fleming, S.M., Frith, C.D. (Eds.), The cognitive neuroscience of metacognition. Springer-Verlag, pp. 293–319.

Gadamer, H.-G., 1996. In: (Gaiger, J., Walker, N., Trans.)., The enigma of health: The art of healing in a scientific age. Stanford University Press.

Haines, D., Wright, J., 2023. Thinking in stories: Narrative reasoning of an occupational therapist supporting people with profound intellectual disabilities' engagement in occupation. Occup Ther Health Care 37 (1), 177–196. https://doi.org/10.1080/07380577.2021.2022260

Hartog, I., Scherer-Rath, M., Kruizinga, R., Netjes, J., Henriques, J., Nieuwkerk, P., et al., 2020. Narrative meaning making and integration: Toward a better understanding of the way falling ill influences quality of life. J Health Psychol 25 (6), 738–754. https://doi.org/10.1177/1359105317731823

Hattie, J.A., Yates, G.C., 2014. Using feedback to promote learning. In: Benassi, V.A., Overson, C.E., Hakala, C.M. (Eds.), Applying science of learning in education: Infusing psychological science into the curriculum. American Psychological Association, pp. 45–58.

Hemphill-Pearson, B.J., 1982. The evaluative process. In: Hemphill-Pearson, B.J. (Ed.), The evaluative process in psychiatric occupational therapy. Charles Slack, pp. 17–26.

Hoffmann, T., Bennett, S., Del Mar, C., 2013. Evidence-based practice across the health professions-e-book, 2nd ed. Elsevier Health Sciences.

Hogarth, R.M., 2014. Deciding analytically or trusting your intuition? The advantages and disadvantages of analytic and intuitive thought. In: Betsch, T., Haberstroh, S. (Eds.), The routines of decision making. Psychology Press, pp. 67–82.

Hopkins, H., Tiffany, E., 1988. Occupational therapy—A problem solving process. In: Hopkins, H.L., Smith, H.D. (Eds.), Willard and Spackman's occupational therapy, 7th ed. Lippincott, pp. 102–111.

Huitt, W., 2003. The information processing approach to cognition. Educational Psychology Interactive 3 (2), 53.

Jeffery, H., Robertson, L., Reay, K.L., 2021. Sources of evidence for professional decision-making in novice occupational therapy practitioners: Clinicians' perspectives. British Journal of Occupational Therapy 84 (6), 346–354.

Kahneman, D., 2011. Thinking, fast and slow. Farrar, Straus and Giroux.

Kielhofner, G., Burke, J., 1983. The evolution of knowledge and practice in occupational therapy: Past, present and future. In: Kielhofner, G. (Ed.), Health through occupation: Theory and practice in occupational therapy. FA Davis, pp. 3–54.

Koch, T., 1996. Implementation of a hermeneutic inquiry in nursing: Philosophy, rigour and representation. J Adv Nurs 24 (1), 174–184. https://doi.org/10.1046/j.1365-2648.1996.17224.x

Krueger, R.B., Sweetman, M.M., Martin, M., Cappaert, T.A., 2020. Occupational therapists' implementation of evidence-based practice: A cross sectional survey. Occup Ther Health Care 34 (3), 253–276. https://doi.org/10.1080/07380577.2020.1756554

Lam Wai Shun, P., Swaine, B., Bottari, C., 2022. Clinical reasoning underlying acute care occupational therapists' assessment of rehabilitation potential after stroke or brain injury: A constructivist grounded theory study. Aust Occup Ther J 69 (2), 177–189. https://doi.org/10.1111/1440-1630.12781

Lau, A.S., Lind, T., Crawley, M., Rodriguez, A., Smith, A., Brookman-Frazee, L., 2020. When do therapists stop using evidence-based practices? Findings from a mixed method study on system-driven implementation of multiple EBPs for children. Adm Policy Ment Health 47 (2), 323–337. https://doi.org/10.1007/s10488-019-00987-2

Lewis, J., Chapparo, C., Mackenzie, L., Ranka, J., 2016. Work after breast cancer: Identification of cognitive difficulties using the Perceive, Recall, Plan, and Perform (PRPP) system of task analysis. British Journal of Occupational Therapy 79 (5), 323–332.

Licht, S., 1947. The objectives of occupational therapy. Occup Ther Rehabil 26 (1), 17–22. https://www.ncbi.nlm.nih.gov/pubmed/20289195

Line, J., 1969. Case method as a scientific form of clinical thinking. Am J Occup Ther 23 (4), 308–313. https://www.ncbi.nlm.nih.gov/pubmed/5803992

MacLeod, M.L.P., McCaffrey, G., Wilson, E., Zimmer, L.V., Snadden, D., Zimmer, P., et al., 2023. Exploring the intersection of hermeneutics and implementation: A scoping review. Syst Rev 12 (1), 30. https://doi.org/10.1186/s13643-023-02176-7

Márquez-Álvarez, L.J., Calvo-Arenillas, J.I., Talavera-Valverde, M.A., Moruno-Millares, P., 2019. Professional reasoning in occupational therapy: A scoping review. Occup Ther Int 2019, 6238245. https://doi.org/10.1155/2019/6238245

Mattingly, C., Fleming, M.H., 1994. Clinical reasoning: Forms of inquiry in a therapeutic practice. FA Davis.

McBee, E., Ratcliffe, T., Picho, K., Schuwirth, L., Artino Jr., A.R., Yepes-Rios, A.M., et al., 2017. Contextual factors and clinical reasoning: Differences in diagnostic and therapeutic reasoning in board certified versus resident physicians. BMC Med Educ 17 (1), 211. https://doi.org/10.1186/s12909-017-1041-x

McKenna, J., Webb, J.A., & Weinberg, A., 2020. A UK-wide analysis of trait emotional intelligence in occupational therapists. International Journal of Therapy and Rehabilitation, 1–13.

Merkebu, J., Battistone, M., McMains, K., McOwen, K., Witkop, C., Konopasky, A., et al., 2020. Situativity: A family of social cognitive theories for understanding clinical reasoning and diagnostic error. Diagnosis (Berl) 7 (3), 169–176. https://doi.org/10.1515/dx-2019-0100

Miciak, M., Lavoie, M.M., Barrington, G.V., 2021. Reflective practice: Moving intention into action. Canadian Journal of Program Evaluation 36 (1), 95–105.

Molineux, M., Baptiste, S., 2011. Emerging occupational therapy practice: Building on the foundations and seizing the opportunities. In: Thew, M., Edwards, M., Baptiste, S., Molineux, M. (Eds.), Role emerging occupational therapy: Maximising occupation-focused practice. Blackwell Publishing, pp. 3–14.

Myers, C.T., 2019. Occupational therapists' perceptions of online competence assessment and evidence-based resources. Am J Occup Ther 73 (2), 7302205090p1–7302205090p8. https://doi.org/10.5014/ajot.2019.029322

National Health & Medical Research Council, 2009. NHMRC additional levels of evidence and grades for recommendations for developers of guidelines NHMRC.

Nott, M.T., Chapparo, C., 2020. Cognitive strategy use in adults with acquired brain injury. Brain Inj 34 (4), 508–514. https://doi.org/10.1080/02699052.2020.1725837

Pelland, M.J., 1987. A conceptual model for the instruction and supervision of treatment planning. Am J Occup Ther 41 (6), 351–359. https://doi.org/10.5014/ajot.41.6.351

Peña, A., 2010. The Dreyfus model of clinical problem-solving skills acquisition: A critical perspective. Med Educ Online 15 (1) https://doi.org/10.3402/meo.v15i0.4846

Råholm, M.B., 2010. Abductive reasoning and the formation of scientific knowledge within nursing research. Nurs Philos 11 (4), 260–270. https://doi.org/10.1111/j.1466-769X.2010.00457.x

Ramsden, P., 2013. Applications of the concepts of strategy and style. In: Schmeck, R.A. (Ed.), Learning strategies and learning style: Perspectives on individual differences. Springer Science, pp. 159–185.

Robertson, L., 2012. Clinical reasoning in occupational therapy. Blackwell.

Rogers, J.C., Holm, M.B., 1991. Occupational therapy diagnostic reasoning: A component of clinical reasoning. Am J Occup Ther 45 (11), 1045–1053. https://doi.org/10.5014/ajot.45.11.1045

Rogers, J.C., Masagatani, G., 1982. Clinical reasoning of occupational therapists during the initial assessment of physically disabled patients. The Occupational Therapy Journal of Research 2 (4), 195–219.

Romiszowski, A.J., 1984. Designing instructional systems. Hogan Page.

Sackett, D.L., Rosenberg, W.M., Gray, J.A., Haynes, R.B., Richardson, W.S., 1996. Evidence based medicine: What it is and what it isn't. BMJ 312 (7023), 71–72. https://doi.org/10.1136/bmj.312.7023.71

Santiago, E.A., Brown, C., Mahmoud, R., Carlisle, J., 2020. Hermeneutic phenomenological human science research method in clinical practice settings: An integrative literature review. Nurse Educ Pract 47, 102837. https://doi.org/10.1016/j.nepr.2020.102837

Scanlan, J., Brentnall, J., Unsworth, C., 2021. Clinical reasoning in occupational therapy practice. In: Brown, T., Bourke-Taylor, H.M., Isbel, S., Cordier, R., Gustafsson, L. (Eds.), Occupational therapy in Australia: Professional and practice issues. Routledge, pp. 174–184.

Scheffer, B.K., Rubenfeld, M.G., 2000. A consensus statement on critical thinking in nursing. J Nurs Educ 39 (8), 352–359. https://doi.org/10.3928/0148-4834-20001101-06

Schell, B.A.B., Gillen, G. (Eds.), 2018. Willard & Spackman's occupational therapy, 13th ed. Wolters Kluwer.

Schell, B.A.B., Schell, J.W., 2018. Clinical and professional reasoning in occupational therapy, 2nd ed. Wolters Kluwer.

Shafaroodi, N., Kamali, M., Parvizy, S., Mehraban, A.H., O'Toole, G., 2014. Factors affecting clinical reasoning of occupational therapists: A qualitative study. Med J Islam Repub Iran 28, 8. https://www.ncbi.nlm.nih.gov/pubmed/25250253

Siegler, R.S., 2007. Cognitive variability. Dev Sci 10 (1), 104–109. https://doi.org/10.1111/j.1467-7687.2007.00571.x

Solman, B., Clouston, T., 2016. Occupational therapy and the therapeutic use of self. British Journal of Occupational Therapy 79 (8), 514–516.

Taylor, R.R., 2020. The intentional relationship: Occupational therapy and use of self. FA Davis.

Thomas, A., Law, M., 2013. Research utilization and evidence-based practice in occupational therapy: A scoping study. Am J Occup Ther 67 (4), e55–e65. https://doi.org/10.5014/ajot.2013.006395

Thompson, B., 2012. Abductive reasoning and case formulation in complex cases. In: Robertson, L. (Ed.), Clinical reasoning in occupational therapy. Blackwell, pp. 15–30.

Unsworth, C., Baker, A., 2016. A systematic review of professional reasoning literature in occupational therapy. British Journal of Occupational Therapy 79 (1), 5–16.

Unsworth, C.A., 2017. Professional reasoning in occupational therapy practice. In: Curtin, M., Adams, J., Egan, M. (Eds.), Occupational therapy for people experiencing illness, injury or impairment: Promoting occupation and participation, 7th ed. Elsevier, pp. 90–104.

VandenBos, G.R., 2007. APA dictionary of psychology. American Psychological Association.

VanderKaay, S., Letts, L., Jung, B., Moll, S.E., 2020. Doing what's right: A grounded theory of ethical decision-making in occupational therapy. Scand J Occup Ther 27 (2), 98–111. https://doi.org/10.1080/11038128.2018.1464060

Watson, L., 2021. The right to know: Epistemic rights and why we need them. Routledge.

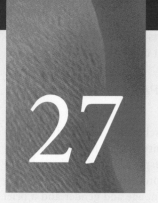

27

CLINICAL DECISION MAKING IN PARAMEDICINE

ROBIN PAP ■ PAUL SIMPSON

CHAPTER AIMS

The aims of this chapter are:

■ to describe the nature of contemporary paramedic practice
■ to outline the context of clinical reasoning within paramedicine
■ to explain models of clinical reasoning relevant to paramedic practice
■ to discuss the effect of cognitive bias on the quality of clinical reasoning
■ to provide strategies for cognitive de-biasing using metacognition and reflective practice.

INTRODUCTION

Paramedic practice throughout the world has undergone a remarkable transformation over the past quarter of a century as the role of the paramedic has responded to changing population health demands. In this chapter we use our experience of these changes in Australia to show how the clinical reasoning required

has been affected. The changing population health demands reflect the increasing prevalence of chronic health problems associated with increasing length of life and initiatives that aim to expand community-based healthcare as a substitute for in-hospital care (Caplan et al., 2012).

Paramedics' professional identity has traditionally centred on management of acute health emergencies including major trauma and cardiac arrest. However, the incidence of these cases in Australia is falling (Boyle et al., 2008; Dyson et al., 2015), largely a result of public health interventions and legislation to change behaviour that is associated with risk for injury or illness. In contrast, paramedics are increasingly caring for older people (Lowthian et al., 2011) with complex healthcare needs and a call to the emergency number is now likely to involve exacerbation of a chronic health condition or injury sustained after a fall.

The changing nature of the cases managed by ambulance services is reshaping the paramedic role. Although paramedics have traditionally functioned in an 'assess, stabilize and transport' paradigm, contemporary models of care now entail advanced patient examination and treatment with a view to determining a clinically appropriate disposition that is as likely to involve referral of the patient to an integrated community-based care pathway as it is transport to an emergency department. Paramedics now also actively engage in health promotion by way of opportunistic counselling for issues relating to management of chronic disease and illness and contribute to injury prevention strategies such as prevention of falls in the elderly by conducting evidence-based risk assessment and screening.

Scope of practice has substantially increased at each end of the spectrum of acuity. In low acuity (but often more complex) contexts, paramedics may perform broad interventions including, but not limited to, wound closure, wound care, falls risk and frailty screening, indwelling urinary catheterization and administration of antibiotics. At the higher end of acuity, paramedic-initiated thrombolysis for STEMI (ST-segment elevation myocardial infarction) and sedation and muscle paralysis for airway management, surgical airways and management of cardiac dysrhythmias have become standards of care in many practice settings.

Finally, the nature of paramedicine practice has evolved and continues to evolve as the discipline in Australia settles into a new era as a registered health profession regulated under the Australian Health Practitioner Regulation Agency (AHPRA) (Gough, 2018). Regulation has promoted expansion of practice settings for paramedics, who are increasingly recognized as valuable members of health professions teams outside the auspices of jurisdictional ambulance services. This is leading to new paradigms of paramedic reasoning and decision making as the traditional model involving a pair of paramedics responding to calls in an ambulance is supplemented by individual practice in nonmobile healthcare settings.

The ability to provide safe and effective healthcare in an increasingly complex and autonomous environment justifies an examination of the nature of clinical reasoning in paramedicine. Given the important influence that clinical decision making has on the delivery of safe and effective care, this chapter describes models of clinical reasoning identified in the health professions literature, the relevance of these models to paramedic practice and the potential effects of cognitive errors and affective bias on clinical decisions and patient outcomes.

THE NATURE OF PARAMEDIC PRACTICE

Paramedics provide unscheduled healthcare to individuals in the community. A call for an emergency ambulance results in a response based on the outcome of the telephone triage process. From that initial call, information about patient age and gender and a brief description of the nature of the problem are available for paramedics to review while travelling to the case.

The initial patient encounter is commonly associated with inaccessible or incomplete health records, limited access to diagnostic tests and competing priorities that include organizational requirements to minimize time spent 'on scene' in order to maximize operational responsiveness. Initial attempts to gather a history and examine a patient are frequently impeded by scene management and situational logistics.

Paramedics must gather data of varying reliability and integrity from several sources to formulate a clinical impression and subsequent treatment plan. Data sources include the patient and others present, which may include friends, relatives and other healthcare professionals. Contextual sources of information include the patient's social environment that may provide evidence of ability to live independently, verification of mechanism of injury or suspicion of illness. Paramedics are required to interpret salient features of the environment in which the clinical encounter takes place to build an impression of the factors that may be associated with the patient's current health status. Finally, the patient's subjective narrative and the paramedic's objective clinical observations complete the data collection process.

Research has described the complexity of paramedic decisions and the multiple levels of system influences that may be associated with increased risk (O'Hara et al., 2015). Decision making by paramedics is characteristically performed in a state of high 'cognitive load', increasing propensity for error (Burgess, 2010). The demands of clinical reasoning compete against multiple priorities that may include maintenance of situational awareness, assessment of safety, counselling and reassurance of bystanders, friends or family and communication with, and coordination of, other emergency service or health-care professionals in what is generally a task-heavy, human-resource-poor environment.

Well-developed clinical reasoning skills, including the ability to self-monitor for factors that may compromise the resulting clinical judgements, are central to the delivery of safe and effective care.

CLINICAL REASONING IN PARAMEDICINE PRACTICE

There is scant research evidence investigating clinical reasoning specific to paramedic practice, with existing studies focussing on decision outcomes rather than the cognitive processes involved in arriving at these decisions (Keene et al., 2022; Perona et al., 2019).

Shaban et al. described theories of decision making in paramedic practice, in a practice environment described as a state of 'constant uncertainty' (Shaban et al., 2004). Earlier research from the United States has identified the importance of critical thinking and diagnostic reasoning skills, with the authors advocating more emphasis on the development of these skills in entry-to-practice paramedic education (Dalton, 1996; Janing, 1994). This research describes the use of inductive and deductive reasoning with an emphasis on the influence that personal beliefs and values can have on the quality of clinical judgements and decisions. Despite arguments for the integration of clinical reasoning and de-biasing strategies within paramedic curricula, there has been little evidence of educational design that aims to enable these skills.

A 2016 survey of Canadian paramedics identified a dominant perception by respondents that they use a rational (conscious) style of thinking over an experiential (intuitive) approach to thinking and problem solving (Jensen et al., 2016). The authors suggest that these styles of thinking correlate with the dual-process theory systems of reasoning (Evans, 2003; see later in the chapter for more detail).

Research and Clinical Reasoning in Paramedicine

Research has proposed that a mix of approaches are used and that these include rule-out worst-scenario, algorithmic thinking and exhaustive thinking, with each of these associated with System 2 thinking (Jensen, 2010). Australian research by Keene et al. studied the effect of

varying likelihood, typicality and answer fluency on the diagnostic impression formed under circumstances designed to replicate the work process of paramedics. They concluded answer fluency and confidence were affected by operational aspects such as concurrent tasks and time pressure (Keene et al., 2022).This absence of substantial research exploring clinical reasoning in the context of paramedicine has led to the extrapolation of theory from other clinical disciplines, most notably emergency medicine. In a generic sense, clinical reasoning involves context-dependent thinking that leads to a clinical judgement, diagnosis, intervention or other action. Clinical reasoning is an essential component of professional competence, which is dependent on technical skills, communication, knowledge and reflection on practice (Epstein and Hundert, 2002).

Core skills involved in safe and effective decision making include the use of appropriate domain-specific knowledge – both propositional knowledge derived from theory and research and nonpropositional knowledge derived from professional and personal experience – and reasoning skills and an ability to reflect on the quality of the individual's cognitive processes and the influence of bias, including affective bias (Croskerry et al., 2010).

The demands occurring during the patient encounter include the complexity of the task, experience and ability of the individual and the delegated responsibility for the task. Decisions associated with a significant level of risk demand a high level of reasoning and problem solving. Reasoning may also be influenced by cultural beliefs and values, risk factors, interpersonal interactions with others on scene and personal beliefs, values and attitudes (Brandling et al., 2017). Overlaying these variables are personal and operational factors such as fatigue (Bartlett et al., 2022; Donnelly et al., 2019). Given the possible consequences of flawed or inadequate thinking and reasoning processes in the prehospital environment, sound clinical reasoning is required to provide safe and effective care for patients.

COGNITIVE STRATEGIES INVOLVED IN CLINICAL REASONING

Although few published studies have described processes of paramedic reasoning and decision making, clinical reasoning strategies described in medicine (Elstein and Schwartz, 2002) and the specialty of emergency medicine will be used as a reference because of similarities in dealing with incomplete information in often hectic and time-poor environments. This literature describes hypothesis testing, inductive reasoning, pattern recognition and the use of heuristics or 'illness scripts' that are based on known descriptions of disease or common features of a particular disease (Kovacs and Croskerry, 1999). These models of reasoning are detailed elsewhere in this book.

One model of reasoning and decision making is known as dual-process theory (DPT) or System 1 and System 2 models of reasoning (Sloman, 1996). System 1 has been described as intuitive decision making, where rapid decisions arise from comparing a familiar pattern of cues with prior examples derived from prior experience (Croskerry, 2009). This style of thinking enables efficient processing of information to form an impression while reducing cognitive load and fits neatly within the context of paramedic decision making. With experience, thinking becomes automatic and a more conscious and analytical form of thinking (System 2) is only engaged when complex, novel or atypical situations are encountered. System 1 has been described as a form of universal cognition (Evans, 2003).

Clinical reasoning in medicine has been shown to involve a System 1 process of reasoning where the clinical features are recognized, resulting in a rapid generation of a hypothesis or definition of the problem. In the emergency medicine setting, a 'recognition primed' model of decision making has been described (Weingart, 2008), which corresponds to the System 1 model of pattern recognition. When the clinical features associated with a patient presentation fail to activate prior recognition because of unusual or atypical clinical findings, a more analytical pathway of clinical decision-making System 2 is likely to be used.

The use of pattern recognition by expert paramedics and the way this differs from novice reasoning can be identified by observing personal (expert versus novice) differences in the approach to the interpretation and classification of a cardiac electrocardiogram (ECG). Given an ECG showing atrial fibrillation, experts can quickly classify the dysrhythmia without the need for extensive analysis. This is largely a function of exposure to many prior examples so that the distinctive pattern of irregular R-R intervals and lack of regular P-wave activity are recognized automatically.

In contrast, novices with knowledge of cardiac electrophysiology but lacking exposure to repeated examples of this dysrhythmia and confirmation of the correct classification may rely on a more analytical and time-consuming dissection of waveform morphology to form a decision regarding the type of dysrhythmia.

ERRORS IN CLINICAL REASONING

Reasoning that underpins the formulation of a diagnosis and subsequent case management plans must be logically sound, defensible and appropriate. This requirement spans all clinical decisions, from the management of minor injury to decisions to withhold or withdraw resuscitation in cases of sudden cardiac arrest. Errors in the field of paramedicine that compromise patient safety or that lead to poor patient outcomes are difficult to find because of limitations of existing reporting practice. A surrogate measure is the incidence of medical indemnity claims in Australia, with paramedics involved in 1.2% of all claims in 2012 to 2013 in Australia (Australian Institute of Health and Welfare, 2014).

A case involving a 50-year-old male reporting a sudden onset of substernal pain that radiates to his left shoulder may initiate a System 1 approach, particularly where the paramedic sees a familiar pattern of clinical signs that may include nonverbal cues. In contrast, a case involving a 22-year-old male reporting a recent onset of chest pain may initiate a System 2 or hypothetico-deductive approach if there is no overt external cause of the pain or when the patient's presentation, including his or her behaviour, is inconsistent with prior examples of nontraumatic chest pain in this age group. The lack of a defining clinical pattern may prompt a more analytical approach to assessment. However, when the pattern of the patient's presentation does not conform to the paramedic's expectations or beliefs about behaviour normally associated with severe pain, judgements about the veracity of the patient's complaint may influence decisions to offer analgesia or refer for further treatment. This may be more likely if the paramedic has developed a model of pain-related behaviour associated with a history of what paramedics have perceived to be 'drug seeking' and drug abuse that has similarities with the current case. Hence, if the patient does not conform to prior exemplars of a 'normal' presentation of acute pain, the diagnosis and management may be compromised by cognitive errors such as 'premature closure' (Croskerry, 2003b), particularly when the diagnosis is influenced by judgements regarding the patient's motives for reporting pain.

Cognitive failures associated with decision making have been collectively referred to as cognitive bias or, more recently, 'cognitive dispositions to respond' (CDR) (Croskerry, 2003b). In addition, the influence of emotions on decision making has been classified as 'affective dispositions to respond' (Croskerry, 2008). The emergency department has been described as a perfect environment for the study of CDR because of the often imperfect information and time limitations that physicians have

to work with, but it could be argued that the setting in which paramedics operate is equally challenging.

CDR that are not recognized and result in an adverse outcome can be considered a cognitive error. Upwards of 30 types of CDR have been described in the literature relating to medical decision making (Croskerry, 2002). Although research investigating CDR in paramedic practice has not been reported, they are highly likely to be relevant and present in paramedic clinical reasoning. For an extensive description of CDR, the reader is referred to the work of Croskerry (2008). Several common CDR factors likely to affect clinical decision making are illustrated in Case Study 27.1.

CASE STUDY 27.1

Factors Influencing Chronic Disease Management

Paramedics are dispatched to a private residence in the inner city. The dispatch information provided to them on the mobile data terminal states that they are responding to a 19-year-old male who is unconscious due to a 'suspected drug overdose'. The paramedics recognize the address and the patient from a previous incident involving a heroin overdose. Whilst en route, one of the paramedics says: 'Here we go again. I wonder how much he's taken this time.' The front door to the residence is unlocked. The interior of the residence is untidy and evidence of what appears to be illicit drug paraphernalia, including syringes, is noted on the kitchen bench. A brief examination involving an attempt to rouse the patient and measurement of his pulse is performed. A rapid heart rate, profuse perspiration and an altered level of consciousness are noted. Considering some key findings consistent with the patient's previous diagnosis, the paramedics form a clinical impression of a narcotic overdose and administer naloxone intramuscularly with no response. Two further doses of naloxone result in no improvement. The paramedics decide to transport the patient to a nearby emergency department. During handover, the triage nurse asks for the blood glucose level (BGL) taken on scene, to which the paramedics report that it was not taken because of the diagnosis of narcotic overdose. A BGL is quickly taken revealing hypoglycaemia of 1.1 mmol/L. After administration of glucose intravenously, the patient's level of consciousness begins to improve.

UNPACKING THE CASE

This incident is rich in flawed clinical reasoning, underpinned by the presence of several CDRs and a failed heuristic decision-making process. 'Anchoring', 'premature diagnostic closure' and 'confirmation bias' are all present to some degree. 'Anchoring' is the common tendency to lock onto early features of a case and not consider or look for other information that might point to another diagnosis. In this example, the call data provided en route and prior knowledge of the address and the patient contributed to the anchoring bias. 'Premature diagnostic closure' is the tendency to terminate the formation of other differential diagnoses as a result of committing to an early diagnosis but without fully confirming it. 'Confirmation bias' results in the clinician neglecting to search for signs or symptoms that might disprove an early clinical impression, tending rather to search for those that will confirm their early impression. This case also illustrates the contextual nature of paramedic clinical reasoning through the powerful influence of the immediate environment and context in which the patient was found. This is a distinct feature of paramedic reasoning, which can be extremely informative and useful on the one hand but cognitively biased on the other and capable of overshadowing the clinical presentation itself.

EDUCATIONAL STRATEGIES TO IMPROVE CLINICAL REASONING

Despite continuing debate about whether it is possible to teach diagnostic reasoning skills (Graber, 2009), there is support for educational design that aims to reduce clinical errors arising from flawed diagnostic reasoning processes (Croskerry et al., 2013). One strategy used to help individuals learn how to monitor their thinking strategies involves the development of self-diagnosis of thinking to enable identification and remediation of thinking errors. Reflection on thinking refers to the conscious assessment of the individual's thinking process or rather it represents thinking about thinking, which is also known as metacognition. Reflection offers the novice the opportunity to be aware of their thinking processes, to understand the effect that cognition has on clinical judgements and to support the transition from novice to expert. Metacognition allows the clinician to think about their thinking while they are thinking, providing self-monitoring in real time at the point where cognitive biases may be actually at play.

When developing the abilities of metacognition and reflective practice, the value of these skills must be evident to the individual, particularly in paramedic practice where technical skills are highly valued by both novices and experts. Students can be taught about metacognition, but its value must be manifest and explicit before students and novice practitioners are likely to accept this skill. Cosby (2011) argues that reflection must be guided by an experienced facilitator or mentor to identify and avoid incorrect conclusions.

REFLECTION POINT

- Reflect on the context in which paramedics conduct clinical reasoning.
- Which clinical, cultural, environmental or situational barriers may exist that would affect the translation of metacognitive education into the ability to be metacognitive in real time when clinical reasoning is occurring?

The development of metacognitive skills can help clinicians to develop strategies for minimizing or avoiding cognitive error, thus 'inoculating' the clinician against error. Prerequisites for effective inoculation are:

- an understanding of error theory, common clinical errors and cognitive de-biasing techniques involving metacognition;
- development of a 'forcing strategy' to prevent common cognitive errors such as anchoring or early diagnostic closure through the use of scenarios or case studies where this error is likely to occur and
- demonstration of a cognitive forcing strategy that is appropriate to the context to avoid error such as, for example a 'clinical pause' or 'clinical time-out' (Croskerry, 2003a).

The use of case-based learning or simulation can be used to develop these skills in the paramedic education setting. Consideration needs to be given to designing learning activities that contain cognitive error traps or that include information about the patient's environment, history and initial presentation that are likely to trigger bias.

As an example, a case contains information about a call to a suburban home to a 25-year-old male with a recent onset of abdominal pain. Stock photographs of the fictional location can be used to create a vignette to illustrate low socioeconomic circumstances. Additional stock photographs can be used to illustrate the patient presentation. Alternatively, actors or standardized patients can be used to play the role of the patient. History may include a 3-hour history of severe (8/10) hypogastric abdominal pain and nausea. The patient volunteers a history of opioid dependence and current medications include methadone. Students should complete the case and then conduct a case debrief with an experienced facilitator, where reasons for actions or decisions can be explored. For example, if the student elects to withhold analgesia, the reasons for the decision should be explored. This process may reveal concerns about the patient's motives for reporting pain. A forcing strategy that may be used in this case is to 'consider the opposite' (Croskerry et al., 2013), where the student is asked to use evidence to rule out the possibility of pain.

Although there is limited evidence of the effectiveness of cognitive de-biasing strategies, the development of strategies that help the clinician to evaluate their thinking to consider alternative explanations for the patient's presentation and to check for the potential influence of emotions or bias on decision making has the potential to reduce clinical errors. In the previous example, the inability to objectively validate and assess pain in others may lead to errors in reasoning, including errors in judging the patient's motives for reporting pain that has no obvious pathological basis. As such, strategies that support personal development of cognitive strategies that reduce the risk for error may reduce the risk for poor clinical judgements and improve the quality of patient care.

SUMMARY

In this chapter we have:

- described contemporary models of paramedic practice
- discussed the context in which clinical reasoning occurs in the discipline of paramedicine
- explored the evidence describing clinical reasoning in paramedicine
- discussed theories of clinical reasoning relevant to paramedicine
- discussed cognitive error in the context of clinical reasoning performed by paramedics
- illustrated the effect of CDR on clinical reasoning
- proposed strategies for enhancing the quality of clinical reasoning through development of metacognition in paramedics.

REFLECTION POINT

Paramedics operate most commonly in a dual-crew capacity.
- Consider the multiple concurrent tasks and functions that must be managed in the initial 10 minutes of a medium-acuity case involving an older person who has fallen and sustained a fractured hip.
- What strategies could be implemented or adopted at the point of care to reduce cognitive load in this scenario?

REFLECTION POINT

- What are the challenges faced by paramedic educators who need to teach clinical reasoning skills to novices? Consider both field education and education in the classroom.

REFERENCES

Australian Institute of Health and Welfare, 2014. Australia's medical indemnity claims 2012–13: Safety and quality of healthcare. (Vol. 15, cat. no. HSE 149.). Canberra, Australia: AIHW.

Bartlett, D., Hansen, S., Cruickshank, T., Rankin, T., Zaenker, P., Mazzucchelli, G., et al., 2022. Effects of sleepiness on clinical decision making among paramedic students: A simulated night shift study. Emerg Med J 39 (1), 45–51. https://doi.org/10.1136/emermed-2019-209211

Boyle, M.J., Smith, E.C., Archer, F.L., 2008. Trauma incidents attended by emergency medical services in Victoria, Australia. Prehosp Disaster Med 23 (1), 20–28. https://doi.org/10.1017/s1049023x00005501

Brandling, J., Kirby, K., Black, S., Voss, S., Benger, J., 2017. Emergency medical service provider decision-making in out of hospital cardiac arrest: An exploratory study. BMC Emerg Med 17 (1), 24. https://doi.org/10.1186/s12873-017-0136-3

Burgess, D.J., 2010. Are providers more likely to contribute to healthcare disparities under high levels of cognitive load? How features of the healthcare setting may lead to biases in medical decision making. Med Decis Making 30 (2), 246–257. https://doi.org/10.1177/0272989X09341751

Caplan, G.A., Sulaiman, N.S., Mangin, D.A., Aimonino Ricauda, N., Wilson, A.D., Barclay, L., 2012. A meta-analysis of "hospital in the home". Medical Journal of Australia 197 (9), 512–519.

Cosby, K., 2011. The role of certainty, confidence, and critical thinking in the diagnostic process: Good luck or good thinking? Acad Emerg Med 18 (2), 212–214. https://doi.org/10.1111/j.1553-2712.2010.00979.x

Croskerry, P., 2002. Achieving quality in clinical decision making: Cognitive strategies and detection of bias. Acad Emerg Med 9 (11), 1184–1204. https://doi.org/10.1111/j.1553-2712.2002.tb01574.x

Croskerry, P., 2003a. Cognitive forcing strategies in clinical decisionmaking. Ann Emerg Med 41 (1), 110–120. https://doi.org/10.1067/mem.2003.22

Croskerry, P., 2003b. The importance of cognitive errors in diagnosis and strategies to minimize them. Acad Med 78 (8), 775–780. https://doi.org/10.1097/00001888-200308000-00003

Croskerry, P., 2008. Cognitive and effective dispositions to respond. In: Croskerry, P., Cosby, K.S., Schenkel, S.M., Wears, R.L. (Eds.), Patient safety in emergency medicine. Lippincott Williams & Wilkins, pp. 219–227.

Croskerry, P., 2009. A universal model of diagnostic reasoning. Acad Med 84 (8), 1022–1028. https://doi.org/10.1097/ACM.0b013e3181ace703

Croskerry, P., Abbass, A., Wu, A.W., 2010. Emotional influences in patient safety. J Patient Saf 6 (4), 199–205. https://doi.org/10.1097/pts.0b013e3181f6c01a

Croskerry, P., Singhal, G., Mamede, S., 2013. Cognitive debiasing 2: Impediments to and strategies for change. BMJ Qual Saf 22 (Suppl 2), ii65–ii72. https://doi.org/10.1136/bmjqs-2012-001713

Dalton, A.L., 1996. Enhancing critical thinking in paramedic continuing education. Prehosp Disaster Med 11 (4), 246–253. https://doi.org/10.1017/s1049023x00043077

Donnelly, E.A., Bradford, P., Davis, M., Hedges, C., Socha, D., Morassutti, P., 2019. Fatigue and safety in paramedicine. CJEM 21 (6), 762–765. https://doi.org/10.1017/cem.2019.380

Dyson, K., Bray, J., Smith, K., Bernard, S., Straney, L., Finn, J., 2015. Paramedic exposure to out-of-hospital cardiac arrest is rare and declining in Victoria, Australia. Resuscitation 89, 93–98. https://doi.org/10.1016/j.resuscitation.2015.01.023

Elstein, A.S., Schwartz, A., 2002. Clinical problem solving and diagnostic decision making: Selective review of the cognitive literature. BMJ 324 (7339), 729–732. https://doi.org/10.1136/bmj.324.7339.729

Epstein, R.M., Hundert, E.M., 2002. Defining and assessing professional competence. JAMA 287 (2), 226–235. https://doi.org/10.1001/jama.287.2.226

Evans, J.S., 2003. In two minds: Dual-process accounts of reasoning. Trends Cogn Sci 7 (10), 454–459. https://doi.org/10.1016/j.tics.2003.08.012

Gough, S., 2018. Welcoming paramedics into the national registration and accreditation scheme, Vol. 15. SAGE Publications Sage UK, London, England. 1–2.

Graber, M.L., 2009. Educational strategies to reduce diagnostic error: Can you teach this stuff? Adv Health Sci Educ Theory Pract 14 (Suppl 1), 63–69. https://doi.org/10.1007/s10459-009-9178-y

Janing, J., 1994. Critical thinking: Incorporation into the paramedic curriculum. Prehosp Disaster Med 9 (4), 238–242. https://doi.org/10.1017/s1049023x00041479

Jensen, J., 2010. *Paramedic clinical decision making*. [Dalhousie University]. Halifax, Nova Scotia.

Jensen, J.L., Bienkowski, A., Travers, A.H., Calder, L.A., Walker, M., Tavares, W., et al., 2016. A survey to determine decision-making styles of working paramedics and student paramedics. CJEM 18 (3), 213–222. https://doi.org/10.1017/cem.2015.95

Keene, T., Pammer, K., Lord, B., Shipp, C., 2022. Fluency and confidence predict paramedic diagnostic intuition: An experimental study of applied dual-process theory. Int Emerg Nurs 61, 101126. https://doi.org/10.1016/j.ienj.2021.101126

Kovacs, G., Croskerry, P., 1999. Clinical decision making: An emergency medicine perspective. Acad Emerg Med 6 (9), 947–952. https://doi.org/10.1111/j.1553-2712.1999.tb01246.x

Lowthian, J.A., Jolley, D.J., Curtis, A.J., Currell, A., Cameron, P.A., Stoelwinder, J.U., et al., 2011. The challenges of population ageing: Accelerating demand for emergency ambulance services by older patients, 1995-2015. Med J Aust 194 (11), 574–578. https://doi.org/10.5694/j.1326-5377.2011.tb03107.x

O'Hara, R., Johnson, M., Siriwardena, A.N., Weyman, A., Turner, J., Shaw, D., et al., 2015. A qualitative study of systemic influences on paramedic decision making: Care transitions and patient safety. J Health Serv Res Policy 20 (Suppl 1), 45–53. https://doi.org/10.1177/1355819614558472

Perona, M., Rahman, M.A., O'Meara, P., 2019. Paramedic judgement, decision-making and cognitive processing: A review of the literature. Australasian Journal of Paramedicine 16, 1–12.

Shaban, R.Z., Wyatt-Smith, C., Cumming, J., 2004. Uncertainty, error and risk in human clinical judgment: Introductory theoretical frameworks in paramedic practice. Australasian Journal of Paramedicine 2 (1), 1–12.

Sloman, S.A., 1996. The empirical case for two systems of reasoning. Psychological Bulletin 119 (1), 3.

Weingart, S.D., 2008. Critical decision making in chaotic environments. In: Croskerry, P., Cosby, K.S., Schenkel, S.M., Wears, R.L. (Eds.), Patient safety in emergency medicine. Lippincott Williams & Wilkins, Philadelphia, pp. 209–212.

28 DECISION MAKING AND CLINICAL REASONING IN OPTOMETRY

CAROLINE FAUCHER ■ CATHERINE SUTTLE

CHAPTER OUTLINE

CHAPTER AIMS

The aims of this chapter are:

- to situate optometry and its scope of practice with respect to other healthcare professions and
- to provide an overview of current clinical decision making and clinical reasoning in optometry.

INTRODUCTION

According to the World Council of Optometry, 'Optometry is a healthcare profession that is autonomous, educated, and regulated (licensed/registered) and optometrists are the primary healthcare practitioners of the eye and visual system who provide comprehensive eye and vision care, which includes refraction and dispensing, detection/diagnosis and management of disease in the eye, and the rehabilitation of conditions of the visual system' (World Council of Optometry, n. d.).

Optometry's scope of practice varies around the world and even within provinces or states of the same country. In some geographical locations, scope of practice is still limited to the provision of spectacles (European Council of Optometry and Optics, 2020). In others (e.g. Australia, United Kingdom), scope of practice has increased considerably over time to a level at which the optometrist's role includes the prescription of therapeutic drugs to treat eye disease (Cooper, 2012; Harper et al., 2016; Kiely and Slater, 2015) and procedures such as ocular surface foreign body removal and punctal plugs insertion (Canadian Association of Optometrists, 2021). Some states of the United States have even expanded the optometric scope of practice to include injections, laser, and other minor surgical procedures (Edwards, 2019; Gibson, 2020). However, comprehensive routine eye and vision examinations remain the main reason to visit an optometrist (American Optometric Association, 2015; Boadi-Kusi et al., 2015; Thite et al., 2015). Although the optometrist's role varies globally, a comprehensive optometric examination includes evaluation of the functional status of the eyes and visual system, assessment of ocular health conditions, establishment of diagnoses, formulation of treatment and management plans and counselling and education of the patient regarding his or her visual and ocular healthcare status (American Optometric Association, 2015). The nature of the eye and vision system is such that many conditions have similar symptoms. Moreover, in asymptomatic patients, comprehensive routine optometric examinations can lead to the detection of a significant number of new eye conditions (including a change in spectacle prescription and new critical diagnosis) and/or result in management changes (Dobbelsteyn et al., 2015; Irving et al., 2016). Therefore, an optometric examination can rarely be driven only by the patient's symptoms (problem-oriented examination). It is rather a thorough investigation of many aspects of vision and eye health (systems examination), embedded in a routine but flexible protocol.

Fig. 28.1 shows the paths that an optometric examination can take, according to the main reason for the encounter. Optometrists have their habitual routine of examination in which they review the oculovisual systems: visual function, refraction, binocular vision and ocular health (Elliott, 2014). Of course, history taking is vital, as many patients presenting for a routine examination, without initially reporting any complaints, finally declare some vision or eye-related symptoms when questioned specifically by their optometrist (Kovarski et al., 2020; Webb et al., 2013). When patients present complex clinical features, optometrists deviate from their routine according to each clinical situation. They are planning, on an ongoing basis, what they will be doing later during the encounter (Faucher et al., 2012). Because a routine optometric examination often leads to incidental findings that were not indicated by the initial reason for the visit, optometrists need to balance the importance of the examination's incidental findings and the patient's expectations or concerns. For example, a patient comes to change her spectacles, but the optometrist uncovers an unsuspected eye disease needing an urgent referral to a specialist. This is a potential site of tension between the patient's and optometrist's respective agendas (Varpio et al., 2007).

This routine aspect of the optometric profession has characteristics in common with some other health professions. Traditional medical textbooks describe very detailed and systematic physical examination of each organ system. Mostly used by students, the value of such a systematic examination may be impractical in clinical settings where time is of the essence (Elliott, 2014; Ramani, 2008). Thus, most published papers or books specifically dedicated to clinical reasoning focus on managing ill patients or patients presenting with complaints. Despite several decades of research on decision making and clinical reasoning in many healthcare professions, optometry remains under-represented and the clinical decision-making literature in optometry is largely focussed on evidence-based practice (EBP) and the effect of training and guidelines (Myint et al., 2014). Only a few articles have specifically focussed on optometrists' or optometry students' clinical reasoning (Corliss, 1995; Faucher et al., 2016; Faucher et al., 2012; Kurtz, 1990; Sundling et al., 2019; Werner, 1989). This chapter provides an overview of decision making and clinical reasoning in optometry.

EVIDENCE-BASED DECISION MAKING IN OPTOMETRY

Clinical reasoning requires critical thinking, which is a way of thinking that is free from bias, suspends judgement and considers different perspectives. It requires not only skills but also an attitude, such that the critical thinker approaches ideas and concepts without bias (da Silva Bastos Cerullo and de Almeida Lopes Monteiro da Cruz, 2010). Clinical knowledge and information from a wide range of sources are also essential to clinical reasoning. The patient's signs, symptoms, preferences and circumstances in addition to knowledge and information from education, colleagues, research and other sources are used throughout the consultation to make clinical decisions with the patient (Faucher et al., 2012; Sundling et al., 2019). The use of experience and information from a range of sources is captured by the concept of EBP, which combines three key factors used in clinical decision making: the practitioner's experience, the patient's circumstances and preferences, and the best available evidence from research (Dawes et al., 2005; Sackett et al., 1996). The clinical decision is made in the environmental context of the practice (Satterfield et al., 2009) and the process may therefore be affected by factors such as Internet access, practice policy and attitudes of colleagues within the practice. Fig. 28.2 illustrates this model, with three key factors contributing to decision making in the practice context.

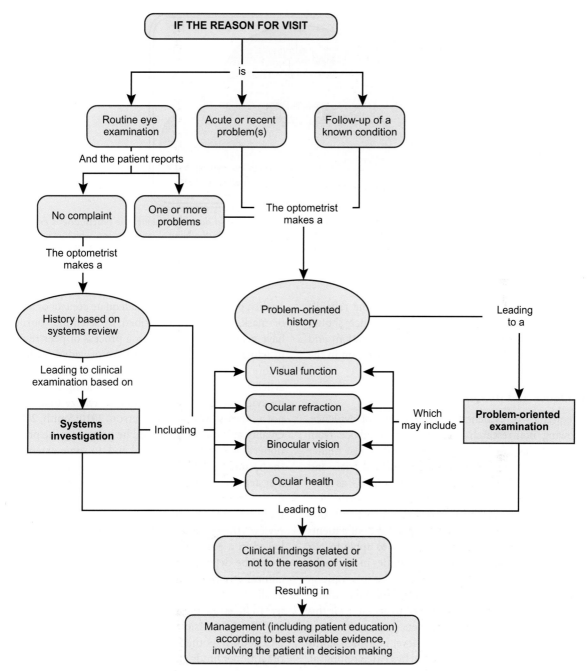

Fig. 28.1 ▧ Categories of reason for an optometric clinical encounter and the type of investigation related to each.

Viewed from this perspective, the quality of clinical decision making depends on the quality of any evidence used. For those clinical questions with relevant research evidence, the optometrist must be aware of its validity or strength, including its relevance and clinical significance for the patient concerned. The model shown in Fig. 28.2 includes the patient's preferences and circumstances, indicating that these should be

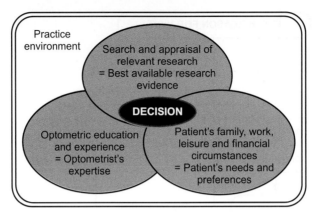

Fig. 28.2 ■ The connection between three key factors in evidence-based clinical decision making: the practitioner's expertise, the patient's preferences and the best available evidence. The decision is made in the clinical environment, which may limit or facilitate the extent to which best evidence is used. (Modified with permission from Satterfield, J.M., Spring, B., Brownson, R.C., et al., 2009. Toward a transdisciplinary model of evidence-based practice. Milbank Q. 87, 368–390. Fig. 5.)

considered in decision making and that the reliability and clinical significance of any evidence should be discussed with the patient so that the patient and practitioner make an informed clinical decision in the context of that patient's situation.

Evidence and Its Quality

Hierarchies of evidence present 'levels' of evidence, showing non-research sources such as advice from colleagues as low level, with case studies just higher than this and with randomized controlled trials and systematic reviews of evidence at higher levels, as illustrated in Table 28.1. This hierarchy reflects the fact that sources such as case studies present us with evidence based on only one or a small number of patients and with results that may be unlikely to apply to our patient. Furthermore, intervention studies in which the researcher and/or patient is aware of the intervention and expected outcome are subject to bias and randomized controlled trials are important to account for this and to provide more reliable evidence of the efficacy of interventions. In addition to the level of evidence, the quality of evidence should be rated by critical appraisal, looking for indicators of bias. This can be achieved using critical appraisal tools such as those made freely available by the Critical Appraisal Skills Programme (2022).

Critical appraisal of this kind is important because a high-level study may be, in some cases, of poor quality, perhaps caused by inadequate control or a lack of masking. Studies described in scientific journals have generally been through a process of peer review in which experts in the area have provided feedback before publication. It might be supposed that the articles passing this process are providing good quality evidence, but it is important to realize that this is not a safe assumption (Henderson, 2010; Smith, 2006). Quality and reliability should be gauged by the practitioner's own critical appraisal and, to some extent, on the basis of the level and type of evidence. For example, a systematic review has been generated by a process designed to minimize bias and is likely to provide more reliable evidence than a traditional literature review (though as indicated earlier, the method followed in a particular review may be flawed and this would be determined by critical appraisal). For some clinical questions, there may be no research evidence at all or the research evidence may be of poor quality. To illustrate these situations and their implications for clinical decision making, Case Studies 28.1 and 28.2 show hypothetical clinical scenarios in which the practitioner finds no evidence (Case Study 28.1) or high-level evidence (Case Study 28.2). In Case Study 28.1, because there is no research evidence, the practitioner must base clinical decision making on information from other sources, experience and existing knowledge, in addition to the patient's preferences. The practitioner advises the patient that although there

TABLE 28.1
Levels of Evidence

Level	Form of Evidence	Description and Examples
High	Systematic review of evidence with or without meta-analysis; evidence-based synopsis of research	Review of research using a wide literature search and a set of criteria to judge research quality. A meta-analysis combines research findings to find a pooled estimate of effect from a large sample.
	Treatment trial with randomization and control	Research in which patients have been randomly allocated to treatment and control groups.
	Treatment trial without control group or with historical control; case-control study; cohort study	Research in which the sample size may be adequate but the control is not or research in which control is not included as part of the study design (e.g. a cohort study).
	Individual case study or small case series	A report of clinical findings in one or a small number of patients.
Low	Recommendation from expert	Advice from a respected colleague, a seminar speaker or author of a continuing education and training article.

CASE STUDY 28.1

Evidence for Clinical Decision Making

Mark is an adult with amblyopia who has found a possible treatment on a website. He tells you that the treatment is a special pair of glasses with flickering, coloured lights presented to either eye. The website suggests a high likelihood of successful treatment of amblyopia and Mark would like to know whether this is worth trying. Your search for research evidence using PubMed and Google Scholar using appropriate key words finds no relevant research. You then access the website Mark was talking about and find no references to research on this method. How do you manage this situation?

CASE STUDY 28.2

Basing Clinical Decision Making and Patient Advice on Evidence

Karen is a 75-year-old patient with mild age-related macular degeneration. She has heard that progression can be slowed by increasing dietary intake of omega 3 fatty acids and asks whether this is correct. A search of the PubMed database and the Cochrane database of Systematic Reviews finds that high-level evidence (a Cochrane systematic review) is available on this clinical topic. It indicates that dietary supplementation with omega 3 fatty acids has no effect on progression of the disease. What advice do you offer Karen?

is no evidence that the method will be harmful, there is also no reliable evidence that this treatment will be effective. In Case Study 28.2, research evidence indicates that dietary supplementation with omega 3 fatty acids has no effect on progression of the disease. The evidence is high level and quality is likely to be high because it has been generated using a method that minimizes bias. Thus, the patient can be advised that this evidence is likely to be reliable and that the supplementation is unlikely to affect disease progression.

Basis of Optometrists' Clinical Decision Making

Optometrists, as with all other healthcare practitioners, have access to a plethora of information on which clinical decisions could be based: continuing education lectures or articles, marketing information on the use of certain diagnostic or therapeutic tools or interventions, advice from colleagues, research-based information in peer-reviewed journals and information in books or other journals. A questionnaire-based study of optometrists in Australia and New Zealand (Suttle et al., 2012) indicates that many rely heavily on undergraduate, postgraduate and continuing education as sources of information on which to base clinical decisions or modifications to their clinical practice, such as use of a new diagnostic technique. Another questionnaire-based study (Lawrenson and Evans, 2013) found that optometrists in the United Kingdom commonly use professional magazines with non-peer-reviewed articles as sources of evidence on which to base lifestyle advice for patients with age-related macular degeneration. More recent research indicates that the main sources of information used by Australian optometrists as a basis for prescribing blue light-blocking spectacle lenses are conference presentations and product information from manufacturers (Singh et al., 2019). In another survey of Australian optometrists, continuing education conferences and events were significant sources of information about clinical decisions on management of childhood myopia (Douglass et al., 2020). The authors also found that optometrists prefer to use preappraised sources of evidence such as systematic reviews over individual research studies, perhaps reflecting the significant work involved in critical appraisal, alleviated to some extent by the critical appraisal tools mentioned earlier.

These findings indicate that optometrists tend to depend on sources other than peer-reviewed published research. A high proportion of optometrists consider that sources such as information from undergraduate, postgraduate, continuing education and manufacturers' product information are acceptable as a basis for their clinical decision making. However, this information is provided through the filter of the educator and may not be critically appraised. The practitioner receiving and using this information may assume that it is of high quality and up-to-date and reliable, but this may not be the case. Peer-reviewed, published research is preferable as a source of evidence because the practitioner can appraise it and gauge its quality before applying it as part of decision making. Intuitively, it seems that the use of more reliable evidence would lead to better patient outcomes, because flawed evidence (e.g. wrongly suggesting high efficacy of a treatment method) would be identified as low quality and treated as such by the practitioner. Surprisingly, there is little high-level evidence on the relationship between EBP and patient outcomes. One study has demonstrated lower patient mortality with EBP than with standard practice (Emparanza et al., 2015). There is not yet, to our knowledge, any such evidence on the effectiveness of EBP in eye care, but the evidence in medicine cited above does suggest that it has a positive effect on health outcomes.

Facilitating EBP

The likelihood that optometrists will find, appraise and use research evidence depends on the time avail-able in the clinical encounter and the clinician's knowledge, skills and beliefs about EBP (Toomey et al., 2021). The time needed for evidence-based decision making may be reduced by systematic reviews focussed on clinical questions, such as those available from the Cochrane Eyes and Vision Group (2024) and the Translating Research into Practice (TRIP (2024)) database. Databases providing free access to preappraised evidence are available for some health disciplines but not yet for optometry. Feasibility and sustainability are challenges for databases of this kind because a great deal of time must be consistently committed by skilled appraisers to provide and maintain up-to-date content. A recent attempt to overcome these problems is crowdsourcing of critical appraisal. An online resource (CrowdCARE, Pianta et al., 2018) has been developed with the aim of teaching critical appraisal skills and building a database of appraised research evidence. Over time, systems such as this may prove helpful as sources of skills and evidence for busy clinicians.

Evidence-based clinical guidelines such as those provided by the College of Optometrists (n. d.) in the United Kingdom provide widely accessed advice based on the best available evidence relevant to certain eye conditions that may be managed by independent prescribing optometrists but do not address a wide range of clinical scenarios. The National Institute for Health and Care Excellence (NICE) (2024) in the United Kingdom provides evidence-based guidance relevant to the investigation and management of a range of conditions, but many optometric clinical encounters would have no relevant guidelines. For example, the blue light filters mentioned earlier have been highly controversial since they have been promoted to patients by some optometry companies without good evidence of their effectiveness (Suttle, 2019). No guidelines address this intervention, but the College of Optometrists does provide a position statement stating that best evidence does not currently support their use (College of Optometrists, 2018). Given a lack of evidence-based guidelines for many optometric clinical questions, it is important that optometrists can critique the evidence presented in continuing education and training seminars or articles. Full details are not usually provided in these situations and the recipient of this evidence would need to find and appraise relevant evidence and any clinical claims. They would therefore need relevant knowledge and skills and these have widely been introduced to optometry teaching curricula (MacDonald et al., 2014) and have been included in some accreditation documents for optometry (Kiely and Slater, 2015), suggesting that optometrists are likely to have some of the required knowledge and skills on graduation. In addition, it may be possible to anticipate some clinical questions, such as whether a new intervention is effective or whether a new diagnostic method has high sensitivity. Thus, barriers, such as time, do limit the extent to which the optometrist can apply EBP, but resources may help and strategies can be adopted to ensure that the practitioner is aware of the best evidence relevant to at least some clinical encounters.

FROM DECISION MAKING TO CLINICAL REASONING

As outlined earlier, clinical decisions need to call on knowledge of the best available evidence and this may need to be sourced and appraised in anticipation, due to time limitations in the clinic. Patients rarely come with classic textbook characteristics. For example, it may be difficult to identify the cause of vision loss, particularly if a patient is seen for the first time: is the vision loss caused by amblyopia, worsening of a retinal disease or a developing cataract? A combination of multiple conditions may complicate the diagnosis. The frequent need for subjective responses from patients also influences clinical results and may render data harder to interpret. Ettinger (1997) has identified six sources of uncertainty in optometry. They are provided in Table 28.2 with examples and strategies for addressing them.

It becomes obvious that, to address those multiple sources of uncertainty in clinical practice, optometrists will have to mobilize several resources and exercise judicious and efficient clinical reasoning.

Scripts Formation and Activation

It is often claimed that the structure of knowledge in memory plays a central role in clinical reasoning. Originating from cognitive psychology, the script theory of reasoning provides a theoretical framework to illustrate how knowledge can be structured for clinical problem solving (Charlin et al., 2000). Scripts are cognitive structures stored in the memory. They contain a complex network of meaningful links among

TABLE 28.2		
Uncertainty in Optometric Clinical Decision Making		
Source of Uncertainty	**Examples or Explanations**	**Strategies for Addressing It**
Limited availability of clinical information	Special populations (limited patient's ability to respond to testing) Invasive procedures (if risks outweigh benefits)	Be familiar with special testing procedures Consider alternative strategies
Limited quality of information	Unreliable responses from patients	Ensure the patient understands Repeat or clarify the directions Use alternative tests
Limited ability to gather definitive information	It is physically impossible to directly inspect every part of the body (e.g. optic chiasm).	Stay up to date Acquire specialized equipment if possible Consider patient referral for certain types of testing
Ambiguity in interpreting clinical data	Reliable data may be subject to interpretation	Consider closer follow-ups Combine multiple tests
Uncertainty in patients' responses to treatment	Efficacy of treatment varies among patients and for the same patient on a different period of time	Monitor patients' response to treatment over time Educate patient about side effects
Examiners' uncertainty	Optometrist's own confidence in generating hypotheses, gathering and analysing data, making diagnoses and choosing treatment plans	Monitor successful cases Reinforce knowledge by additional training, reading and continual education Solicit feedback from clinical experts

clinical features (e.g. enabling conditions, causes and consequences of specific diseases or anomalies) that allow a healthcare practitioner to resolve clinical problems, via diagnosis, investigation or treatment. Scripts develop progressively by applying knowledge through regular practice with patients. To take an example: students in optometry with no clinical experience with glaucomatous patients do possess theoretical (pathophysiological) knowledge about concepts such as physiology of the aqueous humour; intraocular pressure; ocular anatomy; vascularization of the eye; and perception, perimetry and pharmacology. Once in clinical settings, students gradually reorganize what they know about glaucoma into a series of scripts. Meaningful links are created between various pieces of information, particularly regarding diagnosis and treatment. Students' growing experience with diverse cases of glaucoma (various presentations, degrees of severity, rates of progression and responses to treatment) helps them internalize many examples of glaucoma, which enrich any glaucoma script they have already stored. Later, when experienced optometrists recognize cases of glaucoma (script activation), the knowledge required for appropriate case management comes to mind: they will have no need to retrieve pathophysiological details from their long-term memory (Faucher et al., 2016). Keeping up to date with evolving research evidence can also contribute to underpin optometrists' scripts.

Dual-Process Reasoning

Given the multifaceted, complex context of practice and the constantly evolving field of practice, how do optometrists reason during an optometric encounter? Unfortunately, only a few investigators have studied clinical reasoning in optometry. Some authors have adapted medical models to the optometry profession (Corliss, 1995; Ettinger and Rouse, 1997; Kurtz, 1990; Werner, 1989) without conducting any research involving practising optometrists. Part of the answer may be found in work by Faucher et al. (2012). They conducted a qualitative study aiming to make explicit the clinical reasoning processes of optometrists from two contrasting levels of professional development and to highlight the characteristics of clinical reasoning expertise in optometry. Their results are consistent with the script theory of reasoning on several points. They show that

optometrists quickly construct a mental representation of the patient's clinical situation (activation of relevant scripts). Through hypothetico-deductive reasoning, optometrists also anticipate clinical findings throughout the encounter and constantly readjust their initial mental representation of the clinical situation based on any additional clinical findings. According to the script theory of reasoning, this corresponds to the assessment of a fit between activated scripts and the clinical situation (Charlin et al., 2000). Finally, optometrists formulate their management and treatment plan throughout the encounter, not just at the end of it.

These findings show that clinical reasoning in optometry is also consistent with the dual-process theory of reasoning, originating from the cognitive psychology literature (Wason and Evans, 1975) and then proposed to describe clinical reasoning processes (Marcum, 2012; Pelaccia et al., 2011). According to the dual-process theory, clinical reasoning is a multidimensional and complex process involving both nonanalytic and analytic cognitive processes. Nonanalytic processes include tacit or intuitive knowledge, relying on a clinician's previous experience. They are used in an unconscious manner: the clinician automatically recognizes a configuration of signs and symptoms. For example, an optometrist can suspect hyperopia and esotropia as soon as a patient walks in simply by noticing that the patient's spectacles have a magnifying effect on his or her eyes. Analytic processes represent critical thinking and objective analysis that are deliberate and reflective. In the same example, analytic processes will be necessary to put together the clinical findings (patient's history, visual function, refraction, binocular vision, ocular health) to confirm, or not, the presence of hyperopia and esotropia and to make decisions based on the patient's conditions and needs. Those decisions are made throughout the consultation to obtain more information, interpret clinical data, define the problem and to consider treatment and management options (Sundling et al., 2019).

Analytic and nonanalytic processes are intertwined in clinical practice, working in synergy to understand a clinical situation rapidly, to investigate further and to make the appropriate decisions for a given patient. The development of these processes should be fostered and monitored during training and beyond. Again, there is little research evidence about learning clinical reasoning and assessment in optometry. The script concordance test was found to be reliable and capable of discriminating between different levels of optometric students' clinical reasoning (Faucher et al., 2016). More recently, Edgar et al. (2022) adapted, and validated for use in optometry, the Diagnostic Thinking Inventory, used for decades in medical education (Bordage et al., 1990). This self-reflective tool measures two aspects underpinning clinical reasoning: flexibility in thinking and knowledge structure in memory. Further investigation is required, but Edgar et al. (2022) have highlighted the potential of the Diagnostic Thinking Inventory for Optometry for future use. As the scope of practice of this profession rapidly expands, it is crucial to provide students and optometrists with ways to assess and develop their clinical reasoning.

CONCLUSION

Optometrists are primary providers of comprehensive eye and vision care. They usually follow a routine but flexible sequence of examination. Any clinical finding, within normal limits or not, triggers the activation of clinical reasoning processes and leads to the understanding of the clinical situation. Due to time constraints, finding and appraising evidence often occur outside the clinical encounter. Clinical reasoning then helps practitioners to make judgements about the relevance of research and clinical evidence for a specific clinical situation (Higgs et al., 2001). Clinical knowledge, which is essential to clinical reasoning, is constantly enriched by every clinical situation and updated by applying evolving research evidence. Studies suggest, however, that optometrists mostly base their clinical decisions on information from undergraduate, postgraduate and continuing education, rather than on peer-reviewed published research. Further research is needed to assess the effectiveness of EBP in optometry and to understand better the clinical reasoning processes, which are essential to optometrists' actions. Finally, we have to keep an eye on future directions of clinical decision support systems that may assist optometrists in providing more accurate and efficient patient care (Ho et al., 2022), as well as on the eventual applications of artificial intelligence on optometric care. How will these novel technologies influence evidence-based decision making and clinical reasoning in optometry?

REFLECTION POINT

A high proportion of optometrists base their clinical decision making on sources other than peer-reviewed published research.
■ How can we reverse this trend?

REFLECTION POINT

As the scope of practice in optometry increases and optometrists take on more responsibility, there is a need to ensure that the clinical reasoning involved in practice and education is as rigorous as it can be.

SUMMARY

In this chapter, we have outlined that:

■ optometrists are comprehensive eye and vision care providers who have seen their scope of practice expand considerably over time
■ clinical decision-making literature in optometry is largely focussed on evidence-based practice, guidelines and the effect of training
■ optometrists do not base their decisions on peer-reviewed published research as much as they could
■ optometrists' clinical reasoning is consistent with both the dual-process and the script theories of reasoning
■ evidence-based practice, decision making and clinical reasoning need to be investigated further specifically for the optometry profession.

REFERENCES

American Optometric Association, 2015. Evidence-based clinical practice guideline. Comprehensive adult eye and vision examination. American Optometric Association. https://www.aoa.org/AOA/Documents/Practice%20Management/Clinical%20Guidelines/EBO%20Guidelines/Comprehensive%20Adult%20Eye%20and%20Vision%20Exam.pdf

Boadi-Kusi, S.B., Ntodie, M., Mashige, K.P., Owusu-Ansah, A., Antwi Osei, K., 2015. A cross-sectional survey of optometrists and optometric practices in Ghana. Clin Exp Optom 98 (5), 473–477. https://doi.org/10.1111/cxo.12291

Bordage, G., Grant, J., Marsden, P., 1990. Quantitative assessment of diagnostic ability. Med Educ 24 (5), 413–425. https://doi.org/10.1111/j.1365-2923.1990.tb02650.x

Canadian Association of Optometrists, 2021. Optometric scope of practice across Canada. https://opto.ca/sites/default/files/resources/documents/OPTOMETRY%20SCOPE%20ACROSS%20CANADA%20GRID%20-%20Aug%202021.pdf

Charlin, B., Tardif, J., Boshuizen, H.P., 2000. Scripts and medical diagnostic knowledge: Theory and applications for clinical reasoning instruction and research. Acad Med 75 (2), 182–190. https://doi.org/10.1097/00001888-200002000-00020

Cochrane Eyes and Vision Group, 2024. CEV Reviews. https://www.eyes.cochrane.org

College of Optometrists, 2018. Blue blocking spectacle lenses. https://www.college-optometrists.org/clinical-guidance/position-statements/blue-blocking-spectacle-lenses

College of Optometrists. (n. d.). Clinical management guidelines. https://www.college-optometrists.org/clinical-guidance/clinical-management-guidelines

Cooper, S.L., 2012. 1971 – 2011: Forty year history of scope expansion into medical eye care. Optometry 83 (2), 64–73.

Corliss, D.A., 1995. A comprehensive model of clinical decision making. J Am Optom Assoc 66 (6), 362–371.

Critical Appraisal Skills Programme, 2022. *CASP Checklists*. CASP. https://casp-uk.net/casp-tools-checklists/

da Silva Bastos Cerullo, J.A., de Almeida Lopes Monteiro da Cruz, D., 2010. Clinical reasoning and critical thinking. Rev Lat Am Enfermagem 18 (1), 124–129. https://doi.org/S0104-11692010000100019 [pii]

Dawes, M., Summerskill, W., Glasziou, P., Cartabellotta, A., Martin, J., Hopayian, K., et al., 2005. Sicily statement on evidence-based practice. BMC Med Educ 5 (1), 1. https://doi.org/1472-6920-5-1 [pii]

Dobbelsteyn, D., McKee, K., Bearnes, R.D., Jayanetti, S.N., Persaud, D.D., Cruess, A.F., 2015. What percentage of patients presenting for routine eye examinations require referral for secondary care? A study of referrals from optometrists to ophthalmologists. Clin Exp Optom 98 (3), 214–217. https://doi.org/10.1111/cxo.12255

Douglass, A., Keller, P.R., He, M., Downie, L.E., 2020. Knowledge, perspectives and clinical practices of Australian optometrists in relation to childhood myopia. Clin Exp Optom 103 (2), 155–166. https://doi.org/10.1111/cxo.12936

Edgar, A.K., Ainge, L., Backhouse, S., Armitage, J.A., 2022. A cohort study for the development and validation of a reflective inventory to quantify diagnostic reasoning skills in optometry practice. BMC Med Educ 22 (1), 536. https://doi.org/10.1186/s12909-022-03493-6

Edwards, S.L., 2019. Arkansas expands scope of practice for optometrists. TortSource 21 (4), 8–10.

Elliott, D.B., 2014. Evidence-based eye examinations. In: Elliott, D.B. (Ed.), Clinical procedures in primary eye care. Elsevier Saunders, pp. 1–12.

Emparanza, J.I., Cabello, J.B., Burls, A.J., 2015. Does evidence-based practice improve patient outcomes? An analysis of a natural experiment in a Spanish hospital. J Eval Clin Pract 21 (6), 1059–1065. https://doi.org/10.1111/jep.12460

Ettinger, E.R., 1997. Dealing with clinical uncertainty. In: Ettinger, E.R., Rouse, M.W. (Eds.), Clinical decision making in optometry. Butterworth-Heinemann, pp. 39–64.

Ettinger, E.R., Rouse, M.W., 1997. Clinical decision making in optometry. Butterworth-Heinemann.

European Council of Optometry and Optics. (2020). Blue book 2020, trends in optics and optometry – Comparative European data. European Council of Optometry and Optics. https://ecoo.info/wp-content/uploads/2022/02/ECOO_BlueBook_2020-compressed_png.pdf

Faucher, C., Dufour-Guindon, M.P., Lapointe, G., Gagnon, R., Charlin, B., 2016. Assessing clinical reasoning in optometry using the script concordance test. Clin Exp Optom 99 (3), 280–286. https://doi.org/10.1111/cxo.12354

Faucher, C., Tardif, J., Chamberland, M., 2012. Optometrists' clinical reasoning made explicit: A qualitative study. Optom Vis Sci 89 (12), 1774–1784. https://doi.org/10.1097/OPX.0b013e3182776002

Gibson, D.M., 2020. Eye care provider availability for the Medicare population in U.S. states that have expanded optometrist scope of practice. Optom Vis Sci 97 (11), 929–935. https://doi.org/10.1097/OPX.0000000000001599

Harper, R., Creer, R., Jackson, J., Ehrlich, D., Tompkin, A., Bowen, M., et al., 2016. Scope of practice of optometrists working in the UK Hospital Eye Service: A national survey. Ophthalmic Physiol Opt 36 (2), 197–206. https://doi.org/10.1111/opo.12262

Henderson, M., 2010. Problems with peer review. BMJ 340, c1409. https://doi.org/10.1136/bmj.c1409

Higgs, J., Burn, A., Jones, M., 2001. Integrating clinical reasoning and evidence-based practice. AACN Clin Issues 12 (4), 482–490. http://www.ncbi.nlm.nih.gov/pubmed/11759421

Ho, S., Kalloniatis, M., Ly, A., 2022. Clinical decision support in primary care for better diagnosis and management of retinal disease. Clin Exp Optom 105 (6), 562–572. https://doi.org/10.1080/08164622.2021.2008791

Irving, E.L., Harris, J.D., Machan, C.M., Robinson, B.E., Hrynchak, P.K., Leat, S.L., et al., 2016. Value of routine eye examinations in asymptomatic patients. Optom Vis Sci 93 (7), 660–666. https://doi.org/10.1097/OPX.0000000000000863

Kiely, P.M., Slater, J., 2015. Optometry Australia entry-level competency standards for optometry 2014. Clin Exp Optom 98 (1), 65–89. https://doi.org/10.1111/cxo.12216

Kovarski, C., Portalier, S., Faucher, C., Carlu, C., Bremond-Gignac, D., Orssaud, C., 2020. Effects of visual disorders on the academic achievement of French secondary school students. Arch Pediatr 27 (8), 436–441. https://doi.org/10.1016/j.arcped.2020.08.013

Kurtz, D., 1990. Teaching clinical reasoning. Journal of Optometric Education 15 (4), 119–122.

Lawrenson, J.G., Evans, J.R., 2013. Advice about diet and smoking for people with or at risk of age-related macular degeneration: A cross-sectional survey of eye care professionals in the UK. BMC Public Health 13, 564. https://doi.org/10.1186/1471-2458-13-564

MacDonald, K.A., Hrynchak, P.K., Spafford, M.M., 2014. Evidence-based practice instruction by faculty members and librarians in North American optometry and ophthalmology programs. J Med Libr Assoc 102 (3), 210–215. https://doi.org/10.3163/1536-5050.102.3.013

Marcum, J.A., 2012. An integrated model of clinical reasoning: Dual-process theory of cognition and metacognition. J Eval

Clin Pract 18 (5), 954–961. https://doi.org/10.1111/j.1365-2753.2012.01900.x

Myint, J., Edgar, D.F., Murdoch, I.E., Lawrenson, J.G., 2014. The impact of postgraduate training on UK optometrists' clinical decision-making in glaucoma. Ophthalmic Physiol Opt 34 (3), 376–384. https://doi.org/10.1111/opo.12126

Pelaccia, T., Tardif, J., Triby, E., Charlin, B., 2011. An analysis of clinical reasoning through a recent and comprehensive approach: The dual-process theory. Med Educ Online 16, 5890. https://doi.org/10.3402/meo.v16i0.5890

Pianta, M.J., Makrai, E., Verspoor, K.M., Cohn, T.A., Downie, L.E., 2018. Crowdsourcing critical appraisal of research evidence (CrowdCARE) was found to be a valid approach to assessing clinical research quality. J Clin Epidemiol 104, 8–14. https://doi.org/10.1016/j.jclinepi.2018.07.015

Ramani, S., 2008. Twelve tips for excellent physical examination teaching. Med Teach 30 (9-10), 851–856. https://doi.org/10.1080/01421590802206747

Sackett, D.L., Rosenberg, W.M., Gray, J.A., Haynes, R.B., Richardson, W.S., 1996. Evidence based medicine: What it is and what it isn't. BMJ 312 (7023), 71–72. https://doi.org/10.1136/bmj.312.7023.71

Satterfield, J.M., Spring, B., Brownson, R.C., Mullen, E.J., Newhouse, R.P., Walker, B.B., et al., 2009. Toward a transdisciplinary model of evidence-based practice. The Milbank Quarterly 87 (2), 368–390.

Singh, S., Anderson, A.J., Downie, L.E., 2019. Insights into Australian optometrists' knowledge and attitude towards prescribing blue light-blocking ophthalmic devices. Ophthalmic Physiol Opt 39 (3), 194–204. https://doi.org/10.1111/opo.12615

Smith, R., 2006. Peer review: A flawed process at the heart of science and journals. J R Soc Med 99 (4), 178–182. https://doi.org/10.1177/014107680609900414

Sundling, V., Stene, H.A., Eide, H., Hugaas Ofstad, E., 2019. Identifying decisions in optometry: A validation study of the decision identification and classification taxonomy for use in medicine (DICTUM) in optometric consultations. Patient Educ Couns 102 (7), 1288–1295. https://doi.org/10.1016/j.pec.2019.02.018

Suttle, C.M., 2019. Marketing and anecdotal evidence should not guide the delivery of optometric interventions. Ophthalmic Physiol Opt 39 (2), 63–65. https://doi.org/10.1111/opo.12608

Suttle, C.M., Jalbert, I., Alnahedh, T., 2012. Examining the evidence base used by optometrists in Australia and New Zealand. Clin Exp Optom 95 (1), 28–36. https://doi.org/10.1111/j.1444-0938.2011.00663.x [doi]

The National Institute of Health and Care Excellence (NICE), 2024. NICE Guidance. https://www.nice.org.uk/guidance

Thite, N., Jaggernath, J., Chinanayi, F., Bharadwaj, S., Kunjeer, G., 2015. Pattern of optometry practice and range of services in India. Optom Vis Sci 92 (5), 615–622. https://doi.org/10.1097/OPX.0000000000000587

Toomey, M., Gyawali, R., Stapleton, F., Ho, K.C., Keay, L., Jalbert, I., 2021. Facilitators and barriers to the delivery of eye care by optometrists: A systematic review using the theoretical domains framework. Ophthalmic Physiol Opt 41 (4), 782–797. https://doi.org/10.1111/opo.12801

Translating Research Into Practice (TRIP), 2024. Trip medical database. https://www.tripdatabase.com

Varpio, L., Spafford, M.M., Schryer, C.F., Lingard, L., 2007. Seeing and listening - A visual and social analysis of optometric record-keeping practices. Journal of Business and Technical Communication 21 (4), 343–375. https://doi.org/10.1177/1050651907303991

Wason, P.C., Evans, J.S.B.T., 1975. Dual processes in reasoning. Cognition 3 (2), 141–154. https://doi.org/10.1016/0010-0277(74)90017-1

Webb, H., vom Lehn, D., Heath, C., Gibson, W., Evans, B.J.W., 2013. The problem with "problems": The case of openings in optometry consultations. Research on Language and Social Interaction 46 (1), 65–83. https://doi.org/10.1080/08351813.2012.753724

Werner, D.L., 1989. Teaching clinical thinking. Optometry and Vision Science 66 (11), 788–792. https://doi.org/10.1097/00006324-198911000-00011

World Council of Optometry, n.d. WCO's concept of optometry. https://worldcounciloptometry.info/about-us/

29

CLINICAL REASONING IN DIETETICS

RUTH VO ■ MEGAN SMITH ■ NARELLE PATTON

CHAPTER AIMS

The aims of this chapter are:

■ to describe what is known of clinical reasoning within dietetics as portrayed in contemporary literature and
■ to illuminate the sociocultural and physical context of dietetics reasoning through descriptions of dietetic practice models, roles and physical practice settings.

INTRODUCTION

The dietetics profession promotes health and well-being by the application of health and nutrition science for both the prevention and treatment of illness and disease, with individuals, groups and communities. Dietitians in many countries, including the United States, Canada, Australia, New Zealand and the United Kingdom, must hold a minimum of a bachelor's degree and have undertaken hundreds of hours of supervised

practice, with at least 500 hours in Australia and New Zealand (Blair et al., 2022a).

The dominant practice model for clinical dietetics involves dietitians undertaking activities with, and on behalf of, patients about nutrition care and medical nutrition therapy (Andersen et al., 2018). Traditionally, the public hospital sector has been the usual place of employment for clinical dietitians. However, primary care and private clinics are now the fastest growing area of clinical practice in many countries, such as Australia, New Zealand, United Kingdom and the United States (Blair et al., 2022b). Another key and emerging practice setting for clinical dietitians is residential aged care where dietitians can be responsible for delivering quality nutritional care to residents (Romano and Lowe, 2022).

Dietitians' clinical decision making is significantly shaped by the different practice contexts in which they work. Clinical dietitians often work in subspecialties within a hospital setting in parallel with medical specialties (Baird and Armstrong, 1981). Nutrition support is a strong focus of inpatient dietetic services and is involved in a range of subspecialties and practice settings. In most countries, role titles, positions and responsibilities are governed locally and are, therefore, dependent on the institution in which the dietitian practices. In the United States, clinical specialty areas are regulated more closely and dietitians require more assessment and training to gain scope of practice responsibilities and use of titles, e.g. nutrition support dietitian (Corrigan et al., 2021).

Critical thinking and decision making are considered essential practice competencies in clinical dietetics and encompass the ability to use sound clinical judgement and strategic thinking in practice, especially when faced with new opportunities and challenges (Commission on Dietetics Registration, 2021). Interestingly, this highlights a frequent interchangeable use of the terms 'clinical reasoning,' 'critical thinking,' 'clinical judgement' and 'clinical decision making' in the literature and an important need to distinguish between them. The dietetics literature suggests the term 'clinical decision making' refers to the umbrella process of choosing between alternative options that may involve clinical reasoning, critical thinking and clinical judgement (Olsen, 2013; Vo, 2020). Therefore, in this chapter, the term 'clinical decision making' (CDM) is used, except in circumstances where an alternative term is more relevant to the concepts being discussed.

CLINICAL DECISION MAKING IN DIETETICS: A HISTORICAL PERSPECTIVE

Empirical research on the nature of dietitian CDM in any context or setting is very limited. Dietetics research about reasoning and decision making has been focussed on gaining consensus on a standardized and assessable process that dietitians should use to help validate intervention decisions and subsequent patient outcomes (Swan et al., 2017).

Evidence-based practice (EBP) and its core elements of scientific evidence, clinical expertise and patients' values and preferences has been adopted as a guiding principle for dietetic practice. Since EBP has been embraced in dietetics to support decision making (Porter, 1998), a dominant focus of dietitian EBP research has been on quantitative identification and evaluation of dietitians' technical knowledge, critical appraisal of evidence and the degree to which dietitians incorporate evidence into decision making for patients in particular settings (Vogt et al., 2016). This focus has

valued understanding how the dietitian complies with a known standard of knowledge and evidence with the underlying assumption that appropriate use of evidence translates to quality care (Van Horn, 2021).

Internationally, the Nutrition Care Process Model (NCPM) has gradually infiltrated clinical dietetics, offering a standardized care pathway and terminology for health record documentation (Academy of Nutrition and Dietetics, 2022; Swan et al., 2017). The NCPM, developed via expert consensus, is framed as a four-step roadmap for identifying and solving problems in any individual or population-based care setting. The four steps in the model are:

■ nutrition assessment and reassessment
■ nutrition diagnosis
■ nutrition intervention and
■ nutrition monitoring.

The use of the term 'diagnosis' and the emphasis in documenting a standardized approach to 'nutrition diagnosis' is a contemporary shift towards the medical model that was not present within dietetics prior to the NCPM. The most updated version (Swan et al., 2017) has completely removed any mention of clinical judgement. This decision was based on a desire to limit the use of terms that have varied meanings or interpretations aiming to keep the model easy to use within the many contexts where it is applied.

Dietitians have struggled with implementing the NCPM and its associated terminology in practice (Lövestam et al., 2016), suggesting a tension between the reductionist foundations of the NCPM and the highly context-specific nature of patient care. It would seem that CDM, as it occurs in the real world, involves complexities that the NCPM does not capture. The integration of electronic health records, however, has opened up opportunities for dietitians to communicate their CDM formally when documenting nutrition care (Lövestam et al., 2019) and this can be backed up with quantifiable evidence of nutrition treatment.

Since the adoption of the NCPM, two key doctoral projects have explored the nature of CDM in two different groups and contexts within Australian dietetics using an interpretive approach, specifically Gadamer's philosophical hermeneutics. Olsen (2013) focussed on early career dietitians in regional and remote practice settings of Australia and Vo (2020) focussed on experienced dietitians in acute care practice settings. Both of these studies underpin the remaining chapter and are discussed in light of relevant literature within the profession.

COLLABORATIVE CDM IN EARLY CAREER DIETITIANS

Collaborative decision making is sometimes referred to as shared decision making. Collaborative decision making is a model of clinical decision making that includes the patient in a two-way discussion leading to a decision made through mutual deliberation (Charles et al., 1999; Trede and Higgs, 2003).

Olsen (2013) illuminated the core capabilities and conditions required for collaborative decision making (Fig. 29.1) occurring in rural Australia and how these

novice dietitians acquired these capabilities. Core capabilities that are shown to facilitate collaborative decision making include:

- developing self-awareness,
- building caring and trusting relationships,
- establishing and maintaining open and transparent dialogues,
- responding to the given situation,
- identifying and exploring common ground and
- finding time to think and talk.

This research adds to our understanding of how collaborative decision making contributes to dietetic practice in settings such as generalist practice in rural Australia. In these rural settings, practitioners are often working as solo dietitians with limited support.

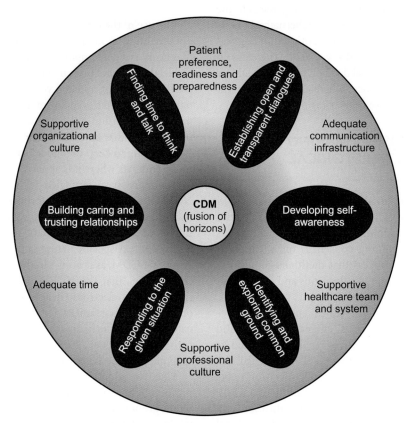

Fig. 29.1 ■ The core capabilities and conditions required for collaborative decision making. *CDM*, Clinical decision making. (With permission from Olsen, M., 2013. Collaborative decision making in early career dietetic practice (PhD thesis). Charles Sturt University, NSW, p. 220.)

Olsen's collaborative decision-making model has various elements in common with the NCPM such as the patient–clinician relationship being central to the process and the emphasis on collaboration and communication (Bueche et al., 2008). The patient–clinician relationship is also dependent on the dietitian's character and ability. The dietitian's approach to engaging with the patient has been revealed as a key aspect of what defines and influences patient-centred care among clinical dietitians (Jones et al., 2021).

While trying to enact a collaborative approach to decision making, dietitians strive to explore client narratives, capabilities and resources before deciding on goals (Al-Adili et al., 2022a). However, dietitians report that there are challenges with managing discrepancies between the feasibility of clinically orientated goals and a patient's personal goals, particularly in chronic disease management settings (Nagy et al., 2020). These challenges highlight gaps in contemporary dietitians' collaborative decision-making skills.

The outpatient practice setting presents specific contextual elements that influence how dietitians successfully engage in collaborative decision making. Tensions between efficiency and effectiveness in primary care settings are influenced by both personal (experience, well-being) and structural (time, financial constraints) factors and client behaviours (engagement, complexity) indicating that technical training is not the only solution to improve collaborative decision making (O'Connor et al., 2019). Dietitians must learn to manage these multidimensional complexities of their practice contexts.

THE MULTIDIMENSIONAL NATURE OF EXPERIENCED DIETITIAN CDM IN THE ACUTE CARE SETTING

The CDM of dietitians in the acute care setting is centred on making clinical decisions to meet the goal of improving individual patients' health. Vo's (2020) doctoral research has informed the development of A Model of the Multidimensional Nature of Dietitian CDM in the Acute Care Setting (Fig. 29.2). The model diagrammatically reflects the nature of making decisions for patient care through a synergistic relationship between five key dimensions:

- Tasks (*Prioritizing, Assessing, Care Planning, Implementing, Monitoring*)
- Interactions
- Reasoning
- Practitioner Factors
- Context (*Clinical Specialty, Resources, Culture, Practice Environment*)

These findings are consistent with other clinical reasoning and CDM models in other professions underpinned by an argument for a multidimensional nonlinear portrayal of CDM (Higgs et al., 2019; Madani et al., 2018). The relationship between these dimensions is continuous with no boundaries depicting a constant interlocking.

Tasks

The dietitian in the acute care setting is focussed on carrying out the core tasks of prioritizing, assessing, care planning, implementing care plans and monitoring patients throughout admission. These tasks are sequential and recurring for which dietitians make decisions about the timing and frequency of patient contact and care. As others have found, care planning for patients involves a collaborative tailoring of the nutrition support prescription with other health professionals (Liljeberg et al., 2021). Monitoring a patient involves both quantitative and qualitative outcomes where qualitative outcomes have been shown to be most significant to patients and yet least represented in standardized medical record systems (Al-Adili et al., 2022b).

The other dimensions of interactions, together with reasoning, practitioner and practice environment, shape how these tasks are carried out. The cognitive tasks involved in dietitian CDM (Vo et al., 2020) are similar to the general steps and description of critical thinking included in the NCPM (Swan et al., 2017) as well as the British Dietitians Association Model and Process depiction of critical reasoning (British Dietetic Association, 2021a).

Interactions

Dietitian CDM is a social phenomenon dependent on effective interactions with others: professionals such as medical practitioners, nurses, allied health professionals as well as patients and their carers. These

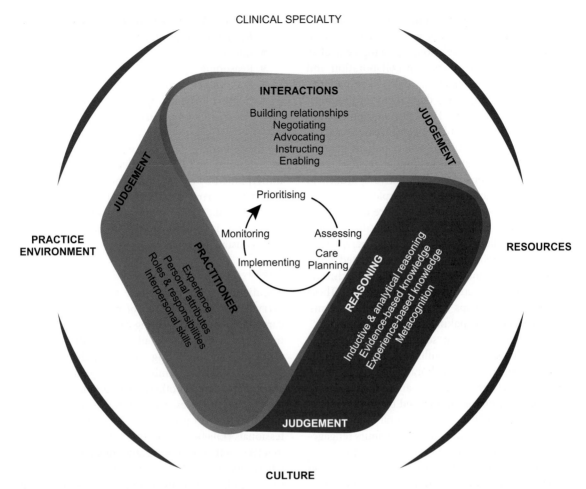

Fig. 29.2 ■ A model of the multidimensional nature of dietitian CDM in the acute care setting. (With permission from Vo, R., Smith, M., Patton, N., 2020. A model of the multidimensional nature of experienced dietitian clinical decision-making in the acute care setting. J. Hum. Nutr. Diet., 33(5), 617.)

interactions are strongly characterized by power relations which dominate dietitian CDM at multiple stages. The power dynamics between dietitians and medical practitioners are particularly significant given the strong influence of medical practitioners within decision-making structures.

Dietitians decide how to respond to power differences depending on the nature of the relationship and context. Dietitians from various clinical practice settings emphasize the impact of interprofessional collaboration on their ability to provide patient-centred care, in particular the level of respect given to the dietitian by various members of the multidisciplinary

team (Jones et al., 2021). Advocacy and negotiation with medical practitioners around nutrition interventions are fundamental to this form of interprofessional work. There is also the interactive work of instructing nursing personnel and, in some cases, patients and caregivers, to facilitate implementation and dissemination of care plans. Then there is the interactive work of empowering patients through collaborative decision making and helping them take some responsibility for their own nutrition and healthcare. While the patient is central to dietitian CDM, it must be remembered that sometimes a patient's condition may prevent them from expressing their values and desires.

In the acute setting, there are few studies that look at relationships between dietitians and patients compared to relationships between patients and other health professionals. There is a need for more studies into the complexities of therapeutic relationships and their effect on patient care (Nagy et al., 2022; Vo et al., 2022). The clinical reasoning involved is one aspect of the therapeutic relationship.

Reasoning

Dietitians need to move fluidly between different reasoning processes based on their knowledge, competence and patients' values and desires. Dietitians' clinical reasoning is typically sophisticated and makes use of clinical judgement. Given the dynamic, complex and uncertain nature of acute care, sound clinical judgement is necessary. Dietitian clinical judgement can be described as:

> 'a sophisticated context-dependent meta-reasoning process directing the nutrition care process that includes and extends beyond logical thinking involving the synthesis and weighing up of various types of information and knowledge enabling the management of complexity, interpersonal interactions and individualised patient care'
> *(Vo et al., 2021, p. 4).*

Experienced dietitians' clinical reasoning is frequently tacit, automatic and incorporating sophisticated pattern recognition, sensitivity, intuition and 'gut feeling'. These abilities contribute to phronesis or practical wisdom. Phronesis is part of the professionalism required to make overall judgements about what is the best course of action for particular patients (Dart et al., 2022b). The formal nutrition assessment process makes use of fast intuitive reasoning as well as analytical thinking, especially hypothetico-deductive reasoning where dietitians are expected to use evidence-based logic. Pattern recognition and intuition can sometimes conflict with the requirement to substantiate decisions as evidence-based. Clinical judgement manages this tension by using metacognitive skills to integrate the different kinds of thinking in a justifiable manner. Metacognition is the awareness and analysis of one's own key decision-making processes (Vo et al., 2020). Metacognition can prompt dietitians to reflect on how

their reasoning may need to change during patient care, according to all the influences involved, internal and external.

Practitioner Factors

Internal influences include individual dietitian attributes such as confidence, empathy, patient-centredness and intrinsic motivation. These can all influence how practitioners apply CDM (Vo et al., 2020). The abilities to build rapport, be persistent yet respectful, and articulate rationales in an efficient and relevant way all contribute to patient care. These characteristics are also considered part of an emerging model of dietitians' professionalism (Dart et al., 2022b).

Interpersonal skills such as assertiveness, the ability to compromise, and social and emotional awareness are also crucial to effective and professional management of power relations with other health professionals (Vo et al., 2020, 2022). The many and various roles and responsibilities of dietitians can also influence the day-to-day nature of CDM, including those not directly related to patient care, for example, team meetings, research projects, record keeping and professional development of oneself and others. A key shaper of the nature of clinical reasoning as it develops over time is the type and amount of clinical experience a dietitian has been exposed to. Dietitians with more experience describe greater confidence to engage in advocating for the patient's nutritional needs (Vo et al., 2020).

Context

Resources, culture, practice environment and clinical speciality can shape and impact the nature and manner of CDM. The acute care setting, as a whole, provides a fast-paced and dynamic environment that influences the nature of CDM. Individual wards and units may share some characteristics but will also have significant differences and these all have an effect on how dietitians are included and supported as part of the multidisciplinary team. The resources (time, budget, therapies) made available to dietitians by the healthcare system and/or hospital all have an influence on what and how patient care decisions are made. This means that dietitians need to be highly adaptable if they are to be effective in their CDM.

Dietitians' CDM is consistently influenced by the particular clinical speciality providing patient care. The attitudes towards nutrition of the other health professionals in a specialty are an important factor, especially the physicians and nurses. Dietitians learn to place a high value on gaining an awareness of the opinions and preferences of each speciality represented in their workload.

REFLECTION POINT

Clinical decision making in dietetics is heavily influenced by physical and sociocultural contextual factors. Think about your most recent patient assessment and identify how your clinical reasoning was influenced by contextual factors such as:

■ your degree of autonomy,
■ who else was involved and their goals,
■ available resources and
■ how the patient made you feel.

How might these factors change your practice in the future?

DEVELOPING DIETITIAN CDM EXPERTISE

A Model of Developing Dietitian CDM Expertise (Fig. 29.3), developed from Vo's doctoral project (Vo, 2020), depicts the crucial relationship between gaining experience that is scaffolded to challenge the dietitian's capability, reflection on this experience and the development of the dietitian's confidence. The model emphasizes key elements that dietitians believe to be influential on their own expertise development. The model shares many themes with how dietetic students develop clinical competencies on placement when explored through the lens of Self-Development Theory (Markwell et al., 2021) and moves beyond traditional skill development models. Most dietetic practice literature has adopted known skill development models (Benner, 1992; Dreyfus and Dreyfus, 1980) and applied them to explain competency development (Andersen et al., 2018; Dietitians Australia, 2021). These models,

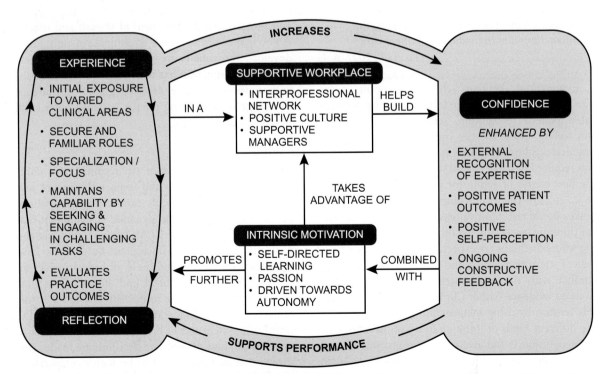

Fig. 29.3 ■ A model of developing dietitian CDM expertise. (With permission from Vo, R., 2020. Experienced dietitian clinical decision making in the acute care setting (PhD thesis). Charles Sturt University, NSW, p. 244).

together with a growing understanding of how dietitian professional identity develops (Snell, 2021), contribute to our current knowledge of CDM expertise development.

Experience

Participation in direct patient care experiences is fundamental to the development of CDM expertise. Challenging experiences are those that create tension between current ability and future capability. These include different phases of experience such as entering specialization and transitioning between jobs, roles and clinical areas. The first couple of years working in acute care dietetics can involve steep learning curves due to engaging with many new and unfamiliar patient care experiences. How dietitians respond to this tension is influential on how CDM expertise is developed from these experiences.

Reflection

Reflection is a thought process dietitians need to engage in during care episodes and throughout practice. Reflection helps dietitians to evaluate the impact of their CDM so that they can enhance their practice. Without reflection, experience could not build expertise. Reflection involves self-awareness during and after decision making and actions, especially when managing interactions with other health professionals where there is a power difference in the relationships. More experienced dietitians view reflection as an ongoing process, not a discrete, one-off activity. Reflection and reasoning help some individuals to consciously check and regulate their thoughts.

Workplace

The contexts in which dietitians work influence how and to what extent they gain confidence and benefit from experience. A positive environment that actively supports dietitians via regular supervision, feedback and the delegation of appropriate autonomy contributes significantly to the development of CDM expertise. Opportunities to learn with, and from, other health professionals are influential on expertise development, facilitated by regular communication of their reasoning as required. Organizational culture, role expectations, policies and resources (time and budgets) influence how

dietitians across different practice settings provide patient-centred care (Jones et al., 2021). Amongst student dietitians, it has been shown that micro-cultures, cohesion, conformity, competition and conflict aversion are influential in shaping a dietitian's emerging professional identity (Dart et al., 2022a).

Intrinsic Factors

A dietitian's level of motivation, specifically intrinsic motivation, supports the development of CDM expertise which is underpinned by a drive to enhance the capabilities that are required to support effective patient care. Motivations also include a desire for greater autonomy, purpose and standing in their professional community. This is in addition to a desire to assist and improve the health of patients. Dietitians demonstrate intrinsic motivation in their clinical practice through passion, dedication and focus and it is a key facilitator of learning from experience.

Confidence

Generally speaking, a dietitian's confidence in making decisions grows over time with increasing experience, autonomy and knowledge in their specific area of practice. Positive patient outcomes related to their decision making, as well as the development of a positive reputation and recognition from the multidisciplinary team, all contribute to increased confidence. Increased confidence contributes to effective advocation and negotiation, as well as a more confident response to dealing with complexity. Williams' (2019) doctoral research highlighted the role of confidence and coaching in developing student competence in diagnostic reasoning. Vo (2020) built on Williams' work by showing how that confidence continues to be significant in enabling further development beyond basic proficiency levels.

Vo's research asserts that dietitian CDM expertise development is a social phenomenon because it is strongly dependent on the practice context. The people within that context can foster the ongoing processes of professional socialization and professional identity development of dietitians. The lens of professional artistry provides a way of integrating all these insights in the CDM of dietitians.

REFLECTION POINT

Practitioner reflection alongside other qualities and dispositions is core to developing expertise in clinical reasoning.

When you are working with patients do you:

- critique your own thinking, e.g. look for assumptions and biases or flaws in your logic;
- examine internal influences on your own critical thinking, e.g. are you tired or distracted or lacking motivation;
- examine the degree of trust established with your patient and the consequent quality of the information being provided;
- identify environmental influences on your thinking, e.g. time constraints and high workloads leading to rushed assessment and treatment and
- identify enablers and hindrances on your confidence within practice.

PROFESSIONAL ARTISTRY IN CLINICAL DIETETICS

Professional artistry is related to a dietitian's expertise and CDM in clinical dietetics. Vo's (2020) Model of Professional Artistry in Clinical Dietetics (Fig. 29.4) illustrates the fundamental qualities and supporting factors that characterize the professional artistry of dietitians. Clinical dietitians who demonstrate professional artistry are *efficient*, *adaptable* and *influential*. Importantly, the model distinguishes professional artistry from expertise or experience level of the dietitian. In comparison, other models refer to advanced or consultant levels of expertise (British Dietetic Association, 2021b), or 'expert' level in the United States (Corrigan et al., 2021). In Australia, the Dietitians Association refers to 'advanced practice' generically, which may or may not include advanced and extended scope of practice such as gastrostomy management (Simmance

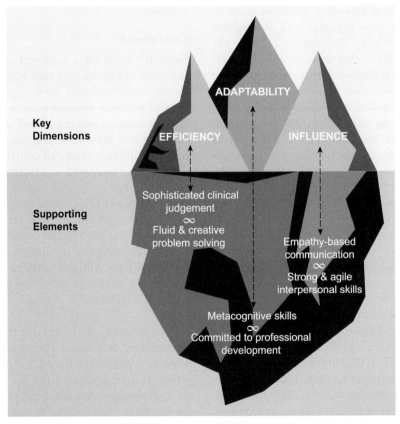

Fig. 29.4 ■ A model of professional artistry in clinical dietetics. (With permission from Vo, R., 2020. Experienced dietitian clinical decision making in the acute care setting (PhD thesis). Charles Sturt University, NSW, p. 270.)

et al., 2019). The advantage of a professional artistry viewpoint is that it enables us to have a different, and hopefully better, understanding of the following components of expertise.

Efficiency

The professional artist practitioner is both efficient and effective in CDM and patient care as a whole because of their sophisticated clinical judgement and fluid and creative problem solving. The clinician's clinical judgement is guided by their significant experience and the development of a strong knowledge network comprised of both scientific and highly tacit experience-based knowledge. This enables dietitians to identify accurately, assess, synthesize and communicate patient information with ease. The dietitian with artistry is able to offer innovative solutions to patient problems using a holistic approach. This entails rapidly creating strategies to overcome difficulties in providing optimal patient care that are tied to the patient's setting, such as resource limitations or difficult interpersonal communication.

Adaptability

The dietitian with professional artistry is adaptable in providing effective patient care and can change themselves and their practice as needed. The practitioner with professional artistry possesses metacognitive skills, ability and commitment to continuous professional development. Metacognitive ability involves habits of reflecting on practice, developing self-awareness and even emotional regulation requiring emotional intelligence (Hutchinson et al., 2018). A dietitian's commitment to professional development includes passion for their work and strong intrinsic motivation that seeks opportunities and takes necessary actions to promote continuous growth and development in their specific professional role.

Influence

Dietitians with professional artistry can consistently influence other people involved with the patient's nutritional care, as well as the patient, to facilitate beneficial outcomes. Influencing patients and other health professionals requires empathy-based communication and excellent interpersonal skills. Empathy-based communication is described as actively building rapport and gaining a shared understanding of the patient's, carers and healthcare team members' concerns and issues. This promotes better advocacy and decision support. Professional artistry includes the ability to interact and communicate with patients in a way that improves each patient's understanding and empowers them to participate in improving their own health. All these features of professional artistry emphasize that clinical dietetics expertise is much more than the simple possession of credentials, specialization and technical skills (Vo, 2020).

SUMMARY

In this chapter, we have:

- contextualized current understanding of clinical decision making in the discipline of clinical dietetics,
- discussed the nature of early career collaborative decision making in rural settings and experienced dietitian CDM in acute hospital settings,
- explored the development of CDM expertise: the interdependence of experience, reflection, confidence, intrinsic motivation and workplace environment and
- explored the role of professional artistry in clinical dietetics: the characteristics of efficiency, adaptability and influence.

REFERENCES

Academy of Nutrition and Dietetics, 2022. Nutrition terminology reference manual (eNCPT): Dietetics language for nutrition care. Retrieved 2 September 2022 from http://www.ncpro.org.

Al-Adili, L., McGreevy, J., Orrevall, Y., Nydahl, M., Boström, A.-M., Lövestam, E., 2022a. Setting goals with patients at risk of malnutrition: A focus group study with clinical dietitians. Patient Education and Counseling 105 (7), 2103–2109. https://doi.org/10.1016/j.pec.2022.02.015

Al-Adili, L., Orrevall, Y., McGreevy, J., Nydahl, M., Boström, A.-M., Lövestam, E., 2022b. Discrepancy in the evaluation of explicit and implicit nutrition care outcomes for patients at risk of malnutrition: A qualitative study. Journal of Human Nutrition and Dietetics 35 (3), 494–503. https://doi.org/10.1111/jhn.12931

Andersen, D., Baird, S., Bates, T., Chapel, D.L., Cline, A.D., Ganesh, S.N., et al., 2018. Academy of Nutrition and Dietetics: Revised 2017 standards of practice in nutrition care and standards of professional performance for registered dietitian nutritionists. Journal of the Academy of Nutrition and

Dietetics 118 (1), 132–140. https://doi.org/10.1016/j.jand.2017. 10.003 e115

Baird, S.C., Armstrong, R.V., 1981. The A.D.A. role delineation for the field of clinical dietetics: 2. Methodology and summary of results. Journal of the American Dietetic Association 78 (4), 374–382.

Benner, P., Tanner, C., & Chesla, C., 1992. From beginner to expert: gaining a differentiated clinical world in critical care nursing. Advances in Nursing Science 14 (3), 13–28. https://doi.org/10.1097/00012272-199203000-00005

Blair, M., Mitchell, L., Palermo, C., Gibson, S., 2022a. Trends, challenges, opportunities, and future needs of the dietetic workforce: A systematic scoping review. Nutrition Reviews 80 (5), 1027–1040. https://doi.org/10.1093/nutrit/nuab071

Blair, M., Palermo, C., Gibson, S., Mitchell, L., 2022b. The Australian and New Zealand dietetics graduate outcomes survey: A cross-sectional study. Nutrition & Dietetics 79 (4), 456–468. https://doi.org/10.1111/1747-0080.12739

British Dietetic Association, 2021a. Model and process for nutrition and dietetic practice. Retrieved July 2024 from https://www.bda.uk.com/practice-and-education/nutrition-and-dietetic-practice/professional-guidance/model-and-process-for-dietetic-practice.html

British Dietetic Association, 2021b. Post registration professional development framework. Retrieved June 2022 from https://www.bda.uk.com/practice-and-education/nutrition-and-dietetic-practice/dietetic-journey.html

Bueche, J., Charney, P., Pavlinac, J., Skipper, A., Thompson, E., Myers, E., 2008. Nutrition care process and model part I: The 2008 update. Journal of the American Dietetic Association 108 (7), 1113–1117. https://doi.org/10.1016/j.jada.2008.04.027

Charles, C., Gafni, A., Whelan, T., 1999. Decision-making in the physician-patient encounter: Revisiting the shared treatment decision-making model. Social Science and Medicine 49 (5), 651–661. https://doi.org/10.1016/s0277-9536(99)00145-8

Commission on Dietetics Registration, 2021. Essential practice competencies for the commission on dietetic registration's credentialed nutrition and dietetics practitioners. 1-38. Retrieved 17 May 2022 from https://admin.cdrnet.org/vault/2459/web///New_CDR_Competencies_2021.pdf

Corrigan, M.L., Bobo, E., Rollins, C., Mogensen, K.M., 2021. Academy of Nutrition and Dietetics and American Society for Parenteral and Enteral Nutrition: Revised 2021 standards of practice and standards of professional performance for registered dietitian nutritionists (competent, proficient, and expert) in nutrition support. Nutrition in Clinical Practice 36 (6), 1126–1143. https://doi.org/10.1002/ncp.10774

Dart, J., Ash, S., McCall, L., Rees, C., 2022a. 'We're our own worst enemies': A qualitative exploration of sociocultural factors in dietetic education influencing student-dietitian transitions. Journal of the Academy of Nutrition and Dietetics 122 (11), 2036–2049.e4. https://doi.org/10.1016/j.jand.2022.03.015

Dart, J., McCall, L., Ash, S., Rees, C., 2022b. Conceptualizing professionalism in dietetics: An Australasian qualitative study. Journal of the Academy of Nutrition and Dietetics 122 (11), 2087–2096.e7. https://doi.org/10.1016/j.jand.2022.02.010

Dreyfus, S.E., Dreyfus, H., 1980. A five-stage model of the mental activities involved in directed skill acquisition. California University Berkeley Operations Research Center [monograph on the Internet]. Available from https://apps.dtic.mil/sti/citations/ADA084551 [Downloaded 1 December 2022]

Dietitians Australia, 2021. National competency standards for dietitians in Australia. Retrieved July 2024 from https://dietitiansaustralia.org.au/media/261

Higgs, J., Jensen, G.M., Loftus, S., Christensen, N., 2019. Clinical reasoning in the health professions, 4th ed. Elsevier Health Sciences.

Hutchinson, M., Hurley, J., Kozlowski, D., Whitehair, L., 2018. The use of emotional intelligence capabilities in clinical reasoning and decision-making: A qualitative, exploratory study. Journal of Clinical Nursing 27 (3-4), e600–e610. https://doi.org/10.1111/jocn.14106

Jones, M., Eggett, D., Bellini, S.G., Williams, P., Patten, E.V., 2021. Patient-centered care: Dietitians' perspectives and experiences. Patient Education and Counseling 104 (11), 2724–2731. https://doi.org/10.1016/j.pec.2021.04.008

Liljeberg, E., Nydahl, M., Lövestam, E., Andersson, A., 2021. A qualitative exploration of dietitians' experiences of prescribing oral nutritional supplements to patients with malnutrition: A focus on shared tailoring and behaviour change support. Journal of Human Nutrition and Dietetics 34 (5), 858–867. https://doi.org/10.1111/jhn.12867

Lövestam, E., Orrevall, Y., Koochek, A., Andersson, A., 2016. The struggle to balance system and lifeworld: Swedish dietitians' experiences of a standardised nutrition care process and terminology. Health Sociology Review 25 (3), 240–255. https://doi.org/10.1080/14461242.2016.1197783

Lövestam, E., Steiber, A., Vivanti, A., Boström, A.M., Devine, A., Haughey, O., et al., 2019. Use of the nutrition care process and nutrition care process terminology in an international cohort reported by an online survey tool. Journal of the Academy of Nutrition and Dietetics 119 (2), 225–241. https://doi.org/10.1016/j.jand.2018.09.002

Madani, A., Gips, A., Razek, T., Deckelbaum, D.L., Mulder, D.S., Grushka, J.R., 2018. Defining and measuring decision-making for the management of trauma patients. Journal of Surgical Education 75 (2), 358–369. https://doi.org/10.1016/j.jsurg.2017.07.012

Markwell, K.E., Ross, L.J., Mitchell, L.J., Williams, L.T., 2021. A self-determination theory analysis of reflective debrief themes about dietetic student placement experiences in hospital: Implications for education. Journal of Human Nutrition and Dietetics 34 (1), 115–123. https://doi.org/10.1111/jhn.12808

Nagy, A., McMahon, A., Tapsell, L., Deane, F., 2020. Developing meaningful client-dietitian relationships in the chronic disease context: An exploration of dietitians' perspectives. Nutrition & Dietetics 77 (5), 529–541. https://doi.org/10.1111/1747-0080.12588

Nagy, A., McMahon, A., Tapsell, L., Deane, F., 2022. The therapeutic relationship between a client and dietitian: A systematic integrative review of empirical literature. Nutrition & Dietetics 79 (3), 303–348. https://doi.org/10.1111/1747-0080.12723

O'Connor, R., Slater, K., Ball, L., Jones, A., Mitchell, L., Rollo, M.E., et al., 2019. The tension between efficiency and effectiveness: a study of dietetic practice in primary care. Journal of Human Nutrition and Dietetics 32 (2), 259–266. https://doi.org/10.1111/jhn.12617

Olsen, M. (2013). Collaborative decision making in early career dietetic practice [Doctoral, Charles Sturt University, Australia.]. https://researchoutput.csu.edu.au/en/publications/collaborative-decision-making-in-early-career-dietetic-practice-3.

Porter, C., 1998. Are we making decisions based on evidence? Journal of the Academy of Nutrition and Dietetics 98 (4), 404–407. http://search.proquest.com/docview/218392423?accountid=34512

Romano, V., Lowe, C.J.M., 2022. The experiences of dietitian's working in care homes in England: A qualitative study. Age and Ageing 51 (2), afac006. https://doi.org/10.1093/ageing/afac006

Simmance, N., Cortinovis, T., Green, C., Lunardi, K., McPhee, M., Steer, B., et al., 2019. Introducing novel advanced practice roles into the health workforce: Dietitians leading in gastrostomy management. Nutrition & Dietetics 76 (1), 14–20. https://doi.org/10.1111/1747-0080.12508

Snell, R. (2021). A longitudinal study on the development of professional identity by dietitians in Australia [Curtin University]. http://hdl.handle.net/20.500.11937/86166.

Swan, W.I., Vivanti, A., Hakel-Smith, N.A., Hotson, B., Orrevall, Y., Trostler, N., et al., 2017. Nutrition care process and model update: Toward realizing people-centered care and outcomes management. Journal of the Academy of Nutrition and Dietetics 117 (12), 2003–2014. https://doi.org/10.1016/j.jand.2017.07.015

Trede, F., Higgs, J., 2003. Re-framing the clinician's role in collaborative clinical decision making: Re-thinking practice knowledge and the notion of clinician–patient relationships. Learning in Health and Social Care 2 (2), 66–73. https://doi.org/10.1046/j.1473-6861.2003.00040.x

Van Horn, L., 2021. Validation of an evidence-based dietetic practice instrument and the association between level of education and use of evidence-based dietetic practices among registered dietitian nutritionists (Publication Number 1078.) [UNF Graduate Theses and Dissertations, University of North Florida]. https://digitalcommons.unf.edu/etd/1078.

Vo, R. 2020. Clinical decision making of experienced dietitians in the acute care setting [Doctoral, Charles Sturt University, Australia]. https://researchoutput.csu.edu.au/en/publications/clinical-decision-making-of-experienced-dietitians-in-the-acute-c/fingerprints/

Vo, R., Smith, M., Patton, N., 2020. A model of the multidimensional nature of experienced dietitian clinical decision-making in the acute care setting. Journal of Human Nutrition and Dietetics 33 (5), 614–623. https://doi.org/10.1111/jhn.12756

Vo, R., Smith, M., Patton, N., 2021. The role of dietitian clinical judgement in the nutrition care process within the acute care setting: A qualitative study. Journal of Human Nutrition and Dietetics 34 (1), 124–133. https://doi.org/10.1111/jhn.12820

Vo, R., Smith, M., Patton, N., 2022. Power, autonomy and interprofessional practice in dietitian clinical decision making: An interpretive study in acute hospitals. Journal of Human Nutrition and Dietetics 35 (1), 124–133. https://doi.org/10.1111/jhn.12917

Vogt, E., Byham-Gray, L., Denmark, R., Touger-Decker, R., 2016. Impact of an evidence-based practice intervention on knowledge and clinical practice behaviors among registered dietitians. Topics in Clinical Nutrition 31 (2), 111–124. https://doi.org/10.1097/TIN.0000000000000061

Williams, K.J., 2019. Reflection, insight, and critical thinking in nutrition diagnostics graduates [Ph.D, Lindenwood University]. ProQuest Central; ProQuest Dissertations & Theses Global. (2175714459).

30

CLINICAL REASONING IN PHARMACY

W. CARY MOBLEY ■ ROBIN MOORMAN-LI

■ ■ ■ ■ ■ ■ ■ ■ ■ ■ ■ ■ ■ ■ ■ ■ ■ ■

CHAPTER OUTLINE

CHAPTER AIMS

The aims of this chapter are:

- to discuss the roles of a systematic patient care process and clinical reasoning in assessing and resolving medication-related problems as part of a collaborative effort to provide patient-centred care
- to provide the reader with a case study example illustrating medication-related problem solving in the Pharmacists' Patient Care Process
- to discuss common sources of error in clinical reasoning.

INTRODUCTION

In a broad sense, clinical reasoning is the reasoning used in clinical problem solving. In other words, it is 'the process of forming conclusions, judgments, or inferences from facts or premises' (Dictionary.com, n.d.) in clinical problem solving. In clinical reasoning, the facts or premises from which decisions are made include signs and symptoms, treatment facts, principles of disease and care, and the practitioner's

understanding of how the patient views their health and quality of life. For a pharmacist, clinical reasoning is centred on solving problems related to medications, which generally involve questions related to the medication appropriateness, effectiveness, safety and adherence. Within these categories, specific types of medication-related problems that pharmacists typically encounter are listed in Box 30.1 (Cipolle et al., 2012). Although clinical problems can vary in different ways (e.g. simple versus complex, acute versus chronic, urgent versus preventative), an important common goal for problem resolution will be an individualized recommendation in accordance with the patient's 'needs, goals, lifestyle, and personal, and cultural values' (Rogers, 1983, p. 36).

With this patient-centred goal in mind, for many clinical problems it may be best that the pharmacist adopts a holistic mindset that visualizes an individual's health as a function of multiple interacting and dynamic systems including the biochemical, cellular, physiological systems that are at the physiological source of ill health, along with the psychological, social and value systems that shape an individual's attitudes and lifestyle (Wilson et al., 2001; Jayasinghe, 2012).

The patient's attitudes and lifestyle can be influential in the development or course of many acute and chronic health problems. For example, an individual's stress or sedentary lifestyle can be important factors in the development and course of various cardiovascular, inflammatory and psychiatric conditions (Schneiderman et al., 2005; Slavich, 2016; Booth et al., 2012). Viewing an individual's health as part of a complete system favours a holistic, integrated approach to clinical reasoning, whereby ideas from different disciplines are integrated to connect different health factors (or determinants) to an individual's health problems. These factors are considered in the creation of a comprehensive plan for the maintenance or improvement of the patient's health.

THE PHARMACIST AS PART OF A COLLABORATIVE TEAM

The pharmacist contributes their unique expertise in medication management as part of a collaborative interdisciplinary effort to maintain or improve a patient's health. In this team approach to healthcare, the knowledge, experience and judgement of practitioners from different disciplines is integrated to make patient-centred healthcare decisions. Given that the assessment and resolution of the patient's health problems will involve understanding the perspectives of patients and of fellow practitioners, it is incumbent on the pharmacist to develop an interdisciplinary mindset. Pharmacists should possess enough insight from other healthcare disciplines to be able to understand the reasoning of their fellow practitioners and to grasp important relationships between their treatment approaches and that of the pharmacist. An interdisciplinary mindset can help the pharmacist work effectively as a member of an interprofessional team dedicated to creating a unified, synergistic and comprehensive plan for achieving health goals for the patient.

CLINICAL PROBLEM SOLVING FOR THE PHARMACIST

There are different models for problem-solving processes related to a patient's medication-related needs, but as with other healthcare professions, the models tend to follow a certain order (Martin et al., 2016; Steiner et al., 2002; Rogers, 1983; American College of Clinical Pharmacology, 2014; Tietze, 2012; Gambrill, 2012). A pharmacist's clinical problem-solving process begins with the gathering and evaluation of information, with goals of understanding the patient's current clinical status and of discovering and explaining drug therapy problems. On the basis of this understanding, the process continues with the generation and selection of strategies to resolve the patient's medication-related problems. The selected strategies are then implemented and monitored for their effectiveness. For this chapter, the Pharmacists' Patient Care Process (PPCP) is the model used to provide a framework to describe pharmacists' clinical problem solving and clinical reasoning. The PPCP is a cyclical process of the following five sequential steps: Collect, Assess, Plan, Implement and Follow-up (see Bennett et al., 2015, for details.) Case Study 30.1 will be used to exemplify the results of each step of the PPCP.

CASE STUDY 30.1

An Introduction

Cally is a 68-year-old female who presents to her primary care physician's (PCP) office with a chief complaint of excessive daytime sedation and continued burning sensations in her feet. Her PCP has referred her to clinical pharmacy services for evaluation of her medications and a recommendation for management of her painful diabetic neuropathy.

The Collection and Assessment of Patient Information

The collection and assessment of patient information is a quest for understanding and explaining the patient's health status and medication-related issues. In this phase, information about the patient is collected, interpreted and evaluated based on the knowledge, experience and reasoning of the pharmacy practitioner. The goal is to create a clear, accurate and comprehensive assessment that will act as the basis for rational medication-related decisions.

Collection

The collection of information may proceed in different ways depending on the nature of the practice and of the clinical encounter. For example, it may begin with a visual cue (e.g. a worried look, a cough or skin discolouration), a verbal description of symptoms by the patient or caregiver, an examination of prescription vials and refill histories, a computer alert during prescription processing, an examination of a medical record or (as in this case) a referral from a physician. Further information may also be gathered in different ways, including direct communication with the patient, communication with caregivers, surrogates and fellow clinicians, and/or by a continued examination of a medical record.

During the collection phase, the pharmacist will systematically, and thoroughly, gather and record subjective and objective information in a manner dictated by the clinical issues and the practice of the pharmacist. Subjective data are commonly described as data provided by the patient or surrogate. Objective data are commonly described as information that is reported, observed or documented by a healthcare provider, can be reproduced, and are fact based. Medication-related information that may be routinely gathered includes a current medication list and information related to the indication, effectiveness, safety and regimen adherence for each medication. Other pertinent information includes age, gender, ethnicity, allergies, lab and other test results, vital signs, physical assessment data, social history and the patient's healthcare goals (Bennett et al., 2015). The pharmacist will also seek to gain the patient's perspectives by ascertaining understandings, beliefs, attitudes and behaviours related to medication

therapy (Cipolle et al., 2012) as well as factors that may present barriers, such as issues of health literacy, distrust or economics (Bennett et al., 2015).

The collection phase may also have a significant diagnostic element as the pharmacist will be on a quest to discover and evaluate potential medication-related problems (such as those listed in Box 30.1), along with their contributing factors. This pharmaceutical diagnosis will typically proceed in a hypothetico-deductive manner, whereby the acquisition of cues leads to a hypothesis of a medication-related problem, which will be tested with a deductive investigation for confirmatory and disconfirmatory information. This information may come from many sources, including how the patient uses the medications; changes in disease status or functional parameters (such as liver or kidney function); symptom onset, severity, aggravating and remitting factors; prescribing or dispensing issues; and social or economic issues. This process may also include judging when a referral or further testing (e.g. laboratory) is warranted. It is important to note that when eliciting information directly from patients, proper communication skills are imperative and include effective wording of the questions, using open-ended questions, active listening skills and developing a good rapport with the patient. The information in Case Study 30.2 summarizes the pharmacist's findings in the Collect step.

Assessment

During the assessment phase, all collected information is meticulously analysed, interpreted and evaluated with a goal of creating a clear, comprehensive and accurate assessment of the patient's health status and medication-related needs. The subjective and objective information is grouped and evaluated for possible relationships in order to hypothesize medication-related problems, which will be confirmed or disconfirmed based on other patient information (Tietze, 2012).

Aside from focussing on the medications, the pharmacist evaluates the patient's function, perceptions of quality of life, current healthcare goals and overall understanding and agreement with the current healthcare plan. Additionally, it is important for the pharmacist to evaluate preventative healthcare issues such as diet concerns, substance use and immunization status to ensure all factors related to medication-related needs have been thoroughly evaluated.

CASE STUDY 30.2

Collect

Cally is a 68-year-old female who presents to the pharmacotherapy clinic at the request of Dr. Jones for evaluation of her current medication regimen and recommendations for her painful diabetic neuropathy. Cally reports a burning sensation in her feet that has become unbearable over the last month. Her description of this pain includes burning pain, with numbness and tingling in both feet. The pain seems to be greater at night rating the pain a 10/10, and averaging about 8/10 during the day. She has decreased her daily activities due to her pain. Her sleep quality has progressively worsened despite the addition of amitriptyline, which she has been taking for about 1 month. She reports that amitriptyline is causing daytime sedation, dry mouth and eyes, increased constipation and periodic episodes of confusion. She is concerned about the constipation, because before amitriptyline she was having a bowel movement once a day with no straining, and now she is having a bowel movement every other day and it is painful to pass. She is hoping these side effects will start to resolve now that she has been taking this medication for a month. She is hoping there are some treatment options which could at least decrease her pain to a 6/10 on average so she can enjoy her daily activities, begin exercising again and improve her overall sleep quality.

Information that was collected about Cally included: current medications (including over-the-counter medications, herbals and dietary supplements), adherence evaluation, past medications and reason for discontinuation, medication allergies, social history (including smoking, alcohol, substance abuse), past medical history, current immunizations, lifestyle habits (including exercise, diet and psychosocial functioning), personal healthcare goals, vital signs and lab results.

When multiple medication-related problems are identified and characterized, they must be prioritized to capture the most urgent issues that could lead to the most immediate negative impact on the patient and thus should receive priority.

The information in Case Study 30.3 summarizes the pharmacist's conclusions in the Assess step for the patient case.

Reasoning in the Collection – Assessment Phase

An assessment is an evaluative process where diagnostic reasoning is applied to collected information to determine the existence and nature of clinical problems, with a particular emphasis on elucidating their aetiology. With this emphasis of determining the causes and contributing factors of medication-related problems, from a reasoning perspective, the assessment phase is largely an explanation-creating phase. To create an explanation, the practitioner infers a working hypothesis (e.g. patient is non-adherent) to explain a set of collected information (e.g. unmet clinical outcomes). The pharmacist then seeks to test the hypothesis deductively by ascertaining further information (e.g. refill history) (Kelley and Hutchins, 2021). With new information, a working hypothesis may be confirmed, or disconfirmed and discarded, and new hypotheses may be inferred and tested. In order to validate a particular explanation as the best explanation and to avoid premature closure on a hypothesis, the pharmacist must purposefully create, test and rule out alternate explanations for the collected information.

The collection-assessment process does not typically continue indefinitely to achieve absolute certainty. Rather, it continues until explanations emerge that can be used to define the patient's clinical status and clinical problems with sufficient adequacy and accuracy that maximizes understanding while minimizing the risks of any remaining uncertainty. Thus, the decision on when to stop the assessment is in part an ethical decision for the practitioner (Rogers, 1983).

Care Plan Development, Implementation and Follow-up: The Therapeutic Phase

With the assessment of the patient's medication-related needs complete, the pharmacist is now able

CASE STUDY 30.3

Assess

1. Uncontrolled painful diabetic neuropathy leading to decreased function, quality of sleep and quality of life. The patient is also experiencing adverse reactions to amitriptyline: daytime sedation, dry mouth and eyes, increased constipation and intermittent confusion. Additionally, amitriptyline is on the Beer's list, which lists drugs that may be inappropriate for use in older adults and those that should be used with caution. The use of amitriptyline in the elderly is not recommended due to adverse drug reactions.

2. Constipation: Adverse drug reaction secondary to anticholinergic effects of amitriptyline.

   Decreased physical activity due to increased pain from diabetic peripheral neuropathy could also be a contributing factor for her constipation.

3. Poorly controlled Type 2 Diabetes: Haemoglobin A1C is currently 9.1%, which exceeds the goal of <7% based on her age and health status. This goal translates to fasting or preprandial glucose levels averaging between 80 and 130 mg/dL.

4. Controlled hypertension and dyslipidaemia: Patient is currently reaching treatment goals. Hypertension: goal <140/90. Lipid levels are acceptable. No adverse drug reactions reported.

---

to create rationally an individualized care plan in collaboration with the patient and other healthcare practitioners.

Planning

Care planning begins by establishing goals of therapy that are defined in terms of measurable outcomes that will be used to measure the effectiveness and safety of recommended interventions (Bennett et al., 2015; Tietze, 2012). Potential medication-related goals include curing or preventing a disease, slowing or halting disease progression, reducing or eliminating signs or symptoms, normalizing laboratory values or providing palliative care (Cipolle et al., 2012). The goals are structured to include observable, measurable and realistic clinical parameters for goal achievement, the desired value or observable change for those parameters, and the expected time frame for their achievement (Cipolle et al., 2012).

With goals of therapy established, the pharmacist proceeds to develop strategies to achieve them. A list of drug and nondrug strategies are generated and evaluated. Some are eliminated and others are selected, with the best strategy selected and alternatives identified (Tietze, 2012). Selection of patient-specific medication interventions involves the weighing of the comparative effectiveness and safety of the options. Multiple patient-specific factors that can influence

the chosen therapy and its outcomes are considered in this decision-making process. These factors include comorbid conditions; therapeutic interventions from other members of the team; patient attitudes, beliefs, healthcare goals and healthcare access; affordability; and the capacity and willingness to comply with the recommendation. Because the patient is at the centre, they are encouraged to be an active participant in this care-planning process and to take responsibility for their own healthcare.

The recommended plan must be acceptable to all parties involved and developed with a collaborative mindset. When the pharmacist is making treatment recommendations, the plan should be evidence based, focussed on clinical goals and should have sound reasoning. As the plan is documented, all clinical goals should be matched to the treatment recommendations and the monitoring parameters that measure the effectiveness of the treatment plan should be clearly indicated. The plan should be clearly written so that every healthcare provider involved in the patient's care can follow the pharmacist's thought pattern. It should include the specific drug, dose, route and duration, as well as the type and frequency of monitoring, any necessary referrals and follow-up instructions to ensure proper monitoring of the patient and achievement of the healthcare goals. Case Study 30.4 summarizes the pharmacist's plan for the patient.

CASE STUDY 30.4

Plan

1. Uncontrolled painful diabetic neuropathy:
   - Goals: Goals include improving pain symptoms and reaching patient set pain goal of 6/10 within 4–6 weeks, improve function, quality of life and sleep within the next month as the treatment regimen is titrated based on patient's response. Minimize adverse drug reactions to the treatment options.
   - Discontinue amitriptyline
   - Start slow titration of gabapentin 300 mg by mouth at bedtime for 1 week, then may increase to 300 mg by mouth two times daily for 1 week, then increase again to 300 mg by mouth three times daily. Titration to continue with goal dosing of gabapentin 600 mg by mouth three times daily to achieve optimal efficacy and tolerability. Monitor for signs of daytime sedation, confusion or peripheral oedema. Evaluate pain levels associated with diabetic peripheral neuropathy (DPN).
   - Encourage proper foot care: Daily examination of each foot to identify cracking, dryness or signs of infection. Stress importance of proper shoe selection.

2. Constipation: Adverse drug reaction secondary to amitriptyline.
   - Goal: Improve symptoms with Bristol stool score of 4 (i.e. like a sausage or snake, smooth and soft) and achieve a daily regular bowel movement within the next 1–4 days without straining. (Note: The Bristol stool scale is a scale that classifies human faeces into seven categories. Type 4 is an average stool that is considered easy to defecate without containing excessive fluid.)
   - Initiate polyethylene glycol 3350 (an osmotic laxative): Mix 17 g in 8 oz of beverage and drink once daily for 3 days then use as needed when Bristol is less than 3 or other symptoms of constipation occur. Hold dose for loose stools. Provide education on Bristol stool chart. Encourage proper hydration, adequate dietary fibre via fruits and vegetables and stress the importance of doing as much exercise as can be tolerated.

3. Poorly controlled Type 2 diabetes
   - Goal: Achieve haemoglobin A1C Goal <7% within the next year to prevent worsening of DPN
   - Refer to PCP to evaluate diabetes medication for adjustment of oral medications to dual therapy to achieve better blood glucose control.
   - Referral for a diabetic education class for improvement of self-management skills

4. Controlled hypertension and dyslipidaemia: Continue current regimen

---

Implementation

Once the developed plan is accepted by the healthcare team, it is imperative to implement it fully. The most important parts of this phase are proper communication to all stakeholders and effective patient education. Thus, the pharmacist will need to possess the cognitive flexibility and empathy to be able to tailor the communication to different individuals involved in planning implementation, including the specific patient, surrogate and/or caregiver to assure optimal understanding and compliance with the plan.

For the patient, the pharmacist will need to use a communication strategy that will enable the assessment of the patient's understanding of their illness and medication plan, as well as the level of motivation and commitment. The pharmacist will need to take the proper amount of time to explain the treatment plan to the patient including not only what the patient will be asked to do, but why this particular plan is deemed the best plan. It is imperative the patient not only understands the entire plan, but also agrees to it. Pharmacists should be keenly aware of communication tips and be well informed on adult education to ensure all information is provided in an effective manner and the patient is not overwhelmed or confused by the information.

Follow-up: Monitoring and Evaluation

The follow-up phase includes the ongoing monitoring and evaluation of the treatment plan. Focussing on the medications, the pharmacist will monitor to ensure treatment efficacy and to determine possible side effects and the patient's overall response and satisfaction with the treatment. During this time, it is also important to continually align the clinical outcomes with the healthcare goals to ensure progress is being made towards achieving these goals. These goals must be continually evaluated to ensure they remain appropriate and achievable because a patient's health can change frequently.

When considering healthcare outcomes to measure, the pharmacist must not only focus on the clinical measures, but must also evaluate the humanistic measures such as patient functioning, ability to participate in self-management and understanding of current medication therapy. Additionally, economic-related measures are important to evaluate including, for example frequency and reasons for emergency room visits and hospitalizations, and overall medication costs. Case Study 30.5 summarizes the pharmacist's follow-up plan (monitoring and evaluation) for the patient.

Reasoning in the Therapeutic Phase

In the therapeutic phase, the practitioner uses the collected information and assessment as the basis, or the premises, to create goals for improvement of the patient's health. In turn, the assessment and goals provide the basis for the generation and selection of therapeutic and monitoring strategies. Thus, therapeutic reasoning in each of these steps involves the generation and substantiation of arguments for what should be done to maintain or improve the patient's health (Kelley and Hutchins, 2021). In the process of therapeutic selection, the pharmacist will use dialectical reasoning and they will argue one therapeutic option against another or in some cases consider an argument for no treatment.

As with other arguments, the proposed strategy must satisfy the basic criteria for valid arguments, namely that its premises (e.g. the assessment and goals) are true and that the conclusion of what to do logically follows (Kelley and Hutchins, 2021). Additionally, the argument for a recommended strategy must be communicated in a way that it can be readily understood and evaluated by each stakeholder. The pharmacist should be able to articulate the evidence on which the recommendation is based and should be able to explain logically how the proposed intervention will affect the underlying pathophysiological processes to achieve the outcomes stipulated in the therapeutic goals and how it may lead to adverse effects (Hawkins et al., 2010).

Ethical reasoning will also be an essential component of therapeutic reasoning, as choices are made in the best interest of and with the consent of the patient whose valued goals must be considered, whose active participation in care planning and implementation

---

CASE STUDY 30.5

Monitor and Evaluate

1. Uncontrolled painful diabetic neuropathy:
   - Improved symptoms based on pain levels, improved function and quality of life, improved sleep quality.
   - Signs and symptoms of side effects upon initiation and slow titration of gabapentin: daytime sedation, confusion.
   - Improved haemoglobin A1C every 3 months following adjustments after follow-up with PCP for diabetes mellitus management, attendance of diabetes self-management skills class.

2. Constipation
   - Bristol stool chart and signs and symptoms of constipation (signs of straining, incomplete evacuation)
   - Frequency of use of polyethylene glycol 3350 to determine whether this should be scheduled.

3. Hypertension/dyslipidaemia
   - Continued control with current regimen, no reports of adverse drug reaction.

is desired, and who is the ultimate change agent for their own health (Rogers, 1983; Hawkins et al., 2010).

Common Sources of Reasoning Errors

Reasoning is our best guide to making decisions about patient care. Therefore, the greater our effort to make valid assertions, arguments and conclusions, the more effective our patient care can be. However, we are fallible and there are many controllable factors that contribute to our fallibility, which we are obligated to recognize and remediate in order to achieve optimal care for our patients. Among these factors are inadequate knowledge and cognitive biases that can undermine our reasoning and are at the source of many of our clinical reasoning errors.

Inadequate Knowledge

Reasoning and all of its elements rely on our understanding of what it is we are reasoning about in order to make accurate interpretations, evaluations, inferences and arguments. This requirement places an onus on the pharmacist to continuously develop a deep, broad, accurate and integrated knowledge base that includes a wide range of concepts, principles and facts. It includes knowledge about diseases and their mechanisms, psychosocial determinants, manifestations, diagnostic elements and morbidity. It includes knowledge about drug and nondrug therapeutic remedies, their mechanisms, risks, benefits, costs and evidentiary support. It also includes knowledge about the practices and perspectives of other healthcare practitioners who join in a collective pursuit of helping the patient to achieve their healthcare goals. This knowledge about what underlies a patient's health and healthcare is integrated with knowledge about the patient (e.g. signs and symptoms) to develop a clear and comprehensive clinical picture and therapeutic plan.

Cognitive Biases

In the process of becoming a competent reasoning clinician, the pharmacist must strive to develop a mindset that excludes the cognitive biases that interfere with the reasoning process and consequently, are often found at the root of many clinical errors. These biases, along with inadequate knowledge, can also lead to suboptimal problem assessment and resolution. There are over 100 potential biases that can affect our reasoning (Croskerry et al., 2013a). Some of the more common examples for pharmacists to be aware of are described here (Croskerry, 2003; Croskerry et al., 2013a; Croskerry et al., 2013b; Scott, 2009).

Anchoring: Relying too heavily on the first piece of information offered. For example, creating an initial impression based on salient features in the patient's initial presentation and failure to adjust this initial impression when warranted by later information.

Ascertainment bias: Prior experiences are used to shape current thinking, leading to seeing what you expect to see.

Availability: Being biased towards more recent information or information that most readily comes to mind when making judgements.

Confirmation bias: Focussing on the signs and symptoms that can confirm a leading diagnostic hypothesis and discounting any data which would counter or refute it.

Fundamental attribution error: The tendency to be inappropriately judgemental and explain illnesses or behaviour on internal factors of a patient, such as personality or disposition, without adequately considering external factors or circumstances.

Premature closure: The process of selecting a hypothesis prior to gathering sufficient information and exploring other valid alternatives.

Representativeness restraint: Judging a situation based on the typical prototype and matching up the current situation to this prototype, leading to a risk of missing an atypical presentation.

When considering this short list of common biases, it is not difficult to envision how a pharmacist can fall victim to them. It is imperative that all healthcare providers, including pharmacists, are keenly aware of these common errors that can negatively impact clinical reasoning and lead to possible negative outcomes for the patient. It is vital to take a step back and look at the entire picture and actively engage in the problem-solving process to allow for appropriate arguments to be developed and evaluated, leading to the best treatment options for the patient.

SUMMARY

In this chapter, we have outlined:

- How pharmacists apply their medication-management expertise and clinical reasoning in clinical problem solving as part of a collaborative effort to achieve effective patient-centred care;
- How pharmacists use clinical reasoning and a systematic patient care process to assess and resolve medication-related problems;
- The contributions of inadequate knowledge and cognitive biases to clinical reasoning errors.

REFERENCES

American College of Clinical Pharmacy, 2014. Standards of practice for clinical pharmacists. Pharmacotherapy 34 (8), 794–797. https://doi.org/10.1002/phar.1438

Bennett, M.S., Kliethermes, M.A., & American Pharmacists Association, 2015. How to implement the pharmacists' patient care process: A systematic approach. American Pharmacists Association. https://pharmacylibrary.com/doi/book/10.21019/9781582122564

Booth, F.W., Roberts, C.K., Laye, M.J., 2012. Lack of exercise is a major cause of chronic diseases. Comprehensive Physiology 2 (2), 1143–1211. https://doi.org/10.1002/cphy.c110025

Cipolle, R.J., Strand, L.M., Morley, P.C., 2012. Pharmaceutical care practice: The patient-centered approach to medication management services, 3rd ed. McGraw-Hill Medical.

Croskerry, P., 2003. The importance of cognitive errors in diagnosis and strategies to minimize them. Academic Medicine 78 (8), 775–780. https://doi.org/10.1097/00001888-200308000-00003

Croskerry, P., Singhal, G., Mamede, S., 2013a. Cognitive debiasing 1: Origins of bias and theory of debiasing. BMJ Quality & Safety 22 (Suppl 2), ii58–ii64. https://doi.org/10.1136/bmjqs-2012-001712

Croskerry, P., Singhal, G., Mamede, S., 2013b. Cognitive debiasing 2: Impediments to and strategies for change. BMJ Quality & Safety 22 (Suppl 2), ii65–ii72. https://doi.org/10.1136/bmjqs-2012-001713

Dictionary.com (n.d.). Reasoning. In: Dictionary.com. Retrieved October 23, 2022, from http://www.dictionary.com/browse/reasoning

Gambrill, E.D., 2012. Critical thinking in clinical practice: Improving the quality of judgments and decisions, 3rd ed. Wiley.

Hawkins, D.R., Paul, R., Elder, L., 2010. The thinker's guide to clinical reasoning. Foundation for Critical Thinking.

Jayasinghe, S., 2012. Complexity science to conceptualize health and disease: Is it relevant to clinical medicine? Mayo Clinic Proceedings 87 (4), 314–319. https://doi.org/10.1016/j.mayocp.2011.11.018

Kelley, D., Hutchins, D., 2021. The art of reasoning, 5th ed. W.W. Norton & Co.

Martin, L.C., Donohoe, K.L., Holdford, D.A., 2016. Decision-making and problem-solving approaches in pharmacy education. American Journal of Pharmaceutical Education 80 (3), 52. https://doi.org/10.5688/ajpe80352

Rogers, J.C., 1983. Eleanor Clarke Slagle Lectureship--1983; clinical reasoning: The ethics, science, and art. The American Journal of Occupational Therapy 37 (9), 601–616. https://doi.org/10.5014/ajot.37.9.60

Schneiderman, N., Ironson, G., Siegel, S.D., 2005. Stress and health: Psychological, behavioral, and biological determinants. Annual Review of Clinical Psychology 1, 607–628. https://doi.org/10.1146/annurev.clinpsy.1.102803.144141

Scott, I.A., 2009. Errors in clinical reasoning: Causes and remedial strategies. BMJ (Clinical Research Ed.) 338, b1860. https://doi.org/10.1136/bmj.b1860

Slavich, G.M., 2016. Life stress and health: A review of conceptual issues and recent findings. Teaching of Psychology (Columbia, Mo.) 43 (4), 346–355. https://doi.org/10.1177/0098628316662768

Steiner, W.A., Ryser, L., Huber, E., Uebelhart, D., Aeschlimann, A., Stucki, G., 2002. Use of the ICF model as a clinical problem-solving tool in physical therapy and rehabilitation medicine. Physical Therapy 82 (11), 1098–1107.

Tietze, K.J., 2012. 'Chapter 7 - Therapeutics planning' Clinical skills for pharmacists, 3rd ed. Mosby. pp. 132–144.

Wilson, T., Holt, T., Greenhalgh, T., 2001. Complexity science: Complexity and clinical care. BMJ (Clinical Research Ed.) 323 (7314), 685–688. https://doi.org/10.1136/bmj.323.7314.685

31

SPEECH PATHOLOGY
Facilitating Clinical Reasoning

BELINDA KENNY ■ RACHEL DAVENPORT ■ ROBYN B. JOHNSON

CHAPTER OUTLINE

CHAPTER AIMS

The aims of this chapter are:

- to provide a framework and tools that speech pathologists may apply to facilitate clinical reasoning and
- to show how speech pathologists may explicitly focus on different reasoning elements to develop and refine their competency in clinical reasoning.

INTRODUCTION

The scope of speech pathology practice is continuing to evolve in response to research evidence, technology, medical advances, government policies and community needs. For example, in Australia, in 2020 the Competency-based Occupational Standards in Speech Pathology (Speech Pathology Association of Australia, 2011) were superseded by Professional Standards (Speech Pathology Australia, 2020) that reflect core areas of competence for practising speech pathologists (SPs). Using the Australian standards as an illustration, clinical reasoning now underpins core competencies across the three identified domains of speech pathology practice. The three domains are 'professional conduct', 'reflective practice and lifelong learning' and 'speech pathology practice'. For example, in reflective practice and lifelong learning, the Professional Standards state, 'We develop our reasoning and decision-making through critical reflection on our practice at an individual, team, organizational and policy level' (Speech Pathology Australia, 2020, p. 13). In speech pathology practice, clinical reasoning is specifically related to the competent synthesis of assessment findings and the judicious application of evidence together with the integration of client, family and community needs required for effective management planning.

Clinical reasoning is also an explicit component of the education of student SPs. The standardized assessment tool, COMPASS (McAllister et al., 2006), for assessing student SPs on clinical placements, which is used in Australia and overseas, includes reasoning as one of the four core professional competency units. Students are required to demonstrate thinking skills and show how they integrate collaborative and holistic viewpoints into their reasoning, i.e. the client and caregivers' views, opinions and wishes, along with current best evidence, which might inform students' decision making. The three components of evidence-based practice (EBP) and International Classification of Functioning, Disability and Health (ICF) frameworks can also assist students and clinicians to integrate information into the reasoning process. Clearly, clinical reasoning is a critical skill for SPs to develop both during their education and their ongoing professional practice. There is an expectation that continuing development of clinical reasoning is essential for maintaining professional competency and adapting to changing workplace demands and community needs.

In some disciplines there is a broad body of research in the area of clinical reasoning outlining how clinicians make decisions (see Chapters 24 and 26) but there has been limited research in this area in speech pathology despite it being a core professional competency (Ginsberg et al., 2016).

In our discipline we have looked at the field of medicine to gain an understanding of how clinical reasoning works in experienced clinicians. Many researchers agree that, for experienced clinicians, clinical reasoning is based on an interaction between an individual's specific knowledge, experience (that is often contextually based) and intuition (Ginsberg et al., 2016; Banning, 2008a, 2008b; Forsberg et al., 2016; Fowler, 1997; Simmons et al., 2003). The issue with these cognitive-based models of clinical reasoning, Pillay and Pillay (2021) argue, is that other contextual and individual factors are ignored. They have put forward a 'contextualized clinical reasoning framework' that... 'recognizes the impact of contextual and personal realities...' (p. 1281). The authors argue that this framework enables healthcare practitioners to practise clinical reasoning in an authentic manner that accounts for 'complexity and diversity of health care contexts globally' (p. 1281). In the following sections, we propose and outline how the ICF model can be used to facilitate clinical reasoning and we use case studies to illustrate how the 'contextualized clinical reasoning framework' can be used to facilitate a different way of approaching developing clinical reasoning with a student and a novice clinician.

ICF AS A FRAMEWORK FOR CLINICAL REASONING

The ICF (World Health Organization, 2001) provides SPs with a framework for professional scope of practice, quality care and intervention (Speech Pathology Association of Australia, 2003). We believe that an ICF framework also provides an effective tool for facilitating clinical reasoning. A key consideration, underpinning SP clinical reasoning, is the importance of communication and swallowing to an individual's health and well-being. The ICF framework makes these components explicit. The framework is also useful in capturing the complexity of other healthcare needs in individuals and communities.

According to the ICF framework, health issues may be classified in two major parts, each comprising specific health components. Part 1 addresses the effects of functioning and disability on an individual's health. Health components underlying functioning and disability include Body Structures (an anatomical component), Functions (a physiological component), Activities (task execution) and Participation (involvement in life situations). Part 2 addresses contextual factors affecting health. The health context may include Environmental Factors (physical, social issues and community attitudes towards communication and swallowing impairment) and Personal Factors (internal factors) (World Health Organization, 2001). Importantly, this biopsychosocial framework shifts professionals' focus from one of handicap to one of facilitating health and well-being. The holistic approach, incorporated within the ICF, can contribute to clinical reasoning and guide person-centred goal setting (Nguyen et al., 2018). Wide application of the ICF framework may support SPs to use effective approaches to clinical reasoning across caseloads to develop, maintain and enhance professional competence.

Applying the ICF framework requires SPs to adopt holistic management for clients with communication and swallowing impairments. Although health is classified under parts and components, the ICF framework presents a dynamic, interactional perspective on health. An underlying assumption is that disease, or disorder, alone does not determine an individual's health outcomes in a simplistic cause/effect relationship. Functional outcomes are influenced by the complex interaction of health components, including the nature of an individual's impairment and environment (Allen et al., 2006). This interactional aspect of healthcare represents a significant move from biomedical to biopsychosocial perspectives on health and resonates with more progressive, participatory models of speech pathology practice, e.g. the Life Participation Approach to Aphasia (Chapey et al., 2000). Developing insights into interactional aspects of health can help SPs transition from clinician-focussed to more person-focussed practice as they consider their clients from a holistic perspective (Forsgren et al., 2022). With continued application of the ICF, clinicians may develop more meaningful goals and activities that meet an individual's communication needs rather than simply dealing with their impairments.

Examples of person-focussed practice are to use the ICF framework as a tool for guiding management approaches with adults with aphasia (Galletta and Barrett, 2014) and children with language impairments (Westby and Washington, 2017). The ICF may also inform outcome measures by addressing the effects of communication and swallowing disorders on participation in everyday life activities (Cunningham et al., 2017; Wallace et al., 2016). When speech pathology clients are perceived as active healthcare decision makers with individual needs, clinicians must change from experts, with all the knowledge, to facilitators who recognize that clients have something important to contribute to their own assessment and management (Brown et al., 2011). For many clients, quality outcomes involve living successfully with a communication or swallowing disorder rather than curing it (Nund et al., 2019). Another benefit of the holistic ICF framework is that it offers a shared language for interprofessional care (Allen et al., 2006).

We believe that the ICF framework may be used for the continuous development of clinical reasoning skills, from professional preparation to practice. As Fig. 31.1 (Johnson et al., 2022) shows, the ICF framework may be readily applied to SPs' knowledge, skills and professional attitudes as they develop along a continuum of competence. Students may master the scientific basics yet struggle to acquire a person-focussed and holistic perspective during assessment and intervention. They may have insight into the importance of functional activities but have limited skills, experience and confidence in planning and delivering coordinated

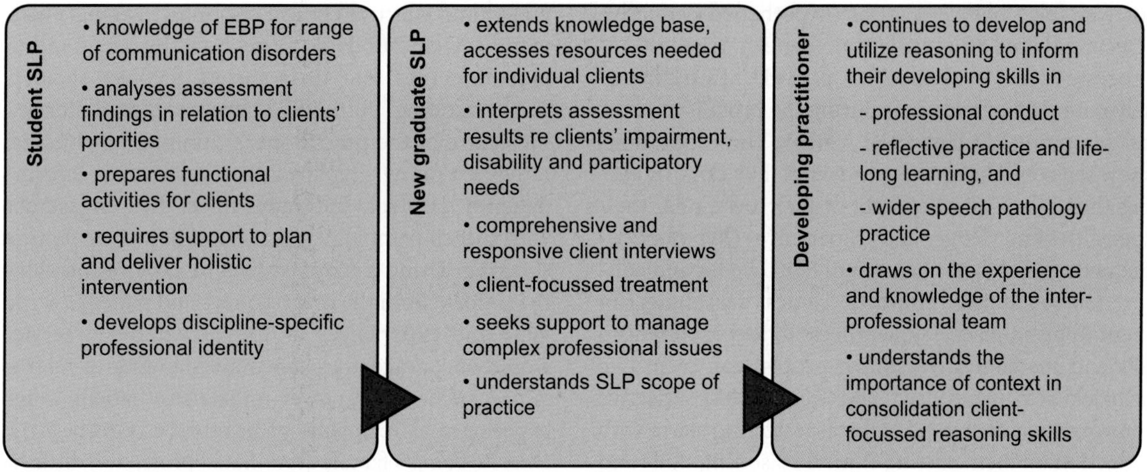

Student SLP
- knowledge of EBP for range of communication disorders
- analyses assessment findings in relation to clients' priorities
- prepares functional activities for clients
- requires support to plan and deliver holistic intervention
- develops discipline-specific professional identity

New graduate SLP
- extends knowledge base, accesses resources needed for individual clients
- interprets assessment results re clients' impairment, disability and participatory needs
- comprehensive and responsive client interviews
- client-focussed treatment
- seeks support to manage complex professional issues
- understands SLP scope of practice

Developing practitioner
- continues to develop and utilize reasoning to inform their developing skills in
  - professional conduct
  - reflective practice and life-long learning, and
  - wider speech pathology practice
- draws on the experience and knowledge of the inter-professional team
- understands the importance of context in consolidation client-focussed reasoning skills

Fig. 31.1 ■ Clinical reasoning in the novice, intermediate and entry-level speech pathology student practice. *EBP*, Evidence-based practice; *SLP*, speech-language pathologist. (With permission from Johnson, R., Kenny, B., Davenport, R., 2022. Speech pathologists' clinical reasoning in the context of the ICF: ICF importance as reasoning develops. figshare. https://doi.org/10.6084/m9.figshare.21737648.v1.)

care. Even strong students benefit from being given the ICF framework as an aid to focus upon clinical reasoning. Adopting an ICF framework may encourage students to 'think like a speech pathologist' and consider the interprofessional, educational and advocacy aspects of their professional roles. For graduates, the ICF also provides a holistic framework for working with individuals, families and communities and developing functional outcome measures.

REFLECTION POINT

Consider how an experienced SP's questioning could focus students on specific components of the ICF:

- Which cranial nerves are impaired and impacting Mrs K's swallowing?
- How can we facilitate Mrs K to have safer and more enjoyable mealtimes?

In the following sections, we suggest strategies to facilitate SPs' clinical reasoning during different stages of the competence continuum.

DEVELOPING AND CONSOLIDATING CLINICAL REASONING

There is no single theory that fully describes the complex nature of clinical reasoning. Experienced practitioners use a combination of approaches, including, for example, 'both analytical (hypothetico-deductive reasoning) and non-analytical (pattern recognition) processes' (Audétat et al., 2013, p. e394). SPs ask themselves a range of questions during the process of clinical reasoning (Delany et al., 2013). These questions show the combination of approaches they can use, asking themselves questions about their own role, their specialist knowledge and experience (hypothetico-deductive) and their clients' individual needs and context (sociocultural). However, clinical reasoning can seem to be an inaccessible process to less experienced SPs and the clinical reasoning process can seem like a 'black box' (McAllister and Rose, 2008). Effective improvement of any SPs' clinical reasoning starts with reflection on their existing clinical reasoning skills and strategies. SPs should aim to continuously develop their ability to see into the 'black box' and understand the clinical reasoning process.

CLINICAL REASONING APPROACHES

Hypothetico-deductive reasoning is a way of making a diagnosis or decision through forming hypotheses from clinical data, comparing it to other evidence (such as theory or experimental data) and refining or rejecting hypotheses until one remains. Novice practitioners almost always need to use this method of clinical reasoning because they have not had the opportunity to build a bank of knowledge and experience required for pattern recognition or forward reasoning as experts do. In contrast, expert practitioners are more likely to tap into their wide experience of cases and clinical clues to come to an accurate hypothesis, often using backward reasoning to check their final hypothesis against the case and its details.

In pattern recognition, practitioners use their specialist knowledge and experience of many case narratives to compare a new client to previous clients with similar difficulties and then apply a similar solution, if possible. As experience increases, knowledge and reasoning become more integrated. It is then possible to see how multiple client behaviours can fit into a range of case narratives. This makes pattern recognition more efficient (in the same way that experienced readers do not sound out every word from the letters but recognize words as whole, meaningful units).

Other forms of reasoning can and should be integrated into effective clinical reasoning. Taking a wider worldview and understanding how the client and the practitioner fit into their society involves sociocultural reasoning. Putting the clients and their stories at the centre of the practitioner's thinking involves narrative reasoning. Exploring the values that inform a patient's worldview and may impact their engagement with speech pathology services might involve feminist thinking. Using a feminist lens to explore the values that inform both the practitioner's and patient's worldview and experiences of speech pathology services would encourage a greater understanding of relevant issues, such as the power imbalances patients might experience as recipients of healthcare (Green, 2012). Despite being a female-dominated profession, little has been written to date about feminist thinking in speech pathology (Skeat et al., 2022). Considering the wider context of the patient, practitioner and the society in which they live involves not only feminist but contextual reasoning (Pillay and Pillay, 2021).

Using one or more of these varying approaches to reasoning can provide holistic depth to practitioners' decision making, both when managing patients and wider career issues (Shapiro et al., 2002). Therefore, when working to problem-solve a student's issues, a holistic approach should be adopted.

SPEECH PATHOLOGY EXAMPLES

Ginsberg et al. (2016) sought to shed light on the thinking of experienced SPs, specifically around diagnostic reasoning. They describe a hierarchy of thinking used by experienced practitioners and suggest a potential stepwise development for less experienced or student SPs to work through this hierarchy. They discovered themes such as 'seeking outside input, rationalizing, hypothesizing, differentiating, summarizing, deferring, comparing, specific planning, general planning and treatment planning' (p. 93). These themes reflect the range of reasoning models used effectively by experienced SPs and align with those described by Delany et al. (2013). More experienced SPs have an essential role in modelling and clearly articulating the process of clinical reasoning to less experienced colleagues and students. This may include helping them to identify structured tasks in the process (such as a hierarchy of questions) if required.

More recently, SPs have explored the complex nature of clinical reasoning by developing multifactorial (Beushausen, 2018) and contextualized (Pillay and Pillay, 2021) clinical reasoning frameworks. Pillay and Pillay (2021) describe SPs as thinking and acting on clinical tasks with patients within the context of macro and micro professional systems. The macrosystems are the broad contexts in which SPs work and clients live, including the legislative, political, socioeconomic and cultural contexts. The microsystems are the immediate surroundings, including local resource availability and the client's personal socioeconomic and educational circumstances. The SP uses the inputs from these systems as well as the essential additional resources of their experience, reflection, peer support, intuition, and collaboration with the wider team to make effective and appropriate decisions around patient care and service provision. This approach fits in well with the ICF because it promotes holistic client care. It provides a

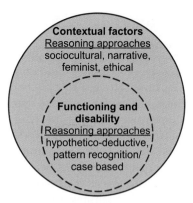

Fig. 31.2 ■ Clinical reasoning approaches and the International Classification of Functioning, Disability and Health. *EBP,* Evidence-based practice; *SLP,* speech-language pathologist. (With permission from Johnson, R., Kenny, B., Davenport, R., 2016. Using the ICF to facilitate development of clinical reasoning (Version 2). figshare. https://doi.org/10.6084/m9.figshare.4235942.v2)

useful framework to help less experienced SPs develop and consolidate their clinical reasoning (Fig. 31.2).

REFLECTION POINT

Focus upon the process of clinical reasoning, not just the outcome.

- Discuss your own thinking and clinical reasoning process or use the questions and themes discussed earlier in the chapter (Delany et al., 2013; Ginsberg et al., 2016).
- Why is hypothetico-deductive reasoning only a beginning?
- What other approaches may facilitate holistic reasoning?

Case Study 31.1 is a synthesis of a clinical educator's (CE) experience working with a novice student. This case illustrates how taking a broader perspective of clinical reasoning is useful, utilizing the contextualized clinical reasoning framework.

ICF AND CLINICAL REASONING IN PRACTICE (CASE STUDY 31.1 ANALYSIS)

Case Study 31.1 presents Val, the experienced clinician, who is used to working in a very client-centred

CASE STUDY 31.1

Supporting a Student

Val is an experienced certified practising SP working in a paediatric setting with preschool children which services clients from diverse backgrounds. She is very experienced in her context but has taken very few students in this particular workplace. This is because she used to believe that students needed some experience under their belts before working in this particular environment. Val is very client-centred in her practice and is sensitive to her clients' contexts and how her own values and thinking impact the care she delivers. Val's thinking has started to change. She now thinks that it is better for students to have early exposure to different environments. This semester Val has taken a 'novice' student, Tash. This is Tash's first placement. On the first day of placement Val sits down with Tash to find out what

Tash's learning goals are and what specific areas she would like to focus on during the placement. Tash's only other clinical experiences thus far have been in the previous semester in the 'Preparation for clinical practice' subject, where she participated in a 'textbook' case history simulation and observed a video of an assessment and therapy session. Tash reported these sessions as really useful and is now keen to see how evidence-based practice is implemented in community organizations such as Val's. Val's practice is driven by multiple complex factors that include, but are not limited to, the use of gold standard evidence. Val would like some suggestions on how to facilitate Tash's clinical reasoning in this context without negating all of the conventional textbook teaching she has learnt at university thus far.

way, factoring in the multiple complexities of the client and context, her own values and beliefs into the way she works. The majority of clinical reasoning models utilized to date have traditionally come from medicine and have taken a reductionist, White, Western, medicalized approach to reasoning and decision making. Val is aware that although this is not the way she practises, it is the way Tash is being largely educated. The developmental framework (Fig. 31.3) we suggest can assist in structuring tasks for Tash, whilst incorporating the contextual factors of the placement and people/families she is working with. Val can manage this complexity for Tash, as she develops her skills, whilst still being exposed to it. Pillay and Pillay's (2021) Contextualized Clinical Reasoning Framework can also provide a 'map' to help guide her work with Tash, so that Tash can incorporate and start to understand how her own values, her views of the world and her position in it influence her thinking from the beginning. This is in contrast to the simplistic view that sensitivity to values is a skill that can be 'bolted on' after graduation. This does not negate what Tash is learning at university, rather it complements it and starts to shape Tash's clinical reasoning to be more sensitive to context.

REFLECTION POINT

■ How might a structured framework such as the Contextualized Clinical Reasoning Framework be useful for CEs and students to help facilitate the development of student reasoning skills?

In the second case study, Alex is a new graduate SP who meets regularly with her manager to help manage the demands of a busy caseload. Consider Alex's clinical reasoning skills in Case Study 31.2.

STRONG CLINICAL REASONING INCLUDES CONSIDERATION OF ALL AREAS OF ICF (CASE STUDY 31.2 ANALYSIS)

The interaction between Alex and her CE suggests that Alex is demonstrating competent skills for a new graduate SP. Key indicators include:

■ Alex's reasoning incorporates an ICF framework. Alex considers the potential effects of Jim's physical and cognitive impairments (Body Functions) following his stroke. Treatment goals are linked to

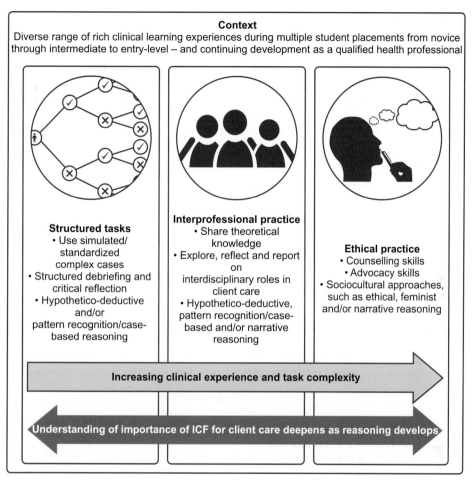

Fig. 31.3 ■ ICF importance as reasoning develops. *ICF*, International Classification of Functioning, Disability and Health. (With permission from Johnson, R., Kenny, B., Davenport, R., 2022. Speech pathologists' clinical reasoning in the context of the ICF: SLP reasoning development. figshare. https://doi.org/10.6084/m9.figshare.21737648.v1)

Jim's functional communication needs (Activities) and facilitation of his social/leisure activities (Participation). Alex includes Jim's wife in the treatment, identifying her need for education about how to communicate with her partner so that she can respond appropriately when Jim tries to communicate at home (Environment). Alex also acknowledges the family's concerns regarding Jim's safety (Environment/Body functions). Alex has attended to Jim's frustration with word finding difficulties and responded by adopting a multimodal intervention approach (Personal/Activities).

■ In keeping with an ICF framework, Alex's concept of her professional role includes discipline-specific intervention, patient and family education, and interdisciplinary teamwork.
■ Alex is demonstrating skills consistent with a contextualized clinical reasoning framework. She is combining an understanding of the client's and family's needs and circumstances with her professional experience, reflection, interdisciplinary collaboration together with support from her manager to make effective management decisions.

CASE STUDY 31.2

Extending a Staff Member's Clinical Reasoning Skills

Lee (manager): Hello Alex. During our last meeting, you raised concerns about how Jim and his family were managing. How did he progress this week?

Alex (new graduate): Overall, well. I focussed on my time management and prioritized key goals. So, Jim still achieved his important goals even though his taxi was late again. I'm learning more about him so I can plan goals and activities that are relevant for Jim. He's more engaged in the therapy and starting to make gains.

Lee: Great, your strategy of involving Jim and his wife with goal setting can help you assign time to the goals that really matter to them. Why do you think his communication is improving?

Alex: Jim was initiating conversation with me about football. He loves this sport! My data show he was 70% successful with nouns and verbs today. Having the online sports results helped. We worked longer on that activity because Jim was so engaged and communicating his messages with speech and gestures. Jim's wife mentioned how much he enjoyed attending football games. It was good to include her in the activity and demonstrate strategies for helping Jim to communicate. She was still 'testing' Jim sometimes. Next time I'll respond more quickly and re-explain our intervention approach when Jim shows frustration.

Lee: Good idea to provide Jim's wife with more education. How could you build on this progress in future sessions with holistic management?

Alex: Communication activities related to Jim's interests in football and fishing. He's not doing those activities yet because his family is worried about his right-sided weakness and memory issues. I need to contact Jim's OT and physio for an update on his other rehabilitation goals.

STRATEGIES FOR EDUCATORS AND MANAGERS: USING THE ICF TO EXTEND CLINICAL REASONING SKILLS

We propose the model in Fig. 31.3 (Johnson et al., 2016) as a framework that will help educators and managers facilitate clinical reasoning with students and staff members with different professional experience and skill levels. This model indicates the importance of supplementing clinical learning experiences with structured tasks, interprofessional collaboration and ethical awareness to enhance clinical reasoning skills.

Structured Tasks

- For students, develop simulated/standardized patients and compile research for complex cases (Sabei and Lasater, 2016). Working in interprofessional teams would further extend students. Miles et al. (2016) found that the students' clinical reasoning skills, among other measures, significantly improved after undergoing interprofessional simulation-based dysphagia training. Some believe that the use of simulated learning environments (SLEs) has much potential for improved clinical reasoning. For example, MacBean et al. (2013) found that the current use of SLEs in speech pathology education was currently limited, but there were many possible benefits. Students can also start to consider their own influence on the clinical reasoning process by using frameworks such as Pillay and Pillay (2021) that draw on situated cognition models of clinical reasoning.

- Educators and managers may explain how deep critical reflection can open the 'black box' of clinical reasoning. Sabei and Lasater (2016) found that using structured debriefing, including critical reflection, facilitated participants to comment on the level of 'their cognitive, affective, and psychomotor performance' (p. 46) in the context of their developing clinical reasoning skills. Students may also use reflective journals to critically review the process and outcomes of their clinical reasoning in new or complex professional scenarios.

- Use structured questions or hierarchies to develop reasoning skills (Delany et al., 2013; Ginsberg et al., 2016); then consider narrative and contextual approaches to extend reasoning.
- Managers and clinicians can use frameworks to guide their own thinking to be more holistic and context sensitive in their care by utilizing frameworks such as Pillay and Pillay (2021).

Interprofessional Tasks

- Set up opportunities for students or new graduates to share theoretical knowledge with students or staff members from the speech pathology team or the wider team.
- Encourage students and staff members to explore the range of roles within the interdisciplinary team and reflect on the way the whole team delivers holistic care.
- Set up interprofessional team tasks because good teamwork skills predict good clinical outcomes (Shrader et al., 2013) and may facilitate contextual reasoning by the team.

Ethical Practice

- Discuss ethical reasoning skills (Kenny et al., 2010; Speech Pathology Australia, 2020) to ensure clinicians understand that effective clinical reasoning is underpinned by sound application of professional codes of ethics. Discussing ethical implications of different intervention options can provide insights into perceived benefits, potential harms, client autonomy and access to quality services.
- Ensure students and new graduates consider using the counselling skills they have learnt. These skills are essential in encouraging clients and carers to comfortably disclose their requirements, both in functional and contextual terms, and thus make full use of available services.
- Discuss the importance of developing advocacy skills because many clients require support to make their requirements known in a range of contexts.

REFLECTION POINT

The challenge for every educator and manager is to customize the use of the ICF and E3BP models to support every clinician in further developing clinical reasoning skills required for work readiness.

SUMMARY

In this chapter, we discussed:

- that, as a profession, we have progressed our understanding of how SPs develop their clinical reasoning skills.
- how clinical reasoning is now a core competency in becoming a graduate speech-language pathologist.
- how we can be more attuned to the complex factors that influence our thinking and reasoning by using frameworks such as the one Pillay and Pillay (2021) propose.
- how using the ICF and E3BP models can assist educators and managers in identifying where staff members' clinical reasoning skills are at developmentally and suggestions for how to develop these skills at various levels (see Fig. 31.3).

We presented practical suggestions to use in everyday clinical situations to support students and extend clinicians' clinical reasoning including:

- structured debriefing,
- utilizing contextual frameworks to facilitate reasoning,
- using student reflection journals,
- overtly modelling own reasoning skills,
- learning in interprofessional teams,
- working through cases and
- simulation.

This information may help educators and managers decide where to begin in order to facilitate the core professional skill of clinical reasoning. We have presented a framework and suggestions for facilitating SPs' clinical reasoning to the next level, as part of a lifelong learning approach that extends from student professional preparation to practising clinicians.

REFERENCES

Allen, C.M., Campbell, W.N., Guptill, C.A., et al., 2006. A conceptual model for interprofessional education: The International Classification of Functioning, Disability and Health (ICF). J. Interprof. Care 20, 235–245.

Audétat, M.C., Laurin, S., Sanche, G., et al., 2013. Clinical reasoning difficulties: A taxonomy for clinical teachers. Med. Teach 35, e984–e989.

Banning, M., 2008a. A review of clinical decision making: models and current research. Journal of Clinical Nursing 17 (2), 187–95. https://doi.org/10.1111/j.1365-2702.2006.01791.x

Banning, M., 2008b. The think aloud approach as an educational tool to develop and assess clinical reasoning in undergraduate students. Nurse Education Today 28 (1), 8–14. https://doi.org/10.1016/j.nedt.2007.02.001

Beushausen, U., 2018. Clinical reasoning in der Sprachtherapie. Sprache·Stimme·Gehör 42 (03), 119–122. https://doi.org/10.1055/a-0625-5896

Brown, K., Worrall, L.E., Davidson, B., et al., 2011. Living successfully with aphasia: A qualitative meta-analysis of the perspectives of individuals with aphasia, family members, and speech-language pathologists. Int. J. Speech Lang. Path 14, 141–155. https://doi.org/10.3109/17549507.2011.632026

Chapey, R., Duchan, J.F., Elman, R.J., et al., 2000. Life participation approach to aphasia: A statement of values for the future. ASHA Leader 5 (3), 4–6. https://doi.org/10.1044/leader.FTR.05032000.4

Cunningham, B.J., Washington, K.N., Binns, A., et al., 2017. Current methods of evaluating speech-language outcomes for preschoolers with communication disorders: A scoping review using the ICF-CY. J. Sp. Lang. Hear. Res 60, 447–464. https://doi.org/10.1044/2016_JSLHR-L-15-0329

Delany, C., Golding, C., Bialocerkowski, A., 2013. Teaching for thinking in clinical education: Making explicit the thinking involved in allied health clinical reasoning. Focus Health Prof. Educ 14, 44.

Forsberg, E., Ziegert, K., Hult, H., Fors, U., 2016. Assessing progression of clinical reasoning through virtual patients: An exploratory study. Nurse Education in Practice 16 (1), 97–103. https://doi.org/10.1016/j.nepr.2015.09.006

Forsgren, E., Åke, S., Saldert, C., 2022. Person-centred care in speech-language therapy research and practice for adults: A scoping review. Int. J. Lang. Com. Dis. 57, 381–402. https://doi.org/10.1111/1460-6984.12690

Fowler, L.P., 1997. Clinical reasoning strategies used during care planning. Clinical Nursing Research 6 (4), 349–61. https://doi.org/10.1177/105477389700600405

Galletta, E.E., Barrett, A.M., 2014. Impairment and functional interventions for aphasia: Having it all. Curr Phys Med Rehabil Rep 2, 114–120. https://doi.org/10.1007/s40141-014-0050-5

Ginsberg, S.M., Friberg, J.C., Visconti, C.F., 2016. Diagnostic reasoning by experienced speech-language pathologists and student clinicians. Contemp. Issues Commun. Sci. Disord 43, 87.

Green, B., 2012. Applying feminist ethics of care to nursing practice. Journal of Nursing & Care 1 (03), 1–4.

Kenny, B., Lincoln, M., Balandin, S., 2010. Experienced speech language pathologists' responses to ethical dilemmas: An integrated approach to ethical reasoning. Am. J. Speech Lang. Pathol 19, 121–134.

Johnson, R., Kenny, B., Davenport, R., 2016. Using the ICF to facilitate development of clinical reasoning (Version 2). figshare. https://doi.org/10.6084/m9.figshare.4235942.v2

Johnson, R., Kenny, B., Davenport, R., 2022. Speech pathologists' Clinical reasoning in the context of the ICF (Version 1). figshare. https://doi.org/10.6084/m9.figshare.21737648.v1

MacBean, N., Theodoros, D., Davidson, B., et al., 2013. Simulated learning environments in speech-language pathology: An Australian response. Int. J. Speech Lang. Pathol 15, 345–357.

McAllister, L., Rose, M., 2008. Speech-language pathology students: Learning clinical reasoning. In: Higgs, J., Jones, M.A., Loftus, S. (Eds.), Clinical reasoning in the health professions, 3rd ed. Elsevier, pp. 397–404.

McAllister, S., Lincoln, M., Ferguson, A., et al., 2006. COMPASS: Competency assessment in speech pathology. Speech Pathology Association of Australia.

Miles, A., Friary, P., Jackson, B., et al., 2016. Simulation-based dysphagia training: Teaching interprofessional clinical reasoning in a hospital environment. Dysphagia 31, 407–415.

Nguyen, T., Stewart, D., Rosenbaum, P., et al., 2018. Using the ICF in transition research and practice? Lessons from a scoping review. Res Dev Disabil 72, 225–239. https://doi.org/10.1016/j.ridd.2017.11.003

Nund, R.L., Brown, B., Ward, E.C., et al., 2019. What are we really measuring? A content comparison of swallowing outcome measures for head and neck cancer based on the International Classification of Functioning, Disability and Health (ICF). Dysphagia 34, 575–591. https://doi.org/10.1007/s00455-019-10005-0

Pillay, T., Pillay, M., 2021. Syncing our global thinking: A framework for contextualized clinical reasoning. Perspectives of the ASHA Special Interest Groups 6 (5), 1281–1290. https://doi.org/10.1044/2021_PERSP-21-00054

Sabei, S.D.A., Lasater, K., 2016. Simulation debriefing for clinical judgment development: A concept analysis. Nurse Educ. Today 45, 42–47.

Simmons, B., Lanuza, D., Fonteyn, M., et al., 2003. Clinical reasoning in experienced nurses. Western Journal of Nursing Research 25 (6), 701–19. https://doi.org/10.1177/0193945903253092

Skeat, J., Attrill, S., Hersh, D., 2022. Feminist research in a female-dominated profession: How can this lens help us to understand ourselves better in speech-language pathology? International Journal of Speech-Language Pathology 24 (5), 484–493.

Shapiro, D.A., Ogletree, B.T., Dale Brotherton, W., 2002. Graduate students with marginal abilities in communication sciences and disorders: Prevalence, profiles, and solutions. J. Commun. Disord 35, 421–451.

Shrader, S., Kern, D., Zoller, J., et al., 2013. Interprofessional teamwork skills as predictors of clinical outcomes in a simulated healthcare setting. J. Allied Health 42, 1E–6E.

Speech Pathology Association of Australia, 2003. Scope of Practice in Speech Pathology. Speech Pathology Association of Australia, Melbourne, VIC.

Speech Pathology Association of Australia, 2011. Competency based occupational standards for speech pathologists: Entry level,

Revised ed. Speech Pathology Association of Australia. https://www.speechpathologyaustralia.org.au/public/libraryviewer?ResourceID=409

Speech Pathology Australia, 2020. *Ethics education package*. https://learninghub.speechpathologyaustralia.org.au/speechpathologyaust/1057-ethics-education-package

Westby, C., Washington, K.N., 2017. Using the International Classification of Functioning, Disability and Health in assessment and intervention of school-aged children with language impairments. Lang Speech Hear Serv Sch 48, 137–152. https://doi.org/10.1044/2017_LSHSS-16-0037 PMID: 28630972.

Wallace, S.J., Worrall, L., Rose, T., et al., 2016. Core outcomes in aphasia treatment research: An e-Delphi consensus study of international aphasia researchers. Am J Speech Lang Pathol 25, S729–S742. https://doi.org/10.1044/2016_AJSLP-15-0150 PMID: 27997949

World Health Organization, 2001. International Classification of Functioning, Disability and Health (ICF). World Health Organization.

32

CLINICAL DECISION MAKING ACROSS ORTHODOX AND COMPLEMENTARY MEDICINE FIELDS

SANDRA GRACE ■ STEPHEN LOFTUS

CHAPTER OUTLINE

CHAPTER AIMS

The aims of this chapter are:

- to discuss the implications for mainstream allopathic practitioners of the widespread use of complementary medicine among their patients
- to discuss the practice of person-centred care that takes into account patients' illness experiences and values their healthcare preferences
- to explore alternative ways of thinking through clinical problems and provide specific examples
- to explore strategies for integrating alternative ways of thinking that combine the strengths of both mainstream allopathic medicine and complementary and alternative medicine.

INTRODUCTION

The goal of clinical reasoning of all healthcare professionals is to identify and articulate patients' health needs and to use specialized knowledge and skills to work out ways to help patients achieve optimal health. To state this seems straightforward and obvious, but it can be problematic. This is because in developed countries the dominant healthcare system is Western medicine, often referred to as allopathic medicine. It has been largely characterized as biomedical, pathology-driven, cure- or disease-oriented, based on the scientific method and using evidence that is predominantly empirical-analytical (Capra, 1983; Hawk, 2005; Hayes, 2007; Uher et al., 2020). Foucault, in his famous work *The Birth of the Clinic* (1994), highlighted the dehumanizing and reductionist aspects of biomedicine. He discussed the rise of allopathic medicine in terms of the 'clinical gaze' that focusses on a pathological view of the body, usually a dead body rather than a living person. From this biomedical viewpoint, health was seen simplistically as the absence of pathology.

Complementary and alternative medicine (CAM) approaches to healthcare have become popular with people who are well and who want fuller explanations about the health and more time with their practitioners (Grace and Higgs, 2010b; Tangkiatkumjai et al., 2020). Advocates of CAM approaches claim that CAM practitioners pay far more attention to what the patient feels and says about their health (Franzel et al., 2013; Uher et al., 2020). One way that the differences between biomedicine and CAM are summarized is to say that biomedicine has a disease focus (what the pathologist looks at) and CAM approaches focus on the illness experience (what the patient goes through). Likewise, biomedicine originally assumed that health was simply absence of pathology, whereas CAM paid more attention to developing the wellness of patients. There is often a much greater holistic view in CAM. As Reeve (an allopathic doctor) put it:

> There is evidence within the complementary and alternative medicine (CAM) literature of individuals undertaking sophisticated and multidimensional assessments of health status and need. For some, explanations of 'dis-ease' within CAM frameworks make more sense of individual illness experiences than a pathological account.
>
> CAM users are not simply dissatisfied with conventional medicine, but make sophisticated assessments of their health needs and the appropriate therapeutic approach needed to address them, drawing on a range of knowledges to support this process.
>
> *(Reeve, 2010, p. 6).*

If we view health and the illness experience from other perspectives, there are far more complex issues than a purely biomedical view assumes. Over recent decades we have seen the emergence of the biopsychosocial model of healthcare, a broadened approach that includes psychosocial aspects of health and illness without sacrificing the traditional biomedical model (Farre and Rapley, 2017). At the same time, Western medicine's responsibility to cure patients of diseases has been reconceptualized as concerned with the importance of cultural, social and psychological influences on health and the patient's experience of health and ill-health (Engel, 1977). For example, health, from the patient's viewpoint, has been described as a sense of 'homelike being-in-the-world' (Svenaeus, 2000, p. 174). There has also been strong recognition of the

role of trauma on physical and mental health and a call for trauma-informed approaches to healthcare. However, structured trauma-informed care has not yet been fully implemented in health disciplines (Goddard et al., 2021; Mersky et al., 2019).

Patient-Centred Care

Clinicians' views of legitimate healthcare are shaped by their education, personal experiences and their own health beliefs, which may be different from those of their patients. The diversity of views means that patients are often willing to call on a surprising range of what they see as health-promoting strategies, including self-directed activities such as physical exercise, meditation and CAM. CAM encompasses a broad domain of healing resources and approaches along with their accompanying theories, evidence and beliefs. Some of the most popular CAMs are acupuncture, chiropractic, homoeopathy, Western herbal medicine, naturopathy, massage therapy, hypnotherapy, traditional Chinese medicine (TCM) and osteopathy. Many patients are also enthusiastic about the use of CAM products such as herbal and homoeopathic medicines and nutritional supplements (Armstrong et al., 2011; Reid et al., 2016).

A significant step forward in our understanding of the prevalence of CAM occurred when Eisenberg et al. (1993) published a paper on the use of unconventional medicine in the United States. This paper reported that one-third of adults in the United States had used at least one unconventional therapy in the previous year, bringing into sharp focus 'one of the most important health consumer trends of the 20th century'(Andrews, 2004, p. 226). Similar growth in CAM use has been observed in other developed countries (Dehghan et al., 2022; Kemppainen et al., 2018). For example, in 2020 it was estimated that 75% of Australians used at least one complementary medicine in the past year, one-third of those to manage a chronic condition (Complementary Medicines Australia, 2020). It is also known that consumers often use CAM in conjunction with other health-promoting strategies, yet most patients do not tell their medical doctors (Ge et al., 2013; Grace et al., 2018; Kelak et al., 2018). Some studies have reported that fewer than 10% of women ask their doctor's advice about using CAM during pregnancy (Forster et al.,

2006; Holst et al., 2009; Hughes et al., 2018). Failure to disclose the totality of their healthcare to their health practitioners could be detrimental to patients who may be ill-informed about safety risks associated with combining some herbal medicines and prescribed drugs. *Hypericum perforatum* (St. John's wort), for example, has been shown to reduce pharmaceutical effectiveness in a range of different drug classes (Nicolusi et al., 2019). A patient taking warfarin is at risk of increased bleeding if they are also taking gingko biloba and a patient on hypoglycaemic therapy who takes Korean ginseng (*Panax ginseng*) is at risk of inadvertently altering their blood glucose levels (Harris et al., 2015).

Given that such a large proportion of the population in Western countries uses CAM (National Center for Health Statistics, 2023), it is important that allopathic medical practitioners have some understanding of all the health measures taken up by their patients. Even if the medical practitioners are opposed to CAM, they need to be conversant with issues associated with the combination of CAM and allopathic medicine (von Conrady and Bonney, 2017). Beyond this, all clinicians need to find and use anything and everything that can reasonably be expected to help their patients achieve optimal health (Saper, 2016), which may include CAM. Person-centred care demands that clinicians focus on the patient, on the patient–practitioner relationship and on what works best for a particular patient at a particular time. Such a focus renders applying labels like 'allopathic medicine' and 'CAM' irrelevant:

> *Ultimately, medicine has a single aim: to relieve human suffering. When measured against this benchmark, different therapies can be seen as either effective or ineffective rather than 'orthodox' or 'unorthodox'. No single professional group has ownership of health, and the best healthcare requires a multidisciplinary approach.*
> **(Cohen, 2004, p. 646)**

Person-centred care also requires doctors to acknowledge and work with their patients' preferences for healthcare. As patients gain greater knowledge of, and agency in, managing their healthcare, it is important to work with what patients know and want. Moreover, being aware of CAM approaches can give clinicians new ways of thinking through clinical problems.

ALTERNATIVE WAYS OF THINKING THROUGH CLINICAL PROBLEMS

Practising person-centred care means taking patients' use of CAM into account, valuing their healthcare choices and being informed about them. This could mean that clinicians may have to learn different ways of thinking through clinical problems based on CAM or collaborating with CAM practitioners in various ways.

The dominant model of clinical reasoning in allopathic medicine is based on a technical rational approach that is grounded in biomedical science, despite claims of the move to a more biopsychosocial model. The current dominance of evidence-based medicine is a good example of this technical rational approach. However, Sackett et al. (2000), pioneers of evidence-based medicine, made it clear that good clinical decision making required the integration of the best available evidence together with the expertise and experience of the practitioner and the wishes and values of the patient. If the patient is a passionate believer in the benefits of CAM, this needs to be part of the clinical decision making that occurs. Because the technical rational approach has a poor vocabulary for articulating both the personal experience of clinicians and the wishes and value systems of patients, these aspects of clinical decision making are often overlooked. This is a major reason for integrating the humanities and social sciences into the curriculum of many health professions. These disciplines have vocabularies and discourses that can enable health professions to think through these wider aspects of healthcare. In the same way, it can be argued that CAM approaches also open up our thinking about what our patients want, need and value so that we can adopt more than one perspective in our attempts to understand and help them. The concept of evidence-informed decision making is relevant here. It recognizes evidence from both scientific studies and practitioner experience and focusses on the mechanisms or processes for implementing evidence-based medicine in clinical practice (Kumah et al., 2022). It draws on the scientific principles of 'proof, reliability and ethical standards' and on evidence based on practitioners' experiences of finding solutions to complex problems (Alla and Joss, 2021). By so doing, the risk of lack of objectivity or of focussing only on evidence that confirms our beliefs is reduced and the quality of care diminished.

In Western medicine, biomedical and/or biopsychosocial practice models predominate, demonstrating the primacy granted to biomedical evidence. By contrast, CAM practitioners draw on a range of different practice models. For example, in homoeopathy most practitioners identify spiritual and energetic dimensions in a meta-physical model of diagnosis and treatment. TCM interprets channels of energy or life force (Qi) as they traverse the body in 12 meridians. The underlying concepts of TCM are illustrated in Box 32.1.

Other CAM practices have produced distinctive models of practice to assess and treat their patients. Australian osteopaths and naturopaths, for example, tend to see patients with complex problems who do not easily fit conventional disease patterns (Grace and Orrock, 2015; Orrock, 2009). Such practitioners have had to be inventive and willing to embrace a wide range of aetiological and treatment possibilities. For example, in osteopathy, patients are initially assessed for red flags (indicators or serious underlying pathology), but if a patient is deemed suitable for osteopathic care, attempts are made to make sense of the patient information by considering a range of practice models. Subjective information collected from patients and objective data from tests and examinations are considered in a context of connected functioning body systems, including biomechanical, biopsychosocial, energy expenditure, neurological, nutritional and respiratory/circulatory (Table 32.1). It is worth noting that osteopathic medicine is accepted as mainstream healthcare practice in some countries such as the United States. Most doctors of osteopathic medicine in the United States practise in primary care, whereas residents from allopathic medical schools often go into specialties (American Medical Association, 2023).

Another CAM approach is that of energetic or vibrational medicine that takes account of critical events in the patient's life, reasoning that emotional trauma may affect the patient's physical health. An 'energetic healer' described her diagnostic process in the following example:

> A patient came in. She had had ulcerative colitis for 10 years. She was 26. It started at 16. She had medical treatment, but it was getting worse, not responding. Before it started, she was fine. I said, 'What happened at 16?' She broke down crying and she told me the whole story. Her grandmother was a control freak, commanding the whole household, having arguments with everyone. And she said, 'I had a big argument with my grandmother one night and the next day my grandmother committed suicide'. So she took all the guilt. Guilt affects the large intestine. I used psychotherapy because that's the quickest way to deal with this and then we did acupuncture. Ten years of treatment and nobody had asked her what happened at the time her troubles started. Nobody checked why she had the problem. They were just treating the symptoms.
>
> *(CAM practitioner)*

Bortoft (2012) refers to *diversity in unity* to emphasize the multiplicity of parts that underpins a holistic view of the world. CAM approaches offer a way to be holistic and at the same time make the most of diverse approaches.

BOX 32.1
UNDERLYING CONCEPTS OF TRADITIONAL CHINESE MEDICINE

- The human body is a miniature version of the larger, surrounding universe.
- Harmony between two opposing yet complementary forces, called yin and yang, supports health and disease results from an imbalance between these forces.
- Five elements – fire, earth, wood, metal and water – symbolically represent all phenomena, including the stages of human life, and explain the functioning of the body and how it changes during disease.
- Qi, a vital energy that flows through the body, performs multiple functions in maintaining health.

(From National Center for Complementary and Integrative Health, 2013. Traditional Chinese medicine: In depth. US Department of Health and Human Services.)

TABLE 32.1	
Diagnostic Models Used in Osteopathic Medicine	
Biomedical	Consideration of signs and symptoms in the context of defined diseases and a need for referral for further medical assessment and management (red flags). This is similar to any primary care practitioner.
Biomechanical	Assessment of the health of the musculoskeletal system, including how the structure (posture) and function are integrated. This is similar to other manual medicine practices and is primarily a mechanical/orthopaedic approach.
Biopsychosocial	Consideration of the psychosocial factors influencing the patient's health, including relational, occupational and financial, and the need for multidisciplinary care. (Mainstream allopathic medicine is now starting to adopt a more biopsychosocial position.)
Energy expenditure	Assessment of whether the patient has optimal energy utilization and consideration of issues that may affect the healing process (e.g. relatively minor mechanical or immune dysfunctions).
Neurological	Assessment of function in the central, peripheral and autonomic nervous systems and the relationship of those systems to all tissues of the body.
Nutritional	Foundational dietary analysis for signs of deficiency or suboptimal nutritional status.
Respiratory/circulatory	Examination of the respiratory mechanism, ensuring that the function of breathing is optimal. Assessment of all tissues of the body for full blood supply and drainage. Assessment of the structural and functional relationship between the two systems.

(From Kuchera and Kuchera, 1994.)

INTEGRATING ALTERNATIVE WAYS OF THINKING WITH MAINSTREAM ALLOPATHIC MEDICINE

Fundamental differences between the underlying philosophies of allopathic medicine and CAM are cited by many as the main barrier to their integration (Mann et al., 2004; Sharp et al., 2018). As described earlier, these differences have been characterized as the biomedical approach of allopathic medicine compared with the more biocultural approach of CAM, or the focus on eliminating the disease-producing agents in allopathic medicine compared with the focus on encouraging the innate ability of the human body to restore itself to health in CAM (Capra, 1983). If one adopts a strictly allopathic pathological focus, then all CAM approaches are likely to be dismissed as unsound and unscientific (Valles, 2020). However, there are now attempts to reconcile CAM approaches with allopathic medicine, evident strongly in the integrative medicine movement that is expanding globally (Seetharaman et al., 2021).

MODELS OF INTEGRATION

Three different relationships between allopathic medicine and CAM have been described: co-existent, co-operative and integrative (Lim et al., 2017) (Fig. 32.1).

Co-existent/Parallel

In the co-existent model, both medical systems work alongside one another with mutual respect, but with little or no interaction. Given the unbridgeable epistemological (i.e. knowledge determination) differences that are sometimes described between CAM and allopathic medicine, this model of parallel systems seems realistic and achievable even for the allopathic practitioners who are opposed to CAM (Lewith and Bensoussan, 2004). Practitioners independently discuss clinical decisions with their patients.

Co-operative

This model refers to the selective incorporation of CAM into allopathic medicine. The most common practice model is one in which allopathic medical practitioners act as primary contact clinicians (with subsequent referral to other providers) (Grace and Higgs, 2010a; Lim et al., 2017). Practitioners make their own clinical decisions but team members may communicate and share patient records. In this model, allopathic medical practitioners tend to be responsible for diagnosis and coordination of healthcare plans. The Australian Government's Chronic Disease Management Plans, for instance, recognize this model in its subsidizing of chiropractic, osteopathy, podiatry, psychology and other allied health treatments for patients with chronic health conditions. Subsidies are

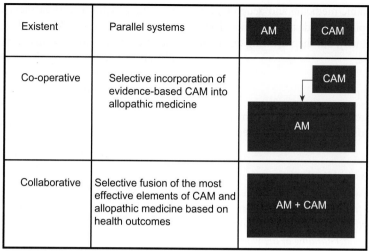

Fig. 32.1 ▪ Models of integration. *AM*, Allopathic medicine; *CAM*, complementary and alternative medicine; *IM*, integrative medicine.

available only if the services are part of enhanced care plans and are supervised by allopathic medical practitioners (Australian Government Services Australia, 2022).

Integrative

In this fully collaborative model, the ideal model described by Lewith and Bensoussan (2004), there is selective fusion of the most effective elements of CAM and allopathic medicine for the optimal health outcomes for patients. Both biomedical evidence and clinical effectiveness are valued. CAM and allopathic practitioners become co-workers with equal input and standing. Decision making is shared and based on consensus of the patient and the healthcare team.

INTEGRATED CLINICAL REASONING

The models of integration of CAM and Western medicine described earlier for clinical practice correspond to models of clinical reasoning integration. According to Lim et al. (2017), integration patterns are likely to be ad hoc and dependent on the particular case. In the co-existent model, clinical decisions are made independently by practitioners and the integration of diagnostic and treatment advice may fall to the patient, particularly if they have chosen not to disclose their use of CAM to their allopathic practitioner (Foley et al., 2019). In the co-operative model practitioners' independent clinical decisions may be discussed with

the patient by a case manager. The fully integrated model involves advice from all members of the healthcare team and takes patients' preferences into account.

There is increasing recognition that some allopathic clinicians readily embrace CAM and have been extensively educated in both allopathic and CAM approaches (Loftus, 2009). Such practitioners can offer insights into how they integrate these approaches in their clinical reasoning. There is a clear preference for using the strengths of allopathic medicine to begin with. The usual practice is to follow standard allopathic protocols with all patients first and ensure there is no pathology (red flags) that should be dealt with by conventional means. If there are no red flags (Loftus, 2009) or if allopathic medicine fails, as it can do, especially in some chronic conditions such as chronic pain, these clinicians may resort to a CAM approach. For example, one allopathic doctor who had extensive training and experience of acupuncture spoke in terms of taking one thinking hat off and putting on another (S. Loftus, 2006, personal communication). This same doctor also related that while undergoing training in acupuncture, he and his medical colleagues would regularly try to 'translate' what they were seeing and doing in the acupuncture clinic into allopathic terms. After several months of trying this, they eventually gave up and concluded that this translation was not realistic. The two ways of conceptualizing the body, health and disease were essentially incompatible. However, this did not dissuade these clinicians from using both allopathic medicine and acupuncture. The two forms are happily used side by side, prioritizing allopathic medicine initially, but then drawing on either approach as appropriate.

REFLECTION POINT

Reflection on clinical reasoning of a general medical practitioner who practises both allopathic medicine and homeopathy:

> I'm certainly aware of the idea that certain facts, certain concepts derive from homoeopathic ideas and certain others derive from what is common mainstream medical thinking. Within my mind these are contained within one sphere of understanding of the world. It's not so much a matter of jumping from one to the other as it is trying to appreciate what that globe actually is from any particular vantage point I happen to be looking at it from and then comparing in my mind which pathways are going to be most useful at that point in time. Some of the more difficult decisions are to do with if I follow one route, if I give this patient an antibiotic now, how will that influence the information gathering that I need to prescribe a homoeopathic remedy that I've been trying to offer for some time? I'm trying to project outcomes based on different interventions and what's going to be most useful for the patient using different possible ways of going about it and whether it's reasonable, perhaps, to use both systems of medicine at the same time. One has to think about a number of factors in making that decision, whether the patient's going to be in close contact with you, how that influences what the best thing to do is. It's rare that the different interventions open to me are in direct competition. It's more a matter of trying to decide what's going to be most useful at any point in time.

Readers: What do you think of these arguments and approaches?

An important challenge facing clinicians in the future is to explore ways in which allopathic medicine and CAM might become integrated in a rigorous manner that respects the strengths of both without jeopardizing the rational foundations of either. We live in a postmodern world and perhaps the integration of CAM is part of what it means to have postmodern healthcare. Modernism is the view, now largely discredited, that there is only one (scientific) way to view anything. This view is exemplified in healthcare by the dominance of biomedical allopathic medicine. A postmodern view accepts that there can be multiple perspectives on anything. The inadequacies of allopathic medicine are evident in the dissatisfaction that some people experience with conventional healthcare in general and its failure to provide satisfactory solutions to chronic conditions in particular (Foley and Steel, 2017; Grace and Higgs, 2010b; Loftus, 2009). This is one of the main reasons why so many people turn to CAM (Armstrong et al., 2011; Mbizo et al., 2018). The other main reason, of course, is that patients want to actively pursue a wellness agenda in their healthcare and lifestyles. Therefore, we need to find new ways of conceptualizing and carrying out the care we provide. As healthcare professionals we also need to admit that much of what we know is empirical and based on our experience of practice, in addition to what we can learn from a formal evidence base.

One step that has been taken in this direction is the development of practice-based evidence. Clinicians can develop new knowledge from their experience of practice itself. There is a realization that the balance between theory and practice is not all one way (that is, from theory to practice) but can be bidirectional. This raises the important questions of how evidence from practice can be theorized, how it is theorized in different systems of thought, and how these systems of thought can inform each other. We can take some lessons from the literature on communities of practice. There are well-known cases where people have had the courage and insight to be boundary crossers between different communities of practice. For example, Schrödinger (1947) wrote a book that brought together physicists and biologists, two groups who previously had little in common. Schrödinger was able to persuade the two groups that they did in fact have a great deal in common and his work is now seen as the start of a new and very successful community of practice, that of molecular biology. Perhaps what we need now are people who are well informed about allopathic medicine and CAM and who can explore ways to bridge the gaps between them. Even if no new community of practice is formed, there is always the

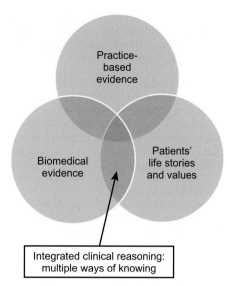

Fig. 32.2 ■ Integrated clinical reasoning.

chance of cross-fertilization of ideas to the benefit of all concerned. The integrated clinical reasoning they undertake will emphasize holism and multiple ways of thinking and knowing, together with what the patient values and brings to the clinical encounter (Fig. 32.2 and Case Study 32.1).

Before integrated clinical reasoning can be widely taken up in clinical practice, it must first be introduced into health professional education, when students are developing their clinical reasoning capabilities. Solutions to 'wicked' clinical problems that require different ways of thinking need to be promoted through case analyses, with role models in communities of practice, and enhanced through work with interprofessional teams and collaborative practice. Most complementary medicine practitioners are primary care practitioners who are available to participate in these teams (Grace, 2012). Their practices are fundamentally holistic in that they draw on the many contexts in which individual health is conceived to assess and treat health conditions and promote health. Their practice wisdom can contribute to primary care that strives to incorporate biopsychosocial and trauma-informed approaches to healthcare. Integrated clinical reasoning that attempts to be evidence-informed, to understand the many contexts of healthcare, and different ways of thinking and knowing, may provide safe and effective healthcare that aligns with what patients want and value.

CASE STUDY 32.1

Multiple Ways of Thinking and Knowing: Cross-Fertilization of Ideas

One homeopathic researcher (and doctor of internal medicine) in a Glasgow teaching hospital, spent a year 'proving' himself to his colleagues. By conducting a poll about what kinds of evidence his colleagues would need to believe that homeopathy is effective, he discovered that more of them would be convinced by 'clinical experience and audit' (grand rounds) than by theoretical adequacy, clinical trials, laboratory evidence or patient reports. So he presented himself at grand rounds armed with video tapes of his successful homeopathic treatment of a man who had intractable cluster headaches for over 3 years (who many of these same colleagues had tried in vain to treat). Over the next few months, his referrals increased dramatically.
(Bayley, 1993, pp. 143–144)

Readers, does this show that homeopaths are not the only ones in medicine whose epistemological foundations are empirical?

SUMMARY

In this chapter, we have explored a number of arguments:

- The attraction of CAM to health consumers has been attributed to its focus on holistic approaches to healthcare compared to the conventional pathological account of diseases found in allopathic medicine. CAM focusses more on a patient's sense of 'dis-ease'.
- CAM offers alternative ways of clinical reasoning and thinking through clinical problems.
- Despite traditional epistemological differences, various collaborations between allopathic medicine and CAM have been developed in many Western countries. Such collaborations provide opportunities to create new practice knowledge, out of which can arise new practice epistemologies based on understanding of how this practice knowledge arises, is used and is developed. Individual clinicians within these collaborations both acquire practice knowledge and contribute to it.
- A distinctive characteristic of the clinical reasoning and practice epistemology of integrative

medicine is the emphasis on holism and multiple ways of thinking and knowing, together with what the patient values and brings to the clinical encounter.

REFERENCES

Alla, K., Joss, N., 2021. What is an evidence-informed approach to practice and why is it important? Australian Institute of Family Studies. Retrieved June 18 from https://aifs.gov.au/resources/short-articles/what-evidence-informed-approach-practice-and-why-it-important.

American Medical Association., 2023. DO vs MD: How much does the medical school degree type matter? American Medical Association. Retrieved June 17 from https://www.ama-assn.org/medical-students/preparing-medical-school/do-vs-md-how-much-does-medical-school-degree-type-matter.

Andrews, G.J., 2004. Sharing the spirit of the policy agenda? Private complementary therapists' attitudes towards practising in the British NHS. Complementary Therapies in Nursing & Midwifery 10, 217–228.

Armstrong, A.R., Thiebaut, S.P., Brown, L.J., 2011. Australian adults use complementary and alternative medicine in the treatment of chronic illness: A national study. Australian and New Zealand Journal of Public Health 35 (4), 384–390.

Australian Government Services Australia, 2022. Chronic disease GP management plans and team care. Australian Government Services Australia Retrieved January 29 from https://www.servicesaustralia.gov.au/chronic-disease-gp-management-plans-and-team-care-arrangements?context=20

Bayley, C., 1993. Homeopathy. Journal of Medical Philosophy 18 (2), 129–145. https://doi.org/10.1093/jmp/18.2.129

Bortoft, H., 2012. Taking appearance seriously: The dynamic way of seeing in Goethe and European thought. Floris Books.

Capra, F., 1983. Turning Point. Harper Collins.

Cohen, M.M., 2004. CAM practitioners and "regular" doctors: Is integration possible? Medical Journal of Australia 180 (12), 645–646.

Complementary Medicines Australia, 2020. Australia's complementary medicines: Industry audit & trends 2020. https://www.cmaustralia.org.au/resources/CMA-industry-presentation-2020.pdf.

Dehghan, M., Ghanbari, A., Heidari, F.G., Shahrbabaki, P.M., Zakeri, M.A., 2022. Use of complementary and alternative medicine in general population during COVID-19 outbreak: A survey in Iran. J Integr Med 20 (1), 45–51. https://doi.org/10.1016/j.joim.2021.11.004

Eisenberg, D.M., Kessler, R.C., Foster, C., Norlock, F.E., Calkins, D.R., Delbanco, T.L., 1993. Unconventional medicine in the United States: Prevalence, costs and pattern use. New England Journal of Medicine 328, 246–252.

Engel, G.L., 1977. The need for a new medical model: A challenge for biomedicine. Science 196 (4286), 129–136. https://doi.org/10.1126/science.847460

Farre, A., Rapley, T., 2017. The new old (and old new) medical model: Four decades navigating the biomedical and psychosocial understandings of health and illness. Healthcare 5 (4), 88. https://doi.org/10.3390/healthcare5040088

Foley, H., Steel, A., 2017. The nexus between patient-centred care and complementary medicine: Allies in the era of chronic disease? Journal of Alternative & Complementary Medicine 23 (3), 158–163. https://doi.org/10.1089/acm.2016.0386

Foley, H., Steel, A., Cramer, H., Wardle, J., Adams, J., 2019. Disclosure of complementary medicine use to medical providers: A systematic review and meta-analysis. Scientific Reports 9, 1573. https://doi.org/10.1038/s41598-018-38279-8

Forster, D., Denning, A., Wills, G., Bolger, M., McCarthy, E., 2006. Herbal medicine use during pregnancy in a group of Australian women. BMC Pregnancy Childbirth 6, 21. https://doi.org/10.1186/1471-2393-6-21

Foucault, M., 1994. The birth of the clinic: An archaeology of medical perception. Vintage.

Franzel, B., Schwiegershausen, M., Heusser, P., Berger, B., 2013. Individualised medicine from the perspectives of patients using complementary therapies: A meta-ethnography approach. BMC Complementary & Alternative Medicine 13, 124. https://doi.org/10.1186/1472-6882-13-124

Ge, J., Fishman, J., Vapiwala, N., Li, S., Desai, K., Xie, S., et al., 2013. Patient-physician communication about complementary and alternative medicine in a radiation oncology setting. International Journal of Radiation Oncology*Biology*Physics 85 (1), e1–e6. https://doi.org/10.1016/j.ijrobp.2012.08.018

Goddard, A., Jones, R.W., Esposito, D., Janicek, E., 2021. Trauma informed education in nursing: A call for action. Nurse Education Today 101, 104880. https://doi.org/10.1016/j.nedt.2021.104880

Grace, S., 2012. CAM practitioners in the Australian workforce: An underutilised resource. BMC Complementary and Alternative Medicine 12, 205.

Grace, S., Bradbury, J., Avila, C., 2018. 'The healthcare system is not designed around my needs': How healthcare consumers self-integrate conventional and complementary healthcare services. Complement Ther Clin Pract 32, 151–156. https://doi.org/10.1016/j.ctcp.2018.06.009

Grace, S., Higgs, J., 2010a. Interprofessional collaborations in integrative medicine. Journal of Alternative & Complementary Medicine 16 (11), 1185–1190.

Grace, S., Higgs, J., 2010b. Practitioner-client relationships in integrative medicine clinics in Australia: A contemporary social phenomenon. Complementary Therapies in Medicine 18 (1), 8–12.

Grace, S., Orrock, P., 2015. Criticality in osteopathic medicine. In: Davies, M., Barnett, R. (Eds.), The Palgrave handbook of critical thinking. Palgrave Macmillan.

Harris, T., Grace, S., Eddey, S., 2015. Adverse events from complementary therapies: An update from the natural therapies workforce survey. Part 2. Journal of the Australian Traditional Medicine Society 21, 162–167.

Hawk, C., 2005. When worldviews collide: Maintaining a vitalistic perspective in chiropractic in the postmodern era. Journal of Chiropractic Humanities 12 (12), 2–7.

Hayes, C., 2007. Back pain: New paradigms in community care. Sydney General Practitioner Conference and Exhibition Primary Care, Sydney Showground, Olympic Park.

Holst, L., Wright, D., Nordeng, H., Haavik, S., 2009. Use of herbal preparations during pregnancy: Focus group discussion among expectant mothers attending a hospital antenatal clinic in Norwich, UK. Complement Ther Clin Pract 15, 225–229. https://doi.org/10.1016/j.ctcp.2009.04.001

Hughes, C.M., Liddle, S.D., Sinclair, M., McCullough, J.E.M., 2018. The use of complementary and alternative medicine (CAM) for pregnancy related low back and/or pelvic girdle pain: An online survey. Complement Ther Clin Pract 31, 379–383. https://doi.org/10.1016/j.ctcp.2018.01.015

Kelak, J.A., Cheah, W.L., Safii, R., 2018. Patient's decision to disclose the use of traditional and complementary medicine to medical doctors: A descriptive phenomenology study. Evidence-Based Complementary & Alternative Medicine 2018, 4735234. https://doi.org/10.1155/2018/4735234

Kemppainen, L.M., Kemppainen, T.T., Reippainen, J.A., Salmenniemi, S.T., Vuolanto, P.H., 2018. Use of complementary and alternative medicine in Europe: Health-related and sociodemographic determinants. Scandinavian Journal of Public Health 46, 448–455. https://doi.org/10.1177/1403494817733869

Kuchera, W.A., Kuchera, M.L., 1994. Osteopathic Principles in Practice. Columbus: Greyden Press. ISBN 1570741514, 9781570741517.

Kumah, E.A., McSherry, R., Bettany-Saltikov, J., van Schaik, P., 2022. Evidence-informed practice: Simplifying and applying the concept for nursing students and academics. British Journal of Nursing 31 (6), 322–330. https://doi.org/10.12968/bjon.2022.31.6.322

Lewith, G., Bensoussan, A., 2004. Complementary and alternative medicine - With a difference. Medical Journal of Australia 180 (11), 585–586.

Lim, E.J., Vardy, J.L., Oh, B.S., Dhillon, H.M., 2017. A scoping review on models of integrative medicine: What is known from the existing literature? Journal of Alternative & Complementary Medicine 23 (1), 8–17. https://doi.org/10.1089/acm.2016.0263

Loftus, S., 2009. Language in clinical reasoning: Learning and using the language of collective clinical decision making [The University of Sydney]. Sydney. http://ses.library.usyd.edu.au/handle/2123/1165

Mann, J., D., Gaylord, S.A., Norton, S.K., 2004. Integrating complementary & alternative therapies with conventional care: Educational resources for health professionals. University of North Carolina.

Mbizo, J., Okafor, A., Sutton, M.A., Leyva, B., Stone, L.M., Olaku, O., 2018. Complementary and alternative medicine use among persons with multiple chronic conditions: Results from the 2012 National Health Interview Survey. BMC Complementary & Alternative Medicine 18, 281. https://doi.org/10.1186/s12906-018-2342-2

Mersky, J.P., Topitzes, J., Britz, L., 2019. Promoting evidence-based, trauma-informed social work practice. Journal of Social Work Education 55, 645–657. https://doi.org/10.1080/10437797.2019.1627261

National Center for Health Statistics, 2023. Statistics on complementary and integrative health approaches. National Center for Complementary and Integrative Health. Retrieved June 17 from https://www.nccih.nih.gov/research/statistics-on-complementary-and-integrative-health-approaches.

Nicolusi, S., Drewe, J., Butterweck, V., Meyer zu Schwabedissen, H.E., 2019. Clinical relevance of St John's wort drug interactions revisited. British Journal of Pharmacology 177 (6), 1212–1226. https://doi.org/10.1111/bph.14936

Orrock, P., 2009. Profile of members of the Australian Osteopathic Association: Part 2 - The patients. Int J Osteopath Med 12 (4), 128–139. https://doi.org/10.1016/j.ijosm.2009.06.001

Reeve, J., 2010. Interpretive medicine: Supporting generalism in a changing primary care world (Occasional paper 88, Issue. R. C. o. G. Practitioners). https://www.ncbi.nlm.nih.gov/pmc/articles/PMC3259801/pdf/OP88_231111.pdf.

Reid, R., Steel, A., Wardle, J., Trubody, A., Adams, J., 2016. Complementary medicine use by the Australian population: A critical mixed methods studies systematic review of utilisation, perceptions and factors associated with use. BMC Complementary & Alternative Medicine 16, 176. https://doi.org/10.1186/s12906-016-1143-8

Sackett, D., Straus, S., Richardson, W., Rosenberg, W., Haynes, R., 2000. Evidence-based medicine: How to practice and teach EBM. Churchill Livingstone.

Saper, R., 2016. Integrative medicine and health disparities. Global Advances in Health and Medicine 5, 5–8. https://doi.org/10.7453/gahmj.2015.133

Schrödinger, E.C., 1947. What is life? The physical aspect of the living cell. Cambridge University Press.

Seetharaman, M., Krishnan, G., Schneider, R.H., 2021. The frontiers of medicine: Frontiers in integrative health and medicine. Medicina 57, 1303. https://doi.org/10.3390/medicina57121303

Sharp, D., Lorenc, A., Feder, G., Little, P., Hollinghurst, S., Mercer, S., et al., 2018. 'Trying to put a square peg into a round hole': A qualitative study of healthcare professionals' views of integrative complementary medicine into primary care for musculoskeletal and mental health comorbidity. BMC Complementary and Alternative Medicine 18, 290. https://doi.org/10.1186/s12906-018-2349-8

Svenaeus, F., 2000. The hermeneutics of medicine and the phenomenology of health: Steps towards a philosophy of medical practice. Kluwer Academic.

Tangkiatkumjai, M., Boardman, H., Walker, D.-M., 2020. Potential factors that influence usage of complementary and alternative medicine worldview: A systematic review. BMC Complement Med Ther 20, 363. https://doi.org/10.1186/s12906-020-03157-2

Uher, I., Cholewa, J., Kunicki, M., Svedova, M., Cimolakova, I., Kchelova, Z., et al., 2020. Allopathic and naturopathic medicine and their object consideration of congruent pursuit. Evidence-Based Complementary & Alternative Medicine 2020, 7525713. https://doi.org/10.1155/2020/7525713

Valles, S., 2020. Philosophy of biomedicine. Stanford Encyclopedia of Philosophy. Retrieved 3 January 2022, from https://plato.stanford.edu/entries/biomedicine/.

von Conrady, D.M., Bonney, A., 2017. Patterns of complementary and alternative medicine use and health literacy in general practice patients in urban and regional Australia. Australian Family Physician 46 (5), 315–320.

PART 5 Pedagogy

This closing section of the book brings together the necessary bridges and synergistic connections that are critical to the development of learners' clinical reasoning (CR) abilities. While it may appear that there are a variety of topics in Part 5 (teaching, learning, clinical education, assessment, curriculum development, leadership and research), these components work synergistically and are essential to taking a holistic view of the pedagogy of CR.

Part 5 provides practical strategies for teaching CR that apply across health professions. Strategies such as focussing on deliberate practice, using higher-order questioning, highlighting the importance of evidence-based practice, learning to use 'think-alouds', deconstructing critical events and reflecting on cognitive biases as teaching tools for fostering learners' lifelong critical thinking skills. We also emphasize that we should establish explicit educational outcome goals for developing adaptive learners who can continue to learn, create knowledge and develop adaptive expertise in making well-reasoned decisions.

Teaching and learning are inseparable, as we do not have evidence of effective teaching without evidence of student learning. Yet, while the evidence for student learning in general comes from assessment, there is no gold standard for assessing whether students have learned CR in particular. No single assessment method can capture the entire process of CR. CR is neither a skill nor an objective activity and there is not one best way of teaching and assessing it. In Part 5, the reader gains a deeper understanding of how current theories addressing both the analytical and nonanalytical processes in CR continually work in conjunction with each other. While there is no perfect measure to assess CR, a less than perfect measure or instrument is preferable to no assessment at all.

CR needs an explicit curriculum structure and a developmental approach for learners. There is no gold standard for curricular design, yet there is an important consideration in creating a roadmap for a CR curriculum that includes broad educational goals and measurable objectives. In Part 5, we have a robust example of CR curriculum development using Kern's six-step model that provides both theoretical and practice considerations for curriculum design. Faculty leaders (or champions) are essential to facilitating the achievement of CR learning outcomes. In Part 5, we also share the perspective and journey of a faculty leader (administrator), highlighting necessary organizational planning for CR, along with considerations for enabling a CR process that is enacted in clinical practice. The connections across teaching, learning and assessment of CR are foundational, but we must always be mindful that learners not only strive to obtain graduate learning outcomes but also ultimately strive to positively impact client outcomes.

The centrality of the development of learners' CR abilities is shared across health professions in addressing the health needs of society. As health professions' education curricula make demands for more content, the need to maintain and enhance learner progression in their development of CR abilities requires leadership and a holistic view of the pedagogy of CR. Research into CR is essential to understanding the processes and conditions for optimal learning and assessment. Learning to research CR is needed and can help inform all aspects of CR – teaching, learning and assessment.

33

TOWARDS A CLINICAL EDUCATION PEDAGOGY FOR DEVELOPING CLINICAL REASONING CAPABILITY

NARELLE PATTON

CHAPTER OUTLINE

CHAPTER AIMS

The aims of this chapter are:

- to examine how healthcare contexts shape students' clinical reasoning capability development during clinical placements
- to apply situated and workplace learning theories to harness rich clinical learning opportunities
- to invite readers to reflect on how their contexts, actions and student dispositions shape clinical reasoning capability development
- to conceptualize clinical reasoning as a complex, dynamic and experiential phenomenon that is embedded in healthcare contexts, embodied in individuals, transformed in action and grounded in an ethical aim to do good for others in unpredictable and challenging situations.

INTRODUCTION

Professional healthcare practices are embedded in practice contexts, embodied in individual practitioner's performances and grounded in an ethical aim to do good for others. Contemporary healthcare settings are undergoing rapid, profound and ubiquitous change (Lehtinen, 2008). Healthcare systems worldwide face increasing demands for accountability in combination with changing patterns of disease and disability, increasing complexity of clients' conditions and expanding locations for health service provision (Patton and Fish, 2016). Clinical reasoning capability, including critical and creative thinking and actions, underpins healthcare professionals' ability to balance these competing demands, to make ethical decisions and to undertake actions for the enhancement of clients' well-being.

Clinical reasoning, core to autonomous and ethical healthcare practice in challenging and dynamic times, is therefore an essential capability to be developed in the next generation of healthcare professionals (Brentnall et al., 2022). To be work ready for a range of dynamic healthcare contexts, graduates need to be equipped to work in a diverse range of settings, including, for example, in teams and online, and to be able to address increasingly complex and chronic healthcare problems (McLaughlin et al., 2019). Consequently, the development of students' clinical reasoning capability is an increasing focus in health professional pre-service education seen by its inclusion as an essential graduate attribute in many health professional programmes and competency in many health professional frameworks (Daniel et al., 2019; Young et al., 2019). However, clinical reasoning capability cannot be developed in academic environments alone because its application is bound to real-life contexts (Croskerry, 2006; Wijbenga et al., 2019). Clinical reasoning is largely developed through students' active engagement in healthcare workplace activities during clinical placements. Therefore, understanding how students learn during clinical placement through engagement with workplace activities is critical to the development of future clinicians who can practise ethically and autonomously while addressing intensifying workplace restraints (Fairbrother et al., 2016). Despite this widely acknowledged importance of clinical reasoning in health education curricula, advancement of pedagogy to develop graduates' capability for clinical reasoning in complex and dynamic healthcare environments is currently limited (Brentnall et al., 2022).

Healthcare professional practices are also inherently human with individual practitioners working to achieve optimum outcomes for people in their unique circumstances. Kemmis and Smith (2008) describe professional practice as morally committed action, informed by theoretical, technical and practical knowledges that constitute traditions in a field. Healthcare professionals are expected to undertake right and considered action to achieve optimum outcomes for people in dynamic and complex circumstances, even if those actions challenge prevailing hegemonic practices. Therefore, turbulent and challenging healthcare contexts require healthcare professionals to have ethical courage, an ability to challenge and change practice respectfully for the better (Jensen and Patton, 2018). Ethical courage and clinical reasoning are inextricably interwoven, with ethical courage dependent on sound clinical reasoning capabilities, including the ability to select optimal actions for the circumstances at hand alongside the courage to undertake selected actions for the good of others. This understanding of the inter-relationship between clinical reasoning and ethical courage illuminates embedded (contextual), embodied (individual and ethical) and transformative (action-oriented) dimensions of clinical reasoning.

This chapter focusses on healthcare students' development of clinical reasoning through clinical practice. In this chapter, clinical reasoning is conceptualized as a complex, dynamic and experiential phenomenon that is embedded in healthcare contexts and practices, embodied in individuals, transformed in action and grounded in an ethical aim to do good with and for others. Clinical reasoning is viewed as a capability that encompasses abilities (critical reasoning skills and practice knowledge) and qualities (ethical courage) that can be used to discern and perform actions in unpredictable and challenging situations.

PEDAGOGICAL UNDERPINNINGS OF CLINICAL EDUCATION

Clinical education is core to the development of healthcare students' professional knowledge, skills and capabilities. The transformative potential of clinical education across a wide range of contexts is well established (Rodger et al., 2008). During clinical placements, students are situated in powerful learning environments that play a critical role in the development of their practice knowledge and skills leading to autonomous healthcare practice (Patton et al., 2018). However, despite the acknowledged centrality of clinical education to healthcare students' preparation for autonomous healthcare practice, there has been little exploration of pedagogical underpinnings of clinical education. Workplaces shape student learning in powerful and significantly different ways to academic environments underscoring the importance of development of specific workplace learning (clinical education) pedagogies (Patton, 2023). Situated and workplace learning theories that acknowledge and harness the significant influence of context alongside student engagement in authentic workplace activities provide a firm foundation for constructing wise clinical education pedagogies that deliberately contribute to clinical reasoning capability development.

Situated learning theory provides a useful way to explore healthcare students' development of clinical reasoning capability during clinical placements. The centrality of environment to learning during clinical education underlines the key contribution of situated learning theories to a better understanding of students' learning during clinical placements (Patton et al., 2013). Lave and Wenger's (1991) situated learning theory outlines a model of workplace learning where learning occurs through opportunities for practice and becoming a full member of a practice community. Lave and Wenger propose that a learner's development of knowledge and skill in practice is a dynamic process realized through a trajectory of increasing levels of participation in workplace activities and communities. This model de-emphasizes notions of mastery and focusses instead on learning resources and opportunities, with learning realized through a novice's gradual movement towards full participation in the community. The contribution of social interaction as part of entering practice communities that embody the development of certain beliefs, behaviours and capabilities has long been acknowledged as an essential part of learning professional healthcare practices (Evans and Rainbird, 2002). More recently, physiotherapy students' development of clinical reasoning capability is identified as occurring through gradually increasing engagement with practical experiences (Wijbenga et al., 2019). Through a focus on workplace resources, relationships and a student trajectory of increasing participation, situated learning theory opens up possibilities for development of distinctive clinical education pedagogies that harness the powerful contributions of workplaces to student learning.

Many contemporary theories of workplace learning are built upon Lave and Wenger's (1991) situated learning theory where the centrality of participation in authentic workplace activities to the quality and quantity of learning undertaken is widely accepted (Boud and Hager, 2012). Workplace learning is a multidimensional phenomenon, which involves complex webs of power, acceptance into a community of practice, and transformation of both learners and practice communities (Patton et al., 2013). Workplaces are often contested spaces with their own hierarchies, relationships and objectives. Therefore, as learning environments, workplaces should be understood as complex negotiations about knowledge use, roles and processes, affordances and engagement (Billet, 2004). During clinical placement, students' status, both as students

and short-term visitors in the workplace, regulates the extent of their participation in workplace activities (Patton, 2018a). As an example, during clinical placements clinical supervisors act as gatekeepers to practise experiences determining the range and amount of client interactions students experience as well as their level of autonomy during those interactions.

Provision of guidance is another significant factor that shapes student learning in workplaces. Learning through participation alone may lead to inappropriate learning with guidance required to make workplace knowledge accessible to students (Boud and Middleton, 2003). As an example, a healthcare student, through observation of a healthcare practitioner alone, may not be able to understand the reasoning processes that underpin that practitioner's actions and may not develop the cognitive processes and knowledge necessary for autonomous clinical reasoning. Whereas clinician explanation of how past experience, cues, heuristics and knowledge guided decision making thereby making tacit cognitive processes explicit can strengthen students' development of clinical reasoning capability. Therefore, key to understanding how students are able to develop clinical reasoning capability in clinical contexts is knowledge of how opportunities for engagement in authentic client activities are made available, the kinds of tasks students are permitted to engage in and the guidance they receive (see Johansson and Boud, 2010).

Development of a full and rich understanding of workplace learning also requires an understanding of how students elect to engage with workplace opportunities (Patton, 2018a). Individuals themselves determine how they engage with and learn through workplace affordances, premised on their values, goals, experiences and brute facts of energy, strength, state of fatigue and emotion (Billett, 2009). For example, under some circumstances, healthcare students may complete placements while continuing to work part-time for financial security, leaving them with less energy to engage with and learn from placement opportunities. Through a focus on the contested nature of workplaces, inclusion of students in authentic workplace activities, provision of guidance and how students elect to engage with learning opportunities, workplace learning theories offer nuanced guidance to the development of distinctive clinical education pedagogies.

Application of situated and workplace learning theories can assist educators to harness the power of clinical education to develop students' practice capabilities. Academics and clinical supervisors are invited to examine critically and potentially to transform their current education practices in light of situated and workplace learning theories. A focus on learners as participants opens up possibilities to enhance clinical education outcomes through examination of how students learn in workplaces, how they are welcomed and accepted in workplaces, invited to undertake meaningful workplace activities, elect to engage in workplace activities and are prepared to participate fully in workplace activities. Identification of a substantial difference between academic and workplace learning environments highlights the criticality of effective student preparation for the significantly different learning that occurs during clinical placements.

REFLECTION POINT

- Academics: Which healthcare workplace factors could be interwoven into curricula to prepare students more authentically for the realities of clinical reasoning in healthcare contexts?
- Clinical educators: What is the impact of your healthcare setting and the guidance you provide on students' development of clinical reasoning capability?

HEALTHCARE AND EDUCATION FORCES SHAPING THE NATURE OF CLINICAL PLACEMENTS

Clinical placements, shaped by healthcare and education demands, are being undertaken in a wider range of health service environments. Health professional shortages, addressed through increasing numbers of health professional programmes and student admissions, have significantly increased demand for clinical placement provision and consequently have led to a shortage of clinical placements (Ardern, 2022). This shortage has generated development of a range of innovative clinical placement experiences including service learning and telehealth placements. In addition, placement shortages have seen many programmes replace clinical placements with simulated activities for early year students with many students not experiencing clinical placements

until the final years of their programmes. The nature of the influence of this wider range of clinical placement contexts needs to be considered in the development of students' clinical reasoning capability.

Service-learning placements are growing in popularity (Patrick et al., 2019) and provide a salient example of clinical placements undertaken in a broad range of contexts. Health service-learning placements can incorporate a variety of elements including collaborative learning, remote supervision, project placements and role-emerging placements across a range of settings such as primary schools, specialist schools, kindergarten networks and homelessness community organizations (Salter et al., 2020). Service-learning placements in nontraditional settings (those outside health services) require academics and placement supervisors to consider how these settings shape students' development of clinical reasoning capability and tailor student preparation and support accordingly.

The COVID-19 pandemic provoked widespread disruption within healthcare organizations and higher education institutions, significantly impacting students and placements (Carolan et al., 2020). The COVID-19 disruption provides another example of how external influences shape students' clinical placements and consequently their clinical learning. The provision of physical healthcare services adapted with many moving away from face-to-face to telehealth appointments (Haines and Berney, 2020). These emergent telehealth modalities became a critical strategy to manage both client services and clinical placement requirements (Nahon et al., 2021). As a consequence of border restrictions, quarantine, health concerns and placement shortages, healthcare students faced uncertainty around placement completion with many experiencing a range of mental health issues (Carolan et al., 2020). Consideration of how COVID-19 affected students' ability to engage with clinical learning opportunities across a range of contexts is required to maximize their clinical learning including development of clinical reasoning capability.

In response to external demands including health professional and placement shortages and the COVID-19 pandemic, a broader range of clinical placements undertaken in varying contexts have been developed and implemented including a proliferation of service learning and project placements outside traditional health service contexts. Deliberate consideration of how this range of contexts combined with students' ability to engage with learning opportunities shape students' development of clinical reasoning capability is required to ensure student learning is maximized in dynamic and difficult times.

CONTEXTUAL INFLUENCES ON CLINICAL REASONING CAPABILITY DEVELOPMENT

Healthcare practices are always situated and inexplicably interwoven with the context within which they occur and therefore must be considered within their contexts (Patton and Higgs, 2018). The understanding that learning is inextricably bound to context is not new. Dewey (1916) described the pervasive and often tacit influence of environment on student learning and identified deliberate construction of appropriate learning environments as a key educator role. Although clinical environments provide powerful and authentic learning contexts for students, our ability to leverage this power is currently hindered by limited exploration of specific clinical education pedagogies underpinned by workplace learning theories. Fine-grained examination of healthcare services as both workplaces and educational contexts is a first step towards opening up pedagogical possibilities to enhance development of students' clinical reasoning capabilities during clinical placements.

Clinical environments have a strong, pervasive and often tacit influence on students' clinical learning and capability development (Patton, 2018b). Each healthcare workplace represents a unique, dynamic, complex (Edwards and Nicholl, 2006) and contested space with its own physical architectures, systems, hierarchies and relationships that are central to healthcare delivery and consequently student learning. Within individual healthcare workplaces, physical (e.g. the level of resource provision), relational (e.g. acceptance), workplace culture (e.g. workplace hierarchies) and temporal (e.g. the fast-paced nature of clinical workplaces) factors have a pervasive and significant influence on student learning during clinical placements.

Physical conditions in health services shape healthcare delivery by creating conditions that enable or constrain certain types of practice (Kemmis and Grootenboer, 2008). Workplace resources in the form of specific equipment and technologies as well as the way workplaces are laid out influence the way practices are enacted and, consequently, pedagogical possibilities for learning (Patton, 2018b). Well-resourced clinical workplaces can facilitate students' ability to formulate and implement a wide range of treatment interventions while less well-resourced clinical workplaces can open up opportunities for students to develop more creative treatment approaches to achieve desired outcomes.

Relational aspects of workplaces are integral, yet often taken for granted, as this workplace dimension powerfully shapes workplace activities and consequently student learning (Markauskaite and Patton, 2019). In clinical workplaces, relational aspects such as a sense of welcome and formation of positive relationships with a range of health service staff can foster students' ability and confidence to ask questions and access practice experiences (Patton, 2018b). A clinical supervisor's workload can also affect how much time supervisors have for supervision activities such as observing student practice, providing feedback and answering questions. As a consequence of high supervisor workload, students can be restricted from engaging in unsupervised clinical practice and instead experience prolonged periods of observation and involvement in nonclinical tasks such as researching conditions (Patton, 2018b).

Workplace culture in the form of contextual guides such as models, cues and access to previously completed or partially completed work significantly influences workplace learning (Rogoff, 1990). Workplace norms and practices have a pervasive and often tacit influence on healthcare students' practice with students experiencing strong pressure to conform to expected practices, for example, completion of medical notes, within healthcare workplaces (Patton, 2018b). When required to complete medical notes, students model their practice on previously completed notes. While students who lack confidence or experience in medical note writing can be particularly reliant on medical notes as contextual guides, all students are generally eager to follow health service protocols (Patton, 2018b). This propensity to follow established practices highlights a susceptibility of students' clinical reasoning to entrenched and often unquestioned workplace practices.

Students are particularly vulnerable to workplace pressures to conform as they occupy a disempowered space in healthcare workplaces. Students are temporary visitors in healthcare workplaces where the primary aim is client care, not student education. Tension between achievement of health service's organizational goals and students' educational goals can result in student education being compromised. As an example, student active participation in a range of complex client treatments can be restricted by clinical supervisors who may be time poor and concerned with their ability to meet service targets. As a consequence, students have little power to disrupt barriers to participation in practice activities and experience a strong need to comply with existing workplace practices (Patton, 2018c). When this occurs, students' development of clinical reasoning capability can be shaped in line with current workplace practices because they are not able to consider and implement a range of alternate treatment approaches.

Temporal dimensions of clinical workplaces also significantly influence student learning, in particular their fast pace and often haphazard nature (Patton, 2018b). Time restraints require students to demonstrate flexibility, adaptability and the ability to formulate alternate treatment plans, often at short notice. When students feel rushed, the quality of their performance and learning can decline (Patton, 2018c).

Clinical workplaces as learning spaces shape healthcare students' clinical learning and provide deeper ways of conceptualizing clinical education and nurturing development of students' clinical reasoning capabilities. Conceptualization of clinical education as situated, multifaceted and fluid learning spaces formed by clinical educator actions, student engagement in practice, student dispositions and workplace influences that strongly shape students' clinical reasoning capability development is represented in Fig. 33.1. This conceptual understanding opens up opportunities for academics, clinical supervisors and students: they can to harness the educational potential of clinical workplaces to facilitate learning during clinical placements and development of wise clinical educational practices.

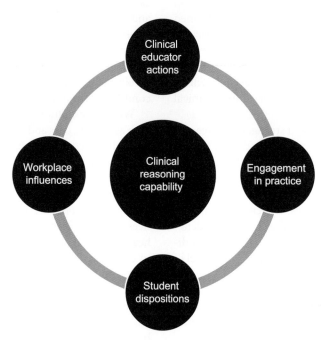

Fig. 33.1 ■ Conceptualization of clinical education as a situated, multifaceted and fluid learning space influencing development of clinical reasoning capability. (Adapted with permission from Patton, N., 2018b. A crucible model for understanding learning in clinical workplace spaces. In: Patton, N., Higgs, J., Smith, M. (Eds.), Developing practice capability: Transforming workplace learning. Brill Sense, Leiden, The Netherlands, pp. 135–148. ISBN 900436692X, 9789004366923.)

REFLECTION POINT

- Academics: How might you prepare students for learning in disempowered spaces during clinical placements?
- Clinical educators: What is the impact of students' disempowered position in health services alongside the 'way things are done here' on their development of clinical reasoning capability?

DEVELOPING CLINICAL REASONING CAPABILITY DURING CLINICAL PLACEMENTS

Healthcare professionals and students are required to make ethical decisions and implement treatments to enhance people's well-being in complex and dynamic healthcare environments (Jensen and Patton, 2018). Clinical reasoning, a tacit skill that critically defines clinician performance and efficacy, is central to ethical decision making. Health profession students' development and application of clinical reasoning capability is inextricably linked with clinical exposure (Wong and Kowitlawakul, 2020) and is directly related to the range of settings and patient categories that students experience within individual healthcare workplaces (Jessee, 2018). Students' clinical reasoning capability is fostered through repetitive and increasing clinical exposure to a wide variety of clients, reflection on those experiences, and ultimately integration of different approaches into their own clinical reasoning approach (Wijbenga et al., 2019). Authentic patient interactions improve students' ability to understand and recall medical conditions and their impact on people's lives, to solve problems and to refine a range of practice skills (Patton, 2018b). During clinical placements, students experience the complexities of practice including the consequences of their clinical reasoning and actions that can be incorporated into their learning (Jensen and Patton, 2018). Development of clinical reasoning capability during clinical placements is irreversibly interwoven with student participation in and reflection on a range of meaningful workplace activities.

Student engagement in clinical activities is a complex and fluid phenomenon regulated by supervisors' and students' dispositions (Patton, 2018b). Supervisors' innate ability to trust students to be safe with patients and students' level of confidence largely determine the level of student engagement in clinical activities. Placement factors such as the presence of other students, provision of adequate time to complete patient activities, encouragement and positive feedback received from placement supervisors, as well as the degree of welcome and acceptance students receive in the workplace positively contribute to building student confidence (Patton, 2018b). Conversely student confidence can be diminished by prolonged periods of passive observation of other therapists, ongoing surveillance and poor-quality practice performance (Patton, 2018b).

Strengthening the quality of clinical placements and, ultimately, the quality of client care depends largely on how clinical supervisors can facilitate the development and application of clinical knowledge and expertise (Tiffen et al., 2014). Apart from facilitating student transition from academic to clinical settings, clinical supervisors can also foster students' critical thinking through provision of clinical experiences and guidance on those experiences (Wong and Kowitlawakul, 2020). Discussion with meaningful feedback that is timely and specific guides purposeful attention to alternate perspectives and engagement in the continuum of reflection (Jessee, 2018). Student learning is further enhanced by individual feedback from the clinical teacher and reflection on the clinical reasoning process, either alone or, even better, together with the clinical instructor or with others (Wijbenga et al., 2019). Despite the acknowledged importance of guidance to students' clinical learning, current health professional shortages and consequent heavy workloads mean that clinicians may not have the time to guide or supervise students in healthcare settings (Jessee, 2018). Ward cultures, including heavy staff workloads which decrease time for students, stand out as a prominent factor that negatively affects student development of clinical reasoning (Wong and Kowitlawakul, 2020). Other barriers stem from a lack of effective teaching pedagogies, unfriendly ward cultures and students' attitudes (Wong and Kowitlawakul, 2020).

To highlight how a wide continuum of student dispositions, clinical supervisor actions and clinical contexts coalesce to shape students' clinical reasoning capability development during clinical placement, Case Study 33.1 provides student composite profiles of two physiotherapy students undertaking their final year placements in an acute care setting.

Re-imagined university curricula that prepare both students and clinical educators to engage in constructive feedback and discussions could harness the potential of clinical placements to transform both student learning and contemporary professional practices (Markauskaite and Patton, 2019). It is only in relational spaces grounded in trust and respect, where a variety of ideas are encouraged and all players are encouraged to enter professional conversations, that meaningful personal, professional and practice community transformations can occur (Patton and Simpson, 2016). Academic curricula, including case studies with role play opportunities, could provide students with the necessary language and confidence to question existing workplace practices respectfully and enable students to share their views (Markauskaite and Patton, 2019). When students are empowered to challenge current practices respectfully, they can be repositioned as drivers of their own learning and opportunities to transform professional practices can be maximized (Markauskaite and Patton, 2019).

CASE STUDY 33.1

Student Clinical Reasoning

Penny is undertaking her final block placement in her home town where she lives with her parents and is a 10-minute walk from the health service where she is undertaking placement. Penny is feeling confident on this placement because her previous placements have gone well and she feels supported by her clinical supervisor who has welcomed her as a valued member of the interprofessional team and encourages her to contribute her ideas regarding client management in team meetings. The nursing staff are approachable and Penny is comfortable discussing her clients' status with them and is consequently aware of any changes to her clients' status and any new treatment approaches that may have been implemented as a result. Penny has a desk in the health professional office and is able to discuss her clients with other health professionals thereby gaining a broader range of perspectives on client management. Her timetable has built in time for researching evidence-based approaches for management of conditions her clients are presenting with. As a result, Penny feels confident in her ability to suggest new evidence-based client management approaches supported by her discussions with colleagues and her research. In this case, Penny's clinical reasoning capability has been actively developed through provision of opportunities to broaden her range of practice approaches through discussion with other clinicians and research as well as her ability to engage with these opportunities.

Peter is undertaking his final block placement a long way from home and has had difficulty securing suitable accommodation and is consequently staying in a caravan park. Peter is feeling anxious about this placement because his previous placement did not go well and he needed a lot of support to meet competency by the end of the placement. Peter is also under considerable financial stress as he has a partner and two young children dependent on his income and he is unable to work while on this placement. He cannot afford to fail this placement as he needs to complete his course on time and begin graduate employment. Peter's clinical supervisor is a very experienced clinician who has worked with the health service for many years and has entrenched practices (e.g. documentation, assessment and treatment strategies) and expects Peter to follow these practices. Peter experiences strong pressure to conform to his clinical supervisor's practices and feels it too risky to suggest alternative strategies (even if he felt they would result in improved client outcomes) because he has limited capacity to research evidence-based approaches and is aware that his clinical supervisor is marking his performance. In this case, Peter's ability to question existing workplace practices has not been actively developed and opportunities to develop his clinical reasoning capability closed down.

In both of these cases, clinical supervisors need to acknowledge individual student circumstances and create learning spaces that encourage students to question, explore a range of treatment approaches and develop their clinical reasoning capability.

SUMMARY

In this chapter, clinical reasoning has been conceptualized as a complex, dynamic and experiential phenomenon that is embedded in healthcare contexts, embodied in individuals, transformed in action and grounded in an ethical aim to do good for others in unpredictable and challenging situations. The significant and complex contribution of health service workplaces to students' development of clinical reasoning capability has been highlighted.

Key points for academics and clinical educators to consider in the development of wise clinical education practices aimed at fostering students' clinical reasoning capability during clinical placements:

- Clinical education is significantly different to academic learning warranting development and implementation of specific pedagogy;
- Situated and workplace learning theories provide a solid platform on which to construct wise clinical education pedagogies;
- Clinical reasoning capability development during clinical placement is strongly shaped by clinical educator actions, student engagement in practice, student dispositions and workplace influences; and
- A focus on students as participants in meaningful and increasingly important workplace tasks opens up possibilities to transform clinical education practice through examination of how students who are accepted into workplaces and invited to undertake workplace activities elect to engage with those activities and are prepared for full participation.

REFERENCES

Ardern, R., 2022. The co-creation of an innovative curriculum model: Balancing lab, simulation, and clinical. Teaching and Learning in Nursing 17, 318–322. https://doi.org/10.1016/j.teln.2022.03.008

Billett, S., 2004. Workplace participatory practices: Conceptualising workplaces as learning environments. The Journal of Workplace Learning 16(6), 312–324. https://doi.org/10.1108/13665620410550295

Billett, S., 2009. Conceptualizing learning experiences: Contributions and mediations of the social, personal and brute. Mind, Culture & Activity 16, 32–47. https://doi.org/10.1080/10749030802477317

Boud, D., Hager, P., 2012. Re-thinking continual professional development through changing metaphors and location in professional practices. Studies in Continuing Education 34 (1), 17–30. https://doi.org/10.1080/0158037X.2011.608656

Boud, D., Middleton, H., 2003. Learning from others at work: Communities of practice and informal learning. Journal of Workplace Learning 15 (5), 194–202. https://doi.org/10.1108/13665620310483895

Brentnall, J., Thackray, D., Judd, B., 2022. Evaluating the clinical reasoning of student health professionals in placement and simulation settings: A systematic review. International Journal of Environmental Research and Public Health 19 (2), 936. https://doi.org/10.3390/ijerph19020936

Carolan, C., Davies, C., Crookes, P., McGhee, S., Roxburgh, M., 2020. COVID 19: Disruptive impacts and transformative opportunities in undergraduate nurse education. Nurse Education in Practice 46, 102807. https://doi.org/10.1016/j.nepr.2020.102807

Croskerry, P., 2006. Critical thinking and decision making: Avoiding the perils of thin-slicing. Annals of Emergency Medicine 48 (6), 720–722. https://doi.org/10.1016/j.annemergmed.2006.03.030

Daniel, M., Rencic, J., Durning, S.J., Holmboe, E., Santen, S.A., Lang, V., et al., 2019. Clinical reasoning assessment methods: A scoping review and practical guidance. Academic Medicine 94 (6), 902–912. https://doi.org/10.1097/ACM.0000000000002618

Dewey, J., 1916. Democracy and education: An introduction to the philosophy of education. McMillan Company.

Edwards, R., Nicholl, K., 2006. Action at a distance. Governmentality, subjectivity and workplace learning. In: Billett, S. Fenwick, T. Sommerville, M. (Eds.), Work subjectivity and learning. Understanding learning through working life, Vol. 6. Springer, Dordrecht, pp. 179–193.

Evans, K., Rainbird, H., 2002. The significance of workplace learning for a 'learning society'. In: Evans, K., Hodkinson, P., Unwin, L. (Eds.), Working to learn transforming learning in the workplace. Kogan Page, London, pp. 7–28.

Fairbrother, M., Nicole, M., Blackford, J., Nagarajan, S., McAllister, L., 2016. A new model of clinical education to increase student placement availability: The capacity development facilitator model. Asia Pacific Journal of Cooperative Education 17, 45–59.

Haines, K.J., Berney, S., 2020. Physiotherapists during COVID-19: Usual business, in unusual times. Journal of Physiotherapy 66 (2), 67–69. https://doi.org/10.1016/j.jphys.2020.03.012

Jensen, G., Patton, N., 2018. Developing capability for ethical courage in clinical workplaces. In: Patton, N., Higgs, J., Smith, M. (Eds.), Developing practice capability: Transforming workplace learning. Brill Sense, Leiden, The Netherlands, pp. 191–198.

Jessee, M.A., 2018. Pursuing improvement in clinical reasoning: The integrated clinical education theory. Journal of Nursing Education 57 (1), 7–12. https://doi.org/10.3928/01484834-20180102-03

Johansson, M., Boud, D., 2010. Towards an emergent view of learning work. International Journal of Lifelong Learning 29 (3), 359–372. https://doi.org/10.1080/02601371003700683

Kemmis, S., Grootenboer, P., 2008. Situating praxis in practice. In: Kemmis, S., Smith, T.J. (Eds.), Enabling praxis: Challenges for education. Sense, Rotterdam, pp. 37–62.

Kemmis, S., Smith, T.J., 2008. Conclusions and challenges in enabling praxis. In: Kemmis, S., Smith, T.J. (Eds.), Enabling praxis: Challenges for education. Sense, Rotterdam, pp. 263–286.

Lave, J., Wenger, E., 1991. Situated learning: Legitimate peripheral participation. Cambridge University Press, Cambridge.

Lehtinen, E., 2008. Discussion: Bridging the individual and social in workplace learning and motivation. International Journal of Educational Research 47, 261–263. https://doi.org/10.1016/j.ijer.2008.07.005

Markauskaite, L., Patton, N., 2019. Learning for employability in the workplace: Developing graduate work capabilities. In: Higgs, J., Crisp, G., Letts, W. (Eds.), Education for employability: Learning for future possibilities. Brill Sense, Rotterdam, Netherlands, pp. 227–236.

Nahon, I., Jeffery, L., Peiris, C., Dunwoodie, R., Corrigan, R., Francis-Cracknell, A., 2021. Responding to emerging needs: Development of adapted performance indicators for physiotherapy student assessment in telehealth. Australian Journal of Clinical Education 9 (1), 17–27. https://doi.org/10.53300/001c.24960

McLaughlin, J.E., Wolcott, M.D., Hubbard, D., Umstead, K., Rider, T.R., 2019. A qualitative review of the design thinking framework in health professions education. BMC Medical Education 19, 98. https://doi.org/10.1186/s12909-019-1528-8

Patrick, C.-J., Valencia-Forrester, F., Backhaus, B., McGregor, R., Cain, G., Lloyd, K., 2019. The state of service-learning. Australia. Journal of Higher Education Outreach & Engagement 23 (3), 185–198. https://openjournals.libs.uga.edu/jheoe/article/view/1528

Patton, N., 2018a. Using practice and workplace learning theories to enhance clinical learning spaces. In: Patton, N., Higgs, J., Smith, M. (Eds.), Developing practice capability: Transforming workplace learning. Brill Sense, Leiden, The Netherlands, pp. 61–68.

Patton, N., 2018b. A crucible model for understanding learning in clinical workplace spaces. In: Patton, N., Higgs, J., Smith, M. (Eds.), Developing practice capability: Transforming workplace learning. Brill Sense, Leiden, The Netherlands, pp. 135–148. ISBN 900436692X, 9789004366923.

Patton, N., 2018c. Clinical learning spaces: Dimensions and character. In: Patton, N., Higgs, J., Smith, M. (Eds.), Developing practice capability: Transforming workplace learning. Brill Sense, Leiden, The Netherlands, pp. 121–134.

Patton, N., 2023. Harnessing the value of authentic work integrated learning experiences in teacher education. In: Winslade, M., Loughland, T., Eady, M.J. (Eds.), Work-integrated learning case studies in teacher education. Springer, Singapore, pp. 49–60.

Patton, N., Fish, D., 2016. Appreciating practice. In: Higgs, J., Trede, F. (Eds.), Professional practice marginalia. Sense, Rotterdam, The Netherlands, pp. 55–64.

Patton, N., Higgs, J., 2018. Professional practice. In: Patton, N., Higgs, J., Smith, M. (Eds.), Developing practice capability: Transforming workplace learning. Brill Sense, Leiden, The Netherlands, pp. 3–14.

Patton, N., Higgs, J., Smith, M., 2013. Using theories of learning in workplaces to enhance physiotherapy clinical education. Physiotherapy Theory and Practice 29, 493–503. https://doi.org/10.3109/09593985.2012.753651

Patton, N., Higgs, J., Smith, M., 2018. Clinical learning spaces: Crucibles for practice development in physiotherapy clinical education. Physiotherapy Theory and Practice 34 (8), 589–599. https://doi.org/10.1080/09593985.2017.1423144

Patton, N., Simpson, M.D., 2016. Harmonising discourse through workplace learning. In: Higgs, J., Trede, F. (Eds.), Professional practice marginalia. Sense, Rotterdam, The Netherlands, pp. 233–240.

Rodger, S., Webb, G., Devitt, L., Gilbert, J., Wrightson, P., McMeekin, J., 2008. Clinical education and practice placements in the allied health professions: An international perspective. Journal of Allied Health 37, 53–62.

Rogoff, B., 1990. Apprenticeship in thinking: Cognitive development in social context. New York. Oxford University Press.

Salter, C., Oates, R.K., Swanson, C., Bourke, L., 2020. Working remotely: Innovative allied health placements in response to COVID-19. International Journal of Work-Integrated Learning 21 (5), 587–600. https://www.ijwil.org/files/IJWIL_21_5_587_600.pdf

Tiffen, J., Corbridge, S.J., Slimmer, L., 2014. Enhancing clinical decision making: Development of a contiguous definition and conceptual framework. Journal of Professional Nursing 30 (5), 399–405. https://doi.org/10.1016/j.profnurs.2014.01.006

Wijbenga, M.H., Bovend'Eerdt, T.J.H., Driessen, E.W., 2019. Physiotherapy students' experiences with clinical reasoning during clinical placements: A qualitative study. Health Professions Education 5, 126–135. https://doi.org/10.1016/j.hpe.2018.05.003

Wong, S.H.V., Kowitlawakul, Y., 2020. Exploring perceptions and barriers in developing critical thinking and clinical reasoning of nursing students: A qualitative study. Nurse Education Today 95, 104600. https://doi.org/10.1016/j.nedt.2020.104600

Young, M., Thomas, A., Gordon, D., Gruppen, L.D., Lubarsky, S., Rencic, J., et al., 2019. The terminology of clinical reasoning in health professions education: Implications and considerations. Medical Teacher 41, 1277–1284. https://doi.org/10.1080/0142159X.2019.1635686

34

LEADING A FACULTY IN IMPLEMENTING CLINICAL REASONING

MEGAN SMITH

■ ■

CHAPTER AIMS

The aims of this chapter are:

- to describe the role of faculty leaders in facilitating the achievement of graduate learning outcomes to impact client outcomes positively
- to propose a framework for the role of faculty level leaders in assuring graduate learning outcomes by engaging in curriculum leadership
- to guide faculty leaders to consider how to apply at scale, and with quality and consistency, contemporary understandings of teaching clinical reasoning derived from research and scholarship.

REFLECTION POINT

- As a faculty leader, where are the opportunities to listen to scholars of clinical reasoning and to understand your role in impacting educational change?

INTRODUCTION: SHARING MY JOURNEY

My introduction to the field of clinical reasoning coincided with the second edition of this book and I began my educational and research journey in the field. At this time, I was developing a deeper understanding of clinical reasoning and decision making through doctoral studies and teaching and considering how my research might shape students' capability to learn how to practise. I was designing scholarly informed curricula and assessments that would test students' reasoning capability. I trusted that my teaching would translate into their practice, leading to the delivery of better-quality healthcare.

My academic career has since progressed through a range of faculty leadership roles as a discipline leader, curriculum designer, head of school of allied health professions, to being the executive dean of a faculty. Preparing this chapter enabled me to reflect on my role transitions and the challenges I have encountered as a leader in promoting and ensuring quality clinical reasoning. As a faculty leader, I have increasingly been focussed on executive and administrative duties and yet central to my purpose is assuring graduate learning outcomes align to our communities' expectations and needs. My reflection on my journey highlights how relevant it is to consider the changing context of health professional education and more broadly higher education. Whereas my initial journey with clinical reasoning commenced with a narrow focus at the teacher–student interface, leadership roles require a broadening of perspective and greater consideration of factors which shape student outcomes, how quality is assured and the extent to which the educational experience ultimately impacts client care and outcomes.

The field of clinical reasoning scholarship continues to deepen our understanding of clinical reasoning and reveals an ever more complex phenomenon applied in an increasingly complex and changing world. Considering clinical reasoning as a complex construct means there is not a single best approach to the teaching and assessment of clinical reasoning and has led to a proliferation of curricula possibilities that are magnified across disciplines (Daniel et al., 2019). However, consistent features suggested are that teaching and assessment methods are authentic, reflect the deeply contextual nature of clinical reasoning (Patton and Christensen, 2019) and require the development of practitioners who are capable of continuing to learn through exposure to complex environments (Christensen and Jensen, 2019).

As an Executive Dean I oversee four schools (organizational units) with responsibilities for teaching and research in the health professions. The health professions in the faculty are listed in Table 34.1. They are distributed across the schools in an organizational structure designed to leverage synergies in teaching approaches, resources and staffing profile. The organizational structure of professions in schools is also practical in terms of feasibly sharing and managing resources.

The university is located in regional New South Wales, Australia, where a high proportion of graduates take up employment in regional, rural and remote settings. The governance and accreditation of health professional education in Australia consists of a combination of formally registered and accredited professions (AHPRA) and self-accrediting professional bodies. The governance of the overall quality of higher education is overseen by Tertiary Education Quality and Standards Agency (TEQSA), which is the regulatory body. The health service sector with which we work consists of Commonwealth-funded primary and community healthcare, aged care and disability services, state-funded hospital and acute care services, and a private healthcare system of hospitals and primary care providers. There is a strong nexus between education providers and the healthcare sector particularly related to clinical placements.

The Australian Healthcare system maintains a generally high standard of care; however, regional differences in healthcare outcomes persist. Most notably, First Nations Australians and Australians living in rural and remote communities experience poorer health outcomes compared with their urban counterparts. The maldistribution of qualified health professionals is a recognized factor in the health inequities with a far greater proportion of qualified health professionals concentrated in metropolitan centres (Australian Institute of Health and Welfare, 2022).

The expectations of graduates for autonomous practice varies by discipline. For example, medicine graduates will undertake supervised internships upon graduation whereas podiatrists are able to be independent first contact practitioners upon graduation. The necessity for graduates to have high-quality clinical reasoning capability is evident particularly where graduates may enter practice in a regional location with a comparative paucity of colleagues and high levels of community need.

TABLE 34.1			
Health Professions in the Faculty of Science and Health			
School of Rural Medicine	**School of Nursing, Paramedicine and Healthcare Sciences**	**School of Dentistry and Medical Sciences**	**School of Allied Health and Exercise Sciences**
Medicine	Indigenous mental health practitioners Nursing Midwifery Paramedicine	Pharmacy Oral health Practitioners Dentistry Nuclear medicine Medical imaging Radiotherapy	Exercise physiologists Physiotherapy Occupational therapy Speech pathology Podiatry

Although much of the work of a faculty leader deals with the administration of courses, units and students, the faculty leader can also play a meaningful role in impacting curricula design and innovation. The case study of the student Mairead has been written to prompt readers to look and question the extent to which faculty leaders hold accountability for graduate outcomes in such a focussed field as clinical reasoning (Case Study 34.1).

Graduation represents a critical juncture between education and quality future healthcare. This juncture comes into acute daily relief for me because I work and live in my regional community where many of our graduates provide direct healthcare for my family. I am afforded a very personal and sobering perspective on the adequacy of preparation for practice of our graduates. For me, being a faculty leader implies a high level of ethical and moral obligation for the quality of

---

CASE STUDY 34.1

Faculty Leaders' Accountability for Graduate Outcomes in Clinical Reasoning

Mairead is a final-year occupational therapy student who has recently completed her last clinical placement. With final assessments now complete, she will shortly join the practice workforce. During her studies she has experienced a curriculum where development of clinical reasoning, as understood by her educators, was designed, taught and explicitly assessed.

As a Faculty Executive Dean, I will shortly sign off on her graduation, a confirmation that she has met the requirements for entry to practice and assurance to the community that she has the skills to provide safe and effective care.

In 'signing off' how do I assure myself Mairead is indeed ready for practice? Is she able to reason clinically as we currently understand best practice to be? Will her preparation for practice carry her forwards adequately as the context for health professional practice continues to change and become more complex?

And what about all of the other students in Mairead's occupational therapy cohort and indeed the faculty as a whole?

---

graduates and for the longer-term legacy of education. This obligation challenges me as a faculty leader, faced with daily managerial concerns such as the availability and distribution of resources, also to be concerned with the details of innovation, equity and impact, applying personal values to leadership, and enacting ethical principles in decision making to meet the needs for quality outcomes (Rao, 2019).

Enabling Clinical Reasoning Curricula Innovation: Applying a Faculty Leaders' Perspective

There continue to be calls for improvements in the explicit teaching of clinical reasoning within educational programmes to prepare students better for practice and meeting complex societal needs. There is a recurrent observation that there is a missing link in the effective translation of research and scholarship into teaching and teaching students to adapt to their practice (Christensen et al., 2019; Cooper et al., 2021; Kavanagh and Szweda, 2017; Parodis et al., 2021; Sudacka et al., 2021). As a body of scholars, we are not confident that advances in understanding about clinical reasoning link to advances in care for patients and clients.

> Capability in learning how to learn from clinical reasoning experiences continues to be a critical missing link between our desired, and our actual, educational outcomes in the context of professional education of today's healthcare professionals.
> **(Christensen and Jensen, 2019, p. 431).**

Whereas in much of the published clinical reasoning literature the focus is on the teacher–student nexus, there is also a call for leaders to pay explicit attention to their obligations to ensure the quality of healthcare provided by graduates (Kavanagh and Szweda, 2017). Christensen and Jensen (2019) draw attention to the risk that occurs when isolated pockets of expertise exist that are less able to bring about 'transformational change than distributed adaptive expertise across individuals, organizations, communities and professions'. Faculty leaders can apply and achieve transformational change at the organizational level to advance curricula innovations in clinical reasoning (Sudacka et al., 2021).

My position is that faculty leaders can shape, influence, and ultimately should, be accountable for health professional graduate outcomes. Although leaders are often positioned at a distance from the teacher–student interface, a framework can be very helpful in this much needed accountability process. I make sense of the role of the faculty leader in assuring graduate outcomes by using a framework which positions curriculum leadership as occurring at different organization levels in a higher education institution Table 34.2. The framework is adapted and developed from work by Fraser (2019) and Vaugh et al. (2022). Fraser (2019) identified that effective educational innovation occurred when multiple levels within the organization act as different types of innovators. Vaugh et al. (2022) extrapolated this further by applying labels of levels micro, meso and macro.

Under this framework, the faculty leader is afforded a hierarchically empowered position with the attendant affordances and accountability for setting policy and strategic direction, enabling resources and opportunities, and setting standards and ensuring their oversight. At the micro level, closest to the student, the teacher–student interaction is where the informed understanding of clinical reasoning as a complex, social-cultural and engaged endeavour occurs and where the shaping of individual learning experiences occurs. Sitting at the meso level is the innovation and decision making of professional academic leaders responsible for curriculum design and leadership to impact cohorts.

A faculty leader applying the three-level framework described in Table 34.2 considers how research and scholarship of clinical reasoning might feed into the decisions and actions reaching down into an organization to best impact student learning and graduate outcomes. Vaugh et al. (2022) illustrate an approach to achieving this in practice, drawing attention to the importance of communicating across and through the

TABLE 34.2

Three-level Framework for Leaders Navigating Curriculum Innovation and Change

Level	Role and Purpose	Understanding of Clinical Reasoning Scholarship	Sphere of Influence
Macro	Faculty leader ■ Direction setting, policymaker and resource enabler	■ Clinical reasoning as one of many elements of curriculum ■ Students are organized in cohorts of disciplines ■ May be limited understanding of detailed relationship of scholarship of clinical reasoning to curriculum planning, design and delivery.	■ Ideas are delegated to others to implement; need to be well informed by lower levels ■ Sets the enabling and constraining context for curricula through authority and decision making ■ High capacity to influence and control outcomes due to resources at their disposal ■ Considers fair and equitable sharing of resource where constraints exist ■ Accountable for multi-professional learning outcomes and governance standards
Meso	Professional leader ■ Cohort and curriculum designers	■ Individuals who consider the broader pedagogy, discipline specific models and educational experience at the cohort level ■ May be informed by research and scholarship	■ Can influence and persuade others of the importance of their ideas and involve them in their implementation ■ Can plan for larger scale and consistency of requirements ■ Coordinate and apply the resources and operational requirements ■ Accountable for cohort learning outcomes ■ Need to set expectations and communicate 'up' for resources
Micro	Lecturers, tutors and facilitators ■ Teaching-student interface	■ Can be informed by understanding of clinical reasoning and application to teaching and assessment approaches ■ Likely to be reflective and reactive to individual students	■ Influence may be limited beyond their own teaching ■ Accountable for individual learning outcomes ■ Work within resources

levels. Using this framework may also reveal where the barriers to effective curriculum implementation and innovation for clinical reasoning may arise. Faculty leaders at the macro level will look to their staff with deep understanding to distil the complex information in ways that it can be communicated into practical requirements. As Vaugh et al. (2022) note, macro leaders need 'complex stakeholder information to be communicated and more easily understood … with the intention of informing decision making and building empathy and alignment'. With the meso level research findings, they need to be packaged into insights and actionable challenge statements which require leaders at this level to reflect deeply on research findings and develop and articulate the insight for daily operational decision making. At the micro level, the research findings need to be captured in a rich but succinct way that increase the likelihood that the findings will be applied to meet the needs of learners and ultimately healthcare consumers.

Planning, Doing and Managing Challenges as the Faculty Leader

Faculty leaders rely upon fingers of influence that reach down into the organization to impact the teaching and assessment of students and assure outcomes. One of the lessons to be learnt as a faculty leader is how to work through others to achieve educational outcomes. Anthony and Antony (2017) describe the academic leader as having special characteristics that distinguish them from leaders in other fields. They describe the academic leader as:

> … *someone with a broad vision of their field, and who has the power to bring the change in their field. They have the ability and capacity to release and engage human potential in the pursuit of a common cause. They must sustain change and this energy must come from within the academic unit, driven by the vision of its leaders.*
>
> **(p. 632)**

My experience is that enacting faculty-wide curricula change is particularly difficult. Staff need not only motivation but training, resources and a combination of drivers and incentives. These drivers can be internal to the organization but also external. My personal leadership example in health professional education is the inclusion of

curricula supporting practice capability with Australian First Nations peoples. The population health differential between First Nations health and the health of non-First Nations Australians is unacceptably wide. A strategy to address the inequity has been to implement educational programs for pre-entry health professionals. Our institution has worked systematically to widen student exposure to the historical context impacting First Nations Australians and First Nations ways of knowing and being. Progress is still being made but this has required leadership at both the individual and policy level to make change. This has been reinforced more recently by drives from Australian professional accrediting bodies who are mandating First Nations content inclusion and practice capability. The impact on positive outcomes for First Nations peoples' health in Australia is still to be realized.

To be successful in achieving the goal of transformational curricular change, leaders need to understand and navigate the concepts of scale, consistency and quality assurance.

Scale

A key difference between the individual teacher and the faculty leader is thinking about the scale of the change or initiative. Whereas much of our theoretical perspective on learning clinical reasoning comes from the lens of the individual practitioner, a faculty leader needs to consider how the learning of many graduates, who will impact the lives of many, will be practically achieved. This need to consider scale and capacity is highly relevant in the current context with growth in demand for skilled health workers. There continues to be constant expansion of training capacity across and within institutions. Frenk et al. (2022) estimate a global doubling of student numbers training to be health professionals in the last 10 years.

The consequence for faculty leaders is to contemplate how to grow capacity often in constrained contexts. Innovation and growth strategies need to be considered by faculty leaders. For example, good clinical reasoning requires students to learn in authentic contexts such as during clinical education placements; however, the size of the practising workforce able to provide supervision can constrain scaling to the number of clinical placements required. Likewise, providing integrated learning experiences in workplace contexts or simulated learning activities are desirable and achievable for small cohorts, but the faculty leader needs to be able to think and plan how these might be delivered for 20 to 100 times the number of students. In my experience, the feasible scaling of curriculum design is not just in number but equivalence of quality that requires skilled leadership. This is an area where desired pedagogies are planned yet can fail to be delivered in practice.

Consistency

This concept of scale reveals another important criterion when planning curricular change in clinical reasoning and that is of consistency across many students. The context of higher education learning is complex and the learning journeys of students are unique. It is impossible to prescribe that each student will have an equal learning experience to reach an equal point in terms of learning to reason clinically upon graduation. As a faculty leader, this critical issue is best viewed through the lens of being an enabler. What conditions need to be put in place to assure that the essential elements for learning occur and for this to remain consistent across students in a discipline and across disciplines? The leader has a pivotal role in overseeing the setting of learning outcomes and then asking the question across the macro to the micro levels of leadership is essential. A faculty leader without access to this information coming from disciplines or without the perspective to see potential challenges within the organization can fail to grasp how to optimize teaching something as complex as clinical reasoning.

Quality Assurance

Part of my development as a faculty leader has been a deeper and broader understanding of the essential value of academic governance in addressing and achieving the challenges in meaningful educational change. Here I refer to governance as the mechanism for assuring consistent, quality decision making both in curricular design and implementation. Academic governance is the mechanism by which the institution and its leaders assure the quality of the educational experience and quality graduate outcomes. Velthuis et al. (2021) described the impact of governance at the micro level and its relationship to macro governance as critical factors in the implementation of curricula change. They identified both the hard factors and soft cultural factors that together shape and influence how change occurs. Governance brings with it accountability and compliance as hard factors align with standards to be met, whereas the soft cultural factors are how these compliance approaches are enacted in practice and can navigate curricular change.

Bendermacher et al. (2021) see quality as an integral element for innovation and essential for leaders in the education of the health professions. The role of leadership behaviours in promulgating a quality culture that leads to organizational change and positive outcomes must be conceptualized more broadly than adherence to rules and compliance. Rather, leaders need to consider the role they play in positively engaging with a vision and commitment to change and improvement. When it comes to the implementation of clinical reasoning curricular change, senior leaders will need to work with leaders at other levels within the organization (meso level) to facilitate a culture that can enact curricular change and innovation in clinical reasoning.

Further Considerations for Curriculum Implementation

With the aforementioned broad considerations in mind, there are focal areas to consider in leading clinical reasoning curricular implementation such as strategic setting of a culture and vision, using policy, distributing resources and specific implementation activities.

Culture and Vision

- Promoting a rich intellectual climate where staff and students are encouraged to reflect and learn from experience
- Advancing discipline-specific reasoning and understanding through research and critical review climate
- Acknowledging the sociocultural construction of learning and innovation
- Fostering a culture of excellence and client-centredness, a sense of purpose and belief in who the outcomes are for

Policy

- Setting policy levers, performance indicators, governance approvals and systems of review and quality assurance

- Identifying and removing barriers to innovation
- Providing informed top-down support that directly impacts staff and students

Resources

- Providing staff and students with access to infrastructure such as simulation and authentic experiences in workplaces in which to practice clinical reasoning
- Providing access to training in content and method to inform teaching and assessment
- Employing staff with a sound understanding of clinical practice
- Enabling adequate resources and facilities for a rich and relevant context of learning
- Ensuring time and support for students to consolidate learning and develop

Implementation

- Implementing curricular design and pedagogies of learning that structure the acquisition of knowledge and models of reasoning
- Providing students with direct experiences of decision making in safe environments with the capacity to learn
- Assuring effective assessment strategies which establish a minimal level or standard required for entry to practice

Navigating the Evolving Context of Higher Education

There are key areas of change in the context of the education of the health professions which continue to develop after the COVID-19 pandemic (Frenk et al., 2022). There are significant health system demands for trained professionals who are ready for an evolving healthcare sector and there is a changing context of higher education for all (leaders, faculty and learners). For example, changes in technology are influencing and enhancing learning and healthcare provision. Although technology-informed changes were already occurring, the pandemic rapidly accelerated expectations and affordances.

The context of higher education is under a constant state of evolution and flux which has also been accelerated by the COVID-19 pandemic. In the education of Australian health professions, there are increased numbers of students with evolving experiences and expectations of higher education and learning. There are financial variations due to changing models of funding, staffing capability and capacity, technology, access to knowledge and places of learning, alignment to a changing healthcare sector, and meeting changing governance and compliance requirements. Faculty leaders in the education of health professions juggle these, often competing, changes as they make decisions to optimize student and graduate outcomes.

Faculty leaders educating health professionals need to navigate the evolving contexts of the health system and health professions education and work towards necessary strategies that integrate, establish and resource critical changes. It is predictable that the context for students learning clinical reasoning within the context of their broader education will become more, not less, complex with multiple moving parts and interdependencies, multiple agents and ideas, and multiple frames of reference.

SUMMARY

This chapter presents the perspective of a faculty leader, in my case an executive dean, who plays a role in planning and enabling the understanding of clinical reasoning to be put into practice. The implications are that leaders need to be invested in the outcome at an ethical and moral level and to care deeply about the impact of understanding for the teachers and the students, but most importantly for the clients. Faculty leaders need to be able to see the organization at all levels and listen to the individuals who can inform them of good practice in clinical reasoning. Likewise, researchers and scholars of clinical reasoning also need to see the educational context at all organizational levels to consider the scale of the implementation of their ideas. In this two-way dialogue between levels within the institution, we must address this complex construct if we want to shape future practice.

In summary, the role of a faculty leader in a faculty of health professions is:

- to understand the higher education context and the context for learning;
- to set a direction aligned to purpose;

- to ensure the pieces are in place and
- to consider how purposeful and scholarly leadership is enacted in practice.

REFERENCES

Australian Institute of Health and Welfare. 2022. Rural and remote health. Australian Government. https://www.aihw.gov.au/reports/rural-remote-australians/rural-and-remote-health

Anthony, S.G., Antony, J., 2017. Academic leadership – Special or simple. International Journal of Productivity and Performance Management 66 (5), 630–637. https://doi.org/10.1108/IJPPM-08-2016-0162

Bendermacher, G.W.G., Dolmans, D.H.J.M., de Grave, W.S., Wolfhagen, I.H.A.P., Oude Egbrink, M.G.A., 2021. Advancing quality culture in health professions education: Experiences and perspectives of educational leaders. Advances in Health Sciences Education: Theory and Practice 26 (2), 467–487. https://doi.org/10.1007/s10459-020-09996-5

Christensen, N., Black, L., Furze, J., Huhn, K., Vendrely, A., Wainwright, S., 2017. Clinical reasoning: Survey of teaching methods, integration, and assessment in entry-level physical therapist academic education. Phys. Ther. 97, 175–186. https://doi.org/10.2522/ptj.20150320

Christensen, N., Jensen, G.M., 2019. Developing clinical reasoning capability - Clinical reasoning in the health professions. In: Higgs, J., Jensen, G.M., Loftus, S., Christensen, N. (Eds.), Clinical reasoning in the health professions, 4th ed. Elsevier Limited, pp. 427–433.

Cooper, N., Bartlett, M., Gay, S., Hammond, A., Lillicrap, M., Matthan, J., et al., 2021. Consensus statement on the content of clinical reasoning curricula in undergraduate medical education. Medical Teacher 43 (2), 152–159. https://doi.org/10.1080/0142159X.2020.1842343

Daniel, M., Rencic, J., Durning, S.J., Holmboe, E., Santen, S.A., Lang, V., et al., 2019. Clinical reasoning assessment methods: A scoping review and practical guidance. Academic Medicine 94, 902–912. https://doi.org/10.1097/ACM.0000000000002618

Fraser, S., 2019. Understanding innovative teaching practice in higher education: A framework for reflection. Higher Education Research & Development 38 (7), 1371–1385. https://doi.org/10.1080/07294360.2019.1654439

Frenk, J., Chen, L.C., Chandran, L., Groff, E.O.H., King, R., Meleis, A., et al., 2022. Challenges and opportunities for educating health professionals after the COVID-19 pandemic. Lancet (London, England) 400 (10362), 1539–1556. https://doi.org/10.1016/S0140-6736(22)02092-X

Kavanagh, J.M., Szweda, C., 2017. A crisis in competency: The strategic and ethical imperative to assessing new graduate nurses' clinical reasoning. Nursing Education Perspectives 38 (2), 57–62. https://doi.org/10.1097/01.NEP.0000000000000112

Parodis, I., Andersson, L., Durning, S.J., Hege, I., Knez, J., Kononowicz, A.A., et al., 2021. Clinical reasoning needs to be explicitly addressed in health professions curricula: Recommendations from a European consortium. International Journal of Environmental Research and Public Health 18, 11202. https://doi.org/10.3390/ijerph182111202

Patton, N., Christensen, N., 2019. Pedagogies for teaching and learning clinical reasoning - Clinical reasoning in the health professions. In: Higgs, J., Jensen, G.M., Loftus, S., Christensen, N. (Eds.), Clinical reasoning in the health professions. Elsevier Limited, pp. 335–344.

Rao, I., 2019. A brief note on the role of ethical leadership in higher education institutions for sustainability. IUP Journal of Management Research 18 (4), 70–79.

Sudacka, M., Adler, M., Durning, S.J., Edelbring, S., Frankowska, A., Hartmann, D., et al., 2021. Why is it so difficult to implement a longitudinal clinical reasoning curriculum? A multicenter interview study on the barriers perceived by European health professions educators. BMC Medical Education 21 (1), 10. https://doi.org/10.1186/s12909-021-02960-w

Vaugh, T., Finnegan-Kessie, T., White, A., Baker, S., Valencia, A., 2022. Introducing strategic design in education (SDxE): An approach to navigating complexity and ambiguity at the micro, meso and macro layers of higher education institutions. Higher Education Research & Development 41 (1), 116–131. https://doi.org/10.1080/07294360.2021.2008325

Velthuis, F., Dekker, H., Coppoolse, R., Helmich, E., Jaarsma, D., 2021. Educators' experiences with governance in curriculum change processes: A qualitative study using rich pictures. Advances in Health Sciences Education 26 (3), 1027–1043. https://doi.org/10.1007/s10459-021-10034-1

35

DEVELOPING A CURRICULUM ON CLINICAL REASONING

THILAN P. WIJESEKERA ▪ STEVEN J. DURNING ▪ ROBERT L. TROWBRIDGE ▪ JOSEPH J. RENCIC

CHAPTER AIMS

The aims of this chapter are:

▪ to define the goals, structure and content involved in developing a health professions curriculum on clinical reasoning and
▪ to describe the types of teaching sessions and educational methods included in a clinical reasoning curriculum.

INTRODUCTION

Diagnostic error is recognized as a significant cause of morbidity and mortality (Ball and Balogh, 2016). Graber et al. estimated that up to 70% of diagnostic errors relate to cognitive processes (Graber et al., 2005). Recent studies have further reinforced that diagnostic reasoning and management reasoning play significant roles in diagnostic error (Raffel et al., 2020). Research of the past 50 years provides significant insight into the cognitive psychology of medical problem solving and decision making (Eva, 2005; Norman,

2005). Thus, with the impetus of diagnostic error that is informed by a greater understanding of the clinical reasoning process, health professions educators seek to explicitly teach the theory and practice of clinical reasoning. Although there are no randomized control trials to guide them, educators continue to apply well-supported theories to develop clinical reasoning curricula. In this chapter, we discuss theoretical and practical considerations in creating a clinical reasoning curriculum.

CURRICULUM DEVELOPMENT

The term curriculum has various definitions, but we define it as the educational content and organization of the teaching of clinical reasoning that prepares learners at a specific level of training to successfully achieve a series of specific objectives (Thomas et al., 2022). There is no uniformly agreed upon number of sessions in a clinical reasoning curriculum and the exact number of sessions will be impacted by the scope of learner's practice, the breadth of content necessary to cover and how the curriculum is structured within the broader health professions programme. There are many approaches to curriculum development including a behavioural approach (i.e. building towards an eventually observable skillset from a learner), a humanistic approach (i.e. incorporating the sociocultural aspects of learner's experience) and a systematic approach (i.e. curriculum engineering) (Hunkins and Ornstein, 2016; Trowbridge et al., 2015). For this chapter, we will apply the systematic approach of Kern's 6-step model (problem identification and general needs assessment; targeted learner needs assessment; goals and objectives; educational strategies; implementation; evaluation and feedback) for recommendations on how to create a clinical reasoning curriculum (Thomas et al., 2022).

STEP 1: PROBLEM IDENTIFICATION AND GENERAL NEEDS ASSESSMENT

Despite its integral nature to every health profession, clinical reasoning can be defined in many different ways (Young et al., 2018). For this chapter, we define clinical reasoning as:

> the cognitive and physical process by which a healthcare professional consciously and subconsciously interacts with the patient and environment to collect and interpret patient data, weigh the benefits and risks of actions, and understand patient preferences to determine a working diagnostic and therapeutic management plan whose purpose is to improve a patient's well-being.
>
> **(Rencic et al., 2016)**

Since clinical reasoning is a complex process involving a breadth of knowledge and skill that also requires extensive experience, building a curriculum for it can be challenging. It is instructive for educators to explore what is being done at a local, regional or national level relative to their own health professions programme (Rencic et al., 2017; Thomas et al., 2022). Not only does doing so help educators understand the ideal approach to a clinical reasoning curriculum at a local level, but it also identifies the gaps in their current approach and feasible options for improvement in the future.

Ideally, a general needs assessment occurs within a diverse group of core educators (e.g. deans, course directors, programme leadership, clinical instructors). Locally, this assessment can range from reviewing diagnostic outcomes (e.g. readmission rates) of learners on different clinical rotations to identifying courses in the institution where clinical reasoning is already being taught (e.g. clinical skills or basic science courses). Nationally, it might include reviewing expectations from accreditation bodies (e.g. Medical Council of Canada, Liaison Committee on Medical Education) or attending educational conferences that disseminate advances in clinical reasoning education. Internationally based organizations, such as the Society to Improve Diagnosis in Medicine (SIDM), have developed 'Competencies to Improve Diagnosis' (Olson et al., 2019). Curriculum development committees should then begin with the 'end in mind', determining developmentally appropriate clinical reasoning educational outcomes (e.g. competencies, milestones, entrustable professional activities) that learners should achieve by course or professional training. The committee should then develop course knowledge, skills and attitudes objectives in alignment with the desired educational outcomes.

STEP 2: TARGETED NEEDS ASSESSMENT

When performing a targeted needs assessment for a curriculum in clinical reasoning, educators should first consider the learners, their specific field, prior training, past performance and attitudes towards clinical reasoning (Thomas et al., 2022). Though the healthcare team includes many providers who work collaboratively, the nature of competency in clinical reasoning varies across fields. Some fields might be more perceptual, others more cognitive, and others more procedural. Specifically, each health profession has unique clinical reasoning responsibilities (i.e. problem-solving and decision-making tasks) that require relevant medical knowledge and abilities. For example, clinical reasoning expectations of a nurse are different from those of a pharmacist, occupational therapist or a speech pathologist. Similarly, the clinical reasoning within specialties of a given health profession also differs as the practice of a surgeon differs significantly from that of a paediatrician.

Beyond the *field and specialty*, it is important to consider learners' *stage of training*. Novice learners (e.g. undergraduate medical education) with limited clinical knowledge and experience benefit from highly guided and scaffolded educational activities focussed on common problems and diseases, controlled clinical experiences (e.g. standardized patients), common cognitive tasks (e.g. differential diagnosis) and more straightforward activities (e.g. clinical problem-solving exercises). More advanced learners (e.g. graduate medical education) might instead benefit from exposure to atypical disease presentations, complex clinical experiences (e.g. real patients with many comorbidities), ambiguous topics (e.g. diagnostic error, treatment thresholds) and more nuanced activities (e.g. morbidity and mortality conferences). The stage of training and degree of learner experience may also impact the preferred learning setting, ranging from classroom to clinic or from individual to large group settings. In addition to learners, other stakeholders to include in a targeted needs assessment include course directors, teachers, patients and administrators (Thomas et al., 2022). Soliciting input from these stakeholders can occur through interviews, focus groups, surveys or even test scores. Using the SWOT analysis framework (i.e. Strengths, Weaknesses, Opportunities, Threats) can be valuable in curriculum design and refinement (Gordon et al., 2000).

REFLECTION POINT

Reflection Questions for Educators

Here are some questions to consider in a needs assessment for your clinical reasoning curriculum:
1. How is clinical reasoning defined by you, your institution and the relevant accreditation bodies in your health profession?
2. Considering their stage of training, what clinical reasoning outcomes are important for your learners?
3. What are realistic times and settings for incorporating clinical reasoning education into your health professions school or training?
4. What are potential barriers for developing a clinical reasoning curriculum at your institution?

STEP 3: GOALS AND OBJECTIVES

Creating a road map for a clinical reasoning curriculum should include broad educational goals and specific measurable objectives by which to achieve them. Broad educational goals might relate to a defined set of competencies (e.g. patient care, medical knowledge, system-based practice) that may include or be included in clinical reasoning (Connor et al., 2020). Other competencies may be more specific to clinical reasoning such as SIDM's 'Competencies to Improve Diagnosis', which has not only individual but team-based and system-related competencies (Olson and Graber, 2020). Objectives should thus be specific and measurable towards supporting and defining a curriculum's educational goals with a potential template being 'who will do how much of what by when' (Thomas et al., 2022). It might be helpful to consider clinical reasoning competencies as end goals (i.e. the desired educational outcome for learners to accomplish) and the objectives as means goals (i.e. actions for learners designed to work towards that desired educational outcome). Educators can develop goals for individual learners as well as the broader curriculum across both educational (e.g. cognitive, attitudinal, skill) and patient care outcomes (e.g. diagnostic error). To inform the writing of specific objectives, educators can lean on foundational clinical reasoning concepts (Table 35.1). Although abstract, cognitive models, theories and terminology provide helpful scaffolds for teachers and learners in the incorporation, application and calibration of knowledge and experience.

Cognitive Model

Although there is no universal model for clinical reasoning, most analytical reasoning models of the diagnostic process of clinical reasoning are based in the scientific method: observations lead to the framing of a question to be answered or a problem to be solved, which leads to hypothesis generation, which leads to the search for evidence to prove one of those hypotheses most likely and the subsequent actions based on this conclusion. Thus, four typically described steps in the clinical reasoning process include data collection, problem representation, generating and prioritizing a differential diagnosis, and management (Bowen, 2006; Thammasitboon et al., 2018). *Data collection* is

	TABLE 35.1	
	Examples of Learning Objectives in a Curriculum	
Clinical Reasoning Component	Educational Objective (Ends)	Educational Objective (Means)
Data collection	Accurately and efficiently collect key clinical findings needed to inform diagnostic hypotheses	By the end of the clinical reasoning course, each student will have taken a hypothesis driven history and physical examination in 5 different patient encounters
Problem representation	Formulate, or contribute to, an accurate problem representation that includes essential epidemiological, clinical and psychosocial information	By the end of the clinical reasoning course, each student will have presented a problem representation on 10 different patient cases
Differential diagnosis	Explain and justify the prioritization of the differential diagnosis by comparing and contrasting each patient's findings and test results	By the end of the clinical reasoning course, each student will have explained a differential diagnosis for 3 case examples on 10 common chief concerns
Management	Engage and collaborate with patients and families, in accordance with their values and preferences, when making a plan for testing and treatment	By the end of the clinical reasoning course, each student will have described a management plan for 5 separate patient cases

the process of identifying relevant historical, physical, laboratory and/or imaging information (Bowen, 2006). *Problem representation* describes how relevant information is synthesized by the clinician, often in the form of a one-line summary of a patient's presentation (Bowen, 2006). *Prioritizing a differential diagnosis* starts with identifying possible diagnoses and then using supporting and refuting information to estimate their likelihood (Thammasitboon et al., 2018). *Management* is the process of identifying possible interventions and implementing them (Cook et al., 2019; Cook et al., 2018). Management reasoning can be further subdivided into testing and therapeutic reasoning. Of note, like the scientific method, it is important to emphasize that clinical reasoning is an iterative and nonlinear process; a healthcare professional may leap unconsciously to a visual diagnosis such as herpes zoster with minimal conscious data collection or problem representation. Furthermore, learners should understand that clinical reasoning is context dependent, meaning that interactions between healthcare professionals, patients and the environment powerfully influence diagnostic and management decisions (Konopasky et al., 2020).

Pertinent Theories

Drawing on the cognitive psychology and educational literature, some notable theories to consider in developing a clinical reasoning curriculum include information processing (e.g. dual process theory, script theory, cognitive load), expertise (e.g. deliberate practice) and situativity (e.g. ecological psychology) (Table 35.2). Dual process theory describes two approaches to thinking: fast or nonanalytical thinking (system 1) and slow or analytical (system 2) thinking (Croskerry, 2009; Kahneman, 2011). Although experts more often use system 1 and novices more often use system 2, it is important that a curriculum include instruction on and provide exercises to improve both (Croskerry et al., 2014; Mamede et al., 2020; Mamede et al., 2010; Trowbridge et al., 2015). In clinical reasoning, cognitive load theory describes the different types of cognitive stressors (e.g. intrinsic, extrinsic, germane load) that can affect working memory for learning and performance (e.g. educational and clinical). For example, a student or trainee would have trouble making the correct diagnosis in a patient presenting with 10 to 15 symptoms and signs because they would have trouble chunking (i.e. organizing information into larger units that can be better stored and accessed through long-term memory) those findings (Young et al., 2014). Situativity theories emphasize the role of context (or the specifics of the situation) and include a broader collection of theories such as situated cognition, ecological psychology, embodied cognition and distributed cognition (Durning and Artino, 2011; Merkebu

TABLE 35.2 Clinical Reasoning Theory Based Educational Strategies	
Theory	**Educational Strategies**
Dual Process Theory	**System 1:** Pattern recognition exercises (e.g. pictures of pathognomonic findings, flashcards with buzzwords for a diagnosis) that focus on rapid diagnosis and management decisions
	System 2: Analytical reasoning exercises (e.g. case conferences) where learners consider pre-test probability, sensitivity/specificity of tests, and reflect on thought process during and after the case
Cognitive Load Theory	**Novice learner:** Focus on typical case presentations of common diseases
	Advanced learner: Include atypical case presentations of common disease and typical presentations of uncommon diseases
Situativity Theory	**Novice learner:** Limit contextual factors in cases, focus more on classroom or simulation experiences
	Advanced learner: Increase contextual factors and complexity in simulated encounters (e.g. time limitations, multiple concurrent tasks); focus more on real clinical encounters
Deliberate Practice Theory	**Volume:** Include numerous simulated and real domain-specific cases of varying difficulty, context and content for problems (e.g. 20 chest pain cases) and diseases (e.g. myocardial infarction, pneumonia)
	Types of exercises: Learners should receive specific and timely feedback on their performance from a teacher or coach (virtual or real) and devise a plan for improvement
Schema	**Cognitive strategies:** Share and encourage learners to build diagnostic frameworks with learners for specific problems (e.g. acute kidney injury framework of pre-renal, intrarenal and post renal causes)
	Mental models: Develop learner's illness scripts by encouraging teachers to ask students to elaborate on their understanding of diseases' epidemiology, pathophysiology and clinical features

et al., 2020). As learners progress, it can be valuable to layer in more contextual complexity (e.g. time limitations, multiple concurrent tasks) to prepare learners for a more realistic practice of clinical reasoning.

Deliberate practice theory proposes that the development of expert performance comes from application of knowledge and a skill in an intentional and coached fashion (Ericsson, 2004). Since curricular time can be limited, it is important to truly be deliberate whenever possible in educational encounters by having the learner reflect (before, during and after the encounter), ideally with some sort of supervisor (Rencic, 2011). Another strategy to overcome the lack of resources is through adaptive expertise, encouraging learners to not only use known solutions but to draw on their knowledge and past experience to solve problems in an unfamiliar situation (Mylopoulos, 2020; Mylopoulos and Kulasegaram, 2018; Mylopoulos et al., 2018). Some of the most valuable tools for developing clinical reasoning are diagnostic frameworks for organizing and approaching information (Vandewaetere et al., 2015). Cognitive strategies help provide a more systematic approach to a problem with examples being rules-of-thumb (e.g. heuristics) or formal guidelines (e.g. treatment protocol). Mental models are more personalized structures for organizing information such as an illness script (i.e. an individual's 'mental file' or understanding of a given condition) (Custers, 2015; Custers et al., 1996).

Emerging Perspectives

Some additional perspectives that are increasingly being highlighted in the clinical reasoning literature and worth considering for incorporating into a curriculum include diagnostic error, uncertainty, Bayesian reasoning, thresholds, metacognition, collaboration and technology. Introducing diagnostic error to any stage can help learners understand the value of a clinical reasoning curriculum and provide important context for other topics and exercises. Uncertainty – defined as a lack of knowledge around a situation – is prevalent in nearly every clinician's practice and can occur in both diagnosis and management (Bhise et al., 2017; Han et al., 2011). Parsing out the teaching aspects of uncertainty can be challenging but often include the approach to complexity and probability or the likelihood of any given option. Encourage learners to become comfortable, but not complacent, with uncertainty while finding ways to approach uncertain situations. One approach to uncertainty is Bayesian (or probabilistic) reasoning, where a clinician considers the pretest probability of multiple diagnoses in a healthcare problem and performs relevant tests that increase or decrease the probability of each possible diagnosis (Brush et al., 2019). As learners understand how to estimate probabilities, their curriculum can correspondingly teach the role of thresholds and the probability where an intervention's risk of harms is equal to its benefits (Pauker and Kassirer, 1980; Stojan et al., 2022). Considerations for a testing or treatment threshold might include, but are not necessarily limited to, intervention factors (e.g. harms, benefits, operator characteristics), disease factors (i.e. risk of harm) and patient factors (e.g. acuity, comorbidities, goals of care) (Abdoler et al., 2020).

Metacognition – an individual's monitoring and regulating of their clinical reasoning – is a potentially helpful cognitive practice. Discussing cognitive biases (e.g. premature closure, anchoring bias, availability bias and confirmation bias) and debiasing strategies to mitigate their effect have been proposed as a means of teaching clinical reasoning and improving its practice. Despite the appeal of this approach, however, there is disagreement over its effectiveness in teaching and improving clinical reasoning abilities (Croskerry et al., 2013; Lambe et al., 2016; Royce et al., 2019; Sherbino et al., 2014). Clinical reasoning is also not practised individually. Thus, collaborative diagnostic reasoning is becoming a more frequently discussed topic in health professions education (Graber et al., 2017). Given the increasingly specialized skillsets of providers, learners should be taught about the roles of other health professions and engage in dialogue with each other to understand their patients (Olson and Graber, 2020). With technology increasingly becoming a core component of medical education and practice of medicine, it would be advantageous for a clinical reasoning curriculum to include some exposure to clinician decision support systems and artificial intelligence, i.e. the use of a digital computational program to facilitate the diagnosis and management of a patient (Pinnock et al., 2020). Because artificial intelligence has shortcomings, largely secondary to the underlying data sets, students should become familiar with how to use these resources as an adjunct to their own clinical reasoning (Lee et al., 2023; Rajpurkar et al., 2018; Sibbald et al., 2022; Strong et al., 2023).

STEP 4: EDUCATIONAL METHODS

There are many different educational methods that can be included in a clinical reasoning curriculum. Some examples of educational methods include, but are not limited to, readings, lectures, small-group learning, demonstration, standardized patients and real patient experiences (Thomas et al., 2022). Some of the advantages and disadvantages of each method in addition to a clinical reasoning example are included in Table 35.3 (Thomas et al., 2022). When choosing educational methods for a clinical reasoning curriculum, it can be helpful to use the four-component instructional design model (4 C/ID) (Vandewaetere et al., 2015). The 4 C/ID posits four key elements of instructional design for developing performance of complex skills: learning tasks, supportive information, procedural information and part-task practice (e.g. problem representation). Using these components effectively with repeated whole-task practice (e.g. diagnosing a standardized patient) in a longitudinal curriculum will lead to complex skill/ability development like clinical reasoning (Vandewaetere et al., 2015).

General Teaching Principles

Guiding principles for the design of sessions in a clinical reasoning curriculum include a focus on patient cases, retrieval practice, learner reflection and feedback (Cooper et al., 2021). Patient cases are valuable because they allow educators to expose learners to conditions and situations that they might encounter in the clinical setting and share frameworks on how to approach them (Guerrasio and Aagaard, 2014; Kassirer, 2010; ten Cate et al., 2017). Cases can vary in the patient characteristics, problems and diseases presented, and clinical reasoning abilities being developed. In the classroom setting, case information is *crafted*, whereas in the clinical setting, patients are *selected* based on a learner's knowledge and skill level. After choosing a focus for a case, the educator has to curate how much clinical information will be provided and when to provide it, which can alter the focus and complexity of the exercise. While real cases can be more

| | **TABLE 35.3** | | |
| | **Clinical Reasoning Educational Methods Examples** | | |
Method	Advantages	Disadvantages	Example
Readings	Low cost, builds medical knowledge, minimal preparation	Passive learning, requires motivation	Article on dual process theory
Lectures	Low cost, large number of learners, structured presentation (particularly valuable for complicated topics)	Passive learning, teacher-centered, dependent on audiovisual methods	Lecture on diagnostic error
Small group learning	Active learning, flexible formats, helps identify learner needs, encourages collaboration and different perspectives	Teacher intensive (can benefit from training), requires base knowledge from learners	Case-based discussion (e.g. morning report) on a patient with chest pain
Demonstration	Efficiency, role modeling	Teacher dependent, variable learner interactions (often passive), difficult to assess learner outcomes	Master clinician rounds with teachers talking out loud through a challenging case
Standardized patients	Better control of teaching material, approximate real life, feedback and reflection opportunities	Requires baseline learner knowledge, requires faculty supervision, time intensive	Observed Structured Clinical Experience (OSCE) with a note (including a differential diagnosis)
Real patient experiences	Highest fidelity to clinical practice, promotes learner motivation and responsibility, feedback and reflection opportunities	Requires baseline learner knowledge, variability of experiences, requires faculty supervision	Student on clinical rotation seeing patient and presenting to healthcare team

memorable, educators should feel empowered to alter details of a real case or even use entirely fictional cases if it better fits their learners' developmental level and the desired level of cognitive load. Educators should also consider the time allotted and the sequence of information, although there is some evidence that presenting an entire case is better for junior learners than serially cued cases (i.e. parts of case revealed sequentially) because it reduces cognitive load (Schmidt and Mamede, 2015).

With cases as the prompt, curriculum developers should encourage retrieval practice in their learners. Retrieval practice activities can begin by having learners, particularly if novice, develop problem lists at a certain stage (or multiple stages) of a case to ensure that they are correctly identifying the relevant information (Cooper et al., 2021). Automaticity of knowledge retrieval in clinical contexts (e.g. the diagnosis 'pops' into the learner's head while talking to a patient) is a hallmark of expertise; therefore learning activities that improve rapid recall are additionally valuable (e.g. digital flash cards, jeopardy game) (Larsen et al., 2009). Reflection can be fostered by having learners

compare and contrast options to better discriminate *what* considerations factored into their decisions (e.g. their differential diagnoses or management plan) and by *how* much (Ark et al., 2007). For example, structured reflection is a form of retrieval practice where learners not only identify alternative diagnoses but also explicitly describe information in a case that supports or refutes that diagnosis (Mamede et al., 2012; Mamede et al., 2014). When learners use self-explanation, particularly for complex patients, they are more likely to understand their patients, to connect clinical to biomedical knowledge and to improve their diagnostic performance (Chamberland et al., 2013; Chamberland et al., 2015). With both retrieval practice and reflection, teacher feedback and modelling are essential (Cooper et al., 2021). Without specific, timely and individualized feedback, learners are unlikely to realize rapid gains in their abilities, especially given the complexity inherent to clinical reasoning.

Teaching in the Classroom

Within the classroom, lectures still have a place in a clinical reasoning curriculum, but it is important to be aware of their strengths and weaknesses (Table 35.3). Lectures can be helpful for efficiently communicating material particularly if limited by teacher availability or time constraints (Friesen, 2011). They can also be helpful conveying challenging concepts that could lead to learner confusion (e.g. introducing and walking through an algorithm for approaching chronic cough). Some best practices for incorporating lectures into a curriculum include making them brief, interactive and case-based. One form of large group session that remains popular is the clinical problem-solving exercise (CPS). During a CPS, an expert clinician is presented an unknown case and asked to explain their clinical reasoning at various intervals, often with questions from the audience or facilitators (Dhaliwal and Sharpe, 2009). Such a session can be modified to require students to solve the case simultaneously providing their answers in audience participation systems or small groups prior to hearing the expert's opinions.

Whether virtual or in-person, small group exercises are the primary and most popular type of session in a clinical reasoning curriculum. Formatted as team-based learning, problem-based learning or case-based conferences (CBC), small group exercises in clinical reasoning usually include a facilitator(s) and fewer than 10 learners who discuss the diagnosis and/or management of a case (ten Cate et al., 2017). A common and popular type of CBC is a type of clinical teaching conference called morning report (Amin et al., 2000). Traditionally held daily and in-person with trainees (e.g. resident physicians), morning report involves a learner presenting a case in a scripted, serial cue fashion (i.e. progressive revealing of information) for colleagues to solve while teachers facilitate (Amin et al., 2000; Ways et al., 1995). Morning report has since been adapted in numerous fashions including virtual and unscripted formats for different types and levels of learners at varying times during the day (Lessing et al., 2020; Murdock et al., 2020). Another important type of CBC is the morbidity and mortality conference, where learners and clinicians debrief on a patient case where an adverse event has occurred to identify possible aetiologies, often including root-cause-analysis techniques (Orlander et al., 2002; Pierluissi et al., 2003). Although cognitive errors are not always identified as a culprit, morbidity and mortality conferences provide a valuable opportunity for interdisciplinary discussions around clinical reasoning and the effect that systems and environment can have on clinical reasoning (George, 2017).

Due to their resource intensity, individualized clinical reasoning teaching sessions are rare in the classroom setting, but useful when available. One-on-one sessions such as low stakes quizzing can be formative and particularly effective in retrieval practice around many different conditions and domains (Green et al., 2018). Some other individual exercises targeting specific parts of the clinical reasoning process include 'thinking base rate' to practice epidemiology, 'highlighter exercise' for identifying important information in a case, or 'playing the role' to explore a learner's illness scripts (Parsons et al., 2022). Oral exams are another opportunity not just to assess but also to teach a learner clinical reasoning. During an oral exam, a teacher can use a case to ask learners relevant scripted or unscripted questions to probe a learner's clinical reasoning and give the feedback as appropriate (Daniel et al., 2019; Memon et al., 2010). The case format can be through a paper vignette or even a standardized patient, the latter of which gives teachers the opportunity to observe a learner's data collection in an authentic but controlled setting. Such simulations exercises can also be in a group or virtual setting, too (Ilgen et al., 2013).

Teaching in the Clinical Setting

Teaching clinical reasoning concurrent with providing patient care necessitates educational choices for teachers before, during and after the clinical encounter. As previously mentioned, teachers should consider their learners' knowledge and experience while being mindful of a patient's complexity before selecting one for their learner. Examples of complexity could include the environment (e.g. a 15-minute encounter in a busy emergency department versus a 30-minute encounter in a private clinic room), the availability of clinical data (i.e. ability of a patient to provide a history or physical exam) or the case itself (e.g. a hospitalized patient with a single, straightforward chief concern versus a clinic patient with five complex agenda items). To facilitate the encounter, teachers could potentially prime the learners by discussing the case in advance or having them look at the chart, although that could lead to cueing and premature closure, respectively.

During the encounter, teachers can choose which level of supervision to provide for their learner. Directly observing a whole encounter can be extremely valuable to understand better a learner's strengths and weaknesses (Daniel et al., 2019). It also provides the teachers the opportunity to fill in and demonstrate areas (e.g. hypothesis-driven history questions) where some learners might struggle in their clinical reasoning. Unfortunately, teachers do not always have the time to fully supervise their learners but can either observe part of an encounter or follow-up afterward. Another option for developing clinical reasoning during an encounter is for multiple learners – at the same or different levels – to potentially interview and examine a patient together.

After a clinical encounter, learners can synthesize their thoughts into an oral and/or written presentation, which can provide rich opportunities for teaching and assessing clinical reasoning (Schaye et al., 2022). Presentations require sufficient time to prepare, ranging from minutes to hours depending on the learner and case. Teachers should provide clear guidelines to their learners on the format and organization of the presentation, so that they can focus on inputting the appropriate information and explaining their clinical reasoning. For example, written presentation formats include a narrative or list format with the former potentially showing improvement in diagnostic accuracy (Payton et al., 2023). While often formatted similarly, case presentations can typically be synthesized more quickly (possibly even immediately after seeing a patient) and provide an opportunity for teachers to engage in real-time discussions with their learners on their clinical reasoning. However, case presentations are time sensitive because clinical data change as patients evolve over time. By contrast, although written presentations take time to complete, they provide an opportunity for teachers to provide feedback at any time. Ideally, the dialogue and feedback occur relatively proximal to the note-writing so that the learner can accurately recall their thoughts at the time of writing. For example, chart-stimulated recall involves teachers reviewing a learner's note from a patient encounter, probing their thought processes, providing feedback and co-creating an action plan to improve performance on future patient encounters (Philibert, 2018; Reddy et al., 2015). Learners can also benefit from keeping patient logs on their clinical encounters with intermittent reflections looking at diagnostic outcomes and errors. Follow-up of patient experiences should be done with their supervisor at the time and potentially a longitudinal coach. Longitudinal coaches who work with learners for several years, which have become more prevalent in health professions education, can be a valuable resource in teaching clinical reasoning given that it is such a complex ability that takes years to develop (Gonzalo et al., 2019; Parsons et al., 2021).

Asynchronous Learning

Because of the limited class time available and the volume of cases necessary to develop clinical reasoning, it can be useful for educators to incorporate asynchronous learning into their curriculum. Asynchronous learning resources can include, but are not limited to, textbooks, journal articles, digital programs or even social media (Manesh and Dhaliwal, 2018). One potential use of these resources could be to explain key theories in clinical reasoning, build general knowledge or provide approaches to important chief concerns (Croskerry et al., 2017; Stern et al., 2015). Another option could be 'worked cases', i.e. written clinical vignettes where senior clinicians have provided their clinical reasoning at various stages of a case (Kassirer et al., 2010; Steinhilber and Estrada, 2017). Recently, 'reason-encoded' databases of common signs, symptoms, labs and imaging have even been created from clinical pathological conferences with natural language processing (Zack et al., 2023). Podcasts such as *The Clinical Problem Solvers, The Curbsiders* and *Core IM* have also become a particularly popular way to teach clinical reasoning through worked cases (Berk et al., 2020).

Virtual patients, i.e. interactive computer programs that simulate real clinical scenarios, are another option for learning clinical reasoning asynchronously (Cook and Triola, 2009). Desirable features in virtual cases include a deep database of clinical scenarios with multiple cases for a given chief concern in addition to distractors to minimize cueing and options for feedback (Manesh and Dhaliwal, 2018). There has been a burgeoning market for virtual patients, both free and proprietary, and educators should evaluate each closely before making the time and monetary investment for their learners. Some examples include *Aquifer, NEJM's Interactive Medical Cases, Teaching Medicine* and *The Human Diagnosis Project* (Abbasi, 2018; Olson et al., 2019; Waechter et al., 2022). There are also public forums for learners to engage in live CPS exercises (e.g. 'virtual morning report') (Murdock et al., 2020). Learners and teachers can even engage with experts in the field through social media (e.g. chats on sites such as X) (Olson and Graber, 2020).

REFLECTION POINT

Reflection Questions for Educators

Here are some questions to consider in a needs assessment for your clinical reasoning curriculum:

1. With your potential clinical reasoning curricular time, which classroom and clinical teaching methods would be realistic and valuable for your learners?
2. How could you supplement your curricular time with asynchronous learning exercises?
3. Which clinical reasoning concepts, theories and perspectives do you want to prioritize for your learners?
4. Who are possible facilitators, coaches and teachers for your educational sessions? What incentives and professional development do they need?

STEP 5: IMPLEMENTATION

In considering implementation, identify resources, obtain support, develop administrative mechanisms and address barriers through a piloting, maintenance and enhancement of a clinical reasoning curriculum (Thomas et al., 2022). Personnel could include academics (e.g. course director[s] and facilitators), administrators and patients (i.e. real or simulated). Curriculum developers should also be mindful of the facilities necessary, which can include classroom space, clinical sites or virtual space. Each of these resources could require different amounts of funding and costs including salary support and protected time. Support can come through internal funding (e.g. deans, department chairs, programme directors) or external funding (e.g. accreditation bodies, grants and philanthropy) with educators tailoring their curricula to those stakeholder expectations (Thomas et al., 2022).

A curriculum's timing (both scheduling and quantity) will play a pivotal role in what should be implemented and how that can be achieved. For example, if the clinical reasoning course is independent, the course leadership will probably have greater flexibility in instructional design, but learners may view the course as less important compared with wider courses (e.g. anatomy, pathophysiology, clinical skills) within the curriculum. On the other hand, if clinical reasoning is integrated into another course, curriculum developers might be able to create a more longitudinal experience with spaced learning and repetition but will probably have to use instructional methods typical of that course. Ideally, a clinical reasoning course is longitudinal with some dedicated elements but will also have threads woven into other related and larger courses. Based on the structure of the curriculum, educators should delineate responsibilities around content (e.g. objectives, materials) and communication (e.g. e-mails, learning management systems), accordingly. Every institution's clinical reasoning curriculum will be different and curriculum developers should work with other stakeholders to create sessions that are realistic to learner needs and resources available.

Prior to piloting the curriculum, educators should anticipate potential barriers including resource limitations (e.g. availability of classrooms or patients), competing demands (e.g. clinical expectations versus teaching) and personal challenges (e.g. conflicts with course leadership on course direction) (Thomas et al., 2022). Some examples of common barriers and potential solutions are included in Table 35.4. Curriculum developers should then begin a pilot with a phase-in of some of the educational sessions (or components of a session) to identify additional barriers and promising findings, while addressing the former and increasing the latter as reasonably possible. After full implementation of the curriculum, educators should continue to find ways to improve and streamline curricular operations. We also strongly believe that the final curriculum should be integrated both horizontally (i.e. within different courses to some degree in the same year) and vertically (i.e. in every year of the training programme) to maximize its impact.

TABLE 35.4

Barriers and Solutions for Teaching Clinical Reasoning

Barrier	Solutions
No gold standard for design	■ Ground educational sessions in theory and curriculum development strategies ■ Employ multiple different types of teaching strategies ■ Engage stakeholders in needs assessment to determine feasible educational methods
Vast scope and/or limited curricular time	■ Teach components, theories and schema for clinical reasoning ■ Utilize different types of asynchronous learning for different case opportunities ■ Incorporate into other associated courses (e.g. basic sciences, clinical skills)
Lack of expert teachers to teach and assess clinical reasoning	■ Create detailed instructor guides for each session and host faculty development sessions ■ Incentivize faculty with salary and professional support (e.g. letters of recommendation) ■ Utilize senior learners (i.e. peer teachers) as instructors

STEP 6: EVALUATION

When evaluating the curriculum, educators should consider the stakeholders (e.g. learners, teachers), content (e.g. educational sessions) and resources (e.g. facilities, equipment) involved in addition to any objectives and associated evaluation methods initially planned (Thomas et al., 2022). Ideally, evaluation is planned in advance and built into certain points of the curriculum to increase the fidelity and yield of the data acquired in addition to facilitating any institutional review board process. There are many different methods for evaluating a clinical reasoning curriculum each with different strengths and limitations with regards to feasibility, reliability and validity. Educators should also be mindful of concerns regarding confidentiality, consent and impact of the evaluation methods on their constituents. Educators should plan how they plan to collect, store and analyse any data they obtain from their evaluations (Thomas et al., 2022). Although beyond the scope of this chapter, assessment of learners' clinical reasoning is an important component of any cur-

riculum. It can also be helpful to get feedback from learners on the effectiveness of and their satisfaction with the chosen educational practices through surveys, interviews and/or focus groups. Similarly, it can also be helpful to get feedback on the teachers about their strengths and areas for improvement for educational sessions. This feedback should be used to improve the curriculum using the institution's existing quality improvement structures (e.g. plan-do-study-act model).

CONCLUSION

Dedicated clinical reasoning curricula are growing across health professions educational programmes with reducing diagnostic error and accreditation body expectations as motivation. Although there is no universally agreed structure for designing a curriculum, it can be helpful to use evidence-based theories adapted to clinical reasoning and standard curriculum design principles. Clinical reasoning curricula should be created and modified based on your learner needs, potential settings, institutional expectations, technological trends and feedback from regularly scheduled curriculum evaluations.

SUMMARY

In this chapter we have presented the following:

■ Clinical reasoning is an important, but complex process, for health professions learners and requires a thoughtful approach to curriculum development.

■ Kern's 6-step model (problem identification and general needs assessment; targeted learner needs assessment; goals and objectives; educational strategies; implementation; evaluation and feedback) can be a helpful approach for clinical reasoning curriculum development.

■ Grounding a clinical reasoning curriculum in a cognitive model, key theories and emerging perspectives can be helpful for developing content.

■ Every clinical reasoning curriculum will be different and curriculum developers should blend classroom, clinical and/or asynchronous educational sessions to fit their learners and resources.

REFERENCES

Abbasi, J., 2018. Shantanu Nundy, MD: The Human Diagnosis Project. JAMA 319 (4), 329–331. https://doi.org/10.1001/jama.2017.13897

Abdoler, E.A., O'Brien, B.C., Schwartz, B.S., 2020. Following the script: An exploratory study of the therapeutic reasoning underlying physicians' choice of antimicrobial therapy. Acad Med 95 (8), 1238–1247. https://doi.org/10.1097/acm.0000000000003498

Amin, Z., Guajardo, J., Wisniewski, W., Bordage, G., Tekian, A., Niederman, L.G., 2000. Morning report: Focus and methods over the past three decades. Acad Med 75 (Suppl 10), S1–S5. https://doi.org/10.1097/00001888-200010001-00002

Ark, T.K., Brooks, L.R., Eva, K.W., 2007. The benefits of flexibility: The pedagogical value of instructions to adopt multifaceted diagnostic reasoning strategies. Med Educ 41 (3), 281–287. https://doi.org/10.1111/j.1365-2929.2007.02688.x

Ball, J.R., Balogh, E., 2016. Improving diagnosis in health care: Highlights of a report from the National Academies of Sciences, Engineering, and Medicine. Annals of Internal Medicine 164 (1), 59–61. https://doi.org/10.7326/M15-2256

Berk, J., Trivedi, S.P., Watto, M., Williams, P., Centor, R., 2020. Medical education podcasts: Where we are and questions unanswered. J Gen Intern Med 35 (7), 2176–2178. https://doi.org/10.1007/s11606-019-05606-2

Bhise, V., Rajan, S.S., Sittig, D.F., Morgan, R.O., Chaudhary, P., Singh, H., 2017. Defining and measuring diagnostic uncertainty in medicine: A systematic review. J Gen Intern Med 33 (1), 1–13. https://doi.org/10.1007/s11606-017-4164-1

Bowen, J.L., 2006. Educational strategies to promote clinical diagnostic reasoning. N Engl J Med 355 (21), 2217–2225. https://doi.org/10.1056/NEJMra054782

Brush J.E. Jr., Lee, M., Sherbino, J., Taylor-Fishwick, J.C., Norman, G., 2019. Effect of teaching Bayesian methods using learning by concept vs learning by example on medical students' ability to estimate probability of a diagnosis: A randomized clinical trial. JAMA Netw Open 2 (12), e1918023. https://doi.org/10.1001/jamanetworkopen.2019.18023

Chamberland, M., Mamede, S., St-Onge, C., Rivard, M.A., Setrakian, J., Lévesque, A., et al., 2013. Students' self-explanations while solving unfamiliar cases: The role of biomedical knowledge. Med Educ 47 (11), 1109–1116. https://doi.org/10.1111/medu.12253

Chamberland, M., Mamede, S., St-Onge, C., Setrakian, J., Bergeron, L., Schmidt, H., 2015. Self-explanation in learning clinical reasoning: The added value of examples and prompts. Med Educ 49 (2), 193–202. https://doi.org/10.1111/medu.12623

Connor, D.M., Durning, S.J., Rencic, J.J., 2020. Clinical reasoning as a core competency. Acad Med 95 (8), 1166–1171. https://doi.org/10.1097/acm.0000000000003027

Cook, D.A., Durning, S.J., Sherbino, J., Gruppen, L.D., 2019. Management reasoning: Implications for health professions educators and a research approach agenda. Acad Med 94 (9), 1310–1316. https://doi.org/10.1097/acm.0000000000002768

Cook, D.A., Sherbino, J., Durning, S.J., 2018. Management reasoning: Beyond the diagnosis. JAMA 319 (22), 2267–2268. https://doi.org/10.1001/jama.2018.4385

Cook, D.A., Triola, M.M., 2009. Virtual patients: A critical literature review and proposed next steps. Med Educ 43 (4), 303–311. https://doi.org/10.1111/j.1365-2923.2008.03286.x

Cooper, N., Bartlett, M., Gay, S., Hammond, A., Lillicrap, M., Matthan, J., et al., 2021. Consensus statement on the content of clinical reasoning curricula in undergraduate medical education. Med Teach 43 (2), 152–159. https://doi.org/10.1080/0142159x.2020.1842343

Croskerry, P., 2009. A universal model of diagnostic reasoning. Acad Med 84 (8), 1022–1028. https://doi.org/10.1097/ACM.0b013e3181ace703

Croskerry, P., Cosby, K., Graber, M.L., Singh, H., 2017. Diagnosis: Interpreting the shadows. CRC Press.

Croskerry, P., Petrie, D.A., Reilly, J.B., Tait, G., 2014. Deciding about fast and slow decisions. Acad Med 89 (2), 197–200. https://doi.org/10.1097/acm.0000000000000121

Croskerry, P., Singhal, G., Mamede, S., 2013. Cognitive debiasing 2: Impediments to and strategies for change. BMJ Qual Saf 22 (Suppl 2), ii65–ii72. https://doi.org/10.1136/bmjqs-2012-001713

Custers, E.J., 2015. Thirty years of illness scripts: Theoretical origins and practical applications. Med Teach 37 (5), 457–462. https://doi.org/10.3109/0142159x.2014.956052

Custers, E.J., Regehr, G., Norman, G.R., 1996. Mental representations of medical diagnostic knowledge: A review. Acad Med 71 (Suppl 10), S55–S61. https://doi.org/10.1097/00001888-199610000-00044

Daniel, M., Rencic, J., Durning, S.J., Holmboe, E., Santen, S.A., Lang, V., et al., 2019. Clinical reasoning assessment methods: A scoping review and practical guidance. Acad Med 94 (6), 902–912. https://doi.org/10.1097/acm.0000000000002618

Dhaliwal, G., Sharpe, B.A., 2009. Twelve tips for presenting a clinical problem solving exercise. Med Teach 31 (12), 1056–1059. https://doi.org/10.3109/01421590902912103

Durning, S.J., Artino, A.R., 2011. Situativity theory: A perspective on how participants and the environment can interact: AMEE Guide no. 52. Med Teach 33 (3), 188–199. https://doi.org/10.3109/0142159x.2011.550965

Ericsson, K.A., 2004. Deliberate practice and the acquisition and maintenance of expert performance in medicine and related domains. Acad Med 79 (Suppl 10), S70–S81. https://doi.org/10.1097/00001888-200410001-00022

Eva, K.W., 2005. What every teacher needs to know about clinical reasoning. Medical Education 39 (1), 98–106. https://doi.org/10.1111/j.1365-2929.2004.01972.x

Friesen, N., 2011. The lecture as a transmedial pedagogical form: A historical analysis. Educational Researcher 40 (3), 95–102.

George, J., 2017. Medical morbidity and mortality conferences: Past, present and future. Postgrad Med J 93 (1097), 148–152. https://doi.org/10.1136/postgradmedj-2016-134103

Gonzalo, J.D., Wolpaw, D.R., Krok, K.L., Pfeiffer, M.P., McCall-Hosenfeld, J.S., 2019. A developmental approach to internal medicine residency education: Lessons learned from the design and implementation of a novel longitudinal coaching program. Medical Education Online 24 (1), 1591256. https://doi.org/10.1080/10872981.2019.1591256

Gordon, J., Hazlett, C., Ten Cate, O., Mann, K., Kilminster, S., Prince, K., et al., 2000. Strategic planning in medical education: Enhancing the learning environment for students in clinical settings. Med Educ 34 (10), 841–850. https://doi.org/10.1046/j.1365-2923.2000.00759.x

Graber, M.L., Franklin, N., Gordon, R., 2005. Diagnostic error in internal medicine. Arch Intern Med 165 (13), 1493–1499. https://doi.org/10.1001/archinte.165.13.1493

Graber, M.L., Rusz, D., Jones, M.L., Farm-Franks, D., Jones, B., Cyr Gluck, J., et al., 2017. The new diagnostic team. Diagnosis (Berl) 4 (4), 225–238. https://doi.org/10.1515/dx-2017-0022

Green, M.L., Moeller, J.J., Spak, J.M., 2018. Test-enhanced learning in health professions education: A systematic review: BEME Guide No. 48. Med Teach 40 (4), 337–350. https://doi.org/10.1080/0142159x.2018.1430354

Guerrasio, J., Aagaard, E.M., 2014. Methods and outcomes for the remediation of clinical reasoning. J Gen Intern Med 29 (12), 1607–1614. https://doi.org/10.1007/s11606-014-2955-1

Han, P.K., Klein, W.M., Arora, N.K., 2011. Varieties of uncertainty in health care: A conceptual taxonomy. Medical Decision Making 31 (6), 828–838. https://doi.org/10.1177/0272989x11393976

Hunkins, F.P., Ornstein, A.C., 2016. Curriculum: Foundations, principles, and issues. Pearson Education.

Ilgen, J.S., Sherbino, J., Cook, D.A., 2013. Technology-enhanced simulation in emergency medicine: A systematic review and meta-analysis. Acad Emerg Med 20 (2), 117–127. https://doi.org/10.1111/acem.12076

Kahneman, D., 2011. Thinking, fast and slow. Macmillan.

Kassirer, J.P., 2010. Teaching clinical reasoning: Case-based and coached. Acad Med 85 (7), 1118–1124. https://doi.org/10.1097/acm.0b013e3181d5dd0d

Kassirer, J.P., Wong, J.B., Kopelman, R.I., 2010. Learning clinical reasoning. Lippincott Williams & Wilkins Health, Baltimore, MD.

Konopasky, A., Artino, A.R., Battista, A., Ohmer, M., Hemmer, P.A., Torre, D., et al., 2020. Understanding context specificity: The effect of contextual factors on clinical reasoning. Diagnosis (Berl) 7 (3), 257–264. https://doi.org/10.1515/dx-2020-0016

Lambe, K.A., O'Reilly, G., Kelly, B.D., Curristan, S., 2016. Dual-process cognitive interventions to enhance diagnostic reasoning: A systematic review. BMJ Qual Saf 25 (10), 808–820. https://doi.org/10.1136/bmjqs-2015-004417

Larsen, D.P., Butler, A.C., Roediger III, H.L., 2009. Repeated testing improves long-term retention relative to repeated study: A randomised controlled trial. Medical Education 43 (12), 1174–1181. https://doi.org/10.1111/j.1365-2923.2009.03518.x

Lee, P., Bubeck, S., Petro, J., 2023. Benefits, limits, and risks of GPT-4 as an AI chatbot for medicine. N Engl J Med 388 (13), 1233–1239. https://doi.org/10.1056/NEJMsr2214184

Lessing, J.N., Wheeler, D.J., Beaman, J., Diaz, M.J., Dhaliwal, G., 2020. How to facilitate an unscripted morning report case conference. Clin Teach 17 (4), 360–365. https://doi.org/10.1111/tct.13111

Mamede, S., Hautz, W.E., Berendonk, C., Hautz, S.C., Sauter, T.C., Rotgans, J., et al., 2020. Think twice: Effects on diagnostic accuracy of returning to the case to reflect upon the initial diagnosis. Acad Med 95 (8), 1223–1229. https://doi.org/10.1097/acm.0000000000003153

Mamede, S., Schmidt, H.G., Rikers, R.M., Custers, E.J., Splinter, T.A., van Saase, J.L., 2010. Conscious thought beats deliberation without attention in diagnostic decision-making: At least when you are an expert. Psychol Res 74 (6), 586–592. https://doi.org/10.1007/s00426-010-0281-8

Mamede, S., van Gog, T., Moura, A.S., de Faria, R.M., Peixoto, J.M., Rikers, R.M., et al., 2012. Reflection as a strategy to foster medical students' acquisition of diagnostic competence. Med Educ 46 (5), 464–472. https://doi.org/10.1111/j.1365-2923.2012.04217.x

Mamede, S., van Gog, T., Sampaio, A.M., de Faria, R.M., Maria, J.P., Schmidt, H.G., 2014. How can students' diagnostic competence benefit most from practice with clinical cases? The effects of structured reflection on future diagnosis of the same and novel diseases. Acad Med 89 (1), 121–127. https://doi.org/10.1097/acm.0000000000000076

Manesh, R., Dhaliwal, G., 2018. Digital tools to enhance clinical reasoning. Med Clin North Am 102 (3), 559–565. https://doi.org/10.1016/j.mcna.2017.12.015

Memon, M.A., Joughin, G.R., Memon, B., 2010. Oral assessment and postgraduate medical examinations: Establishing conditions for validity, reliability and fairness. Adv Health Sci Educ Theory Pract 15 (2), 277–289. https://doi.org/10.1007/s10459-008-9111-9

Merkebu, J., Battistone, M., McMains, K., McOwen, K., Witkop, C., Konopasky, A., et al., 2020. Situativity: A family of social cognitive theories for understanding clinical reasoning and diagnostic error. Diagnosis 7 (3), 169–176. https://doi.org/10.1515/dx-2019-0100

Murdock, H.M., Penner, J.C., Le, S., Nematollahi, S., 2020. Virtual morning report during COVID-19: A novel model for case-based teaching conferences. Med Educ 54 (9), 851–852. https://doi.org/10.1111/medu.14226

Mylopoulos, M., 2020. Preparing future adaptive experts: Why it matters and how it can be done. Med Sci Educ 30 (Suppl 1), 11–12. https://doi.org/10.1007/s40670-020-01089-7

Mylopoulos, M., Kulasegaram, K., Woods, N.N., 2018. Developing the experts we need: Fostering adaptive expertise through education. J Eval Clin Pract 24 (3), 674–677. https://doi.org/10.1111/jep.12905

Mylopoulos, M., Steenhof, N., Kaushal, A., Woods, N.N., 2018. Twelve tips for designing curricula that support the development of adaptive expertise. Med Teach 40 (8), 850–854. https://doi.org/10.1080/0142159x.2018.1484082

Norman, G., 2005. Research in clinical reasoning: Past history and current trends. Med Educ 39 (4), 418–427. https://doi.org/10.1111/j.1365-2929.2005.02127.x

Olson, A., Rencic, J., Cosby, K., Rusz, D., Papa, F., Croskerry, P., et al., 2019. Competencies for improving diagnosis: An interprofessional framework for education and training in health care. Diagnosis (Berl) 6 (4), 335–341. https://doi.org/10.1515/dx-2018-0107

Olson, A.P., Graber, M.L., 2020. Improving diagnosis through education. Academic Medicine 95 (8), 1162. https://doi.org/10.1097/ACM.0000000000003172

Olson, A.P.J., Singhal, G., Dhaliwal, G., 2019. Diagnosis education – An emerging field. Diagnosis 6 (2), 75–77. https://doi.org/10.1515/dx-2019-0029

Orlander, J.D., Barber, T.W., Fincke, B.G., 2002. The morbidity and mortality conference: The delicate nature of learning from error. Acad Med 77 (10), 1001–1006. https://doi.org/10.1097/00001888-200210000-00011

Parsons, A.S., Clancy, C.B., Rencic, J.J., Warburton, K.M., 2022. Targeted strategies to remediate diagnostic reasoning deficits. Acad Med 97 (4), 616. https://doi.org/10.1097/acm.0000000000004244

Parsons, A.S., Kon, R.H., Plews-Ogan, M., Gusic, M.E., 2021. You can have both: Coaching to promote clinical competency and professional identity formation. Perspectives on Medical Education 10 (1), 57–63. https://doi.org/10.1007/s40037-020-00612-1

Pauker, S.G., Kassirer, J.P., 1980. The threshold approach to clinical decision making. New England Journal of Medicine 302 (20), 1109–1117. https://doi.org/10.1056/NEJM198005153022003

Payton, E.M., Graber, M.L., Bachiashvili, V., Mehta, T., Dissanayake, P.I., Berner, E.S., 2023. Impact of clinical note format on diagnostic accuracy and efficiency. J Health Inf Manag 0 (0). https://doi.org/10.1177/18333583231151979

Philibert, I., 2018. Using chart review and chart-stimulated recall for resident assessment. J Grad Med Educ 10 (1), 95–96. https://doi.org/10.4300/jgme-d-17-01010.1

Pierluissi, E., Fischer, M.A., Campbell, A.R., Landefeld, C.S., 2003. Discussion of medical errors in morbidity and mortality conferences. JAMA 290 (21), 2838–2842. https://doi.org/10.1001/jama.290.21.2838

Pinnock, R., McDonald, J., Ritchie, D., Durning, S.J., 2020. Humans and machines: Moving towards a more symbiotic approach to learning clinical reasoning. Med Teach 42 (3), 246–251. https://doi.org/10.1080/0142159x.2019.1679361

Raffel, K.E., Kantor, M.A., Barish, P., Esmaili, A., Lim, H., Xue, F., et al., 2020. Prevalence and characterisation of diagnostic error among 7-day all-cause hospital medicine readmissions: A retrospective cohort study. BMJ Qual Saf 29 (12), 971–979. https://doi.org/10.1136/bmjqs-2020-010896

Rajpurkar, P., Irvin, J., Ball, R.L., Zhu, K., Yang, B., Mehta, H., et al., 2018. Deep learning for chest radiograph diagnosis: A retrospective comparison of the CheXNeXt algorithm to practicing radiologists. PLoS Med 15 (11), e1002686. https://doi.org/10.1371/journal.pmed.1002686

Reddy, S.T., Endo, J., Gupta, S., Tekian, A., Park, Y.S., 2015. A case for caution: Chart-stimulated recall. J Grad Med Educ 7 (4), 531–535. https://doi.org/10.4300/jgme-d-15-00011.1

Rencic, J., 2011. Twelve tips for teaching expertise in clinical reasoning. Med Teach 33 (11), 887–892. https://doi.org/10.3109/0142159X.2011.558142

Rencic, J., Durning, S., Holmboe, E., Gruppen, L., 2016. Assessing competence in professional performance across disciplines and professions. In: Wimmers, P.F., Mentkowski, M. (Eds.), Innovation and change in professional education. Springer.

Rencic, J., Trowbridge, R.L., Fagan, M., Szauter, K., Durning, S., 2017. Clinical reasoning education at US medical schools: Results from a national survey of internal medicine clerkship directors. J Gen Intern Med 32 (11), 1242–1246. https://doi.org/10.1007/s11606-017-4159-y

Royce, C.S., Hayes, M.M., Schwartzstein, R.M., 2019. Teaching critical thinking: A case for instruction in cognitive biases to reduce diagnostic errors and improve patient safety. Acad Med 94 (2), 187–194. https://doi.org/10.1097/acm.0000000000002518

Schaye, V., Miller, L., Kudlowitz, D., Chun, J., Burk-Rafel, J., Cocks, P., et al., 2022. Development of a clinical reasoning documentation assessment tool for resident and fellow admission notes: A shared mental model for feedback. J Gen Intern Med 37 (3), 507–512. https://doi.org/10.1007/s11606-021-06805-6

Schmidt, H.G., Mamede, S., 2015. How to improve the teaching of clinical reasoning: A narrative review and a proposal. Med Educ 49 (10), 961–973. https://doi.org/10.1111/medu.12775

Sherbino, J., Kulasegaram, K., Howey, E., Norman, G., 2014. Ineffectiveness of cognitive forcing strategies to reduce biases in diagnostic reasoning: A controlled trial. CJEM 16 (1), 34–40. https://doi.org/10.2310/8000.2013.130860

Sibbald, M., Monteiro, S., Sherbino, J., LoGiudice, A., Friedman, C., Norman, G., 2022. Should electronic differential diagnosis support be used early or late in the diagnostic process? A multicentre experimental study of Isabel. BMJ Qual Saf 31 (6), 426–433. https://doi.org/10.1136/bmjqs-2021-013493

Steinhilber, S., Estrada, C.A., 2017. Exercises in clinical reasoning: A retrospective. J Gen Intern Med 32 (1), 1–2. https://doi.org/10.1007/s11606-016-3906-9

Stern, S.D., Cifu, A.S., Altkorn, D., 2015. Symptom to diagnosis. McGraw-Hill Education LLC, New York, NY.

Stojan, J.N., Daniel, M., Hartley, S., Gruppen, L., 2022. Dealing with uncertainty in clinical reasoning: A threshold model and the roles of experience and task framing. Med Educ 56 (2), 195–201. https://doi.org/10.1111/medu.14673

Strong, E., DiGiammarino, A., Weng, Y., Basaviah, P., Hosamani, P., Kumar, A., et al., 2023. Performance of ChatGPT on free-response, clinical reasoning exams. medRxiv. https://doi.org/10.1101/2023.03.24.23287731

ten Cate, O., Custers, E.J., Durning, S.J., 2017. Principles and practice of case-based clinical reasoning education: A method for preclinical students, Vol. 15. Springer.

Thammasitboon, S., Rencic, J.J., Trowbridge, R.L., Olson, A.P., Sur, M., Dhaliwal, G., 2018. The assessment of reasoning tool (ART): Structuring the conversation between teachers and learners. Diagnosis 5 (4), 197–203. https://doi.org/10.1515/dx-2018-0052

Thomas, P.A., Kern, D.E., Hughes, M.T., S.A, T., Chen, B.Y., 2022. Curriculum development for medical education: A six-step approach, 4th ed. Johns Hopkins University Press.

Trowbridge, R.L., Rencic, J.J., Durning, S.J., 2015. Teaching clinical reasoning. American College of Physicians.

Vandewaetere, M., Manhaeve, D., Aertgeerts, B., Clarebout, G., Van Merriënboer, J.J., Roex, A., 2015. 4C/ID in medical education: How to design an educational program based on whole-task learning: AMEE Guide No. 93. Med Teach 37 (1), 4–20. https://doi.org/10.3109/0142159x.2014.928407

Waechter, J., Allen, J., Lee, C.H., Zwaan, L., 2022. Development and pilot testing of a data-rich clinical reasoning training and assessment tool. Acad Med 97 (10), 1484–1488. https://doi.org/10.1097/acm.0000000000004758

Ways, M., Kroenke, K., Umali, J., Buchwald, D., 1995. Morning report. A survey of resident attitudes. Arch Intern Med 155 (13), 1433–1437. https://doi.org/10.1001/archinte.155.13.1433

Young, J.Q., Van Merrienboer, J., Durning, S., Ten Cate, O., 2014. Cognitive load theory: Implications for medical education: AMEE Guide No. 86. Med Teach 36 (5), 371–384. https://doi.org/10.3109/0142159x.2014.889290

Young, M., Thomas, A., Lubarsky, S., Ballard, T., Gordon, D., Gruppen, L.D., et al., 2018. Drawing boundaries: The difficulty in defining clinical reasoning. Acad Med 93 (7), 990–995. https://doi.org/10.1097/acm.0000000000002142

Zack, T., Dhaliwal, G., Geha, R., Margaretten, M., Murray, S., Hong, J.C., 2023. A clinical reasoning-encoded case library developed through national language processing. J Gen Intern Med 38 (1), 5–11. https://doi.org/10.1007/s11606-022-07758-

36

TEACHING CLINICAL REASONING TO PRECLINICAL MEDICAL STUDENTS

PATRICK NEWMAN ▪ GURPREET DHALIWAL ▪ SIRISHA NARAYANA ▪ DENISE CONNOR

CHAPTER AIMS

The aims of this chapter are:

- to describe the key elements, learning goals and teaching strategies for an integrated clinical reasoning curriculum for preclinical medical students
- to emphasize an approach for aligning a clinical reasoning curriculum with the developmental stage of learners, building in complexity as students near clinical training.

INTRODUCTION

Traditionally, medical schools have not explicitly taught clinical reasoning. Rather, they imparted medical knowledge and then offered opportunities for students to apply that knowledge in examinations, simulations and patient care. In recent years, there has been an increasing appreciation of the importance of explicit instruction as a means to cultivate exceptional clinical reasoning (National Academies of Science, Engineering, and Medicine [NASEM], 2015) and an increasing number of medical schools now teach students how clinicians reason through patients' clinical problems.

Clinical reasoning is a procedure akin to tying a surgical knot or auscultating the heart and it requires the same longitudinal instruction, practice, coaching and formative feedback. In this chapter, we outline a curriculum for clinical reasoning for preclinical medical education that accomplishes the following goals:

- Introduces the science of reasoning, fosters use of the vocabulary of reasoning and provides a map of the reasoning process (Understanding Reasoning section)
- Integrates reasoning practice with both medical knowledge acquisition and clinical skill building (Integration section)
- Builds on the foundational frameworks of reasoning by introducing more advanced topics relevant to the clinical environment such as clinical uncertainty, diagnostic error and management reasoning (Advanced Topics in Reasoning section)

UNDERSTANDING REASONING

Introducing the concepts of reasoning gives students a rationale for engaging with the curriculum and understanding reasoning as a set of defined, discrete steps that can be described, practised and improved upon over time.

Modes of Reasoning

Modern perspectives on the science of reasoning place emphasis on clinical reasoning as both an internal cognitive process (specific processes occurring in the mind of a healthcare provider) and a contextual, sociocultural activity (where judgement is influenced by social, cultural and environmental factors) (Bleakley, 2021; Bowen, 2006; Daniel et al., 2020; Torre et al., 2020). Instruction that begins with internal cognitive theories of clinical reasoning can provide an approachable framework to introduce key terminology and themes.

Cognitive psychology proposes two intertwined reasoning modes: intuitive and analytic (Eva, 2005). Intuitive reasoning, also known as 'pattern recognition', describes a subconscious, rapid process. Analytic reasoning describes a deliberate, systematic, slower process. Teachers should avoid setting up a false hierarchy between these strategies because either mode can result in diagnostic success or error. Combined reasoning (merging intuition and analysis) can be introduced as a strategy to mitigate error (e.g. performing a diagnostic time-out after a diagnosis is made and asking 'what else could this be?') (Ark et al., 2006; Lambe et al., 2016; Norman et al., 1999).

Learning Goals

After the introduction, students should be able to compare and contrast intuitive versus analytic reasoning and describe the benefits of combined reasoning.

Teaching Strategies

Students' familiarity with reasoning modes can be developed through sessions that:

- Showcase a clinician thinking aloud while analysing a case. After the expert discusses a segment of clinical data, a teacher offers a metacognitive commentary, describing the cognitive processes underlying the expert's reasoning (e.g. pointing out intuitive versus analytic reasoning). The *Journal of General Internal Medicine*'s Exercises in Clinical Reasoning Series provides a useful illustration of this approach (Henderson et al., 2010).

Language of Reasoning

In all complex fields, students and teachers require a shared vocabulary to communicate effectively. Reasoning terms provide a shared language for examining how students and practising clinicians can think about, discuss and learn from clinical problems (Dhaliwal and Ilgen, 2016). Orientation to the language of reasoning should include the concepts elaborated in Table 36.1.

By learning how to translate patients' stories into medical terminology, students can begin to communicate their reasoning precisely to other clinicians. Semantic qualifiers enable students to re-cast patients' stories into refined clinical problems that can be more easily solved (Fig. 36.1).

The concept of problem representation has been extended in the clinical reasoning literature to capture both the early mental abstraction of the problem and the summative assessment statement. However, because early problem representation serves a different role in the reasoning process than the later summative assessment (i.e. early problem representation shapes the hypothesis-driven history and physical exam whereas the summative assessment shapes communication with other clinicians), it can be helpful to separate these concepts.

Learning Goals

After exposure to reasoning terminology, students should be able:

- to demonstrate accurate transformation of the components of patients' stories into abstract medical terminology using semantic qualifiers (e.g. 'shortness of breath with walking that has been getting worse' becomes 'progressive dyspnoea on exertion') and
- to apply problem representations, summative assessments, schemas, illness scripts and prioritized differential diagnoses in the diagnostic process.

Teaching Strategies

Ask students to identify active problems from written, live or video patient histories and use medical terms and semantic qualifiers to describe each problem. Peer and facilitator feedback can highlight the utility of the problem representation in guiding additional data gathering.

TABLE 36.1

Reasoning Vocabulary

Reasoning Concept	Definition	Purpose	Example
Semantic transformation	Translation of specific characteristics of the clinical data set into medical terminology	■ Acculturation ('talking like a doctor') ■ Emphasizes compare/contrast of illness scripts by use of opposing semantic qualifiers	■ 'It started suddenly last night' becomes 'acute' ■ 'All of the joints in my arms and legs are aching' becomes 'symmetrical polyarthralgia'
Problem representation	Abstracted essence of a patient's clinical issue using medical terms and semantic qualifiers	■ Triggers knowledge stored as illness scripts, which continuously informs additional data acquisition	■ Young man with acute, painless monocular blindness ■ Older adult with chronic tobacco use and episodic gross haematuria
Assessment (summative problem representation)	Summary statement or 'one-liner', positioned at the start of the A&P	■ Highlights features of a patient's H&P that justify a "most likely" diagnosis ■ Contextualizes key elements of a patient's abstracted problem	■ 48-year-old woman on immunosuppressive agents with chronic productive cough, fevers, progressive dyspnoea, and left upper lobe rhonchi
Diagnostic schema	A systematic approach or framework for thinking through a complex clinical problem	■ Links mechanistic thinking and pathophysiology with clinical syndromes ■ Offers analytic approaches to developing differential diagnoses for complex problems	■ Acute kidney injury can be broken down into prerenal, intrinsic, or postrenal causes
Illness script	Mental model of disease featuring: predisposing conditions (epidemiology/risk factors); time course/tempo; clinical features (signs/symptoms); mechanism of disease	■ Organizes medical knowledge about a diagnosis around the most relevant features and key categories ■ Emphasizes features that differentiate one diagnosis from other illnesses	■ An early script for vasovagal syncope may include: often in young, healthy patients; hyperacute, short duration; premonitory symptoms of nausea, pallor, diaphoresis; transient hypotension caused by bradycardia and/or vasodilation from a sensory stimulus
Prioritized differential diagnosis	Organizes potential diagnoses as most likely, can't miss, less likely and least likely with a rationale for ranking	■ Encourages 'thinking aloud' to justify *prioritized* diagnostic thinking by comparing/contrasting potential diagnoses	■ The most likely diagnosis is migraine based on the subacute onset, unilateral and pulsatile qualities, with photophobia and vomiting ■ Also possible but less likely is tension headache, given that there can be some overlap in symptoms and some migraine sufferers experience pain on both sides of the head ■ A less likely but 'can't miss' diagnosis is a subarachnoid haemorrhage (SAH). However, SAH is usually sudden onset with accompanying neurological deficits

Encourage students to notice when clinicians use medical terminology versus everyday language. Students can reflect on how technical language influences problem solving, while also considering the importance of everyday language for patient communication.

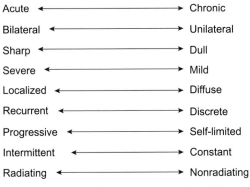

Fig. 36.1 ▪ Examples of opposing semantic qualifiers.

Map of the Reasoning Process

Understanding the discrete steps of reasoning (Fig. 36.2) can help teachers and students identify areas needing additional practice.

REFLECTION POINT

For the map of the reasoning process to have the greatest impact, teachers in both the preclinical and clinical domains must use a shared language to describe their thinking process and to critique students' work.

- Consider how you would develop and implement a faculty development programme at your institution with the aim of spreading the language of reasoning beyond reasoning-focussed didactics.
- How would such a faculty development campaign look at your institution?
- Who are the key stakeholders you would need to engage to implement this campaign?

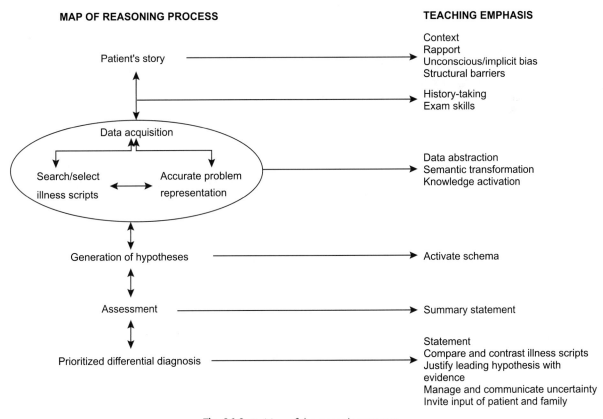

Fig. 36.2 ▪ Map of the reasoning process.

Learning Goals

Learning goals should align with students' development. At the foundational level, students should be able:

- to abstract the key attributes of patients' chief concerns, including onset, chronology and severity and use them to create succinct problem representations,
- to identify relevant data pertaining to the chief concern (e.g. history of diabetes is relevant to a foot infection),
- to identify relevant contextual information that pertains to the problem representation (e.g. recent international travel),
- to identify matches and mismatches between a patient's presentation and the typical features of candidate illness scripts.

Prior to starting clerkships, students should be able:

- to identify the most likely, cannot miss and less likely diagnoses when analysing cases,
- to defend selection of a most likely diagnosis based on the clinical data set,
- to explain why other diagnoses are less likely based on the clinical data set,
- to describe how the likelihood of a diagnosis is affected by pretest probability, base rate and incremental data, leading to a post-test probability,
- to apply diagnostic approaches (schemas) for commonly encountered clinical problems.

Teaching Strategies

- Case-based sessions prompt students to link history and examination findings with diagnostic considerations and pathophysiology while they develop diagnostic approaches to common clinical problems.
- Cases in the preclinical curriculum should focus on common presentations and diseases, not rare ones (e.g. the approach to dyspnoea should be developed through the juxtaposition of pneumonia and heart failure, not granulomatosis with polyangiitis and sarcoidosis).

When students reach the clerkships, atypical presentations and rare diagnoses can be introduced and anchored to students' foundation of prototypical clinical presentations (Kassirer, 2010).

- Cases should progress from simple paper cases in which a complete data set is provided to serial cue cases in which students must request necessary data, to SP cases in which students must gather data. This gradual increase in complexity and cognitive demands can help to maximize learning while avoiding overwhelming working memory with novel data and tasks (Schmidt et al., 2015).
- Cases presented near the end of preclinical education should include opportunities to apply Bayesian reasoning (e.g. for diagnoses with accessible data about pre-test probability and test characteristics such as streptococcal pharyngitis (Centor criteria, throat swab test characteristics)). Teachers can emphasize both the limitations of applying quantitative approaches and reference the more qualitative Bayesian thinking that clinicians utilize in the real world (e.g. assigning 'low', 'intermediate' or 'high' pre-test probability) (McGee, 2002; Medow and Lucey, 2011).

Students should consolidate clinical reasoning concepts by:

- writing evolving problem representations at several steps of a case (e.g. after the HPI, after the medical history, after the examination). Teachers should facilitate discussion at each step and point out how the evolving problem representation influences further data gathering,
- working with peers to create a schema delineating the categories of disease (e.g. pre-renal/intrinsic/postrenal) that guides the approach to a common clinical problem (e.g. acute kidney injury),
- defending their diagnostic considerations and prioritization orally and in writing, as they will in the clinical environment.

Patient cases focussing on rare diagnoses or atypical presentations are often used for teaching in the clinical setting. However, typical, straightforward patient cases are the highest yield for early learners who are just beginning to build their illness scripts for common diagnoses.

- Which clinical syndromes in your specialty are fundamental for students to understand?

INTEGRATION

Integrating reasoning principles with medical knowledge acquisition, clinical skill building and communication training enables students to scaffold their early knowledge, put the reasoning framework into practice and develop links between the cognitive and behavioural skills needed to solve clinical problems.

Integration With Medical Knowledge Acquisition

Preclinical students' early knowledge structures can influence their ability to develop differential diagnoses in clinical encounters. Teaching students to organize their knowledge as a library of schemas can enhance their ability to analyse patients who present with symptoms, not assigned diagnoses (Stern et al., 2014; Cammarata and Dhaliwal, 2023). Emphasizing compare/contrast thinking helps students select which information to encode in their early illness scripts. For instance, as students think through the problem of acute chest pain and appreciate the need to differentiate pulmonary embolism (PE) from angina, they may recognize the value of exacerbating features of the pain (e.g. pleuritic in PE versus exertional in angina) in their diagnostic thinking and emphasize these distinguishing features as they develop and refine the relevant illness scripts (Lisk et al., 2016a, 2016b; Woods, 2007).

Learning Goals

Students engaged in an integrated reasoning curriculum should be able:

- to outline illness scripts for common diagnoses (Custers, 2015),

- to describe the defining (must be present) and differentiating (discriminate between related diagnoses) features of two to three scripts relevant to a given problem representation (e.g. gout and osteoarthritis both cause knee pain, but only gout would have a synovial white blood cell count greater than 25,000 WBC/µL) (Bowen, 2006).

Teaching Strategies

To achieve these learning outcomes, we suggest several strategies:

- Focus on compare/contrast learning (Lucey, 2015). For example, instead of delivering didactic content focussed on a single diagnosis, use a compare/contrast learning strategy such as an illness script grid (Table 36.2) that requires students to consider simultaneously two or three competing diagnoses for a given clinical syndrome with an emphasis on differentiating characteristics (Stern et al., 2014),
- Present two patient cases of migraine and headache within a single session and ask students to identify defining/differentiating features in the original data sets (Table 36.3),
- Link medical knowledge content covered in reasoning sessions (motor weakness) with the basic science curriculum (neuroanatomy).

Integration With Hypothesis-Driven Data Collection

Integration of clinical skill building with reasoning encourages the replacement of the 'thorough historical and physical examination (H&P)' with the 'hypothesis-driven H&P'. In the former, students check off a long list of manoeuvres regardless of a patient's problem. In the latter, students engage their diagnostic reasoning and make intentional decisions about how to focus their data gathering (e.g. focussing on gathering data with defining and discriminating power) (Allen et al., 2016).

Learning Goals

Students should be able:

- to show how divergent findings on physical examination affect diagnostic thinking for

TABLE 36.2
Example Illness Script Grid

Compare/Contrast Illness Script Grid for the Clinical Syndrome of Transient Loss of Consciousness

Diagnosis	Vasovagal Syncope	Seizure	Arrhythmia
Predisposing conditions (risk factors, epidemiology)	Triggers: strong emotions, stress (e.g. pain, venipuncture)	Metabolic abnormalities (electrolyte disturbances, renal failure); brain lesions (cancer, stroke)	Ischemia, electrolyte abnormalities, channelopathies
Time course, pattern	Hyperacute, Short duration	Hyperacute Can be prolonged duration	Hyperacute, Short duration
Clinical features	Premonitory symptoms include nausea, diaphoresis, pallor Occurs when sitting/standing, recovery when supine	Premonitory symptoms (may have aura) (e.g. déjà vu) or nonspecific symptoms (e.g. dizziness, paraesthesia) Prolonged recovery (postictal state) with confusion	Minimal premonitory symptoms (may have palpitations) Injury common (sudden, without bracing for a fall) Quick recovery, no prolonged confusion
pathophysiology/ mechanism of disease	Neural reflex → hypotension from bradycardia or peripheral vasodilation from faulty neural signal	Abnormal neuronal firing in the brain (hyperexcitability, hypersynchrony)	Abnormal cardiac rhythm → decreased cardiac output → poor perfusion of brain

TABLE 36.3
Traditional Versus Compare/Contrast Approach to Clinical Learning

Traditional Approach	Compare/Contrast Approach
Disease based (e.g. migraine)	Clinical syndrome based (e.g. headache)
1 patient case	2–3 related patient cases
Build, reinforce, elaborate medical knowledge about a diagnosis	Identify features that differentiate common causes of a clinical syndrome

Based on Stern, S., Cifu, A., Altkorn, D., 2014. Symptom to diagnosis: An evidence-based guide. McGraw-Hill Professional, New York: NY.

a clinical syndrome (e.g. presence/absence of hypervolaemia in a dyspnoeic patient),

■ to demonstrate use of historical questions and examination manoeuvres that differentiate among candidate diagnoses during information gathering with a standardized patient (SP) (e.g. ask about time to peak intensity of acute headache; assess for presence/absence of cervical lymphadenopathy with sore throat).

Teaching Strategies

■ Utilize clinical vignettes which contextualize physical examination skill development by 'pausing' before the exam to consider how certain findings would modify the differential diagnosis,

■ Integrate reasoning concepts into data-gathering sessions (e.g. when taking the history of the present illness with SPs, take time to ask students to articulate their working problem representation and reflect on how the problem representation activates diagnostic considerations and informs additional data gathering),

■ Expose students to H&Ps performed by experts and provide a parallel clinical reasoning narration; the experts reason aloud as they acquire new information in the history and then plan, execute and interpret examination manoeuvres.

Integration With Patient-Centred and Interprofessional Communication

Clinical reasoning is a contextually situated, socially mediated activity, involving interactions between the patient and the entire diagnostic team (Daniel et al., 2020; Torre et al., 2020).

Integration of clinical reasoning concepts with curricula on patient-centred communication can demonstrate how skills in interviewing patients and in sharing thinking with patients during the process facilitates the co-creation of diagnosis. Conversely, examples of difficulties in communication can illustrate how communication issues can adversely impact the diagnostic process.

Integration with curricula on interprofessional collaboration can highlight the many capabilities and skills of members of different health professions, with an emphasis on how effective communication can improve diagnostic accuracy by harnessing the entire healthcare team.

Learning Goals

Students should:

- appreciate the link between patient-centred communication and diagnostic accuracy,
- demonstrate use of skills such as open-ended questions and empathic and summarizing statements (e.g. 'to make sure I'm understanding correctly, I'd like to summarize what I've heard so far; can you let me know if I've missed anything or got anything wrong?'),
- describe strategies that promote effective interdisciplinary and interprofessional teamwork, facilitate open and respectful dialogue among team members and minimize structural hierarchies that can impede communication.

Teaching Strategies

Authentic patient stories are a powerful means to link communication with diagnosis. Sessions can do the following:

- Feature panels in which patients highlight occasions when they were not able to share their complete clinical story with providers because of negative feelings engendered during the visit (e.g. discomfort, shame), and compare with encounters when they were able to share important information because of positive rapport and trustworthiness established (Aper et al., 2015);
- Include SP feedback on how the patient–provider interaction either facilitated or impaired disclosure of historical details. SPs require additional training to modify how they disclose information based on the quality of the rapport built by the student;
- Bring together students across health professions for case-based, role-play of interprofessional

communication (e.g. nursing, medical student and pharmacy students practise solving a case together after their own independent analysis). Include time for discussion of how communication facilitated or hampered patient care within the context of a simulated case;

- Invite experienced members of other healthcare professions to participate in discussions of clinical reasoning alongside physicians;
- Provide examples of real-world cases in which engagement of a large diagnostic team was critical to reach the correct diagnosis and emphasize which communication strategies made this possible.

REFLECTION POINT

Effective integration of reasoning into existing curricula requires collaboration among many stakeholders.

- Who are the stakeholders at your institution within both the basic and clinical sciences?
- How would you engage these educational leaders to intentionally create clear linkages between traditional content and new reasoning-focussed content?

ADVANCED TOPICS IN REASONING

Once students understand the elements of diagnostic success, they can be introduced to advanced concepts in clinical reasoning, such as diagnostic uncertainty, diagnostic error and management reasoning. Acknowledging the entire spectrum of diagnostic performance requires nurturing students' self-efficacy while simultaneously instilling humility and a commitment to continuous self-improvement (Simpkin and Schwartzstein, 2016; Sommers and Launer, 2014). Diagnostic error should be introduced as a quality and safety issue rooted in cognitive, social/structural and systems factors (NASEM, 2015).

Normalizing Uncertainty

Openly discussing uncertainty early in medical education and demonstrating that experts grapple with this issue allows students to reflect more intentionally on uncertainty throughout their training and professional lives. Diagnostic uncertainty is best explored after students have developed a solid foundation with the reasoning framework, but before entering immersive clinical training. Students should begin to recognize uncertainty within clinical cases and communicate it with patients and colleagues. Familiarizing students with the language of probability and base rates can be a useful adjunct to discussions about uncertainty (Maserejian et al., 2009). Additionally, students may benefit from learning about frameworks for discussing and communicating uncertainty (e.g. the diagnostic 'safety net' to engage patients in anticipatory guidance about red flag symptoms, 'scenario planning' which highlights likely outcomes for patients, including worst case scenarios, and models that help clinical teams juxtapose diagnostic certainty against diagnostic accuracy) (Meyer et al., 2021; Moulder et al., 2022; Santhosh et al., 2019).

Learning Goals

Students should be able:

- to describe sources of uncertainty in diagnosis (e.g. patients with atypical presentations) and
- to communicate about diagnostic uncertainty and next steps with patients and colleagues.

Teaching Strategies

- Introduce a simulated case where students must convey diagnostic uncertainty to a colleague in written and oral formats;
- Role-play shared decision making with SPs when a clear diagnosis is lacking;
- Involve an SP in shared decision making about next steps in the face of diagnostic uncertainty (e.g. the role of a therapeutic trial);
- Hold panel presentations with clinicians from many practice settings discussing their experiences with uncertainty;
- Offer insight into the effect of uncertainty on patients (e.g. patients whose diagnoses remained elusive for an extended time are invited to discuss the effect of uncertainty on their quality of life);
- Present authentic cases in which a definitive diagnosis is not identified;
- Consider developing assessments where open-ended questions have more than one right answer to model the reality of uncertainty in clinical practice (Moulder et al., 2022);
- Students can role-play how to convey uncertainty to patients and colleagues;
- Students can practice using frameworks and tools to name explicitly, reflect upon and communicate uncertainty (Santhosh et al., 2019; Santhosh et al., 2022; Wolpaw et al., 2009).

Diagnostic Error

Students should develop the capacity to recognize circumstances and thought processes that may contribute to diagnostic errors, which encompass inaccurate diagnoses, inappropriate diagnostic delays and inadequate communication of diagnoses to patients. To acquire this skill, students need practice in retrospectively analysing errors using a systematic approach for classifying diagnostic errors.

Cognitive errors are an effective way to engage students with the fallibility of human judgement and inaccuracies in assessing diagnostic probabilities, which influence the diagnostic process. Although an exhaustive survey of cognitive errors can be overwhelming and counterproductive for early learners, introducing a few common forms of cognitive error (e.g. anchoring, diagnostic momentum) in a case-based fashion can provide students with awareness about the universal susceptibility to mistakes.

The impacts of implicit bias (unconscious social bias related to stereotyping) and systems-level factors such as structural racism on the diagnostic process should also be introduced as important contributors to diagnostic error (Braveman et al., 2022). Discussions about strategies for moving towards equity in diagnosis are critical to pair with identifying the problem of diagnostic disparities. These conversations can be particularly burdensome for students who come from communities that experience discrimination in healthcare. Expert consultation and a trauma-informed medical education approach should be considered when designing curricular sessions focussed on disparities to avoid causing unintended harm to learners (Brown et al., 2021). Facilitators with expertise in hosting conversations related to racism and other forms of oppression are also critical for the success of discussion sections.

Learning Goals

Students should be able:

- to describe a framework for the causes of diagnostic errors (e.g. systems, cognitive, no fault) (Graber et al., 2005),
- to describe situations that may increase the risk for diagnostic error (e.g. multitasking, emotionally charged encounters, fatigue) (Johns et al., 2009; NASEM, 2015; Schmidt et al., 2017),
- to describe three common cognitive tendencies (e.g. premature closure, anchoring, availability bias) and recognize examples in clinical vignettes,
- to explain the concept of diagnostic disparities, describe the impacts of implicit bias (e.g. related to racism or sexism) and systems-level/structural oppression on diagnosis, and propose a potential strategy to address these issues.

Teaching Strategies

During discussions of errors, care must be taken to create a growth-oriented learning environment and to set a constructive, rather than a blaming, tone. Strategies include:

- Sessions presenting information about disparities in diagnosis (e.g. related to racism, sexism) (Goyal et al., 2021; Haeri et al., 2011; Kawas et al., 2021; Moy et al., 2015; Olbert et al., 2018; Tsoy et al., 2021);
- Sessions exploring individual-level implicit bias and its potential impact on the diagnostic process, and systems-level aspects of oppression (e.g. inaccurate readings of pulse oximetry across the full range of skin tones) and their impact on diagnosis (Sjoding et al., 2020);
- Patient panels or video testimonials discussing the impacts of diagnostic error (NB: it can be helpful to include trigger warnings when sharing personal stories of harm);
- Facilitated discussions using written, live or video patient vignettes to explore common causes of cognitive error, situations at high risk of error and the impact of implicit bias and structural oppression (Aquifer, 2024; Reilly et al., 2013);
- Sessions in which students discuss cases of diagnostic error and undertake an analysis of

underlying cognitive, social/structural and systems factors;

- NB: When featuring sessions focussed on implicit bias and structural oppression such as racism, it is critical to undertake expert consultation to reduce the risk of causing unintended harm to learners who have themselves experienced oppression.

Strategies to Reduce Risk of Error

Introducing uncertainty and error without sharing strategies to deal with these issues can be counterproductive and negatively affect students' self-efficacy. Offering insight into how clinicians manage these issues establishes a problem-solving mindset that can carry students forwards into their professional lives.

Discussion of the potentially negative effect of cognitive biases such as anchoring should be balanced with acknowledgement that heuristics, or mental shortcuts, are valuable problem-solving tools (Dhaliwal, 2017). Rather than leaving students with the impression that all heuristics should be avoided, teachers can emphasize the importance of engaging in circumspection, recognizing when a heuristic is being used and using reflective practice to check a diagnosis arrived at quickly, particularly when faced with complex cases (Mamede et al., 2008). Teachers should also point out that excessively analytic approaches can lead to inappropriate overweighting of distracting features during the reasoning process.

Deliberate individuation of patients (e.g. learning about what makes a patient unique, counteracting the tendency to categorize patients within stereotyped social groups), perspective-taking and the conscious cultivation of empathy can be introduced as tools to combat implicit bias (Boscardin, 2015). Courses should also explore systems-level interventions needed to combat the impact of racism and other forms of oppression on the diagnostic process. For example, ensuring exam findings across the full spectrum of skin tones are included in didactics and clinical resources is a systems-level intervention that can reduce disparities in diagnosis (UCSF, n.d.).

Learning Goals

Students should be able:

- to recognize situations that are particularly vulnerable to common cognitive biases,

- to demonstrate the use of combined intuitive and analytic reasoning strategies in a clinical case (Ark et al., 2006; Eva et al., 2007),
- to describe mechanisms for reducing the risk for error in high-risk situations (e.g. fatigue, hand-offs) (Johns et al., 2009; NASEM, 2015; Starmer et al., 2014),
- to reflect on implicit bias and describe ways of deliberately individuating patients,
- to propose strategies for combatting systems-level racism, sexism and other forms of oppression that impact the diagnostic process.

Teaching Strategies

- Case-based sessions can facilitate students' abilities to define common forms of cognitive error and identify situations where they may be at risk (e.g. recent missed diagnosis influencing judgement in current case) (Graber et al., 2012);
- A panel of providers can discuss their experiences with system factors that increase the risk for error, such as confusing electronic health record interfaces, and describe their practices for reflection after diagnostic errors;
- Case presentations in which a diagnostic error is made because of inadequate knowledge (e.g. presuming wheezing was pathognomonic for an asthma exacerbation) can open discussion into how clinicians learn from these experiences and revise their illness scripts accordingly;
- Videos demonstrating the effect of body language and differential responses to patient questions can be provocative tools for generating discussion about the effect of implicit bias on patient–provider communication during the diagnostic process.

REFLECTION POINT

Discussion of uncertainty and error in the preclinical domain should be followed by ongoing openness to these discussions in the clinical setting. Otherwise, the 'hidden curriculum' will quickly reverse students' perceptions of which topics are acceptable for discussion. Consider whether your institution currently has a climate that encourages or discourages dialogue about uncertainty and error. If these subjects are met with resistance, how might you embark on institutional culture change? Reflect on what might be the first steps to expand your institutional culture to include meaningful discussion about experiences with uncertainty and cognitive error.

A Primer on Management Reasoning

Management reasoning describes the process of making decisions about patient care after diagnosis. While diagnostic reasoning is a classification task, management reasoning is an optimization task, which calls for the consideration of many factors including patient preferences, costs of care and system limitations. Therapeutic reasoning is a subset of the management decision-making process that pertains to the selection of a treatment. The mental schemas clinicians may activate in therapeutic decision making have been referred to as 'management scripts' (Abdoler et al., 2020; Parsons et al., 2020). These scripts may be taught as a starting point for different syndromes. After scripts are activated, management options are selected. Options are influenced by probability of disease, benefits and harms of a therapy (which requires consideration of 'threshold', e.g. is the probability of lung cancer in a patient with concerning symptoms high enough to consider a biopsy?), shared decision-making, high-value care considerations and tolerance of clinical uncertainty (Wijesekera et al., 2022).

Learning Goals

Preclinical students should be able:

- to develop initial management scripts for common syndromes and
- to identify common patient and systems factors that influence management strategies.

Teaching Strategies

- Students can begin completing management script templates for common conditions or diagnoses for different patients.
- Teachers can challenge learners to consider various scripts or options for management by altering case details and re-visiting the appropriate management approaches.

- When teaching about a diagnosis, teachers can describe the specific treatments that a clinician might perform in order to confirm a preliminary diagnosis or evaluate alternative diagnostic possibilities (e.g. a therapeutic trial of diuretics for a patient with dyspnoea and lower extremity oedema to determine whether heart failure may be contributing) (Parsons et al., 2020).

REFLECTION POINT

We have suggested a comprehensive and integrated reasoning curriculum. However, incremental curriculum change is often more feasible.
- Which learning goals and learning strategies would you target first?
- How would you adapt these learning strategies to your institutional context?
- What would be your elevator pitch to key stakeholders to gather support for launching a curricular innovation focussed on reasoning at your institution?

CONCLUSION

Diagnostic reasoning is an intricate and complex skill and students should be afforded an opportunity to understand and practice this process before undertaking it in the clinical setting. Instruction should start at the beginning of medical school and be integrated throughout the curriculum, with increasing complexity and uncertainty introduced along the way.

With an explicit reasoning map, students can analyse their own reasoning, mark their progress and set goals for improvement.

As students move from the preclinical domain to patient care, they can continue to use this language to organize their learning in the infinitely more complex clinical world. Clinical faculty should be supported and equipped with the same language of reasoning and frameworks imparted to students and should have opportunities to practise giving actionable feedback on the reasoning process that links with the reasoning framework.

A reasoning curriculum has the potential to empower students to see diagnostic thinking as a process that can be deliberately improved throughout one's training and career. Patients will benefit from being cared for by

thoughtful physicians who embrace the importance of reflection and self-improvement in the diagnostic process, who are aware of the risk for error and who can identify and manage uncertainty in a patient-centred manner. Developing a longitudinal, integrated reasoning curriculum is a challenging and rewarding process for educators who believe that clinical reasoning is one of the most important procedures in medicine.

SUMMARY

In this chapter, we have outlined:

- Content for preclinical medical student education focussed on understanding reasoning,
- An approach for integration of a reasoning curriculum with other elements of students' education, such as medical knowledge acquisition, history-taking and communication skills, and
- Ways to build upon foundational clinical reasoning frameworks that will help prepare students for continued learning in the clinical environment.

REFERENCES

Abdoler, E.A., O'Brien, B.C., Schwartz, B.S., 2020. Following the script: An exploratory study of the therapeutic reasoning underlying physicians' choice of antimicrobial therapy. Academic Medicine 95 (8), 1238–1247. https://doi.org/10.1097/ACM.0000000000003498

Allen, S., Olson, A., Menk, J., et al., 2016. Hypothesis-driven physical examination curriculum. Clinical Teacher 14 (6), 417–422. https://doi.org/10.1111/tct.12581

Aper, L., Veldhuijzen, W., Dornan, T., et al., 2015. 'Should I prioritize medical problem-solving or attentive listening?': The dilemmas and challenges that medical students experience when learning to conduct consultations. Patient Education and Counseling 98 (1), 77–84. https://doi.org/10.1016/j.pec.2014.09.016

Aquifer. (2024). *Aquifer diagnostic excellence*. Aquifer. https://aquifer.org/courses/aquifer-diagnostic-excellence/.

Ark, T.K., Brooks, L.R., Eva, K.W., 2006. Giving learners the best of both worlds: Do clinical teachers need to guard against teaching pattern recognition to novices? Academic Medicine: Journal of the Association of American Medical Colleges 81 (4), 405–409. https://doi.org/10.1097/00001888-200604000-00017

Bleakley, A., 2021. Re-visioning clinical reasoning, or stepping out from the skull. Medical Teacher 43 (4), 456–462. https://doi.org/10.1080/0142159X.2020.1859098

Boscardin, C.K., 2015. Reducing implicit bias through curricular interventions. Journal of General Internal Medicine 30 (12), 1726–1728. https://doi.org/10.1007/s11606-015-3496-y

Bowen, J.L., 2006. Educational strategies to promote clinical diagnostic reasoning. New England Journal of Medicine 355 (21), 2217–2225. https://doi.org/10.1056/NEJMra054782

Braveman, P.A., Arkin, E., Proctor, D., et al., 2022. Systemic and structural racism: Definitions, examples, health damages, and approaches to dismantling. Health Affairs (Millwood) 41 (2), 171–178. https://doi.org/10.1377/hlthaff.2021.01394

Brown, T., Berman, S., McDaniel, K., et al., 2021. Trauma-Informed Medical Education (TIME): Advancing curricular content and educational context. Academic Medicine 96 (5), 661–667. https://doi.org/10.1097/ACM.0000000000003587

Cammarata, M., Dhaliwal, G., 2023. Diagnostic schemas: Form and function. Journal of General Internal Medicine 38 (2), 513–516. https://doi.org/10.1007/s11606-022-07935-1

Custers, E.J., 2015. Thirty years of illness scripts: Theoretical origins and practical applications. Medical Teacher 37 (5), 457–462. https://doi.org/10.3109/0142159X.2014.956052

Daniel, M., Durning, S.J., Wilson, E., et al., 2020. Situated cognition: Clinical reasoning and error are context dependent. Diagnosis (Berlin) 7 (3), 341–342. https://doi.org/10.1515/dx-2020-0011

Dhaliwal, G., 2017. Premature closure? Not so fast. BMJ Quality & Safety 26 (2), 87–89.

Dhaliwal, G., Ilgen, J., 2016. Clinical reasoning: Talk the talk or just walk the walk? Journal of Graduate Medical Education 8 (2), 274–276. https://doi.org/10.4300/JGME-D-16-00073.1

Eva, K.W., 2005. What every teacher needs to know about clinical reasoning. Medical Education 39 (1), 98–106. https://doi.org/10.1111/j.1365-2929.2004.01972.x

Eva, K.W., Hatala, R.M., LeBlanc, V.R., et al., 2007. Teaching from the clinical reasoning literature: Combined reasoning strategies help novice diagnosticians overcome misleading information. Medical Education 41 (12), 1152–1158. https://doi.org/10.1111/j.1365-2923.2007.02923.x

Goyal, M.K., Chamberlain, J.M., Webb, M., et al., 2021. Pediatric Emergency Care Applied Research Network (PECARN). Racial and ethnic disparities in the delayed diagnosis of appendicitis among children. Academic Emergency Medicine 28 (9), 949–956. https://doi.org/10.1111/acem.14142

Graber, M.L., Franklin, N., Gordon, R., 2005. Diagnostic error in internal medicine. Archives of Internal Medicine 165 (13), 1493–1499. https://doi.org/10.1001/archinte.165.13.1493

Graber, M.L., Kissam, S., Payne, V.L., et al., 2012. Cognitive interventions to reduce diagnostic error: A narrative review. BMJ Quality & Safety 21 (7), 535–557. https://doi.org/10.1136/bmjqs-2011-000149

Haeri, S., Williams, J., Kopeykina, I., et al., 2011. Disparities in diagnosis of bipolar disorder in individuals of African and European descent: A review. Journal of Psychiatric Practice 17 (6), 394–403. https://doi.org/10.1097/01.pra.0000407962.49851.ef

Henderson, M., Keenan, C., Kohlwes, J., et al., 2010. Introducing exercises in clinical reasoning. Journal of General Internal Medicine 25 (1), 9. https://doi.org/10.1007/s11606-009-1185-4

Johns, M.M., Wolman, D.M., Ulmer, C., 2009. Resident duty hours: Enhancing sleep, supervision, and safety. National Academies Press, Washington, DC. https://nap.nationalacademies.org/catalog/12508/resident-duty-hours-enhancing-sleep-supervision-and-safety

Kassirer, J.P., 2010. Teaching clinical reasoning: Case-based and coached. Academic Medicine 85 (7), 1118–1124. https://doi.org/10.1097/acm.0b013e3181d5dd0d

Kawas, C.H., Corrada, M.M., Whitmer, R.A., 2021. Diversity and disparities in dementia diagnosis and care: A challenge for all of us. JAMA Neurology 78 (6), 650–652. https://doi.org/10.1001/jamaneurol.2021.0285

Lambe, K.A., O'Reilly, G., Kelly, B.D., et al., 2016. Dual-process cognitive interventions to enhance diagnostic reasoning: A systematic review. BMJ Quality & Safety 25 (10), 808–820. https://doi.org/10.1136/bmjqs-2015-004417

Lisk, K., Agur, A.M., Woods, N.N., 2016a. Examining the effect of self-explanation on cognitive integration of basic and clinical sciences in novices. Advances in Health Sciences Education Theory and Practice 22 (5), 1–13. https://doi.org/10.1007/s10459-016-9743-0

Lisk, K., Agur, A.M., Woods, N.N., 2016b. Exploring cognitive integration of basic science and its effect on diagnostic reasoning in novices. Perspectives on Medical Education 5 (3), 147–153. https://doi.org/10.1007/s40037-016-0268-2

Lucey, C.R. (2015). Clinical problem-solving: Dr. Lucey (UCSF public online course content). Vimeo. https://vimeo.com/album/2358328.

Mamede, S., Schmidt, H.G., Penaforte, J.C., 2008. Effects of reflective practice on the accuracy of medical diagnoses. Medical Education 42 (5), 468–475. https://doi.org/10.1111/j.1365-2923.2008.03030.x

Maserejian, N.N., Lutfey, K.E., McKinlay, J.B., 2009. Do physicians attend to base rates? Prevalence data and statistical integration in the diagnosis of coronary heart disease. Health Services Research 44 (6), 1933–1949. https://doi.org/10.1111/j.1475-6773.2009.01022.x

McGee, S., 2002. Simplifying likelihood ratios. Journal of General Internal Medicine 17 (8), 646–649. https://doi.org/10.1046/j.1525-1497.2002.10750.x

Medow, M.A., Lucey, C.R., 2011. A qualitative approach to Bayes' theorem. Evidence-Based Medicine 16 (6), 163–167. https://doi.org/10.1136/ebm-2011-0007

Meyer, A., Giardina, T.D., Khawaja, L., et al., 2021. Patient and clinician experiences of uncertainty in the diagnostic process: Current understanding and future directions. Patient Education and Counseling 104 (11), 2606–2615. https://doi.org/10.1016/j.pec.2021.07.028

Moy, E., Barrett, M., Coffey, R., et al., 2015. Missed diagnoses of acute myocardial infarction in the emergency department: Variation by patient and facility characteristics. Diagnosis (Berlin) 2 (1), 29–40. https://doi.org/10.1515/dx-2014-0053

Moulder, G., Harris, E., Santhosh, L., 2022. Teaching the science of uncertainty. Diagnosis (Berlin) 10 (1), 13–18. https://doi.org/10.1515/dx-2022-0045

National Academies of Sciences, Engineering, and Medicine [NASEM], 2015. Improving diagnosis in health care. National Academies Press, Washington, DC. https://nap.nationalacademies.org/catalog/21794/improving-diagnosis-in-health-care

Norman, G.R., Brooks, L.R., Colle, C.L., et al., 1999. The benefit of diagnostic hypotheses in clinical reasoning: Experimental study of an instructional intervention for forward and backward reasoning. Cognition and Instruction 17 (4), 433–448. https://doi.org/10.1207/S1532690XCI1704_3

Olbert, C.M., Nagendra, A., Buck, B., 2018. Meta-analysis of Black vs. White racial disparity in schizophrenia diagnosis in the United States: Do structured assessments attenuate racial disparities? Journal of Abnormal Psychology 127 (1), 104–115. https://doi.org/10.1037/abn0000309

Parsons, A.S., Wijesekera, T.P., Rencic, J.J., 2020. The management script: A practical tool for teaching management reasoning. Academic Medicine 95 (8), 1179–1185. https://doi.org/10.1097/ACM.0000000000003465

Reilly, J.B., Ogdie, A.R., Von Feldt, J.M., et al., 2013. Teaching about how doctors think: A longitudinal curriculum in cognitive bias and diagnostic error for residents. BMJ Quality & Safety 22 (12), 1044–1050. https://doi.org/10.1136/bmjqs-2013-001987

Santhosh, L., Chou, C.L., Connor, D.M., 2019. Diagnostic uncertainty: From education to communication. Diagnosis 6 (2), 121–126. https://doi.org/10.1515/dx-2018-0088

Santhosh, L., Rojas, J.C., Garcia, B., et al., 2022. Cocreating the ICU-PAUSE tool for intensive care unit-ward transitions. ATS Scholar 3 (2), 312–323. https://doi.org/10.34197/ats-scholar.2021-0135IN

Schmidt, H.G., Mamede, S., Penaforte, J.C., 2015. How to improve the teaching of clinical reasoning: A narrative review and a proposal. Medical Education 49 (10), 961–973. https://doi.org/10.1111/medu.12775

Schmidt, H.G., van Gog, T., Schuit, S.C., et al., 2017. Do patients' disruptive behaviors influence the accuracy of a doctor's diagnosis? A randomized experiment. BMJ Quality & Safety 26 (1), 19–23.

Simpkin, A.L., Schwartzstein, R.M., 2016. Tolerating uncertainty: The next medical revolution? New England Journal of Medicine 375 (18), 1713–1715. https://doi.org/10.1056/NEJMp1606402

Sjoding, M.W., Dickson, R.P., Iwashyna, T.J., et al., 2020. Racial bias in pulse oximetry measurement. New England Journal of Medicine 383 (25), 2477–2478. https://doi.org/10.1056/NEJMc2029240

Sommers, L.S., Launer, J., 2014. Clinical uncertainty in primary care. Springer, New York.

Starmer, A.J., Spector, N.D., Srivastava, R., et al., 2014. Changes in medical errors after implementation of a handoff program. New England Journal of Medicine 371 (19), 1803–1812. https://doi.org/10.1056/NEJMsa1405556

Stern, S., Cifu, A., Altkorn, D., 2014. Symptom to diagnosis: An evidence-based guide. McGraw-Hill Professional.

Torre, D., Durning, S., Rencic, J., et al., 2020. Widening the lens on teaching and assessing clinical reasoning: From "in the head" to "out in the world. Diagnosis 7 (3), 181–190. https://doi.org/10.1515/dx-2019-0098

Tsoy, E., Kiekhofer, R.E., Guterman, E.L., et al., 2021. Assessment of racial/ethnic disparities in timeliness and comprehensiveness of dementia diagnosis in California. JAMA Neurology 78 (6), 657–665. https://doi.org/10.1001/jamaneurol.2021.0399

UCSF. (n.d.). Inclusive skin color project. UCSF. https://guides.ucsf.edu/c.php?g=1081119&p=9159811.

Wijesekera, T., Parsons, A., Abdoler, E., et al., 2022. Management reasoning: A toolbox for educators. Academic Medicine 97 (11), 1724. https://doi.org/10.1097/ACM.0000000000004796

Wolpaw, T., Papp, K.K., Bordage, G., 2009. Using SNAPPS to facilitate the expression of clinical reasoning and uncertainties: A randomized comparison group trial. Academic Medicine 84 (4), 517–524. https://doi.org/10.1097/ACM.0b013e31819a8cbf

Woods, N.N., 2007. Science is fundamental: The role of biomedical knowledge in clinical reasoning. Medical Education 41 (12), 1173–1177. https://doi.org/10.1111/j.1365-2923.2007.02911.x

37

TEACHING CLINICAL REASONING IN NURSING EDUCATION

TRACY LEVETT-JONES ▪ JACQUELINE PICH ▪ NICOLE BLAKEY

CHAPTER OUTLINE

CHAPTER AIMS

The aims of this chapter are:

- to present a suite of teaching and learning strategies that can be used by clinical educators[1] to facilitate the development of nursing students' clinical reasoning skills
- to highlight the relationship between clinical reasoning and patient outcomes.

INTRODUCTION

The importance of clinical reasoning in healthcare cannot be overstated, with a body of research attesting to the relationship between clinical reasoning skills and patient outcomes (Alyahya et al., 2021). Although nursing students generally learn the purpose and process of clinical reasoning in on-campus activities, clinical placements provide authentic, rich and dynamic opportunities for engagement in learning experiences that can enhance this cognitive skill set (Levett-Jones, 2022). This chapter provides a suite of teaching and learning strategies that can be used by educators to facilitate the development of nursing students' clinical reasoning skills; these include: autonomous practice, deliberate practice, higher-order questioning, evidence-based practice, think aloud, deconstruction of critical events and reflection on cognitive biases. These strategies are interlinked and progress in complexity, but each has a focus on patient safety.

PROVIDING OPPORTUNITIES FOR AUTONOMOUS PRACTICE

Junior students, and sometimes even those who are more senior, often depend on their educator or mentor

---

[1] In this chapter, the term 'educator' refers to anyone who provides clinical teaching to nursing students, including those who are formally appointed (e.g. university-employed facilitators) and those who are informally allocated (e.g. preceptors or mentors).

to identify patient problems, plan care and delegate tasks. This approach does not allow students to engage independently in higher-order thinking about their practice. An effective teaching strategy to enhance students' capacity for autonomous clinical reasoning is to ask them to imagine that they are the registered nurse who is fully responsible for the patient's care. This approach challenges students to make sense of clinical data in order to develop a nursing diagnosis and to learn to navigate uncertainty and grapple with complex clinical decisions rather than immediately deferring to their educator or mentor. Students can be asked to explain which cues/patient information they collect and why, how they make sense of the data, the thinking that underpins their decision making and their rationales for care.

When students are lacking in confidence or unwilling to offer a nursing diagnosis or related nursing actions, educators can encourage them to simply 'take a guess', even if they are wrong. Similarly, when caring for patients with complex co-morbidities and multiple management goals, students can be challenged to prioritize their nursing actions. For example, the educator could ask the student to identify and justify their immediate nursing priorities for the care of a person with a pain score of 7 out of 10 on a numerical rating scale, an oxygen saturation level of 88% or a blood glucose level of 3.0 mmol/L. Additionally, asking students to predict 'what might happen if no action were taken in this situation' prompts them to 'think ahead' and anticipate potential outcomes, depending on a particular course of action taken or omitted. These active learning strategies encourage learners to 'step up' when caring for patients and can enhance their clinical reasoning skills (Bristol et al., 2019).

REFLECTION POINT

- What are some of the main challenges that you have encountered in clinical settings when attempting to teach nursing students to become competent and confident in clinical reasoning?
- What strategies have you used to overcome these challenges?

FOCUSSING ON DELIBERATE PRACTICE

Deliberate practice (DP) is critical to the development of clinical reasoning skills. Although expertise is sometimes assumed to be an outcome of exposure, experience and knowledge, research demonstrates only a weak relationship between these factors and actual performance (Bathish et al., 2018) For example, once an elite sportsperson reaches a level of expertise, more experience will not, by itself, result in further improvement. However, if their coach provides opportunities for DP by ensuring that every practice session has a specific purpose, improvement in targeted areas is more likely.

Similarly, individualized opportunities for purposeful, repetitive and systematic practice can be designed to improve nursing students' performance in specific aspects of clinical reasoning.

DP is most effective when educators provide:

- well-defined learning goals related to discrete aspects of clinical reasoning,
- immediate feedback that is clear and specific,
- adequate time for problem solving and
- opportunities for repeated practice to gradually refine specific aspects of clinical reasoning performance (Mabry et al., 2020).

Educators frequently report that, although nursing students typically manage the initial stages of clinical reasoning (for example, collecting cues/information) confidently, they often struggle with higher-order thinking skills. Although students may be able to assess a person's vital signs, fluid balance and oxygen saturation level accurately, they often find synthesizing and making sense of this information to be more challenging. By designing opportunities for DP, educators can focus on more challenging skills such as cue clustering, forming a nursing diagnosis and planning appropriate nursing actions, ultimately enhancing each learner's overall clinical reasoning ability.

USING HIGHER-ORDER QUESTIONING

The use of higher-order questions is key to the development of the critical-thinking and clinical-reasoning skills that are integral to nursing practice (Falcó-Pegueroles et al., 2021). However, a number of studies have reported that in their interactions with students, educators predominantly use low-level questions, centred on knowledge and comprehension (Phillips et al., 2017). Knowledge-based questions, according to Bloom's Taxonomy, represent the lowest category in the cognitive domain and require only simple recall of information. Although these types of lower-level questions are important to learning, the use of higher-order questions that require analysis, synthesis and evaluation is crucial to clinical reasoning (Farmer et al., 2021).

Low-level questions can be answered by simple recall of previously learned information and are often framed using terms such as 'what', 'when', 'who', 'which', 'define', 'describe', 'identify', 'list' and 'recall'. Other characteristics of low-level questions include the use of closed questions that will elicit a yes or no response, questions that elicit recall of factual information, and leading questions that provide clues in their wording as to the answer required. By comparison, higher-order questions probe students' understanding and reasoning by asking them to critique, analyse, synthesize or evaluate their actions (Box 37.1).

EMPHASIZING THE IMPORTANCE OF EVIDENCE-BASED PRACTICE

A sound evidence base is critical to clinical reasoning. Without evidence to inform practice, nursing diagnoses and decisions may be based on little more than 'hunches' and anecdotes. Although best practice guidelines and articles should inform students' decision making, role modelling by educators is essential if students are to value evidence-based literature. When asking students to provide an evidence-based rationale for their decisions, educators can encourage them to access contemporary literature by undertaking a quick but highly focussed Internet-based search. When educators encourage students to use this approach to address specific and complex patient problems, it demonstrates that accessing evidence-based literature is both feasible and valuable (Skela-Savič et al., 2020). Additionally, educators can ask students to discriminate among different levels of evidence, emphasize the importance and value of different sources of evidence

---

BOX 37.1
LEVELS OF QUESTIONS – AN EXEMPLAR

EXAMPLES OF QUESTIONS RELATED TO HAND HYGIENE

The clinical facilitator has concerns about a student's compliance with hand hygiene requirements and wants to test her understanding.

Low-level question: 'What are the five moments of hand hygiene?'

This leads the student to the answer by jogging her memory about the five moments required. The student is likely to frame the answer with the information given in the question; however, there is no way of knowing if the student understands the importance of the five moments. In this way, the student can hide their lack of understanding.

Mid-level question: 'Can you tell me about the policy that relates to hand hygiene?'

This question is better in that it is not leading in nature; however, it is designed to elicit an answer based on the student's memory or recall of the policy rather than an ability to apply the policy to their practice.

High-level question: 'Can you critique your hand hygiene practice with reference to the relevant policy?'

This question also requires the student to recall their knowledge of the hand hygiene policy. However, by asking them to critique their practice, the student must evaluate their hand hygiene performance to determine whether or not they have complied with the policy.

Higher-level question: 'Whilst wearing gloves and attending your patient, you collected clean linen from the linen trolley. Can you critique your actions and the implications'?

This question takes a moment of practice that is related to a lapse in hand hygiene; however, there is no mention of hand hygiene. The student must first critique their actions to make the link to hand hygiene, then critique their practice with respect to the relevant policy/guidelines, and lastly consider the implications of their actions for patient safety.

(e.g. empirical studies, clinical expertise, patient's values and preferences) and help students to develop an understanding of terms such as 'rigor', 'validity', 'reliability' and 'feasibility'. Most important, when educators role-model or facilitate the use of evidence-based resources, they are teaching students that clinical reasoning is a scientific and rigorous process that requires intelligence, integrity and a commitment to lifelong learning.

LEARNING TO THINK ALOUD

The think-aloud (TA) approach is both a teaching and a research strategy. In nursing education, TA can be used to engage students in the process of clinical reasoning by encouraging them to verbalize their thinking while attempting to analyse and solve clinical problems (Verkuyl et al., 2018). The aim of TA is for educators to gain access to students' thought processes, including their train of thought, ability to make connections and identify relationships, and application of prior learning to problem solving. TA also provides a diagnostic opportunity to gain insights into any difficulties being encountered by learners in regards to clinical reasoning (Banning, 2008).

When facilitating TA, educators can prompt students to verbalize their thoughts and the rationales underpinning their actions as they engage in critical thinking and problem solving. This enables errors in the student's clinical reasoning to be identified and rectified and 'faulty' clinical reasoning patterns to be remediated (Pinnock et al., 2015). The specific information that is gained from the TA process is highly useful. Too often, educators can identify when a student is not thinking critically, but without deep insights into their thinking processes, it is difficult to understand why. Thus, the insights generated from TA can lead to the provision of structured and targeted learning support (e.g. using deliberate practice) designed to improve clinical reasoning skills (Altalhi et al., 2021).

The TA strategy can be used in a classroom setting and in simulation, but it is equally suited for use in the clinical environment. When facilitating, TA educators may need to remind the student to keep talking aloud and prompt them to explain their thinking where required. The use of words such as 'describe' can help orient the student and subtle prompts such as 'what are you thinking now?', 'why are you thinking that?' and 'can you talk me through that thought process?' can be used as occasional reminders if students stop verbalizing their thoughts. It is also valuable for educators to role-model TA when demonstrating patient care activities. This clarifies what is expected of students and gives them insights into the thinking processes of expert clinicians. Although the TA approach can be time-consuming, it can lead to a significant improvement in students' clinical reasoning skills and confidence (Todhunter, 2015).

In a professional environment with real-time demands, it is maybe necessary to wait until the end of an activity before reviewing the thinking processes and outcomes. Retrospective TA can also be a useful strategy for improving clinical reasoning. Questioning after retrospective TA should aim to elicit students' thinking and to ensure that they understood the rationale behind their actions. Therefore, closed questions that require a yes or no response should be avoided as should questions that are leading in nature. For example, asking the student 'At what blood pressure reading would you withhold metoprolol?' would be considered leading because this question provides the link between the medication and its indication for use and helps orient the student in their thinking. A better question would be 'Can you carefully describe your thinking as you administered Mr Smith's medications?' Educators should be aware that when engaging in retrospective TA, periods of silence are appropriate, as they allow students the opportunity to gather their thoughts if needed (see Case Study 37.1).

CASE STUDY 37.1

Example of the Use of the Think-Aloud Strategy

Betty Dobson is a 75-year-old patient who was admitted with a fractured wrist after an unwitnessed fall at home 2 days ago. She is complaining of feeling a bit lightheaded and dizzy and tells the nursing student caring for her that she is too tired to get out of bed today. The nursing student moves to collect a sphygmomanometer. The educator prompts the student to think aloud and explain her reasoning. The student explains that the patient's symptoms may be caused by hypotension, so she wants to take the patient's blood pressure to confirm this. The student takes the blood pressure and obtains a reading of 98/60 mmHg. She asks the patient how much she has been drinking, explaining to her educator that dehydration can be a cause of hypotension. The educator might then prompt the student to explain the link between hypotension and dehydration and to consider other clinical issues that can cause dehydration.

DECONSTRUCTING CRITICAL EVENTS

Deconstructing critical events during debriefing fosters critical thinking and informs clinical reasoning (Dreifuerst, 2012). This teaching strategy involves students working in groups to deconstruct a critical event using the clinical reasoning cycle as the organizing framework. Students work systematically through the cycle using a table or a mind map to help them record and organize the patient information. In a similar approach to the TA method, students need to articulate their thoughts and the rationales behind their decision making. The complexity of the clinical exemplars used can increase as the students' progress in their nursing programmes so that students can continually extend their clinical reasoning skills.

Mind maps provide students with a strategy for integrating critical thinking and problem-solving skills (Wu and Wu, 2020). The advantages of mind mapping include its free-form and unconstrained structure, the generation of unlimited ideas and links, promotion of creativity and encouragement of brain-storming (Alsuraihi, 2022). In order for meaningful learning to occur, students must link new information with their existing knowledge. The multisensory nature of mind maps, which can incorporate colour and pictures, also facilitates the transfer of information from short- to long-term memory (see Case Study 37.2).

REFLECTING ON COGNITIVE BIASES

Retrospective analyses of critical incident reports have identified that cognitive errors rather than a lack of knowledge are the major cause of errors in healthcare (Alyahya et al., 2021). Decision making is a complex process and generally an intuitive or an analytical approach is used (this is sometimes referred to as dual-process theory) (Croskerry, 2003). Intuitive decision making is used repetitively in our everyday lives and when at work. It is a largely unconscious thought-processing system that is fast, mostly effective but also prone to failure (Melin-Johansson et al., 2017). Intuitive thinking is typically 'hardwired' to save time and mental effort, especially when we are familiar (or overly familiar) with a task, when there are time constraints and when there is a real or perceived need to take shortcuts. It is sometimes characterized by an

---

CASE STUDY 37.2

Example of a Mind-Mapping Activity

Jacob Chikuhwa is a 75-year-old patient who is 1 day post-op after major surgery for oesophageal cancer. He has IV fluids running at 80 mL per hour and a patient-controlled analgesia (PCA) of morphine. At 0700 hours, his vital signs were temperature 37°C, pulse rate 110 beats per minute (weak and thready), respiratory rate 20 breaths per minute and blood pressure 110/55 mmHg. His urine output is averaging 10 to 15 mL per hour. In groups, create a mind map that illustrates the pathophysiology related to Mr. Chikuhwa's current situation and the related thinking processes. See Fig. 37.1 for an example of a mind map.

'I've got this … I've seen it a hundred times' attitude. By contrast, analytical decision making is a conscious process that is generally reliable, safe and effective, but it is also slow and deliberate (Croskerry, 2003).

Clinical educators have a responsibility to help nursing students become aware of cognitive factors that affect their clinical reasoning, for example:

- the hardwired tendency for intuitive thinking the risk of cognitive overload – studies have shown that an average of only seven units of information can be held in the working memory (Miller, 1956)
- the tendency to make errors when thinking is affected by fatigue, stress, prejudice and preconceptions (Croskerry et al., 2013).

REFLECTION POINT

- Can you recall any personal or professional experiences in which your cognitive biases impacted your clinical reasoning?
- What did you learn from this experience?
- How could you use your experience to inform or improve your teaching?

One way of raising learners' awareness is through the provision of opportunities for reflection on and in practice. This allows for metacognition, or thinking about thinking, by stepping away from the immediate

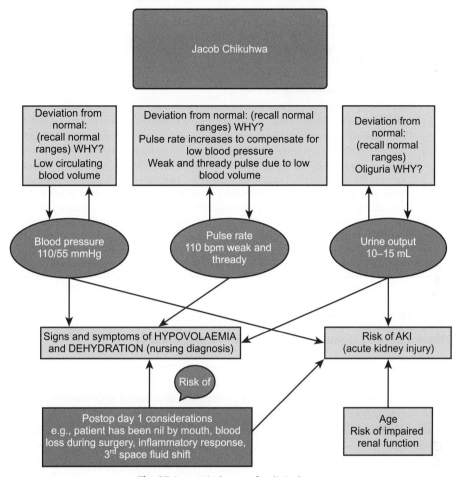

Fig. 37.1 ■ Mind map of a clinical case.

problem to examine and reflect on one's thinking or to re-examine a clinical situation after it has passed.

Both intuitive and analytical thinking, irrespective of level of nursing experience, can be influenced by cognitive biases. These types of thinking errors are one of the major causes of inaccurate clinical reasoning and consequently adverse patient outcomes. Educators must help students to become familiar with various types of cognitive biases (Table 37.1) and to consider how their clinical reasoning can be clouded by negative stereotypes, preconceptions and prejudices.

Educators should be alert to situations where students demonstrate thinking errors that are influenced by cognitive biases; for example, comments such as 'he is drug seeking, he doesn't really have pain' (fundamental attribution error), 'she is 85 … so confusion is not at all surprising' (ascertainment bias); and 'I'm sure' (overconfidence bias). These thinking errors interfere with effective clinical reasoning and are therefore a risk to patient safety. Educators should question (and even challenge) students when they are concerned about their cognitive biases and use these as opportunities for 'just in time teaching'. These situations can also be used to prompt students to reflect on and consider the basis to their flawed perceptions and thinking processes.

REFLECTION POINT

■ With reference to Table 37.1 and Case Study 37.3, how could you facilitate students' reflection on practice in a way that encourages and enables them to identify their own cognitive biases?

TABLE 37.1

Examples of Cognitive Biases That Affect Clinical Reasoning

Cognitive Bias	Definition
Anchoring	The tendency to lock onto salient features in the patient's presentation too early in the clinical reasoning process and failing to adjust this initial impression in the light of later information. Compounded by confirmation bias.
Ascertainment bias	When a nurse's thinking is shaped by prior assumptions and preconceptions, for example, ageism, stigmatism and stereotyping.
Confirmation bias	The tendency to look for confirming evidence to support a nursing diagnosis rather than look for disconfirming evidence to refute it, despite the latter often being more persuasive and definitive.
Diagnostic momentum	Once labels are attached to patients, they tend to become stickier and stickier. What starts as a possibility gathers increasing momentum until it becomes definite and other possibilities are excluded.
Fundamental attribution error	The tendency to be judgemental and blame patients for their illnesses (dispositional causes) rather than examine the circumstances (situational factors) that may have been responsible. Psychiatric patients, those from minority groups and other marginalized groups tend to be at risk of this error.
Overconfidence bias	A tendency to believe we know more than we do. Overconfidence reflects a tendency to act on incomplete information, intuition or hunches. Too much faith is placed on opinion instead of carefully collected cues. This error may be augmented by anchoring.
Premature closure	The tendency to apply premature closure to the decision-making process, accepting a diagnosis before it has been fully verified. This error accounts for a high proportion of missed diagnosis.

Adapted from Croskerry, P., 2003. The importance of cognitive errors in diagnosis and strategies to minimize them. Acad. Med., 78(8), 775–780.

CASE STUDY 37.3

A Reflection About Cognitive Biases by a Third-Year Nursing Student

A 52-year-old male patient, John (pseudonym), was brought into the emergency department by the police and the local mental health team. John was in breach of his community treatment order. On presentation, John had slurred speech, was unable to stand or walk unassisted and was very aggressive. A code black was called after the triage nurse was punched and the attending nurse was bitten whilst obtaining a blood pressure. The emergency medical officer and two security personal responded, with John being restrained and sedation administered.

I had been asked to obtain a patient history. However, upon presentation I had already labelled John as an alcoholic who was homeless and suffering from some sort of mental illness. I didn't see the purpose of taking a full patient history and thought that we just needed to sober him up and then release him back to the mental health team. The clinical reasoning errors that influenced my attitude and thinking included fundamental attribution error (I believed the patient's illness and situation were self-inflicted as a result of his decision to drink) and overconfidence bias and unpacking principle (I did not believe this patient had any real medical issues because of my labelling him as an alcoholic). As a result of my assumptions, I did not collect a thorough history or assessment of this patient and disregarded the real medical and social problems that he was presenting with.

John was homeless and had been for the past 6 years, since his wife, daughter and two grandchildren had been killed in a car accident; he was simply unable to function anymore. Three years ago, John had come to the attention of the mental health team and he was diagnosed with an anxiety disorder, delusions, paranoia and panic attacks; he was also misusing alcohol and drugs; however, he had been clean and sober for the past 18 months. It was later established that John had a blood alcohol reading of zero. He was diagnosed with severe dehydration and a mild cerebrovascular haemorrhage.

I was fortunate to have been supervised throughout this experience so my personal judgements did not endanger this patient. However, this has been an invaluable experience for me as I have learnt that you need to treat every patient individually without judgement and a thorough history is essential to understand what may be affecting the patient's health status. I will endeavour to remember this in the future and not allow my biases to cloud my thinking.

Source: Levett-Jones, T., Sundin, D., Bagnall, M., et al., 2010. Learning to think like a nurse. Handover – Hunter N. Engl. Nurs. J. 3, 15–20.

SUMMARY

In this chapter, we have explored seven creative strategies for facilitating the development of nursing students' clinical reasoning skills:

- providing opportunities for autonomous practice,
- focussing on deliberate practice,
- using higher-order questioning,
- emphasizing the importance of evidence-based practice,
- learning to think aloud,
- deconstructing critical events and
- reflecting on cognitive biases.

Each of these strategies can be used to address students' specific learning needs in relation to clinical reasoning and to foster lifelong critical thinking habits.

REFLECTION POINT

- Can you think of any upcoming opportunities to apply some of the suggestions in this chapter to your clinical teaching?
- What actions would you need to take to prepare for this teaching and to optimize effectiveness of the selected activity?

REFERENCES

Altalhi, F., Altalhi, A., Magliah, Z., Abushal, Z., Althaqafi, A., Falemban, A., et al., 2021. Development and evaluation of clinical reasoning using "think aloud" approach in pharmacy undergraduates – A mixed-methods study. Saudi Pharmaceutical Journal 29 (11), 1250–1257. https://doi.org/10.1016/j.jsps.2021.10.003

Alsuraihi, A.A., 2022. The effect of implementing mind maps for online learning and assessment on students during COVID-19 pandemic: A cross sectional study. BMC Medical Education 22 (1), 169. https://doi.org/10.1186/s12909-022-03211-2

Alyahya, M.S., Hijazi, H.H., Alolayyan, M.N., Ajayneh, F.J., Khader, Y.S., Al-Sheyab, N.A., 2021. The association between cognitive medical errors and their contributing organizational and individual factors. Risk Management and Healthcare Policy 14, 415–430. https://doi.org/10.2147/RMHP.S293110

Banning, M., 2008. The think aloud approach as an educational tool to develop and assess clinical reasoning in undergraduate students. Nurse Education Today 28 (1), 8–14. https://doi.org/10.1016/j.nedt.2007.02.001

Bathish, M., Wilson, C., Potempa, K., 2018. Deliberate practice and nurse competence. Applied Nursing Research 40, 106–109. https://doi.org/10.1016/j.apnr.2018.01.002

Bristol, T., Hagler, D., McMillian-Bohler, J., Wermers, R., Hatch, D., Oermann, M.H., 2019. Nurse educators' use of lecture and active learning. Teaching and Learning in Nursing 14 (2), 94–96. https://doi.org/10.1016/j.teln.2018.12.003

Croskerry, P., 2003. The importance of cognitive errors in diagnosis and strategies to minimize them. Academic Medicine 78 (8), 775–780. https://doi.org/10.1097/00001888-200308000-00003

Croskerry, P., Singhal, G., Mamede, S., 2013. Cognitive debiasing 1: Origins of bias and theory of debiasing. BMJ Quality & Safety 22 (Suppl 2), ii58–ii64. https://doi.org/10.1136/bmjqs-2012-001712

Dreifuerst, K.T., 2012. Using debriefing for meaningful learning to foster development of clinical reasoning in simulation. The Journal of Nursing Education 51 (6), 326–333. https://doi.org/10.3928/01484834-20120409-0

Falcó-Pegueroles, A., Rodríguez-Martín, D., Ramos-Pozón, S., Zuriguel-Pérez, E., 2021. Critical thinking in nursing clinical practice, education and research: From attitudes to virtue. Nurs Philos 22 (1), e12332–n/a. https://doi.org/10.1111/nup.12332

Farmer, R.W., Saner, S., Weingartner, L.A., Rabalais, G., 2021. Questioning Aid for Rich, Real-Time Discussion (QARRD): A tool to improve critical thinking in clinical settings. MedEdPORTAL 17, 11132. https://doi.org/10.15766/mep_2374-8265.11132

Levett-Jones, T. (Ed.), 2022. Clinical reasoning: Learning to think like a nurse, 3rd ed. Pearson, Sydney.

Mabry, J., Lee, E., Roberts, T., Garrett, R., 2020. Virtual simulation to increase self-efficacy through deliberate practice. Nurse Educator 45 (4), 202–205. https://doi.org/10.1097/NNE.0000000000000758

Melin-Johansson, C., Palmqvist, R., Rönnberg, L., 2017. Clinical intuition in the nursing process and decision-making—A mixed-studies review. Journal of Clinical Nursing 26 (23-24), 3936–3949. https://doi.org/10.1111/jocn.13814

Miller, G., (1956). "Human memory and the storage of information," in IRE Transactions on Information Theory, vol. 2, no. 3, pp. 129–137, September 1956, https://doi.org/10.1109/TIT.1956.1056815

Phillips, N.M., Duke, M.M., Weerasuriya, R., 2017. Questioning skills of clinical facilitators supporting undergraduate nursing students. Journal of Clinical Nursing 26 (23-24), 4344–4352. https://doi.org/10.1111/jocn.13761

Pinnock, R., Young, L., Spence, F., Henning, M., Hazell, W., 2015. Can think aloud be used to teach and assess clinical reasoning in graduate medical education? Journal of Graduate Medical Education 7 (3), 334–337. https://doi.org/10.4300/JGME-D-14-00601.1

Skela-Savič, B., Dobnik, M., Kalender-Smajlović, S., 2020. Nurses' work characteristics and self-assessment of the work environment—Explorative cross-sectional study. Journal of Nursing Management 28 (4), 860–871. https://doi.org/10.1111/jonm.13010

Todhunter, F., 2015. Using concurrent think-aloud and protocol analysis to explore student nurses' social learning information communication technology knowledge and skill development. Nurse Education Today 35 (6), 815–822. https://doi.org/10.1016/j.nedt.2015.01.010

Verkuyl, M., Hughes, M., Fyfe, M.C., 2018. Using think aloud in health assessment: A mixed-methods study. The Journal of Nursing Education 57 (11), 684–686. https://doi.org/10.3928/01484834-20181022-10

Wu, H.Z., Wu, Q.T., 2020. Impact of mind mapping on the critical thinking ability of clinical nursing students and teaching application. Journal of International Medical Research 48 (3), 0300060519893225.

38

INTERPROFESSIONAL PROGRAMMES TO DEVELOP CLINICAL REASONING

ROLA AJJAWI ▪ ROSEMARY BRANDER ▪ JILL E. THISTLETHWAITE

CHAPTER OUTLINE

CHAPTER AIMS

The aims of this chapter are:

- to clarify key concepts in relation to interprofessional education (IPE), collaborative practice and clinical reasoning
- to integrate research and practice knowledge in relation to IPE and clinical reasoning
- to have a greater understanding of how to develop collaborative clinical reasoning.

INTRODUCTION

Clinical reasoning (CR) is a key capability for healthcare professionals. Although there is overlap between how CR is conceptualized and taught across professions, there are differences arising from variations in professionals' roles, responsibilities and scope of practice. A recent scoping review identified diversity across health professions in their operationalizations of CR, for example the nursing literature prioritized it as a skill, medicine as diagnosis and allied health as contextual (Young et al., 2020), while dentistry predominantly focussed on therapeutic reasoning (Khatami et al., 2019). Collaborative clinical reasoning (CCR) is defined as when 'two or more healthcare team members negotiate diagnostic, therapeutic, or prognostic issues of an individual patient resulting in an illness or treatment plan' (Kiesewetter et al., 2017, p. 123). How information is represented by individual team members and exchanged within a team influences CCR (Kiesewetter et al., 2017).

Interprofessional education (IPE) is recommended as a method of 'learning together to work together' (WHO, 2010). Additionally, IPE together with collaborative practice (CP) is regarded as a World Health Organization's priority for universal health coverage (WHO, 2022). In this chapter, we focus on the rationale

---

BOX 38.1
DEFINITIONS OF IPE, IPL AND CP

- Interprofessional education (IPE): Occasions when two or more professions learn with, from and about each other to improve collaboration and the quality of care (Centre for the Advancement of Interprofessional Education (CAIPE), 2002).
- Interprofessional learning (IPL): 'Learning arising from interaction between members (or students) of two or more professions. This may be a product of formal IPE or happen spontaneously in the workplace or in education settings' (Freeth et al., 2005, p. 15).
- Collaborative practice (CP): In healthcare, CP occurs when multiple health workers from different professional backgrounds provide comprehensive services by working with patients, their families, carers and communities to deliver the highest quality of care across settings (WHO, 2010, p. 7).

---

for IPE and its feasibility as a means of helping students develop CR in preparation for working collaboratively and in teams. Key terms are defined in Box 38.1.

WHAT IS IPE?

Early advocates of IPE realized the illogicality of each health profession being educated in a silo with little interaction with other professions (e.g. Barr, 1996). They argued that uniprofessionally trained practitioners typically move into a healthcare system in which clients interact with a diverse range of providers but with little experience of this way of working. Clients with complex needs and chronic conditions require a team-based or collaborative approach to diagnosis and management because one profession does not typically have the capability to do everything necessary. The rationale for IPL is therefore to facilitate such interactions through providing students with a grounding and experience in teamwork and its theory. Activities to help develop CCR are a good platform for achieving IPL outcomes. Students require time to observe and discuss their own and other professionals' approaches to decision making, undertake the interprofessional negotiation that may be required and, together with the client's input, reach consensus for a plan of care.

The push to incorporate IPE into university-based prequalification healthcare professional education

programmes has gained momentum because accreditation bodies in many countries have included IPL outcomes or competencies in their standards. A problem, however, is that these outcomes are frequently expressed in different words without agreement across all professions. This can hinder planning educational activities as each profession tries to meet its own requirements. Language may also be a barrier to successful implementation of IPE; even agreeing on terminology, such as patient, client or service-user, may be difficult. However, when delivered effectively, IPE can foster an understanding of the broad range of healthcare professions, the ways in which they interact with clients and how they complement each other. IPL activities are likely to be more successful in achieving these outcomes if there is interdependence (genuine contribution of each profession involved), embodiment (learners experience what it is like to work collaboratively within their professions and with others through authentic activities) and facilitators are skilled interprofessionally (Maddock et al., 2023).

LEARNING OUTCOMES

Frameworks defining IPL outcomes have been published (Thistlethwaite et al., 2014; IPEC, 2016). The WHO (2022) framework for universal healthcare includes competencies related to the practice philosophy of teamwork as one of six competency domains that 'health workers should integrate into their practice to contribute towards the provision of quality health services' (p. 13). There is commonality in terms of broad outcomes (Box 38.2), which may be used for developing IPL activities focussing on CCR. It is important for learners to be aware of what they are expected to achieve, not only in terms of subject content (e.g. diagnostic reasoning categories) but also 'with, from and about' their peers from the professions involved. The rationale for IPE and its importance for clinical practice need to be discussed with learners.

IPL ACTIVITIES FOR CLINICAL REASONING

Practitioners need to develop the skills to engage in CCR; they must be able to discern which professions,

---

BOX 38.2
BROAD AREAS OF IPL OUTCOMES AND THEIR RELEVANCE TO CLINICAL REASONING

- Interprofessional communication: Enabling professionals to discuss and agree on, from the data they have gathered, the nature of the condition and the goals of care.
- Interprofessional working: Working with one or more other professionals to achieve their goals in partnership with the client and family.
- Responsibilities and role clarification: An important part of the understanding necessary to plan care.
- Team functioning: Achieving the goals requires optimal team working and respect.
- Collaborative and shared leadership: Agreement among the professionals and the client on the leadership required, which may change, throughout the care path.
- Interprofessional conflict resolution: Necessary when professionals' data and care plans differ with recognition that constructive conflict may lead to better care and outcomes.
- Professional values and ethical practice throughout.

---

specialists and community partners are required for successful diagnosis and care. Therefore, developing an understanding of CR with respect to collaborative competencies across professions and sectors at an early stage of career development is an asset. This needs to occur across a variety of contexts in increasingly complex ways.

LEARNING THROUGH STRUCTURED OPPORTUNITIES IN THE CLASSROOM

Activities that promote discussion and shared thinking about a real or hypothetical client case are ideal IPL opportunities for promoting CR. Many examples exist in the literature grounded in problem-based (e.g. Lestari et al., 2019), case-based (e.g. Hanum et al., 2023) and team-based learning (e.g. Fatmi et al., 2013) and role play (e.g. Berger et al., 2022). In these collaborative inquiry–constructed approaches, students exchange ideas, identify knowledge deficits, clarify roles and responsibilities, agree on solutions and develop care plans. They learn with each other

about specific client presentations, the roles of other healthcare professionals in exploring clients' stories and caring for clients, and improve their understanding of other healthcare professional values, semantics, roles and contributions – all important for CCR.

The design of cases and scenarios can be quite sophisticated. For example, Jorm et al. (2016) used complexity theory to deliver IPL activities for 1220 healthcare students through developing complicated client cases that required more than simple application of each student's profession-specific knowledge. These cases were designed so that they provided a context for meaningful interaction. The issue of scenario realism, the degree to which a scenario is likely to be similar to participants' experiences in real life, has been found to be crucial for student engagement (van Soeren et al., 2011). To achieve this aim, case scenarios must be interprofessional. Realistic clinical scenarios allow participants to practice their profession-specific knowledge in an interprofessional context. Client scenarios can be extended beyond the classroom into simulated settings, where aspects of realism and fidelity may be more closely maintained.

LEARNING THROUGH SIMULATION

CCR simulation can provide learners with opportunities to develop competence in skills required for successful collaboration. Learning through simulation has the potential to enable students and clinicians to analyse their own actions critically, reflect on skills and critique the clinical decisions of others (van Soeren et al., 2011). One such activity is the Health Care Team Challenge (HCTC) in which students form interprofessional teams that participate in a friendly competition. Students are provided with a client case and are asked to develop a client-centred collaborative plan of care, reinforced with evidence and best practice, which they present to a judging panel and audience. The educational process centres on group learning with authentic teamwork over time (Newton et al., 2013).

The HCTC process is rigorous, following stipulated competition rules occurring at local, regional, national and international levels. Students develop knowledge of their own and each other's roles and abilities within the team and for the unique simulated case. They can develop high-level teamwork skills, for example, in

CASE STUDY 38.1

Preparing for Team Work

Your IPL group, consisting of students from medicine, nursing, nutrition, pharmacy and physiotherapy, is asked to consult with Rosie, a 77-year-old attending the community clinic to which you are attached. Rosie has been referred for help with pain and poor mobility caused by osteoarthritis in both knees. Her body mass index is 31, and she is taking medication for type 2 diabetes, hypertension and chronic pain. This is the first time you have worked together in this group. Before meeting Rosie, how do you prepare to work as a team? What do you hope to learn from this encounter and what is the value of collaborating with students from other health professions? If you are the educator facilitating the interprofessional care plan, how might you help students to understand different professional groups' perspectives on diagnosis and care?

conflict resolution and collaborative leadership, as they work together through the client's case and negotiate a best plan of care. Students become more knowledgeable about common healthcare regulatory issues and anticipate safety issues for service users and for healthcare workers. Together they build trust, dispel professional stereotypes and strengthen their competence for CP. When feasible, the patient (or client)/family representatives are involved in the care plan, may give feedback on team performance and/or may be part of the judging team.

In other examples, speech pathology and dietetics students have participated in interprofessional simulation workshops to treat patients with clinical dysphagia. Students gained confidence, preparedness, knowledge and improved their CR scores (Miles et al., 2016). Debriefs prompted discussions of clinical decisions with their peers and the vignettes were developed by an interprofessional team (see Case Study 38.1).

VIRTUAL IPL

Virtual learning has burgeoned over the past few years in the global pandemic environment (Ingels et al., 2022) mirroring real-life practice. Students have had the opportunity to participate in virtual real-life interprofessional teams (Zhang et al., 2022), as well as virtual simulation teams (Showstark et al., 2023; Holland et al., 2022) during their IPL. Consequently, theory development and evaluation of virtual IPL is necessary. Early work indicates that it may be a useful tool to scaffold learning toward interprofessional workplace experiences (Azim et al., 2022). The link between virtual IPL and developing CCR needs to be further explored.

WORKPLACE-BASED LEARNING

Prequalification learners frequently tell us that application of interprofessional principles in the workplace is difficult. Higgs et al. (2008) described the development of CR ability as integrating theoretical and clinical knowledge to make sense of clinical findings. This ability can then help develop practice wisdom that incorporates the understanding of complex social interactions, ethical subtleties and individual situations and context.

Learning spaces, which bridge workplace and classroom learning, have been extended in creative ways to facilitate the development of practice wisdom, which takes considerable time and exposure to clinical realities. Hearing about experiences from authentic interprofessional teams provides a 'reality check' and enables students to extend their imaginations into, and further their understandings of, clinical practice. Through critical discussion and reflection with each other, plus guided faculty and clinician facilitation, students can sort through domains such as individual and team roles, communications and actions taken, and propose questions and alternative solutions for the scenarios presented.

Learning in Hospitals

Examples of hospital-based IPL include interprofessional student-led outpatient and hospital clinics and interprofessional training wards (IPTWs). These settings have been found to increase students' understanding of their future professional roles and those of other professions, highlighting the value of teamwork for client care (Falk et al., 2013). They have positive long-term effects on interprofessional socialization and collaboration (Mink et al., 2021). The proximity among students, sharing of responsibility and authentic tasks have been found to enable CP and development of professional knowledge, for example, through round-table discussions of client care, negotiations and decision making about specific clients. Students on an IPTW can work to clarify how the variety of professional roles and understandings of care contribute to the team, the care plan and ultimately the welfare of the client.

CR has been found to be an important factor in the success of an IPTW and the development of interprofessional care plans (Visser et al., 2019). IPTWs have raised awareness of unexpected issues where students experienced dissonance between the reality of CP and expectations of their own professional role (Falk et al., 2013). Being able to discuss and guide students' expectations is important for optimizing their engagement and learning. The supervising clinicians on IPTWs ideally work with students from other professions as well as their own. They have been shown to be able to scaffold the CR of all students by modelling interprofessionality, facilitating reflections on care and ensuring that all students feel able to participate in discussions (Visser et al., 2020).

Learning in the Community Through Community Engagement, Partnerships and Service

A mutually beneficial approach, centred on both student and community needs, has demonstrated successful learning outcomes (Brander et al., 2015a). For example, students who were scheduled for placements in primary care clinics were organized to spend time together to review and discuss educational modules about compassion in primary care purposefully created for IPL. This opportunity encouraged students to develop CR skills related to CP and compassion in the primary care context, which they could extrapolate to other healthcare contexts (Donnelly et al., 2016). Interprofessional student-run free clinics (SRFC) in underserved areas in the United States allowed learners to provide hands-on care. Evaluations indicate that students working in SRFC perceive that their CR skills improve as well as their attitudes to working in teams (Seif et al., 2014) and CP skills (Hu et al., 2018).

Community engagement and community partnerships are inextricably linked for the creation of useful and accountable learning opportunities. A variety of IPL experiences with real healthcare teams, across a variety of contexts, will assist students to develop CR in preparation for demanding healthcare careers. In addition, interprofessional faculty and clinicians working together to deliver educational initiatives are provided with robust prospects to role-model the realization of collaboration, reveal some of the hidden curriculum and facilitate learners' professional behaviour growth. Fig. 38.1 shows the different IPE models of interaction.

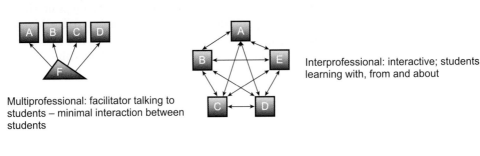

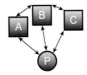

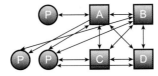

Multiprofessional: facilitator talking to students – minimal interaction between students

Interprofessional: interactive; students learning with, from and about

Students interviewing a patient together

IP training ward or clinic: students interacting with patients and each other

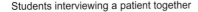

Fig. 38.1 ■ Examples of multiprofessional and interprofessional (IP) activities. *A, B, C, D, E,* students from different health professions; *F,* facilitator; *P,* patient.

LEARNING ABOUT COLLABORATIVE LEADERSHIP

Collaborative leadership is a more complex form of leadership that has emerged to better fit with collaborative client-centred care and the realities of current-day regulations and practice. Collaborative leaders 'engage one another in such a way that leaders and followers raise one another's levels of motivation and morality and nurture interdependencies among multiple parties' (VanVactor, 2012, p. 555) for the achievement of collective goals and successful outcomes. Four key leadership competencies of collaborative teams have been identified: being authentic, empowering, facilitating and sustaining (Brander et al., 2015b).

Dow et al. (2013) suggested a framework to assist with curriculum planning for CP for healthcare workers, which includes the development of leadership. First, 'leadership and followership', described as being co-produced by the healthcare workers, requires the ability to move between leading and following roles. Second, 'locus and formality of leadership' is demonstrated by the ability to modify leadership behaviours based on a leader's relationship to the team and the formality of leadership required for any unique situation (Dow et al., 2013, p. 954). Dow et al. (2013) claim that learners, at all levels who develop CR and skills related to these concepts, will be better team members and leaders. Learning experiences, from the classroom to simulation to the clinic, are important to develop the needed team competencies for successful outcomes in healthcare professional learners.

CHALLENGES OF IPE

Introducing and sustaining IPL activities is challenging. Descriptions of IPE frequently cite problems as being logistical, including large numbers of learners in undergraduate programmes across multiple departments and schools; timetabling as each healthcare professional course has its own system and clinical placements; curriculum space; and varying supervisory requirements. With committed educators and careful planning, logistics may be overcome and there are many examples of innovative ways of doing this. In our experience, the major barriers are professional hierarchies, lack of understanding of IPE and what it may achieve, and concerns about professional identity and scope of practice. Further development and adoption of virtual IPL opportunities has been shown to mitigate some of these barriers (Showstark et al., 2023). It is important that everyone involved in IPE development agrees on learning outcomes and/or competencies to be achieved, activities necessary for that achievement, the type and timing of assessment and what faculty development and commitment is required.

Professionals typically approach client problems based on profession-specific ways of knowing because of professional socialization into particular ways of thinking, talking and being (Ajjawi and Higgs, 2008). This poses specific challenges in relation to IPL for the development of CR. A multicentre European study exploring the difficulties of implementing a longitudinal CR curriculum identified collaboration issues, lack of interprofessional communication and disagreement about the concept as three barriers to overcome (Sudacka et al., 2021). Healthcare professional educators may, therefore, need to discuss how CR is conceived by different professions and what implications this has for IPE. Students working interprofessionally may need to move from their usual professional responsibilities to negotiate and make decisions collectively for the care of the client (Falk et al., 2013). These 'boundary zones' can be sites of struggle, where educator support and debrief are essential.

REFLECTION POINT

- How might you identify that a student is struggling with CCR?
- How could you tackle this?

FACULTY DEVELOPMENT

A robust programme of faculty development for IPE is necessary to enable staff to acquire attributes required for effective interprofessional facilitation (see Reflection Point about the attributes for effective interprofessional facilitation.). Such development should be devised and delivered by an interprofessional group. As IPL activities for CR may take place within a range of locations, faculty development is a complex process. An interprofessional educator should be attuned to the dynamics of IPL and skilled in optimizing learning opportunities while valuing each participating profession's experience and expertise (Barr, 1996).

A study into educators facilitating IPE programmes found that not all brought positive attitudes towards other professions (Croker et al., 2016). Interprofessional facilitators need to develop awareness of how students are interacting and be able to involve students in feedback dialogue about team processes and their roles, responsibilities and language. The facilitator may need to challenge stereotyping, encourage students to challenge this themselves and compare group work to develop students' quality judgements. It is important that all professions involved feel able to contribute and that no one profession dominates discussions. Focussing students on client needs, rather than specific professional roles, can be valuable for educators to break down boundaries through shared negotiation and decision making.

REFLECTION POINT

Reflect on the attributes below for effective interprofessional facilitation:

- How do these match your own experiences and capacity?
- How might you tackle these in a faculty development programme?
  - Knowledge of the rationale/evidence for IPE
  - Commitment to IPE
  - Knowledge of roles, responsibilities and scope of practice of healthcare professionals
  - Understanding of teamwork theory
  - Understanding of CP/CCR and what it looks like in the workplace
  - Understanding of professional identity development and its effect on interprofessional practice
  - Skills in negotiation and conflict resolution

SUMMARY

- There are differences in the way clinical reasoning is conceptualized and taught across professions arising from variations in professionals'

knowledge, roles, responsibilities and scope of practice.
- The development of clinical reasoning requires students to observe and discuss their own and other professional's approaches to decision making and the negotiation that may be required interprofessionally (with the client) to agree on a management plan and carry it out.
- Learning to reason interprofessionally can be taught through the formal (e.g. case-based learning, simulation) and the practice (e.g. community placements and IPTWs) curriculum, both in-person and virtual IP teams. Vignettes need to be interprofessional and demonstrate real-world complexity.
- Making the reasoning focus explicit allows for discussion and exploration of how others think in practice.
- The role of the educator is complex and nuanced, with specific faculty development required.

REFERENCES

Ajjawi, R., Higgs, J., 2008. Learning to reason: A journey of professional socialisation. Advances in Health Sciences Education: Theory and Practice 13 (2), 133–150. https://doi.org/10.1007/s10459-006-9032-4

Azim, A., Kocaqi, E., Wojkowski, S., Uzelli-Yilmaz, D., Foohey, S., Sibbald, M., 2022. Building a theoretical model for virtual interprofessional education. Medical Education 56 (11), 1105–1113. https://doi.org/10.1111/medu.14867

Barr, H., 1996. Ends and means in interprofessional education: Towards a typology. Education for Health 9, 341–352.

Berger, S., Krug, K., Goetz, K., 2022. Encountering uncertainty and complexity in decision-making: An observational study of clinical reasoning among medical and interprofessional groups of health care students. Journal of Interprofessional Care 37 (2), 262–271. https://doi.org/10.1080/13561820.2022.2061928

Brander, R., Bainbridge, L., Van Dijk, J., Paterson, M., 2015a. Transformative continuing interprofessional education and professional development to meet patient care needs: A synthesis of best practices. In: Orchard, C., Bainbridge, L. (Eds.), Interprofessional client-centred collaborative practice: What does it look like? How can it be achieved? Nova, pp. 113–130.

Brander, R., MacPhee, M., Careau, E., Tassone, M., Verma, S., Paterson, M., et al., 2015b. Collaborative leadership for the transformation of health systems. In: Forman, D., Jones, M., Thistlethwaite, J. (Eds.), Leadership and collaboration: Further developments for interprofessional education. Palgrave MacMillan, pp. 153–166.

Centre for the Advancement of Interprofessional Education (CAIPE), 2002. About CAIPE. https://www.caipe.org/about.

Croker, A., Wakely, L., Leys, J., 2016. Educators working together for interprofessional education: From "fragmented beginnings" to being "intentionally interprofessional". Journal of Interprofessional Care 30 (5), 671–674. https://doi.org/10.1080/13561820.2016.1181613

Donnelly, C., Brander, R., Watson, S., O'Riordan, A., Murphy, S., Chapman, C. (2016). *Teaching compassionate care in primary care using enhanced online delivery methods.* The Canadian Conference for Medical Educators, Montreal, Canada. Abstract #OF 1–3, p. 103.

Dow, A.W., DiazGranados, D., Mazmanian, P.E., Retchin, S.M., 2013. Applying organizational science to health care: A framework for collaborative practice. Academic Medicine 88, 952–957.

Falk, A.L., Hult, H., Hammar, M., Hopwood, N., Dahlgren, M.A., 2013. One site fits all? A student ward as a learning practice for interprofessional development. Journal of Interprofessional Care 27 (6), 476–481. https://doi.org/10.3109/13561820.2013.807224

Fatmi, M., Hartling, L., Hillier, T., Campbell, S., Oswald, A.E., 2013. The effectiveness of team-based learning on learning outcomes in health professions education: BEME Guide No. 30. Medical Teacher 35 (12), e1608–e1624. https://doi.org/10.3109/0142159X.2013.849802

Freeth, D., Hammick, M., Reeves, S., Koppel, I., Barr, H., 2005. Effective interprofessional education: Development, delivery and evaluation. Blackwell Publishing.

Hanum, C., Findyartini, A., Soemantri, D., 2023. Collaborative clinical reasoning learning using an integrated care pathway in undergraduate interprofessional education: An explorative study. Journal of Interprofessional Care 37 (3), 438–447. https://doi.org/10.1080/13561820.2022.2086221

Higgs, J., Jones, M.A., Titchen, A., 2008. Knowledge, reasoning and evidence for practice. In: Higgs, J., Jones, M.A., Loftus, S., Christensen, N. (Eds.), Clinical reasoning in the health professions, 3rd ed. Elsevier Health Sciences, pp. 151–161.

Holland, A., deGravelles, P., Knight, D., Dickinson, K., Neill, K., Morris, D., et al., 2022. The haunted house experience: Developing a home health assessment training utilizing an interprofessional, interinstitutional virtual simulation. Journal of Allied Health 51 (2), 65E–69E.

Hu, T., Cox, K.A., Nyhof-Young, J., 2018. Investigating student perceptions at an interprofessional student-run free clinic serving marginalised populations. Journal of Interprofessional Care 32 (1), 75–79. https://doi.org/10.1080/13561820.2017.1363724

Ingels, D.J., Zajac, S.A., Kilcullen, M.P., Bisbey, T.M., Salas, E., 2022. Interprofessional teamwork in healthcare: Observations and the road ahead. Journal of Interprofessional Care 37 (3), 338–345. https://doi.org/10.1080/13561820.2022.2090526

Interprofessional Education Collaborative (IPEC), 2016. Core competencies for interprofessional collaborative practice: 2016 update. The National Academies Press.

Jorm, C., Nisbet, G., Roberts, C., Gordon, C., Gentilcore, S., Chen, T.F., 2016. Using complexity theory to develop a student-directed interprofessional learning activity for 1220 healthcare students. BMC Medical Education 16 (1), 199. https://doi.org/10.1186/s12909-016-0717-y

Khatami, S., Macentee, M., Loftus, S., 2019. Clinical reasoning in dentistry. In: Higgs, J., Jensen, G.M., Loftus, S., Christensen, N. (Eds.), Clinical reasoning in the health professions, 4th ed. Elsevier, pp. 261–270.

Kiesewetter, J., Fischer, F., Fischer, M.R., 2017. Collaborative clinical reasoning—A systematic review of empirical studies. Journal of Continuing Education in the Health Professions 37 (2), 123–128. https://doi.org/10.1097/CEH.0000000000000158

Lestari, E., Stalmeijer, R.E., Widyandana, D., Scherpbier, A., 2019. Does PBL deliver constructive collaboration for students in interprofessional tutorial groups? BMC Medical Education 19 (1), 360. https://doi.org/10.1186/s12909-019-1802-9

Maddock, B., Dārziņš, P., Kent, F., 2023. Realist review of interprofessional education for health care students: What works for whom and why. Journal of Interprofessional Care 37 (2), 173–186. https://doi.org/10.1080/13561820.2022.2039105

Miles, A., Friary, P., Jackson, B., Sekula, J., Braakhuis, A., 2016. Simulation-based dysphagia training: Teaching interprofessional clinical reasoning in a hospital environment. Dysphagia 31 (3), 407–415. https://doi.org/10.1007/s00455-016-9691-0

Mink, J., Mitzkat, A., Krug, K., Mihaljevic, A., Trierweiler-Hauke, B., Götsch, B., et al., 2021. Impact of an interprofessional training ward on interprofessional competencies - A quantitative longitudinal study. Journal of Interprofessional Care 35 (5), 751–759. https://doi.org/10.1080/13561820.2020.1802240

Newton, C., Bainbridge, L., Ball, V.A., Wood, V.I., 2013. Health care team challenges: An international review and research agenda. Journal of Interprofessional Care 27 (6), 529–531. https://doi.org/10.3109/13561820.2013.800848

Seif, G., Coker-Bolt, P., Kraft, S., Gonsalves, W., Simpson, K., Johnson, E., 2014. The development of clinical reasoning and interprofessional behaviors: Service-learning at a student-run free clinic. Journal of Interprofessional Care 28 (6), 559–564. https://doi.org/10.3109/13561820.2014.921899

Showstark, M., Joosten-Hagye, D., Wiss, A., Resnik, C., Embry, E., Zschaebitz, E., et al., 2023. Results and lessons learned from a virtual multi-institutional problem-based interprofessional learning approach: The VIPE program. Journal of Interprofessional Care 37 (1), 164–167. https://doi.org/10.1080/13561820.2022.2040453

Sudacka, M., Adler, M., Durning, S.J., Edelbring, S., Frankowska, A., Hartmann, D., et al., 2021. Why is it so difficult to implement a longitudinal clinical reasoning curriculum? A multicenter interview study on the barriers perceived by European health professions educators. BMC Medical Education 21 (1), 575. https://doi.org/10.1186/s12909-021-02960-w

Thistlethwaite, J., Forman, D., Matthews, L.R., Rogers, G.D., Steketee, C., Yassine, T., 2014. Competencies and frameworks in interprofessional education: A comparative analysis. Academic Medicine 89, 869–874.

van Soeren, M., Devlin-Cop, S., MacMillan, K., Baker, L., Egan-Lee, E., Reeves, S., 2011. Simulated interprofessional education: An analysis of teaching and learning processes. Journal of Interprofessional Care 25 (6), 434–440. https://doi.org/10.3109/13561820.2011.592229

VanVactor, J.D., 2012. Collaborative leadership model in the management of health care. Journal of Business Research 65 (4), 555–561. https://doi.org/10.1016/j.jbusres.2011.02.021

Visser, C.L.F., Kusurkar, R.A., Croiset, G., ten Cate, O., Westerveld, H.E., 2019. Students' motivation for interprofessional collaboration after their experience on an IPE ward: A qualitative analysis framed by self-determination theory. Medical Teacher 41 (1), 44–52. https://doi.org/10.1080/0142159X.2018.1436759

Visser, C.L.F., Croiset, G., Wouters, A., Kusurkar, R., 2020. Scaffolding clinical reasoning of healthcare students: A qualitative exploration of supervisors' perceptions on an obstetric IPE ward. Journal of Medical Education and Curricular Development 7, 1–9.

World Health Organization, 2010. Framework for action on interprofessional education and collaborative practice Health Professions Network Nursing and Midwifery Office. World Health Organization, Geneva.

World Health Organization, 2022. Global competency and outcomes framework for universal health coverage. Health Workforce UHL, WHO, Licence: CC BYNC-SA 3.0 IGO.

Young, M.E., Thomas, A., Lubarsky, S., Gordon, D., Gruppen, L.D., Rencic, J., et al., 2020. Mapping clinical reasoning literature across the health professions: A scoping review. BMC Medical Education 20 (1), 107. https://doi.org/10.1186/s12909-020-02012-9

Zhang, W.J., Mansour, D.Z., Lee, M., 2022. Interprofessional education and older adults in the shared virtual classroom: Lessons learned during the COVID-19 pandemic. Journal of Gerontological Nursing 48 (8), 52–56. https://doi.org/10.3928/00989134-20220630-04

39

TEACHING CLINICAL REASONING IN PARAMEDICINE

RYAN K. BATENHORST

CHAPTER OUTLINE

CHAPTER AIMS

The aims of this chapter are:

- to describe effective pedagogical approaches for teaching clinical reasoning
- to determine pedagogical strategies for integrating simulation into teaching clinical reasoning
- to apply strategies for incorporating evidence-based practices
- to discuss the value of interprofessional collaboration in paramedicine and clinical reasoning education
- to analyse effective strategies for incorporating clinical reasoning into paramedicine education
- to examine challenges and future directions of integrating clinical reasoning into paramedicine education.

INTRODUCTION

Clinical reasoning is a cognitive process used by healthcare professionals, such as doctors, nurses and paramedics, to analyse patient data, make diagnoses, develop treatment plans and ultimately provide patient care. Paramedicine clinical reasoning is a complex cognitive and metacognitive process (Markum, 2012) paramount to patient care in paramedicine practice. *Reasoning* is a process that relates to thought processes, the arrangement of ideas and the assessment of experiences to reach conclusions (Banning, 2008). In the clinical context, paramedics draw on their specific scientific knowledge and clinical experience and integrate that with what is known about the specific situation and patient. They must analyse and synthesize all this information and differentiate its usefulness and application to the patient. This process leads to an informed decision about patient management (Ross et al., 2023).

In paramedicine, clinicians regularly encounter complex patients with multiple co-morbidities across the biopsychosocial spectrum (Edwards et al., 2015; Ross, 2021). These episodes often need to be defined, with management only sometimes fitting into a right or wrong category. An essential process for paramedics

435

is to develop clinical reasoning skills that incorporate their knowledge of pathologies and their previous experiences, combined with the patient presentation, to determine treatment pathways. Paramedics also generally work in the out-of-hospital setting where episodes of care can occur in uncontrolled environments with time pressures (Jennings et al., 2009). These circumstances add cognitive load to clinicians trying to collect, process and make sense of complex information (Ross, 2021). It involves assessing and interpreting a patient's condition based on information such as vital signs, patient history and physical examination findings. The process is dynamic and continuously evolving as new information becomes available. Practical clinical reasoning allows paramedics to prioritize interventions, to determine the most appropriate course of action and to deliver optimal patient care in a time-sensitive, high-stress environment.

Paramedicine clinical reasoning relies on information gathering, analysis and synthesis to arrive at a working diagnosis and implement a suitable treatment plan. Practical clinical reasoning allows paramedics to deliver timely and appropriate patient care in emergencies, which can ultimately improve patient outcomes. Continuous training, experience and an evidence-based approach are essential for enhancing paramedics' clinical reasoning skills and ensuring the best possible care for patients in their most vulnerable moments (Ross et al., 2023).

EFFECTIVE PEDAGOGICAL APPROACHES

Teaching clinical reasoning to paramedicine students is a critical aspect of their education. Clinical reasoning directly impacts paramedicine students' ability to make quick and accurate decisions in emergencies. Clinical reasoning should not be seen as 'just a technical skill' that could be checked off, but it includes knowledge, problem solving, as well as other noncognitive attributes that are all visible in practice (Trowbridge et al., 2015). The authors noted that a more effective pedagogical approach to teaching clinical reasoning skills to paramedicine students is to build from clinical or simulated clinical authentic learning experiences (Andersson et al., 2019). A number of pedagogical strategies are described here and summarized in Table 39.1.

Effective teaching of clinical reasoning requires a balance and integration of theoretical knowledge, hands-on experience and opportunities for self-directed learning through debriefing and reflection on those experiences. By incorporating these pedagogical strategies, educators can help paramedicine students become confident and competent in their decision-making abilities, preparing competent clinicians who create increased positive outcomes for patients.

SIMULATION-BASED CLINICAL EDUCATION

Simulation-based education represents the use of high-fidelity simulation scenarios that replicate real-life emergencies. Simulations provide a safe environment for students to practise their clinical reasoning skills and receive instructor feedback. Simulation is a primary teaching modality and consistently used to educate and train paramedics. Simulation is inherently effective at teaching clinical skills and building student competence in particular areas (Wheeler and Dippenaar, 2020). Similarly, simulation effectively provides paramedicine students with experiences and opportunities to learn in varied environments using differing techniques (Holmboe et al., 2018; Knox et al., 2015). These experiences allow students to apply the relevant skills and knowledge when faced with actual patients (Wheeler and Dippenaar, 2020).

Strategies for Using Simulation in Paramedic Education

Simulation is an increasingly important strategy in health professions education. The term *simulation* can be interpreted in a variety of ways. However, in this context, it describes techniques that imitate prehospital patient situations and are designed to demonstrate procedures, decision making and critical thinking (Jeffries, 2005).

The increasing trend in simulation use in health professions education has many benefits. Notably, simulation allows standardization and consistent replication of patient conditions, it can provide a solution for overcoming limitations of clinical opportunities (e.g. low-frequency encounters) and it can provide an opportunity for students to develop their skills without subjecting actual patients to risk (Rodgers, 2007). Evidence from several

TABLE 39.1
Pedagogical Strategies

Case-based learning	Educators utilize actual or simulated case studies to engage students in problem-solving scenarios that represent real-world emergencies. This strategy allows students to apply their knowledge to real-world situations using critical thinking skills gained from knowledge and previous experiences (McLean, 2016).
Oral case scenarios	Students engage in oral case scenarios when students verbalize treatment strategies for routine and complex patient encounters. This strategy helps students visualize strategies to address patient complaints, allows educators to identify areas of weakness and gaps in knowledge and application, and identifies patterns of weakness among cohorts of students (Thalluri & Penman, 2013).
Concept mapping	In this pedagogical strategy, students create visual representations of a patient presentation, assessment, differential diagnoses and treatment plans. Concept maps help organize to build what they know as they develop a visual representation or structure of their knowledge and facilitate connections they are making between different aspects of patient care (Bilton et al., 2017).
Reflection strategies	After encountering a case or participating in a simulation, educators can challenge paramedic students to reflect back on their performance and decision making as part of a debriefing strategy. Self-reflection and self-assessment can enhance metacognition and allows students to identify areas for improvement in knowledge or experience gaps (Swanwick et al., 2019).
Collaborative learning environments	Paramedics often work in teams, and learning to communicate and reason together effectively is crucial for successful patient care. Johnston et al. (2014) wrote that academics could work horizontally across disciplines to employ interprofessional experiences in simulation as an educational tool to teach vital communication skills. Therefore, when paramedicine is housed in institutions along with other health professions, there are many opportunities for interprofessional education and collaborative practice.
Guided discovery	In this strategy, instead of providing students with all the answers, educators guide them through a series of questions to explore different aspects of a case, identifying comprehension and knowledge gaps. This method stimulates critical thinking and encourages students to seek relevant information independently through a guided approach (Makoolati et al., 2021).
Field experience through clinical rotations	Observing and participating in actual emergencies under preceptor supervision allows students to learn from experienced practitioners and gain practical insights. In most cases, preceptors are not educators. Thus, they may need to be made aware of the objectives of the clinical rotation and the expectations of the academic institution in which the student is enrolled. Clinical rotations should have intended outcomes that trained preceptors facilitate and these need to be communicated with preceptors before the rotation commences. Students should also be engaged in patient care and allowed to develop a differential diagnosis and compose a treatment plan for each patient encounter.
Debates and case discussions	Educators can organize debates on controversial topics in prehospital care or facilitate discussions about challenging cases to encourage students to explore multiple perspectives and potential solutions. Educators can also construct debates and discussions based on the objectives of the current topic presented in the coursework. This strategy encourages students to arrive for class prepared to debate or discuss topics associated with the current coursework or patient complaints being presented.

healthcare disciplines has shown that simulation can improve knowledge and skill performance (Cook et al., 2013; Simon et al., 2012; Wyatt et al., 2004). One study found that paramedicine student error rates were reduced when simulation was used to instruct specific programme components (Motola et al., 2013). Simulation-based education provides standardization and consistency for more reliable assessment of learner performance whereas traditional clinical learning experiences often rely on chance encounters (Hayden et al., 2014; Holmboe et al., 2018).

While such evidence of learning enhancement provides sufficient justification to support the use of simulation in initial paramedic education, a growing body of evidence supports the use of simulation as a substitute for selected clinical experiences. Several studies have reported that replacing a portion of clinical requirements with simulation is equal to or, in some cases, more effective than an equivalent clinical experience (Hall et al., 2005; McGaghie et al., 2011; Salzman et al., 2007; Watson et al., 2012). This evidence is critical for emergency medical services education, given the documented challenges of achieving targeted clinical and field skills and required assessments for paramedicine students (Westgard et al., 2013) and the limited number of opportunities to perform advanced airway management on real patients (Johnston et al., 2006; Mishra and Koehler, 2006).

Simulation is often used in clinical experiential education, but there are also effective strategies for integrating simulation into a paramedicine curriculum that include the following:

- Design realistic scenarios: Create simulation scenarios that closely mimic real-life emergencies paramedics might encounter or have encountered. Use high-fidelity manikins, standardized patients or a combination to make the simulations as authentic as possible. Construct the scenarios to align with the learning objectives and progress in complexity as students advance.
- Student designed scenarios: Allow students to create and present scenarios as a team to the class. Assign students patient conditions or a specific complaint and allow them to create a scenario based on the specific patient complaint. This allows students to be creative while making them think critically regarding the scenario details, physiology and pathology of the patient complaint or disease process. Then have the students who constructed the scenario select their patient, team and team leader and conduct the scenario.
- Active participation: Engage students actively in the simulation process. Assign roles to different students, allowing them to rotate through various responsibilities, such as team leader, partner, bystander, family member, law enforcement officer or patient. Active participation allows students to experience patient encounters from different perspectives.
- Prebriefing and debriefing: Before starting the simulation, provide a prebriefing session where you set the context and objectives. After the simulation, conduct a debriefing session to discuss the students' performance, decisions made and outcomes. Encourage students to reflect on their actions and thought processes during the simulation. Encourage discussion about what went well, what could have been better and why

(Wilson and Asbury, 2019). Another strategy is to record the simulation sessions and to play them back during debriefing. These recordings allow students to reflect on their performance objectively through active discussion while identifying improvement areas.
- Incorporate decision-making challenges: Introduce unexpected developments and challenges during the simulation to reflect the unpredictable nature of real-life emergencies. These unexpected variables require students to think critically, to adapt their approach and to make informed decisions under pressure.
- Interprofessional collaboration: Explore opportunities to involve students from other health professions disciplines (e.g. nursing, medicine, pharmacy, physical therapy) in the simulations. This fosters teamwork, communication and an understanding of each other's roles in patient care. Patient hand-offs, as well as patient reports, are valuable experiences to engage students. Each discipline has different objectives in its treatment regimen. Engaging students in these crucial areas of the patient care continuum is an essential skill in interprofessional collaboration (Furseth et al., 2016; Herge and Hass, 2023).
- Self-directed learning: Encourage students to engage in self-directed learning and study beyond the simulation sessions. Provide them with additional resources, such as medical journals, case studies and online learning materials, to deepen their understanding of clinical reasoning. Paramedicine students must be encouraged to become lifelong learners by learning how to read and interpret research (Williams et al., 2013).
- Promote evidence-based practice: Discuss and demonstrate the importance of using evidence-based guidelines in their decision-making process. Encourage students to support their clinical reasoning with relevant research. Require students to support their treatment modalities by citing relevant research and encourage an evidence-based environment backed by the latest research, driven by students' literature review (McKenna et al., 2015).

The integration of simulation-based clinical education presents an invaluable opportunity to enhance the teaching of clinical reasoning in paramedic education. By providing students with realistic scenarios that represent or were actual emergencies, learners can develop their decision-making skills in a safe and controlled environment. The experiential learning gained through simulation fosters confidence, critical thinking and practical problem-solving abilities, ultimately preparing paramedicine students to deliver the highest quality of care to patients in the field (Williams et al., 2016).

INCORPORATING EVIDENCE-BASED PRACTICE

Incorporating evidence-based practice (EBP) in paramedicine clinical reasoning education is essential to ensure that future paramedics are equipped with the latest, most effective and safest practices in prehospital care. By integrating EBP into their training, paramedicine students can develop critical thinking skills, improve patient outcomes and contribute to the profession's advancement (Mudderman et al., 2020).

Although students spend a great deal of time in classrooms and learn didactic knowledge that includes EBP, statistics and exposure to the critical thinking concepts, students or clinicians might not readily apply the newly learned skills or transfer their newfound knowledge to practice. To assist in transferring and applying skills, educators must learn and use active learning strategies that facilitate the knowledge transfer and application to clinical reality (Barrett et al., 2018; Musolino and Jensen, 2020).

The paramedic education curriculum should include dedicated EBP modules or courses. These courses should cover the principles of EBP, understanding research methodologies and how to appraise critically and to apply research findings in science, medicine and paramedicine. Educators also help students see the importance of online databases and journals where they can access the latest research relevant to prehospital care. Access can be achieved through partnerships with academic institutions, medical libraries or online platforms granting access to peer-reviewed articles. If the programme is part of an academic institution, students should have orientation and access to libraries and peer-reviewed databases to access research (Wilson et al., 2021).

Journal clubs and research projects can also be effective strategies to inspire students to delve into research. Educators can organize regular journal clubs where students can discuss and critique recent research articles. These meetings of like-minded students can foster a culture of critical thinking and allow students to stay current with the latest developments in prehospital care. Research projects encourage students to engage in research related to science, medicine and paramedicine. This research could be through small-scale studies, audits or quality improvement projects. Involvement in research helps students understand the research process and its impact on patient care.

By incorporating EBP into paramedicine student clinical reasoning education, educators can foster a generation of competent and knowledgeable paramedics who provide the best possible care to their patients based on the latest scientific evidence.

Integrating Technology Into Clinical Reasoning Education

Integrating technology into clinical reasoning education for paramedicine students can significantly enhance their learning experience and prepare them for real-world scenarios (Birtill et al., 2021). Virtual reality (VR) and augmented reality (AR) technology can be utilized to immerse students in virtual medical environments (Holmboe et al., 2018). These tools can enable students to visualize complex anatomical structures, to practice procedures and to interact with virtual patients, enhancing their clinical decision-making abilities. The emergence of AR and mixed reality (MR) modalities has increased the potential of simulation in paramedicine education and the integration of AR/MR into education programmes should be underpinned by sound learning design. Research continues to emerge regarding the most effective pedagogical strategies for utilizing this advanced technology in paramedic education (Birtill et al., 2021).

Assessing Paramedicine Student Clinical Reasoning

Assessing paramedicine students' clinical reasoning is essential to ensure students have the necessary skills and knowledge to provide safe and effective patient care. Clinical reasoning is not a generic skill but requires working knowledge that is connected to problem solving in the clinical situation. There is no gold standard for the clinical reasoning process and finding ways to have clinical scenarios along with structure and feedback can be helpful (Trowbridge et al., 2015). Here are some potentially effective methods to assess paramedicine students' clinical reasoning:

- Scenario-based assessments: Present paramedicine students with realistic patient scenarios that they might encounter in the field. These scenarios can be created through written case studies, simulated patient encounters or role-playing exercises. Observe how students gather information, prioritize interventions and make decisions based on the available data.
- Student-created scenarios: Present a student with a patient with a specific medical complaint or traumatic injury. Allow the student to be creative and use critical thinking strategies to create a patient scenario that has both logical sequence and pathophysiological accuracy (see Box 39.1).
- Objective structured clinical examinations (OSCEs): OSCEs are practical exams that assess various clinical skills, including clinical reasoning. Stations can be created to test the student's ability to assess patients, to develop treatment plans and to manage emergencies. Trained examiners evaluate the student's performance based on specific

criteria. Programmes can also use multiple examiners as additional personnel serving as both team members and examiners or add additional examiners to help increase interrater reliability (Cazzell and Howe, 2012).

- Critical thinking and problem-solving questions: Include scenarios in cognitive exams or quizzes that require students to apply their clinical reasoning abilities. These questions prompt students to analyse patient information and devise an appropriate intervention. This preparation will assist students in learning at a higher application level of Bloom's Taxonomy that will prepare them for certification and licensure examinations (Assaly and Smadi, 2015).
- Reflective writing or journalling: Educators can assign students to keep a reflective journal to document their clinical rotations experiences. Journalling can help them process their clinical reasoning and identify areas for improvement. Additionally, reviewing and providing feedback on these reflections can aid in their development.
- Preceptor and instructor feedback: Regularly solicit feedback from preceptors and instructors who supervise the students during clinical rotations. These professionals can provide valuable insight into the student's clinical reasoning abilities and offer constructive feedback for improvement.
- Small group discussions: Encourage students to participate in small group discussions where they can present cases and discuss their clinical reasoning with peers. These discussions foster collaborative learning and allow students to learn from each other's perspectives (Sinnayah et al., 2019).
- 1-minute paper: Present a patient complaint relative to the course's objectives or the material just presented and give students 1 minute to write as much information as they know about the topic, the patient's condition or the material presented. This paper will give educators valuable insight into patterns in knowledge gaps or overall comprehension of the material (Anderson and Burns, 2013).
- PMIQ: PMIQ is another valuable tool for assessing student learning by identifying knowledge gaps and comprehension of the material. In a PMIQ assessment of student learning, educators have students write on paper vertically the letters PMIQ.

BOX 39.1
STUDENT CASE STUDY PRESENTATIONS

1. Select a patient interaction that was particularly interesting or pertinent to the current objectives of the course.
2. Present the case from the perspective initially of the patient's presentation.
3. Present the patient's chief complaint, medical history and interventions performed.
4. Present the background of the call and any known outcomes (students should be encouraged to explore the patient outcomes for educational purposes).
5. Present the patient continuum of care, whether the patient was admitted, required surgical or significant medical interventions, patient outcome and the pathophysiology of the patient's disease process.
6. Cite and present any research or pertinent literature on the patient's presentation, condition or treatment modality.

Then spell out *P* for Pluses, *M* for Minuses, *I* for Interesting and *Q* for questions. Then the educator must explain that pluses are for things students seemed to learn or now know due to the lecture or activity. Minuses are things that students feel that they have not grasped after the activity. *I* is for things the students found interesting, meaning perhaps they are interested but may not understand everything. Lastly, for *Q*, students are invited to use this category for areas of the lecture or activity where they still have questions. This assessment of student learning gives students and educators a nonthreatening, nonstressful means to assess items students have learned, are approaching learning, do not quite understand, or simply have questions about. Whether the student has missed something in the learning or is not grasping the concept at all, it gives educators the ability to assess student learning in real time with valid data (Sharma et al., 2020).

Overall, a comprehensive assessment of paramedicine student clinical reasoning should involve a combination of practical scenarios, written exams, reflective exercises and real-world observations. These assessment tools do not have to be high-stakes or stressful tests. They can be simple, nonthreatening tools given to students with the objective of measuring whether learning is occurring and how well students grasp the material. By utilizing various assessment methods, educators can better measure each student's clinical reasoning abilities and provide valuable data to educators where knowledge gaps may exist.

INTERPROFESSIONAL COLLABORATION

Case Study 39.1 illustrates several elements of both critical thinking and vital communication and collaboration that resulted in a positive outcome for a patient with a positionally life-threatening medical condition. In this scenario, several elements of interprofessional communication and collaboration exist. They are:

- Interprofessional communication between dispatch and the paramedics,
- Communication and collaboration between paramedics (Jon and Heath),

---

CASE STUDY 39.1

Interprofessional Communication and Collaboration in Paramedicine

MEDIC 1131 RESPOND NONEMERGENT TO A PATIENT COMPLAINING OF WEAKNESS

Medic 1131 and Engine 41 responding. Upon arrival, the paramedics find the patient lying in bed on a warm spring afternoon, complaining of generalized weakness. The patient explains to the paramedics, Jon and Heath, that he had been working outside all afternoon on this oddly warm day in early spring. The patient has no other medical problems and takes no medications. Heath then reaches for the patient's wrist to feel for a pulse. As Heath touches the man's arm, a strange look emerges on Heath's face. He looks at Jon with a puzzled look and says 'we should apply the monitor'. The patient's heart rate is slow. The paramedics applied the heart monitor and discovered the patient had a complete heart block.

At that point, the paramedics decided to obtain a 12-Lead ECG to better analyse the patient's heart rhythm and look for patterns of infarction or heart attack. At that point, the patient looks at the paramedics, identifies himself as a physician and inquires about what the paramedics see on the heart monitor. At that point, Heath calls to dispatch and requests another unit for transport as Jon steps into the other room to contact the hospital to notify the cardiac catheterization lab (Cath lab) that they would be transporting a confirmed ST elevated myocardial infarction (STEMI), i.e. heart attack, patient.

As Jon is contacting the hospital, Heath is explaining to the patient, Dr Smith, that his weakness is probably caused by a low heart rate due to a third-degree heart block because he is having a heart attack. Just then, the additional paramedic unit arrives and Heath gives a quick report to them and then asks them to get the stair chair to move the patient from the upstairs bedroom downstairs to the awaiting ambulance.

Just as the additional paramedics arrive with the stair chair to move Dr Smith to the waiting ambulance, Jon returns from notifying the hospital of the STEMI alert patient and that they are approximately 12 minutes out. As Dr Smith is loaded into the ambulance by the additional paramedics, Jon prepares his IV equipment. As Jon starts Dr Smith's IV, he instructs the other paramedics to obtain a repeat set of vital signs and administer 324 mg of aspirin to help break up any blockage that has occurred, causing the heart attack.

En route, Dr Smith's blood pressure and heart rate remain critically low. Jon then contacts the hospital again to update them on the patient's condition and that they are approximately 5 minutes away. The nurse from the hospital in the Emergency Department instructs the paramedics to bypass the emergency department and go directly to the Cath lab, where the team is waiting for their arrival.

Upon arrival at the hospital, the paramedics are met by Emergency Department nurses and the Cath lab team, who are waiting for the paramedics and Dr Smith. The paramedics and the Cath lab team then accompany Dr Smith to the Cath lab, where he is prepared for cardiac catheterization and stent placement. During the walk to the Cath lab, paramedics Heath and Jon report to the Cath lab team, informing them of Dr Smith's complaints, their findings concerning his heart rate and rhythm, his 12-Lead results, and his medical history. They also inform the Cath lab team that the patient Dr Smith is also a physician and that his wife is on her way to the hospital from her work. The entire team of paramedics and Cath lab staff then move Dr Smith to the surgical table and he is moved into the Cath lab for his procedure. The Cath lab staff thanks the paramedic team for a job well done and because of their quick critical thinking, it is likely that there is minimal damage done to the patient's heart muscle as a result of the heart attack.

- Interprofessional communication between paramedics and the patient, Dr Smith,
- Communication between the paramedics and Dr Smith's wife,
- Interprofessional communication and collaboration between paramedics Jon and Heath and the additional unit paramedics,
- Interprofessional communication and collaboration between Jon and the initial hospital contact alerting them of a STEMI alert,
- Interprofessional communication and collaboration between the ER staff and the Cath lab team,
- Interprofessional communication and collaboration between Jon and the additional unit

paramedics caring for Dr Smith for the transport to the hospital,
- Interprofessional communication and collaboration between Jon and the ER staff for the radio update on Dr Smith's condition,
- Interprofessional communication and collaboration between the paramedics and the Cath lab staff as they give them a report on Dr Smith's condition.

This scenario represents how vital interprofessional communication and collaboration are in paramedicine. Effective communication and collaboration can mean the difference between life and death. Interprofessional collaboration and clinical reasoning are vital for paramedicine students as they play a crucial role in pre-hospital care. Collaboration and reasoning improve patient outcomes, communication and healthcare delivery (Furseth et al., 2016).

Strategies for Interprofessional Collaboration

Interprofessional collaboration refers to the cooperative effort of healthcare professionals from different disciplines working together to provide comprehensive care to patients. In the context of paramedicine students, this involves partnering with other healthcare providers such as nurses, physicians, emergency medical technicians (EMTs) and other health professionals, not to mention bystanders, patients and their families (Furseth et al., 2016).

The Interprofessional Education Collaborative (Interprofessional Education Collaborative, 2023) has developed core competencies for interprofessional collaborative practice encompassing four domains of competence (values and ethics, roles and responsibilities, communication, and teams and teamwork). These domains, including interprofessional communication, are seen as essential for safe, high-quality and accessible, patient-centred care.

Students become more comfortable interacting and communicating with other team members during clinical interprofessional scenarios. Johnston et al. (2014) found that large-scale IPE simulation was an effective tool for developing communication skills and understanding roles that has helped students develop a shared understanding between disciplines (Johnston et al., 2014).

Given the high-stress, emotional context that is part of prehospital work, particularly with trauma, paramedics need these critical aspects of interprofessional collaboration communication, respect, teamwork and conflict resolution. Effective communication is essential for sharing patient information, exchanging ideas for patient care management and ensuring seamless coordination during patient interactions. Paramedicine students must be able to communicate clearly and concisely, both in verbal and written forms. Recognizing and respecting the expertise and roles of other healthcare members fosters a collaborative environment. Paramedicine students must learn to collaborate with other clinicians, to value input and to seek to understand their perspectives (Williams and Webb, 2015).

Collaborative teams work cohesively, pooling their knowledge and skills to solve problems and deliver optimal care. Paramedicine students should actively participate in team discussions, contribute to areas where they have had experience and learn to collaborate in various clinical and simulated clinical experiences. They should work in teams of collaborative health professionals with instructors who simulate working with team members with more experience and knowledge and with EMT students with less experience and knowledge. Allowing students to work in teams with clinicians outside paramedicine allows students to work with people unfamiliar to them, similar to that of a multidisciplinary emergency department or a prehospital public scene. In interprofessional collaboration, decisions are made collectively, considering input from all team members. Paramedicine students should be willing to engage in shared decision making and be open to feedback (Rutherford-Hemming and Linder, 2023).

Conflicts may arise in a team environment and paramedicine students need to develop skills to manage and resolve conflicts constructively and professionally. Conflict resolution is not only part of medicine but also a large part of paramedicine, both within the team and in managing the patients. There can be unruly bystanders, patients and patient family members and some scenes are unsafe or can become unsafe. *Conflict resolution* is a valuable skill and every paramedicine student should have the opportunity to explore strategies and tactics to enhance conflict resolution skills.

CLINICAL REASONING

For paramedics, Lord and Simpson (2019) wrote that clinical reasoning involves the ability to provide safe and effective healthcare in an increasingly complex and autonomous environment. Thus, clinical reasoning is an essential skill in paramedicine, used by qualified paramedics and students for data collection, problem identification, differential diagnoses, decision making and reflective practice.

Regularly reflecting on past cases and experiences can help paramedics improve clinical reasoning skills. Thompson et al. (2020) wrote that critical self-evaluation is fundamental to professional health roles. Reflective practice is now a recognized feature of the professional capabilities of registered paramedics in Australia, which has implications for both education and industry when determining competency. The authors argued that sustainable reflective practice skills should appear earlier and include opportunities for active student involvement in decisions regarding their learning. Thompson et al. (2020) then concluded that students readily embraced the principles of reflective practice and could effectively contribute to high-level decisions regarding their work despite having only recently commenced the programme. In addition, the high levels of broad agreement suggest that reflective practice and critical thinking-based assessments have an important role in paramedicine.

The collaboration between paramedicine students and other healthcare professionals can enhance the quality of clinical reasoning and patient care. Different perspectives and areas of expertise contribute to a comprehensive assessment of the patient's condition and enable better decision making (Gibbons et al., 2022).

Paramedicine students should actively engage in team discussions, share their clinical findings and seek input from other professionals. Simultaneously, they should absorb the insights provided by other team members to refine their clinical reasoning abilities. Overall, interprofessional collaboration and clinical reasoning empower paramedicine students to become proficient, compassionate and effective prehospital care providers, improving patient outcomes and contributing to increased positive patient outcomes (Andersson et al., 2019).

CHALLENGES AND FUTURE DIRECTIONS

In paramedicine education, clinical reasoning is critical in preparing competent and skilled paramedics who can make sound decisions in emergencies. However, like any educational process, it comes with challenges and evolving future directions.

Challenges include:

- Time constraints: Paramedic education programmes often have limited time to cover a vast range of knowledge and skills. Allocating sufficient time to teach and practice clinical reasoning can be challenging (Mudderman et al., 2020).
- Varied experience levels: Paramedicine students come from diverse backgrounds and may have varying levels of healthcare experience. Tailoring teaching strategies to accommodate these differences can be challenging but is essential.
- Limited clinical exposure: While paramedicine students undergo clinical placements, the volume and variety of cases they encounter might need to be increased to develop robust clinical reasoning skills.
- Integration of theoretical and practical knowledge: Connecting theoretical concepts with real-world patient encounters can be challenging, especially in nonurban areas. Students may need help to apply classroom knowledge to actual situations; however, integrating theoretical concepts into practical and real-world applications can help bridge knowledge and experience gaps.
- Rapidly evolving healthcare landscape: Paramedicine is subject to constant science, research and technology advancements. There are also constant advancements in best practices, scope of practice and skill utilization. The evolution of paramedicine towards professionalism is backed up by the growth of its own body of knowledge (Olaussen et al., 2021). These advancements will create challenging environments to ensure educational content remains aligned with current trends and the latest research.
- Individual learning styles: Students have diverse learning preferences and traditional didactic approaches may only effectively engage some learners in developing clinical reasoning abilities.

Therefore, educators need to find ways to engage students in their own learning, stimulate critical thinking and make clinical applications.
- Assessment: Evaluating clinical reasoning can be subjective and have a decreased likelihood of interrater reliability. Traditional assessment methods may need to be adjusted to capture and assess the complexity of decision making in real-life scenarios (Brentnall et al., 2022).

Future directions include:

- Active learning approaches: Odum et al. (2021) wrote the student-centred nature of active learning contrasts with the instructor-centred atmosphere of lecture-based pedagogies. Lecture-based instructional approaches view the learner as a passive recipient of the instructors expertise, whereas active learning pedagogies perceive the learner as an engaged participant in the learning process (Sabagh and Saroyan, 2014).
- Technology integration: VR and AR simulations can provide realistic and safe practice environments for paramedicine students to refine their clinical reasoning skills. The emergence of AR and MR modalities has increased the potential of simulation in paramedicine education. However, integrating AR/MR into education programmes should be underpinned by sound learning design. Research continues to emerge regarding the most effective uses of this advanced technology (Birtill et al., 2021).
- Interprofessional education: Collaborative training with other healthcare professionals, such as nurses and physicians, can expose paramedicine students to different perspectives and improve their ability to work in a team-based environment.
- Peer learning and mentoring: Creating opportunities for peer-to-peer learning and mentorship programmes can facilitate the exchange of clinical experiences and promote a culture of continuous improvement.
- Reflective practice: Encouraging paramedicine students to engage in reflective practices, such as debriefing after simulated scenarios or real patient encounters, can help them identify knowledge gaps and areas for improvement in their clinical reasoning process.

- Research and evidence-based teaching: Continued research into effective teaching methods for clinical reasoning and evidence-based instructional design can inform the development of more efficient pedagogical approaches.

CONCLUSION

Incorporating comprehensive training in clinical reasoning is an indispensable component of paramedic education. As frontline healthcare providers, paramedics encounter diverse and challenging situations where rapid, accurate decision making can mean the difference between life and death. When clinical reasoning is integrated into their educational curriculum, aspiring paramedics can enhance their ability to think critically, analyse complex patient presentations and formulate appropriate treatment plans. Moreover, this emphasis on clinical reasoning fosters a deeper understanding of patient care, instils confidence and promotes ongoing professional development. As the healthcare landscape continues to evolve, equipping paramedics with robust clinical reasoning skills promotes optimal patient outcomes and reaffirms their crucial role as indispensable members of the healthcare team. By nurturing this essential cognitive skill, paramedic education will prepare future generations of highly competent and compassionate paramedics.

SUMMARY

In this chapter, we have discussed:

- Teaching clinical reasoning in paramedic education requires a multifaceted approach
- Effective pedagogical strategies for teaching clinical reasoning in paramedic education
- Simulation education strategies for engaging students at a higher level of learning
- Incorporating evidence-based practice as an effective pedagogical strategy for teaching clinical reasoning in paramedic education
- The value of interprofessional collaboration in paramedic education
- Challenges and future directions of teaching clinical reasoning in paramedic education.

Overall, by focussing on active learning, clinical simulation, evidence-based practice, interprofessional collaboration and continuous development, paramedic education can enhance the clinical reasoning abilities of future paramedics.

REFERENCES

Anderson, D., Burns, S., 2013. One-minute paper: Student perception of learning gains. College Student Journal 47 (1), 219–227. https://link.gale.com/apps/doc/A345882743/AONE?u=googlescholar&sid=bookmark-AONE&xid=a20b2f7a

Andersson, U., Maurin Söderholm, H., Wireklint Sundström, B., Andersson Hagiwara, M., Andersson, H., 2019. Clinical reasoning in the emergency medical services: An integrative review. Scandinavian Journal of Trauma, Resuscitation and Emergency Medicine 27, 1–12. https://doi.org/10.1186/s13049-019-0646-y

Assaly, I.R., Smadi, O.M., 2015. Using Bloom's taxonomy to evaluate the cognitive levels of master class textbook's questions. English Language Teaching 8 (5), 100–110. https://doi.org/10.5539/elt.v8n5p100

Banning, M., 2008. Clinical reasoning and its application to nursing: Concepts and research studies. Nurse Education in Practice 8 (3), 177–183. https://doi.org/10.1016/j.nepr.2007.06.004

Barrett, J.L., Denegar, C.R., Mazerolle, S.M., 2018. Challenges facing new educators: Expanding teaching strategies for clinical reasoning and evidence-based medicine. Athletic Training Education Journal 13 (4), 359–366. https://doi.org/10.4085/1304359

Bilton, N., Rae, J., Logan, P., Maynard, G., 2017. Concept mapping in health sciences education: Conceptualizing and testing a novel technique for the assessment of learning in anatomy. MedEdPublish 6 (3): 1–17. https://doi.org/10.15694/mep.2017.000131

Birtill, M., King, J., Jones, D., Thyer, L., Pap, R., Simpson, P., 2021. The use of immersive simulation in paramedicine education: A scoping review. Interactive Learning Environments 31 (4), 2428–2443. https://doi.org/10.1080/10494820.2021.1889607

Brentnall, J., Thackray, D., Judd, B., 2022. Evaluating the clinical reasoning of student health professionals in placement and simulation settings: A systematic review. International Journal of Environmental Research and Public Health 19 (2), 936. https://doi.org/10.3390/ijerph19020936

Cazzell, M., Howe, C., 2012. Using objective structured clinical evaluation for simulation evaluation: Checklist considerations for interrater reliability. Clinical Simulation in Nursing 8 (6), e219–e225. https://doi.org/10.1016/j.ecns.2011.10.004

Cook, D.A., Brydges, R., Zendejas, B., Hamstra, S.J., Hatala, R., 2013. Mastery learning for health professionals using technology-enhanced simulation: A systematic review and meta-analysis. Academic Medicine 88 (8), 1178–1186. https://doi.org/10.1097/ACM.0b013e31829a365d

Edwards, M.J., Bassett, G., Sinden, L., Fothergill, R.T., 2015. Frequent callers to the ambulance service: Patient profiling and impact of case management on patient utilisation of the ambulance service. Emergency Medicine Journal 32 (5), 392–396. https://doi.org/10.1136/emermed-2013-203496

Furseth, P.A., Taylor, B., Kim, S.C., 2016. Impact of interprofessional education among nursing and paramedic students. Nurse Educator 41 (2), 75–79. https://doi.org/10.1097/NNE.0000000000000219

Gibbons, C., Landry, V., Boudreau, S., 2022. Interprofessional collaboration competencies of nursing students, nurse practitioner students, and paramedics in a simulated palliative home care setting: A pilot study. Quality Advancement in Nursing Education-Avancées en formation infirmière 8 (4), 3. https://doi.org/10.17483/2368-6669.1340

Hall, R.E., Plant, J.R., Bands, C.J., Wall, A.R., Kang, J., Hall, C.A., 2005. Human patient simulation is effective for teaching paramedic students endotracheal intubation. Academic Emergency Medicine 12 (9), 850–855. https://doi.org/10.1197/j.aem.2005.04.007

Hayden, J.K., Smiley, R.A., Alexander, M., Kardong-Edgren, S., Jeffries, P.R., 2014. Supplement: The NCSBN National Simulation Study: A longitudinal, randomized, controlled study replacing clinical hours with simulation in prelicensure nursing education. Journal of Nursing Regulation 5 (2), C1–S64. https://doi.org/10.1016/S2155-8256(15)30062-4

Herge, E., Hass, R., 2023. Patient-centered simulation: Practicing interprofessional teamwork with standardized patients. Journal of Interprofessional Care 37 (2), 272–279. https://doi.org/10.1080/13561820.2022.2069089

Holmboe, E., Durning, S., Hawkins, R., 2018. Evaluation of clinical competence, 2nd ed. Elsevier.

Interprofessional Education Collaborative. 2023. IPEC Core Competencies for Interprofessional Collaborative Practice: Version 3. Washington, DC: Interprofessional Education Collaborative.

Jeffries, P.R., 2005. A framework for designing, implementing, and evaluating: Simulations used as teaching strategies in nursing. Nursing Education Perspectives 26 (2), 96–103. PMID: 15921126

Jennings, P.A., Cameron, P., Bernard, S., 2009. Measuring acute pain in the prehospital setting. Emergency Medicine Journal 26 (8), 552–555. https://doi.org/10.1136/emj.2008.062539

Johnston, B.D., Seitz, S.R., Wang, H.E., 2006. Limited opportunities for paramedic student endotracheal intubation training in the operating room. Academic Emergency Medicine 13 (10), 1051–1055. https://doi.org/10.1197/j.aem.2006.06.031

Johnston, T., MacQuarrie, A., Rae, J., 2014. Bridging the gap: Reflections on teaching interprofessional communication to undergraduate paramedic and nursing students. Australasian Journal of Paramedicine 11, 1–10. https://doi.org/10.33151/ajp.11.4.2

Knox, S., Cullen, W., Dunne, C., 2015. A national study of continuous professional competence (CPC) amongst pre-hospital practitioners. BMC Health Services Research 15, 532–542. https://doi.org/10.1186/s12913-015-1197-1

Lord, B.A., Simpson, P.M., 2019. Clinical decision making in paramedicine. In Higgs, J., Jensen, G.M., Loftus, S., Christensen, N. (Eds.), Clinical reasoning in the health professions, pp. 295–301.

Makoolati, N., Amini, M., Raisi, H., Yazdani, S., Razeghi, A., 2021. The effectiveness of Guided Discovery Learning on the learning and satisfaction of nursing students. Hormozgan Medical Journal 18 (6), 490–496. https://civilica.com/doc/1912926

Marcum, J.A., 2012. An integrated model of clinical reasoning: Dual-process theory of cognition and metacognition. Journal of Evaluation in Clinical Practice 18 (5), 954–961. https://doi.org/10.1111/j.1365-2753.2012.01900.x

McGaghie, W.C., Issenberg, S.B., Cohen, M.E.R., Barsuk, J.H., Wayne, D.B., 2011. Does simulation-based medical education with deliberate practice yield better results than traditional clinical education? A meta-analytic comparative review of the evidence. Academic Medicine: Journal of the Association of American Medical Colleges 86 (6), 706. https://doi.org/10.1097/ACM.0b013e318217e119

McKenna, K.D., Carhart, E., Bercher, D., Spain, A., Todaro, J., Freel, J., 2015. Simulation use in paramedic education research (SUPER): A descriptive study. Prehospital Emergency Care 19 (3), 432–440. https://doi.org/10.3109/10903127.2014.995845

McLean, S.F., 2016. Case-based learning and its application in medical and health-care fields: A review of worldwide literature. J Med Educ Curric Dev, 3. https://doi.org/10.4137/JMECD.S20377

Mishra, P., Koehler, M.J., 2006. Technological pedagogical content knowledge: A framework for teacher knowledge. Teachers College Record 108 (6), 1017–1054. https://doi.org/10.1111/j.1467-9620.2006.00684.x

Motola, I., Devine, L.A., Chung, H.S., Sullivan, J.E., Issenberg, S.B., 2013. Simulation in healthcare education: A best evidence practical guide. AMEE Guide No. 82. Medical Teacher 35 (10), e1511–e1530. https://doi.org/10.3109/0142159X.2013.818632

Mudderman, J., Nelson-Brantley, H.V., Wilson-Sands, C.L., Brahn, P., Graves, K.L., 2020. The effect of an evidence-based practice education and mentoring program on increasing knowledge, practice, and attitudes toward evidence-based practice in a rural critical access hospital. JONA: The Journal of Nursing Administration 50 (5), 281–286. https://doi.org/10.1097/NNA.0000000000000884

Musolino, G., Jensen, G., 2020. Clinical reasoning and decision making in physical therapy: Facilitation, assessment, and implementation. Slack.

Olaussen, A., Beovich, B., Williams, B., 2021. Top 100 cited paramedicine papers: A bibliometric study. Emergency Medicine Australasia 33 (6), 975–982. https://doi.org/10.1111/1742-6723.13774

Odum, M., Meaney, K., Knudson, D.V., 2021. Active learning classroom design and student engagement: An exploratory study. Journal of Learning Spaces 10 (1), 27–42. http://libjournal.uncg.edu/jls/article/view/2102

Rodgers, D.L., 2007. High-fidelity patient simulation: A descriptive white paper report. Healthcare Simulation Strategies 10 (4), 68–77.

Ross, L.J., 2021. The structured clinical approach. In: Paramedic principles and practice: A clinical reasoning approach, 2nd ed. Elsevier, pp. 137–141.

Ross, L., Semaan, E., Gosling, C.M., Fisk, B., Shannon, B., 2023. Clinical reasoning in undergraduate paramedicine: Utilisation of a script concordance test. BMC Medical Education 23 (1), 1–7. https://doi.org/10.1186/s12909-023-04020-x

Rutherford-Hemming, T., Linder, G., 2024. Exploring the frameworks, needs, and barriers of interprofessional education and simulation in emergency medicine. Simulation in Healthcare:

Journal of the Society for Medical Simulation 19 (1), 47–51. https://doi.org/10.1097/SIH.0000000000000712

Sabagh, Z., Saroyan, A., 2014. Professors' perceived barriers and incentives for teaching improvement. International Education Research 2 (3), 18–40. https://doi.org/10.12735/ier.v2i3p18

Salzman, J.G., Page, D.I., Kaye, K., Stetham, N., 2007. Paramedic student adherence to the National Standard Curriculum recommendations. Prehospital Emergency Care 11 (4), 448–452. https://doi.org/10.1080/10903120701536701

Sharma, H.L., Priyamvada, P., Chetna, C., 2020. PMI (Plus-Minus-Interesting): An attention-directed strategy for enhancing creative thinking among elementary school students. Mukt Shabd Journal 9 (6), 2376–2394.

Simon, E.L., Lecat, P.J., Haller, N.A., Williams, C.J., Martin, S.W., Carney, J.A., et al., 2012. Improved auscultation skills in paramedic students using a modified stethoscope. The Journal of Emergency Medicine 43 (6), 1091–1097. https://doi.org/10.1016/j.jemermed.2012.01.048

Sinnayah, P., Rathner, J.A., Loton, D., Klein, R., Hartley, P., 2019. A combination of active learning strategies improves student academic outcomes in first-year paramedic bioscience. Advances in Physiology Education 43 (2), 233–240. https://doi.org/10.1152/advan.00199.2018

Swanwick, T., Forrest, K., O'Brien, B.C., 2019. Understanding medical education: Evidence, theory, and practice. 3rd ed. Wiley-Blackwell; Association for the Study of Medical Education. Hoboken, NJ. ISBN: 9781119373858

Thalluri, J., Penman, J., 2013. Case scenario oral presentations as a learning and assessment tool. Journal of the World Universities Forum 5 (3), 51–62. https://doi.org/10.18848/1835-2030/CGP/v05i03/56803

Thompson, J., Couzner, L., Houston, D., 2020. Assessment partnerships from the start: Building reflective practice as a beginning paramedic student competency. Australasian Journal of Paramedicine 17, 1–8. https://doi.org/10.33151/ajp.17.750

Trowbridge, R., Rencic, J., Durning, S., 2015. Teaching clinical reasoning. American College of Physicians, Philadelphia, PA.

Watson, K., Wright, A., Morris, N., McMeeken, J., Rivett, D., Blackstock, F., et al., 2012. Can simulation replace part of clinical time? Two parallel randomised controlled trials. Medical Education 46 (7), 657–667. https://doi.org/10.1111/j.1365-2923.2012.04295.x

Westgard, B.C., Peterson, B.K., Salzman, J.G., Anderson, R., Buldra, M., Burnett, A.M., 2013. Longitudinal and regional trends in paramedic student exposure to advanced airway placement: 2001–2011. Prehospital Emergency Care 17 (3), 379–385. https://doi.org/10.3109/10903127.2013.764949

Wheeler, B., Dippenaar, E., 2020. The use of simulation as a teaching modality for paramedic education: A scoping review. British Paramedic Journal 5 (3), 31–43. https://doi.org/10.29045/14784726.2020.12.5.3.31

Williams, B., Abel, C., Khasawneh, E., Ross, L., Levett-Jones, T., 2016. Simulation experiences of paramedic students: A cross-cultural examination. Advances in Medical Education and Practice 7 (1), 181–186. https://doi.org/10.2147/AMEP.S98462

Williams, B., Boyle, M., Winship, C., Brightwell, R., Devenish, S., Munro, G., 2013. Examination of self-directed learning readiness of paramedic undergraduates: A multi-institutional study. Journal of Nursing Education and Practice 3 (2), 102. https://doi.org/10.5430/jnep.v3n2p102

Williams, B., Webb, V., 2015. A national study of paramedic and nursing students' readiness for interprofessional learning (IPL): Results from nine universities. Nurse Education Today 35 (9), e31–e37. https://doi.org/10.1016/j.nedt.2015.05.007

Wilson, A., Asbury, E., 2019. Improving simulation debriefing in paramedic education: The paramedic debrief model. Australasian Journal of Paramedicine 16, 1–10. https://doi.org/10.33151/ajp.16.656

Wilson, A., Howitt, S., Holloway, A., Williams, A.M., Higgins, D., 2021. Factors affecting paramedicine students' learning about evidence-based practice: A phenomenographic study. BMC Medical Education 21, 1–12. https://doi.org/10.1186/s12909-021-02490-5

Wyatt, A., Fallows, B., Archer, F., 2004. Do clinical simulations using a human patient simulator in the education of paramedics in trauma care reduce error rates in preclinical performance? Prehospital Emergency Care 8 (4), 435–436. https://doi.org/10.1016/j.prehos.2004.06.005

40

DEVELOPING CLINICAL REASONING CAPABILITY

NICOLE CHRISTENSEN ■ GAIL M. JENSEN

CHAPTER AIMS

The aims of this chapter are:

- to explore the concept of capability as an adaptive learning outcome
- to discuss a proposed model of clinical reasoning capability
- to explore the relationship of competence and capability in clinical reasoning and development of adaptive expertise
- to discuss future implications for educators of tomorrow's healthcare professionals.

INTRODUCTION

The work of the health professions is inherently complex and, more often than not, situated in what Schön (1987) famously described as a 'swampy' and uncertain practice environment. The challenge for educators is to prepare learners for practice that includes both routine and novel or unexpected practice encounters.

Most health professions today have recognized the need to establish competency-based educational standards for performance outcomes at each level of education to minimize the unwarranted variability in learning outcomes and subsequent lack of consistency in quality of care for the patients and the society they serve (Lucey et al., 2018; Timmerberg et al., 2022). Competence has been defined as what the learner is able to do in real, authentic practice (Holdsworth and Thomas, 2021; Timmerberg et al., 2022). The risk of adopting a narrow focus on prescribed learning outcomes in either academic or clinical learning settings is that educators and learners can lose sight of the importance of also developing capability as a central learning outcome (Holdsworth and Thomas, 2021; Kaslow et al., 2022; O'Connell et al., 2014).

This chapter focusses on the development of health professionals capable of clinical reasoning in the 'swampy' and uncertain environments mentioned by Schön. Under conditions of uncertainty, true experts in the practice of healthcare have the capability to engage in collaborative clinical reasoning leading to wise judgements. These are also people whose knowledge base is continually evolving. Why is that? This chapter addresses important concepts about the development of thinking and learning skills that underlie clinical reasoning and the development of clinical reasoning capability, essential to the preparation of practitioners for the constantly changing and uncertain practice of healthcare.

CAPABILITY AS A LEARNING OUTCOME

The concept of *capability*, described in the higher education literature originally by Stephenson (1998), comprises a particular set of attributes and abilities. While competence has been focussed on what a learner can do in the present, capability implies a future-oriented focus on learners' practice (Holdsworth and Thomas, 2021; Stephenson, 1998). Capability is a key outcome for graduates of higher education, enabling them to contribute to the work of their professions more effectively and substantively and by extension, contribute to the betterment of health in broader society. Capability is a demonstrable and justifiable confidence and ability to interact effectively with other people and to undertake tasks in known and unknown contexts, both now and in the future (Stephenson, 1998). Capability is demonstrated through:

- confident, effective decision making and associated actions in practice,
- confidence in the development of a rationale for decisions made,
- confidence in working effectively with others and
- confidence in the ability to navigate unfamiliar circumstances and learn from the experience.

In addition to development of justifiable confidence in one's own effectiveness as a collaborator and a decision maker, in both known and unknown contexts, capability is also characterized by a motivation to develop one's own knowledge intentionally and continuously, through reflective learning in clinical practice (Doncaster and Lester, 2002). Capabilities can therefore be considered to enhance competence, broadening a learner's focus towards continual experiential learning throughout their professional career

(Kaslow et al., 2022). This aspect of capability as an educational outcome aligns well with another concept with roots in the education and expertise literature: the adaptive learner.

Adaptive Learners

Adaptive learners are described as able to thrive in changing environments by learning in and for practice and adapting as necessary (Cutrer et al., 2017; Cutrer et al., 2020; Mylopoulos, 2020). Characteristic of these individuals is their engagement in continuous learning and self-improvement. Adaptive learners achieve this through active self-monitoring and critical reflection, integrated with actively sought external feedback. They are motivated and skilled in learning from their experiences to change and grow. When needed, they can innovate, enabling themselves to continue to perform well when encountering complex, uncertain and novel situations (Cutrer et al., 2017; Schumacher et al., 2013). The justifiable confidence, or self-efficacy, of a capable individual in their ability to make well-reasoned decisions collaboratively, in both known and unknown circumstances, is the result of adaptive learning. This, in turn, is related to transformative learning.

Transformative learning theory (Cranton, 2006; Mezirow, 2009) is a branch of constructivist learning theory that can provide a foundation for educational strategies that facilitate clinical reasoning capability in learners. In healthcare education these strategies are often based on clinical reasoning experiences. Transformative learning takes place when a learner uses a prior understanding to construct a new or revised interpretation to guide future action, thereby transforming themselves through the emergence of new knowledge and understanding (Mezirow, 2009). This view meshes well with the way adaptive learners are thought to generate new knowledge to make wise decisions.

Holdsworth and Thomas (2021) recently described capability as an overarching concept that includes competence and that is integral to transformative learning. Their expanded view of capability integrates development of knowledge and competence required to 'explore the assumptions, biases, and the limitations of existing practice' (Holdsworth and Thomas, 2021, p. 1469). This critical reflection on one's own assumptions leading to development of new ways of understanding is a hallmark of transformative learning

(Cranton, 2006). Capability and competence, then, go hand-in-hand in the development of transformative learning and in the development of adaptive expertise.

REFLECTION POINT

1. As a student, do you recognize attributes in yourself that fit with descriptions of capable, adaptive learners? What aspects of the description of a capable, adaptive learner do you feel you need to develop further?
2. As an educator, how can you intentionally design learning activities to develop capability?

CLINICAL REASONING CAPABILITY

Building on the model of capability as a desirable outcome for higher education, Christensen et al. (Christensen et al., 2008b; Christensen, 2009; Christensen & Nordstrom, 2013) described clinical reasoning capability as confidence in the ability to effectively integrate key thinking and learning skills to make sense of and learn collaboratively from clinical experiences, in both known and unknown clinical contexts (Fig. 40.1). The model of clinical reasoning capability is informed by an understanding of the key characteristics of the clinical reasoning of physiotherapist experts and identified gaps between these experts and the clinical reasoning of novices (Christensen et al., 2008a; Christensen, 2009; Edwards et al., 2004). The model proposed four key areas of thinking and experiential learning skills, directly related to descriptions of skills inherent in the clinical reasoning of expert physiotherapists across all practice settings. These skill sets, linked to the development of excellence as both a clinical reasoner and an experiential learner, are: reflective thinking, critical thinking, complexity thinking and dialectical thinking (Christensen et al., 2008a, 2008b; Christensen, 2009).

These proposed clinical reasoning capability skills are consistent with the literature on capability, especially the emphasis on coping with new and previously unknown contexts (Doncaster and Lester, 2002; Kaslow et al., 2022; Stephenson, 1998).

However, these skills are not intended to represent a definitive or exhaustive list of all aspects of thinking and learning important to developing excellence in clinical reasoning. For example, although not the focus of this chapter, other more affective qualities of

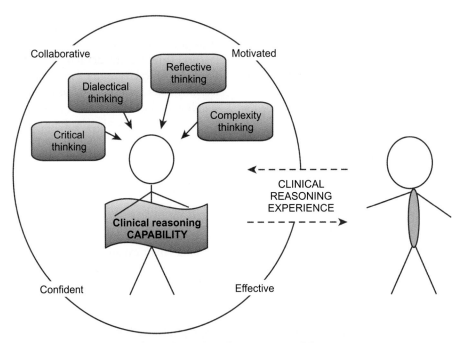

Fig. 40.1 ■ Clinical reasoning capability.

experienced clinical reasoning such as emotional intelligence have become a focus of research more recently (e.g. Chaffey et al., 2012; Marcum, 2013). Physical therapists use of movement provides another example of where clinical reasoning research benefits from a broader lens. Christensen and colleagues (2023) explored how therapists use movement as a component of clinical reasoning and found that communicating with patients not only about, but also through, movement is central to their reasoning, providing context for interpreting patients' participation, activity restrictions and for maximizing function.

Essential Thinking and Experiential Learning Skills for Clinical Reasoning Capability

Descriptions of each of the thinking and experiential learning skill sets proposed to be essential to the development of clinical reasoning capability follow.

Reflective Thinking

Reflective thinking is thinking about a situation in order to make sense of it. In clinical reasoning this involves evaluating the influence of all relevant aspects of the situation and individuals involved (e.g. clinician, patient, clinical setting, resources available, time constraints, etc.). Reflection allows for interpretation of experience. The thinker also attempts to know the 'why' of a situation by subjectively and objectively reconsidering the context in order to bring to light the underlying assumptions used to justify beliefs (Mezirow, 2000). When reflective thinking calls into question the adequacy of the clinician's knowledge, the clinician is prompted to learn something new and/or revise prior knowledge. Schön (1987) describes various moments in time when reflection is integral to making sense of, and eventually improving, practice: reflection-on-action, reflection-for-action and reflection-in-action. As applied to a clinical reasoning encounter, reflection-on-action occurs after the clinical action is completed and involves cognitive organization of experiences to make sense of what happened. Reflection-for-action involves planning for future encounters by thinking back on past experiences. This includes reflecting on the adequacy of the knowledge available to the clinical reasoner during those past encounters, identifying and actively seeking to fill any gaps in existing knowledge, and making links between past experiences and anticipated future events.

Reflection-in-action occurs in the midst of an experience and allows for modification of clinical reasoning by 'thinking on your feet' in order to best adapt to an emerging understanding of a situation. In order to use reflection-in-action successfully to modify decision making in the moment, a clinician must be able to readily access contextually relevant knowledge from memory. This is closely related to the idea of metacognition (Higgs et al., 2008; Marcum, 2012; Ng et al., 2022; Schön, 1987), which is self-awareness and monitoring of one's own thinking while in action. Wainwright and colleagues (2010) describe how reflection at different times in relation to a clinical encounter was used by both novice and experienced clinicians. Their research findings include the observation that novices less commonly used reflection-in-action and when it was used, it focussed mainly on the patient's performance. More experienced clinicians reflected in action more often and were focussed not only on the patient's performance but also on self-monitoring of their own reasoning in action. These findings highlight the importance of facilitation of reflection and evaluation of one's reasoning as essential to developing expertise in clinical reasoning.

Critical Thinking

Critical thinking is intimately linked to reflective thinking and involves the disciplined process of actively conceptualizing, synthesizing, analysing and evaluating information; this information can be gathered or generated from observation, experience, interaction, reasoning and reflection and acts as a guide towards action (Paul and Elder, 2006). In this context, critical thinking is conceived of as a way of thinking about thinking with an emphasis on questioning and clarifying erroneous assumptions. It is a skill that promotes learning from and about thinking. In this way, similar to reflective thinking, critical thinking is also linked to metacognition.

In the context of clinical reasoning capability, critical thinking applies to both the examination and management of a particular patient's clinical presentation and to the critical evaluation of one's own thinking or reasoning used to engage in, interpret and synthesize that patient's clinical information (Christensen et al., 2008b; Christensen, 2009). Critical thinking also attempts to bring to light blind spots or gaps in knowledge that may be adversely affecting a clinician's clinical reasoning in a given context. Critical thinking has an important role in exploring the potential for biases, incorrect assumptions, inadequate knowledge and detecting unconscious errors of interpretation in clinical reasoning.

Complexity Thinking

Complexity thinking acknowledges the dynamic inter-dependencies at work between the many elements and players influencing a given situation (Plsek and Greenhalgh, 2001). Therefore, complexity thinking is linked to the recognition and consideration of the relative weighting of all relevant internal (within the person) and external (the context in which the person is functioning) factors influencing a given clinical presentation (Christensen et al., 2008b; Christensen and Nordstrom, 2013). Skilled clinical reasoning has been shown to be, in part, characterized by this ability to see and appropriately address all influences (both biological and psychosocial) at play in a particular clinical presentation, leading to a plan of care that clinician and patient can mutually accept (Edwards et al., 2004). The ability to see a situation from multiple frames of reference is a key aspect of complexity thinking in clinical reasoning, including ethical reasoning. Both students and practitioners must be able to use analytical as well as interpretative skills in managing uncertain situations, often characterized by multiple perspectives and/or pathways to resolution.

Capability in clinical reasoning is also characterized by motivation and skill in learning from clinical experiences (Christensen et al., 2008b; Christensen, 2009). Consistent with a complexity science perspective on learning, clinical experience alone is not enough to bring about learning; rather, experience is viewed as a trigger, or an opportunity, for learning to emerge from interactions with other individuals (Davis and Sumara, 2006). Complexity thinking, therefore, is also a key element that enables a capable clinician to consider and appreciate the importance and implications of establishing a collaborative relationship with the patient. Collaboration is an essential component of clinical reasoning, both as solo practitioners and as members of interprofessional healthcare teams, because of the complex, interactive, social systems through which decisions emerge. This collaborative interaction between participants in clinical reasoning is an important hallmark of clinical reasoning capability (Christensen et al., 2008b; Christensen, 2009).

Complexity thinking allows us to integrate an understanding of both the physical and biological aspects of a patient's presentation together with the psychosocial and behavioural aspects, as well as the contexts of healthcare systems and wider communities, in a comprehensive biopsychosocial approach. Interestingly, Alhadeff-Jones (2012) proposed that a trigger for transformative learning is a recognition of some of the challenges raised by the complexity inherent in particular contexts such as collaborative clinical reasoning. Alhadeff-Jones also proposed that complexity thinking can be 'a method of learning involving human error and uncertainty... taking into consideration both the individual and collective experiences grounding any activity' (p. 190). In this way, complexity thinking is again closely linked to collaborative clinical reasoning and the learning that can emerge for all involved. Complexity thinking is also consistent with the dialectical reasoning approach observed in the reasoning of experts (Edwards and Jones, 2007).

Dialectical Thinking

The clinical reasoning of experts, as described by Edwards and Jones (2007), is characterized by a fluidity of reasoning between deductive thinking and inductive thinking within each of the clinical reasoning strategies (Edwards et al., 2004). Dialectical thinking is seen when expert physiotherapists move in their reasoning between contrasting biological and psychosocial poles in a fluid and seemingly effortless manner. This dialectical thinking ability is necessary for a holistic understanding that considers the clinical presentation of a patient's problem(s) in the context of the patient as a person and is consistent with a biopsychosocial approach to clinical reasoning (Edwards and Jones, 2007). Development of dialectical thinking allows clinicians to achieve a more complex and contextual understanding of situations both impacting, and impacted by, a patient's presentation. Dialectical thinking and complexity thinking can be seen as interdependent and promote capability in clinical reasoning. This is because capability includes effectiveness in working with others to achieve collaborative and productive working relationships (Doncaster and Lester, 2002; Stephenson, 1998). An advanced reasoning ability is the perception of what is important information and being able to interpret its implications for all aspects of the biopsychosocial approach. This ability needs to be developed through practice and assistance.

REFLECTION POINT

1. As a student, are you aware of using all four of the thinking and experiential learning skill sets that capable clinical reasoners use in their clinical reasoning? What ideas do you have to strengthen your skills and integrate them into your clinical reasoning?

2. As an educator, what are the thinking and experiential learning skill sets you tend to focus on developing in students when facilitating clinical reasoning development? What learning activities can you create to strengthen the skill sets you have tended not to focus on in the past?

FACILITATING CLINICAL REASONING CAPABILITY AND ADAPTIVE EXPERTISE

The interdependence between clinical reasoning ability and the development of clinical knowledge is a well-known dimension of expertise. Experts are those who both know a lot and are skilled at learning from their clinical experiences. Expertise is not a static concept or a goal that one reaches passively through accumulation of years of experience or achievement of credentials. The foundations are the continual learning and innovative problem solving that are crucial to wise decision making in conditions of uncertainty. This type of expertise has been termed adaptive expertise and can only be achieved through adaptive learning (Mylopoulos et al., 2016; Mylopoulos, 2020).

Adaptive expertise is described as a 'context appropriate, balanced cluster of learning oriented, self-regulatory, and metacognitive processes that moderate and mediate the application of abilities and previously acquired knowledge to problem solution, future knowledge acquisition, and ultimately effective leadership' (Birney et al., 2012, p. 563). Adaptive expertise demands flexibility in knowledge structures and performance

to respond effectively in novel situations and is highly metacognitive (Cutrer et al., 2020; Hatano et al., 1986). Therefore, there are clear connections to the aspects of capability described previously. These are the thinking and experiential learning skills essential to clinical reasoning capability and the notion of adaptive expertise development in the context of learning in, and from, clinical reasoning experiences.

FUTURE IMPLICATIONS

Our challenge is to foster the development of the adaptive learner. Calls for explicit curricular focus on the promotion and development of adaptive learners have been well argued in the current literature (Jensen et al., 2017a; Jensen, 2022; Mylopoulos et al., 2016). Capability in learning how to learn from clinical reasoning experiences continues to be a critical missing link between our desired, and our actual, educational outcomes in the context of professional education of today's healthcare professionals.

Our understanding of capability has been changing from what learners are competent to do now to an ability to adapt and innovate as they progress through their careers. However, this understanding appears to be more prominent in some professions (and some parts of the world) than others (Kaslow et al., 2022; O'Connell et al., 2014). Links to the concepts of adaptive learning and adaptive expertise are not commonly included in these discussions, although some overlap is evident in some concepts that are discussed.

Jensen and colleagues (2017a, 2017b) characterized excellence in professional and postprofessional education in their national study of physiotherapy education in the United States. Their findings described ways in which creative teachers provided learning contexts for their students that promoted the developmental skills, attributes and dispositions that characterize an adaptive and capable learner.

These included:

- placing students early on in their curriculum into situations where they could safely struggle and experiment in complex and uncertain practice situations;
- providing practice-based learning environments with multiple teachers and learners at multiple

levels of development and professional education, all engaged in frequent feedback exchanges, reciprocal teaching and learning processes, and mutual inquiry around complex, uncertain clinical problems and situations; and

■ fostering a culture of excellence, continuous feedback and improvement and transparency in the goals and intended outcomes for all learning activities.

While Jensen and colleagues' study focussed on excellence in education as a whole, their findings are clearly relevant to creating optimal contexts within which learners can be encouraged to develop clinical reasoning capability. Indeed, one of the recommendations these authors put forward, to promote intentional educational excellence across education programmes, is that the profession develop a longitudinal view and strategy for development of clinical reasoning that spans from professional entry through to postgraduate education and is continued throughout a learner's career (Jensen et al., 2017a). Adaptive learners are nurtured in authentic, complex, practice-based learning environments across the developmental continuum from novice to expert; it is precisely these environments that can promote the development of justifiable (i.e. can be tested and proven) confidence in their abilities to reason their way through any situation they encounter. Although novices cannot be directly taught to be expert clinical reasoners, they can be taught to rely on their thinking and experiential learning skills to guide them while in action. Critical reflection on their reasoning experiences can reveal areas ripe for new knowledge development. Encouragement to embrace and engage in discussions of clinical reasoning with explicit attention to complexity thinking and the interplay between inductive and deductive reasoning inherent in dialectical thinking can go a long way towards development of capability in clinical reasoning.

Essential to the development of capability in clinical reasoning is facilitation of, and provision of, formative feedback about a learner's critical self-reflection abilities, when evaluating their own clinical reasoning performance. Self-directed learning, an essential value and behaviour exhibited by both capable and adaptive learners, builds on the ability to self-assess one's own performance critically; this is a precursor to development of flexible (adaptive) expertise (Birney et al., 2012).

Ultimately, as healthcare educators and students, we should be working towards the establishment of explicit educational outcome goals (competencies) for development of adaptive learners, capable in clinical reasoning. Explicit integration of capabilities into competency-based education approaches could guard against the tendencies to focus only on what can be done in the present, in predictable known practice contexts (Kaslow et al., 2022). This would, eventually, be very likely to increase the number of practitioners who would go on to develop adaptive expertise. As Bransford and colleagues (2009) explain, isolated pockets of expertise hold less potential to bring about transformational change than distributed adaptive expertise across individuals, organizations, communities and professions. If we can shift our focus in professional education to the development of excellent adaptive learners who are capable in clinical reasoning, we can transform for the better the inequitable experiences of varying quality of care that our patients are living through today.

SUMMARY

In this chapter we have outlined:

■ qualities and attributes that characterize capable, adaptive learners, who are motivated and justifiably confident in their abilities to make sound, collaborative decisions and to learn and adapt in known and unknown situations;
■ the thinking and experiential learning skill sets that must be integrated into reasoning in order to optimize clinical reasoning capability; these comprised reflective thinking, critical thinking, complexity thinking and dialectical thinking;
■ the role of clinical reasoning capability in development of adaptive expertise and the implications for educators of health professionals.

REFLECTION POINT

1. As a student, are you given feedback about how well you are able to self-reflect critically on your

clinical reasoning? Can you think of how to improve your capability in this area?

2. As an educator, do the learning activities you provide for learners include intentional opportunities to reason clinically in novel (new to them), complex situations? How do you facilitate the development of critical self-reflection and self-directed learning in the practice setting?

REFERENCES

Alhadeff-Jones, M., 2012. Transformative learning and the challenges of complexity. In: Taylor, E.W., Cranton, P., Associates, The handbook of transformative learning: Theory, research, and practice. Jossey-Bass Wiley, San Francisco, CA, pp. 178–194.

Birney, D.P., Beckmann, J.F., Wood, R.E., 2012. Precursors to the development of flexible expertise: Metacognitive self-evaluations as antecedences and consequences in adult learning. Learning and Individual Differences 22 (5), 563–574. https://doi.org/10.1016/j.lindif.2012.07.001

Bransford, J., Mosborg, S., Copland, M.A., Honig, M.A., Nelson, H.G., Gawel, D., et al., 2009. Adaptive people and adaptive systems: Issues of learning and design. In: Hargreaves, A., Lieberman, A., Fullan, M., Hopkins, D. (Eds.), Second international handbook of educational change, part 1. Springer, Dordrecht, The Netherlands, pp. 825–856.

Chaffey, L., Unsworth, C.A., Fossey, E., 2012. Relationship between intuition and emotional intelligence in occupational therapists in mental health practice. American Journal of Occupational Therapy 66 (1), 88–96. https://doi.org/10.5014/ajot.2012.001693

Christensen, N., 2009 Development of clinical reasoning capability in student physical therapists, Doctor of Philosophy Thesis, University of South Australia, Adelaide, South Australia, available at http://trove.nla.gov.au/work/36257790.

Christensen, N., Jones, M., Edwards, I., Higgs, J., 2008a. Helping physiotherapy students develop clinical reasoning capability. In: Higgs, J., Jones, M., Loftus, S., Christensen, N. (Eds.), Clinical reasoning in the health professions, 3rd ed. Butterworth Heinemann Elsevier, London, UK, pp. 389–396.

Christensen, N., Jones, M., Higgs, J., Edwards, I., 2008b. Dimensions of clinical reasoning capability. In: Higgs, J., Jones, M., Loftus, S., Christensen, N. (Eds.), Clinical reasoning in the health professions, 3rd ed. Butterworth Heinemann Elsevier, London, UK, pp. 101–110.

Christensen, N., Nordstrom, T., 2013. Facilitating the teaching and learning of clinical reasoning. In: Jensen, G.M., Mostrom, E. (Eds.), Handbook of teaching and learning for physical therapists, 3rd ed. Butterworth-Heinemann Elsevier, St. Louis, MO, pp. 183–199.

Christensen, N., Black, L., Gilliland, S., Huhn, K., Wainwright, S., 2023. The role of movement in physical therapist clinical reasoning. Physical Therapy 103 (12), 1–10. https://doi.org/10.1093/ptj/pzad085

Cranton, P., 2006. Understanding and promoting transformative learning: A guide for educators of adults, 2nd ed. Jossey-Bass Wiley, San Francisco, CA.

Cutrer, W.B., Miller, B., Pusic, M., Mejicano, G., Mangrulkar, R., Gruppen, L., et al., 2017. Fostering the development of master adaptive learners: A conceptual model to guide skill acquisition in medical education. Academic Medicine 92 (1), 70–75. https://doi.org/10.1097/ACM.0000000000001323

Cutrer, W., Pusic, M., Gruppen, L., Hammoud, M., Santen, S., 2020. The master adaptive learner. The AMA MedEd Innovation Series. Elsevier, Philadelphia, PA.

Davis, B., Sumara, D., 2006. Complexity and education: Inquiries into learning, teaching, and research. Lawrence Erlbaum Associates, Mahwah, NJ.

Doncaster, K., Lester, S., 2002. Capability and its development: Experiences from a work-based doctorate. Studies in Higher Education 27 (1), 91–101. https://doi.org/10.1080/03075070120099395

Edwards, I., Jones, M., 2007. Clinical reasoning and expert practice. In: Jensen, G., Gwyer, J., Hack, L., Shepard, K. (Eds.), Expertise in physical therapy practice, 2nd ed. Saunders Elsevier, St. Louis, MO, pp. 192–213.

Edwards, I., Jones, M., Carr, J., Braunack-Mayer, A., Jensen, G.M., 2004. Clinical reasoning strategies in physical therapy. Physical Therapy 84 (4), 312–330. https://doi.org/10.1093/ptj/84.4.312

Hatano, G., Inagaki, K., Stevenson, H., Azuma, J., Hakuta, K., 1986. Two courses of expertise. In: Child development and education in Japan. WH Freeman and Company, New York, NY. 262–272.

Higgs, J., Fish, D., Rothwell, R., 2008. Knowledge generation and clinical reasoning in practice. In: Higgs, J., Jones, M., Loftus, S., Christensen, N. (Eds.), Clinical reasoning in the health professions, 3rd ed. Butterworth Heinemann Elsevier, London, UK, pp. 163–172.

Holdsworth, S., Thomas, I., 2021. Competencies or capabilities in the Australian higher education landscape and its implication for the development and delivery of sustainability education. Higher Education Research & Development 40 (7), 1466–1481. https://doi.org/10.1080/07294360.2020.1830038

Jensen, G.M., Hack, L., Nordstrom, T., Gwyer, J., Mostrom, E., 2017a. Part 2: Excellence in physical therapist education: A call to reform. Physical Therapy 97 (9), 875–888. https://doi.org/10.1093/ptj/pzx062

Jensen, G.M., Nordstrom, T., Mostrom, E.M., Hack, L.M., Gwyer, J., 2017b. A national study of excellence and innovation in physical therapist education: Part 1 – design, methods, and results. Physical Therapy 97 (9), 857–874. https://doi.org/10.1093/ptj/pzx061

Jensen, G.M., 2022. Physical therapy education through the lens of the master adaptive learner 24th Pauline Cerasoli lecture. Journal of Physical Therapy Education 36 (4), 348–358. https://doi.org/10.1097/JTE.0000000000000260

Kaslow, N.J., Farber, E.W., Ammons, C.J., Graves, C.C., Hampton-Anderson, J.N., Lewis, D.E., et al., 2022. Capability-informed competency approach to lifelong professional development. Training and Education in Professional Psychology 16 (2), 182–189. https://doi.org/10.1037/tep0000392

Lucey, C.R., Thibault, G.E., ten Cate, O., 2018. Competency-based, time-variable education in the health professions: Crossroads. Academic Medicine 93 (35), S1–S5. https://doi.org/10.1097/ACM.0000000000002080

Marcum, J.A., 2012. An integrated model of clinical reasoning: Dual-processing theory of cognition and metacognition. Journal of Evaluation in Clinical Practice 18 (5), 954–961. https://doi.org/10.1111/j.1365-2753.2012.01900.x

Marcum, J.A., 2013. The role of emotions in clinical reasoning and decision making. Journal of Medicine and Philosophy 38 (5), 501–519. https://doi.org/10.1093/jmp/jht040

Mezirow, J., 2000. Learning to think like an adult: Core concepts of transformation theory. In: Mezirow, J. (Ed.), Learning as transformation: Critical perspectives on a theory in progress. Jossey-Bass, San Francisco, CA, pp. 3–33.

Mezirow, J., 2009. Transformative learning theory. In: Mezirow, J., Taylor, E.W., Associates, Transformative learning in practice: Insights from community, workplace, and higher education. Jossey-Bass Wiley, San Francisco, CA, pp. 18–31.

Mylopoulos, M., Brydges, R., Woods, N.N., Manzone, J., Schwartz, D.L., 2016. Preparation for future learning: A missing competency in health professions education. Medical Education 50 (1), 115–123. https://doi.org/10.1111/medu.12893

Mylopoulos, M., 2020. Preparing future adaptive experts: Why it matters and how can it be done. Medical Science Educator 30 (S1), S11–S12. https://doi.org/10.1007/s40670-020-01089-7

Ng, S., Forsey, J., Boyd, V., Friesen, F., Langlois, S., Ladonna, K., et al., 2022. Combining adaptive expertise and (critically) reflective practice to support the development of knowledge, skill, and society. Advances in Health Sciences Education 27, 1265–1281. https://doi.org/10.1007/s10459-022-10178-8

O'Connell, J., Gardner, G., Coyer, F., 2014. Beyond competencies: Using a capability framework in developing practice standards for advanced practice nursing. Journal of Advanced Nursing 70 (12), 2728–2735. https://doi.org/10.1111/jan.12475

Paul, R., Elder, L., 2006. The miniature guide to critical thinking: Concepts & tools, 4th ed. The foundation for critical thinking, Santa Rosa, CA.

Plsek, P.E., Greenhalgh, T., 2001. Complexity science: The challenge of complexity in health care. British Medical Journal 323, 625–628. https://doi.org/10.1136/bmj.323.7313.625

Schumacher, D., Englander, R., Carraccio, C., 2013. Developing the master learner: Applying learning theory to the learner, the teacher, and the learning environment. Academic Medicine 88 (11), 1635–1645. https://doi.org/10.1097/ACM.0b013e3182a6e8f8

Schön, D., 1987. Educating the reflective practitioner. Jossey-Bass Inc. Publishers, San Francisco, CA.

Stephenson, J., 1998. The concept of capability and its importance in higher education. In: Stephenson, J., Yorke, M. (Eds.), Capability and quality in higher education. Kogan Page, London, UK, pp. 1–13.

Timmerberg, J.F., Chesbro, S.B., Jensen, G.M., Dole, R.L., Jette, D.U., 2022. Competency-based education and practice in physical therapy: It's time to act! *Physical Therapy*, 102, pzac018. https://doi.org/10.1093/ptj/pzac018.

Wainwright, S.F., Shepard, K.F., Harman, L.B., Stephens, J., 2010. Novice and experienced physical therapist clinicians: A comparison of reflection is used to inform the clinical decision-making process. Physical Therapy 90 (1), 75–88. https://doi.org/10.2522/ptj.20090077

41 LEARNING TO COMMUNICATE CLINICAL REASONING

ROLA AJJAWI ■ JOY HIGGS

CHAPTER OUTLINE

CHAPTER AIMS

The aims of this chapter are:

- to reflect on core processes of communicating clinical reasoning
- to consider strategies for learning to communicate clinical reasoning
- to reflect means and strategies on learning to communicate clinical reasoning
- to look at the importance of context in developing clinical reasoning.

INTRODUCTION

Clear and effective communication of clinical reasoning is essential for all healthcare professional practice, especially in the current healthcare climate. The increasing requirements associated with the pandemic have set up extra demands on communication and made the work of both clinicians and patients more difficult. Active consumer involvement is more important than ever before and highlights the importance of clear communication and collaborative decision making. Poor communication can lead to discontinuity of care, compromise of patient safety and patient dissatisfaction (Vermeir et al., 2015).

REFLECTION POINT

Often students in health science courses focus on learning knowledge and skills.
- Do you?
- Does your course help you learn about doing clinical reasoning and communicating it?
- How well are you able to communicate your reasoning?
- What are the challenges you experience in communicating your reasoning?

Healthcare professionals are accountable for their decisions and service provision to various stakeholders, including clients, families, health sector managers, policy makers and colleagues. An important aspect of this accountability is the ability to articulate clearly and to justify management decisions. Beyond this, communication of clinical reasoning is necessary for novice healthcare professionals to develop their clinical reasoning and the ability to communicate this reasoning appropriately to the various people they deal with and are responsible to in their clinical practice encounters. In this chapter, we present the core processes of communicating clinical reasoning along with ways that learning in these areas can be enhanced through classroom and workplace learning. This is supported by a synthesis of research investigating how healthcare professionals develop the ability to unpack and communicate their clinical reasoning and a discussion of ideas for teachers regarding supporting students' learning and faculty development initiatives.

COMMUNICATION OF CLINICAL REASONING

Communicating clinical reasoning may be verbal (either face-to-face or via telehealth) or written (such as in handover or referral letters and email). Perhaps more radical, communication of clinical reasoning is also embodied, constituted through perception, bodies, eye-gaze and gestures where situated bodily processes constitute cognition (Gallagher and Payne, 2015; Øberg et al., 2015).

Because of its rapid, complex and often subconscious or intuitive nature, practitioners and students cannot easily recall and explain the fine details and nuances of their own reasoning. Also, clinical reasoning is not a single process; it varies with expertise, discipline and individual practice models. However, it is possible to 'slow down' and systematically examine some of the processes involved in reasoning to reflect on them more clearly, thereby facilitating articulation of clinical reasoning.

For instance, novices frequently use and are taught a more analytical form of reasoning such as hypothetico-deductive reasoning and are encouraged to 'think aloud' about the various alternative possibilities (of differential diagnosis, investigation options, treatment alternatives, prognosis pathways and client choices). These approaches are useful to build sound reasoning practices that avoid errors such as quickly choosing the most obvious answer/solution or failing to carefully consider the pros and cons of different treatment decisions in relation to the client's particular context. Talking aloud or explaining our reasoning also helps check our knowledge and understanding of what is going on, both in relation to the clinical situation and the client's life and well-being.

REFLECTION POINT

In Part 4 of this book, the various chapters consider how reasoning is conducted and interpreted in different professions.
- Have a look at the chapters most relevant to your situation and reflect on how your disciplinary perspective influences your reasoning and how you communicate it.
- How do other disciplinary perspectives influence the reasoning of practitioners in these disciplines?

Effective communication of clinical reasoning involves a depth of knowledge and understanding of clinical reasoning and the factors involved in and influencing the decision-making process. Practitioners, both novice and experienced, must draw on multiple forms of knowledge (formal, professional/experiential, embodied and personal) to inform the content and process of communicating reasoning. In addition, communication of clinical reasoning in practice is multifactorial, requiring cognitive and metacognitive processing of many factors about the co-communicator(s), the message to be communicated and the environmental context in which the communication takes place. In all of this, we need to remember that communication cannot be thought of as a discrete skill that can be learned separate from the underlying thinking and content (Ajjawi and Higgs, 2012).

REFLECTION POINT

Metacognition is 'thinking about what you are thinking about'. This is an invaluable skill and process to bring into your reasoning and communicating. For instance, when you are talking with a child, parent or colleague, how do you change your language? And even in the process of speaking, you can ask yourself:
- Have I got my thinking right about what the recipient can understand and what is important to them?
- How well do you understand, monitor and adapt the language you use in different circumstances?

We subscribe here to a view of clinical reasoning as socially mediated activity or practice (Koufidis et al., 2021). This differs to reasoning as cognitive activity. Within the socially mediated activity view, language is not simply a mental representation of preexisting thoughts and real-life objects (as in the cognitive paradigm). Instead, it is the 'fabric of social interaction' (Koufidis et al., 2021, p. 445). Language constructs identities and frames of thinking. Therefore, articulating reasoning does not completely reflect actual reasoning processes but represents a (re)construction and (typically) a simplification of the more complex, rapid and multilayered processes that operate in practice. These communications are constructed in ways that are perceived as being most relevant to the audience, context and purpose of the communication. With experience, clinical reasoning becomes almost 'second nature' and requires effort to bring these circumstances and processes of reasoning to consciousness, often after the event as a post-hoc rationalization or justification and reporting of the decisions reached. We also see the role of culture at play in these stories. For example, Peters et al. (2017) showed that physicians drew on expected cultural narrative structures of evidence-based medicine where they downplayed the role of intuitive reasoning, instead preferencing rational-analytical type language.

LEARNING TO COMMUNICATE CLINICAL REASONING: WHAT'S INVOLVED?

There has been limited research in the health sciences into how healthcare professionals learn to communicate clinical reasoning in practice. Learning such a complex skill begins at university and continues after graduation in practitioners' chosen career paths. In this chapter, we are taking a broad view of learning as becoming (e.g. becoming a nurse and learning to think and practise like a nurse), where individuals and their social cultures are enmeshed, with each influencing and changing the other (Hager et al., 2012). This reframing of the nature of learning combines construction and a sense of belonging, where individuals construct and reconstruct their understanding, knowledge, skills and practices entailing shifts in 'habitus' and identity. Similarly, the contexts in which learning takes place are constructed and reconstructed (Hager and Hodkinson, 2009).

BOX 41.1
A MESSAGE TO EDUCATORS

Educating students, in particular, prompts practitioners to break down more automated reasoning to first principles to reduce the complexity of reasoning for students and to provide a structure upon which the students could start to develop their own illness scripts. This dual mode of performance (what practitioners think/do and how they explain it more simply to students) is a necessity because of the nature of expert–novice differences in clinical reasoning and the dynamic nature of communication (Ajjawi and Higgs, 2012). Further, from the perspective of the rhetoric and language of clinical reasoning, this reconstruction can be seen as a tool for persuading others (clients, families, students, peers) and oneself of the cogency of the underlying reasoning and the actual decisions made (Nugus et al., 2009), sensitive to particular cultures and contexts.

Learning is neither simply the acquisition of knowledge and skills nor a straightforward process of participation and socialization. Students and novice practitioners need to learn how to learn differently in classroom, online and workplace learning situations and to consider what this means for their developing professional identity. For instance, in practical classes they can 'try out' their reasoning and get feedback without any consequences for clients and it is safer to say 'I don't know'. In workplaces when working, reasoning and communicating with genuine clients, it is a challenging task to deal simultaneously with unfamiliar situations (and possibly make mistakes and have to change their decisions) and maintain the trust of clients and ensure client safety (Box 41.1).

Learning the Context of Clinical Reasoning

Thinking occurs in some sort of context, yet it is easy to forget about context in clinical reasoning. For each patient it is the context that shapes the way they inhabit that space or represents that way of being in the space. This can be older or younger manifestations of a condition, a person who speaks the local language or someone who has a speech disorder, or someone who has no rights to the common privileges shared by patients. The Internet is a source of information (not necessarily reliable). Chapter 2 draws our attention to the context and sources of healthcare. 'Making sense of "what is going on with this patient" necessitates reading the context in which the encounter is unfolding and deliberating a path of response justified in that specific context' (Koufidis et al., 2022, p. 109). Situating the patient in various settings (e.g. ICU) can add different factors such as time pressure to the task of teaching clinical reasoning or require inventiveness and imagination on the part of the teacher (Richards et al., 2020).

Researching Reasoning and Communication

In our own research into clinical reasoning (Ajjawi and Higgs, 2008, 2012), we looked at aspects of learning how to reason and how to communicate reasoning. This research highlighted the interplay between individuals and their learning culture. Practitioners talked about the opportunities they had in their everyday work to use their prior knowledge to practise communication of clinical reasoning with a wide variety of people, which aided in the development of their communication ability. These opportunities were often unplanned and revolved around 'authentic contribution' in work practices, communicating with clients about their conditions and management plans, helping students develop their own reasoning and communicating in team meetings and continuing professional development activities.

Participants spoke about their learning journeys as being supported and developed through the practices of their communities. Learning the practices of the community takes place through engagement in actions and interactions that are embedded in the culture and history forming the practice. Such learning and the emphasis on the cultural learning process can be seen as essential parts of the broader concept and process of professional socialization (Abrandt Dahlgren et al., 2004), which is based on learning the particular profession's socially constructed norms, values and beliefs through interaction within workplace and cultural situations. This is so specific as to encompass specific words or sequences of words that situate the clinician as a member of a particular group with shared meanings and goals – so-called 'tokens of membership' (Peters et al., 2017).

Implications for University Curricula

Communication skills training is a central component of health professions curricula, required by regulatory bodies. Communication of clinical reasoning with different stakeholders (clients, families, colleagues, supervisors) should be an explicit goal of health professions curricula and its place in formal curricula needs to be clearly defined. Experiential learning strategies are typically recommended for communication skills curricula, such as simulation, modelling and case discussion (Rider and Keefer, 2006), plus inbuilt opportunities for peer, teacher and internal (self) feedback. Other creative endeavours include narrative journalling and storytelling about clients' journeys (Charon, 2001). Blogging in fieldwork education has also been used as a means of promoting reflection and self-regulation of clinical reasoning in final-year physiotherapy students (Tan et al., 2010). Findings from experimental research with medical students highlight how self-explanation can be used to improve diagnostic accuracy and performance, with best results documented for the group who also listened to a near-peer's self-explanation of the same case (Chamberland et al., 2015). Common to these strategies is the opportunity for active processing and articulation of clinical reasoning.

One study examined a subject developed to teach second-year medical students the important link between communication and clinical reasoning (Windish et al., 2005). The subject ran for 6 weeks and used mainly experiential learning methods such as role play, videotaped encounters and feedback through self-reflection, peers and faculty. Compared with a control group, the experimental group scored higher in establishing rapport as rated by the standardized patients and elicited more psychosocial history items in communication. Evaluation feedback on the course indicated that 95% of the participants considered integrated learning of communication and clinical reasoning to be beneficial. Windish et al. (2005) claimed that this integration allowed students to understand the important relationship between the biomedical and psychosocial aspects of patient care. The value of this research lies in recognition of the need to teach both processes in parallel and to make explicit the important link between reasoning and communication.

An approach common to medical education that seeks to strengthen diagnostic reasoning that adopts the principles of active processing and reflection is called *deliberate reflection* (Mamede and Schmidt, 2023). This pedagogical approach involves presenting students with a case and asking them to generate

BOX 41.2
A MESSAGE TO EDUCATORS

What is your role in learning or fostering learning about reasoning and communication of reasoning within the formal and informal curriculum? How might you give or seek feedback comments on these capabilities?

diagnostic hypotheses. Students are then encouraged to verify a particular hypothesis by its supporting presenting signs and symptoms (identified in the case information). They are then asked to falsify the hypothesis by what is absent or contradictory. This is repeated for each alternative hypothesis and students are then asked to rank the most likely diagnosis. This approach helps students to develop relationships between a particular disease and its concomitant signs and symptoms and has been found to improve the accuracy of diagnostic reasoning (Mamede and Schmidt, 2023). If carried out in a group, the discussion generated among peers would be valuable for learning how to communicate these relationships. Deliberate reflection could be built into the curriculum and could be modelled for students by academics and healthcare professionals via articulation of thought processes. Students could be encouraged to evaluate their practice and that of others against rubrics, which explicate standards. Seeking feedback is important to help calibrate judgements and improve the quality of clinical reasoning (Box 41.2).

Implications for Workplace Learning

Workplaces lend themselves to helping students learn to communicate clinical reasoning particularly because they are places where clinicians engage in authentic practices and experience the consequences of practice interventions that can be sound or unsound, beneficial or harmful and relevant to the client or not. Strategies for learning about reasoning and communication are many and varied, including observation and feedback, modelling, bedside teaching encounters, self-reflection, peer learning and case discussion. Individuals need to seek out opportunities to observe senior practitioners and educators and to seek feedback from various people, including their clients and peers. Discussions about learners' perceptions of their learning compared with observations of and by teachers at university or seniors in the workplace may aid

the development of learners' critical self-assessment skills (Paschal et al., 2002).

Research highlights the valuable role of mentors and role models in the development of communication abilities, particularly in the professional development of novice practitioners (Ajjawi and Higgs, 2008, 2012). This development may be spurred by generating regular opportunities for new graduates to discuss their reasoning about their clients and to ask questions of the senior practitioners. Learners could be supported to choose their communication role models based on alignment with their personal identities (Denniston et al., 2019). Incorporating self-explanation and prompt questions between learners at different levels is another strategy (Chamberland et al., 2015) amenable to workplace learning situations where students from different year levels work with new graduates and more experienced colleagues. Seniors, educators and facilitators need to be aware of their professional responsibilities in guiding and mentoring novice practitioners. These professional responsibilities extend beyond the possession of formal knowledge and technical skills to include attitudes, values and beliefs of senior colleagues or role models, which strongly influence the development of students' professional identities. This role transcends what is articulated explicitly; it encompasses the behaviour and values that embody a profession. These may be implicit or tacit and remain highly influential in professional development.

Research into bedside teaching as an essential mode of workplace learning provides important insight into the communication of clinical reasoning. Bedside teaching brings together distinct but overlapping activity systems of patient care and student education (Ajjawi et al., 2015). In this way, bedside teaching encounters offer important opportunities for students to learn how to communicate clinical reasoning through observation, modelling, practice, feedback and assessment. However, in trying to educate students while caring for their clients, practitioners may inadvertently exclude their clients through the use of jargon, bodily positioning and referring to them, for instance, in the third person or as an object or disease (Ajjawi et al., 2015). Similarly, students often report feeling confused when communicating clinical reasoning, as to whether they should be performing for the client and/or performing for the clinical educator, who is often also their assessor.

When students adopt this latter genre of communication of clinical reasoning, they also tend to adopt jargon, refer to clients in the third person and shift their gaze away from their clients, therefore excluding them from the clinical communication, as they talk *about* rather than *with* clients (Elsey et al., 2016). Being clear about expectations within bedside teaching encounters, being careful with language and engaging both students and clients within the communication, that is, privileging the student–client relationship, ensures that all actors are included in the interaction. The time after the consultation can then be utilized by clinical educators and students to discuss particular decisions made with the patient and the underlying reasoning in more depth.

REFLECTION POINT

- What is your experience when you are working in student–client–educator situations?
- How do you deal with the competing priorities of learning and client care?
- Do your reasoning, communication and actions change because there is a clinical educator observing and/or assessing you?

Implications for Faculty Development

Although clinical educators broadly see communication skills as essential for student–client communication, there is less recognition of the need for learning about communication of the students' developing reasoning. Clinical educators have been found to focus on procedural aspects of gathering information and communicating a management plan as necessary for student–client communication (Woodward-Kron et al., 2012) and excluding the communication of reasoning. This is disappointing because encouraging students to make their thinking explicit would be an effective strategy to help them improve their clinical reasoning and their communication of it (Ajjawi and Higgs, 2008). Perhaps going unnoticed is the clinical educators' role in modelling this communication to the students and the importance of seeing clinical workplaces as ideal for opportunistic learning. We can never predict all the possibilities and unexpected occurrences in the workplace that provide opportunities for learning.

Understanding the powerful influence of the workplace culture on learning enables practitioners to adopt a critical and reflective stance with regard to the activities of their workplaces. This understanding also encourages them to be strategic in their learning and professional development and to be active agents in choosing both what is learned and the process of learning within the community. Therefore, healthcare professionals (novice and experienced alike) need to combine giving deliberate attention to their work activities with self-monitoring, rather than relying on unreflective and unchallenged routine and habit. Monitoring communication performance in terms of self-awareness and reflective capacity is considered a feature of skilled communication (Verheijden et al., 2023).

According to de Cossart and Fish (2005), three main processes that develop good reflective practice are: (a) following a rigorous process for reflection (that is particular to each individual), (b) engaging in dialogue with teachers and peers (including talking and writing as key means of developing reflection) and (c) recognizing ethical and moral obligations to clients and colleagues (e.g. maintaining confidentiality). These could be key processes used within faculty development initiatives, for instance, around client cases and/or for mentoring relationships. In their faculty development programme, Delany and Golding (2014) explored how to make thinking visible by identifying and then 'repackaging' the thinking steps used by experts when they engage in clinical reasoning in 'thinking routines'. These thinking routines consisted of short, repeatable actions that unpack lines of thinking and provide heuristics or 'tools' for enabling and promoting this thinking. Clinical educators are encouraged first to identify the types of knowledge they are privileging, the cognitive processes they are using and the connections they are making in their mind. They then refine this thinking to concrete steps or thinking routines that capture the specific clinical context. These steps help to make the structure of clinical educators' thinking visible, a necessary precondition to developing clinical reasoning.

SUMMARY

In this chapter we have:

- argued that communication cannot be thought of as a discrete skill that can be learned separate

from the underlying thinking (reasoning and decision making) and content of practice: it is multifactorial and context-specific;
- discussed strategies that promote this learning, including practice, deliberate reflection, modelling, role-play, self-appraisal and feedback;
- encouraged readers to engage in reflection and explicit learning about how to communicate clinical reasoning and remember that developing these abilities is the responsibility of individuals, universities and the workplace and
- emphasized the importance of context in teaching clinical reasoning.

REFLECTION POINT

Having read this chapter, now consider:
- What have you learned that you can use to help develop your or your students' reasoning, and how can this be communicated?

REFERENCES

Abrandt Dahlgren, M., Richardson, B., Sjostrom, B., 2004. Professions as communities of practice. In: Higgs, J., Richardson, B., Abrandt Dahlgren, M. (Eds.), Developing practice knowledge for health professionals. Butterworth-Heinemann, pp. 71–88.

Ajjawi, R., Higgs, J., 2008. Learning to reason: A journey of professional socialisation. Advances in Health Sciences Education 13 (2), 133–150. https://doi.org/10.1007/s10459-006-9032-4

Ajjawi, R., Higgs, J., 2012. Core components of communication of clinical reasoning: A qualitative study with experienced Australian physiotherapists. Advances in Health Sciences Education 17 (1), 107–119. https://doi.org/10.1007/s10459-011-9302-7

Ajjawi, R., Rees, C., Monrouxe, L.V., 2015. Learning clinical skills during bedside teaching encounters in general practice: A video-observational study with insights from activity theory. Journal of Workplace Learning 27 (4), 298–314. https://doi.org/10.1108/JWL-05-2014-0035

Chamberland, M., Mamede, S., St-Onge, C., Setrakian, J., Bergeron, L., Schmidt, H., 2015. Self-explanation in learning clinical reasoning: The added value of examples and prompts. Medical Education 49 (2), 193–202. https://doi.org/10.1111/medu.12623

Charon, R., 2001. Narrative medicine: A model for empathy, reflection, profession, and trust. JAMA 286 (15), 1897–1902. https://doi.org/10.1001/jama.286.15.1897

Delany, C., Golding, C., 2014. Teaching clinical reasoning by making thinking visible: An action research project with allied health clinical educators. BMC Medical Education 14 (1), 20. https://doi.org/10.1186/1472-6920-14-20

Denniston, C., Molloy, E.K., Ting, C.Y., Lin, Q.F., Rees, C.E., 2019. Healthcare professionals' perceptions of learning communication in the healthcare workplace: An Australian interview study. BMJ Open 9 (2), e025445. https://doi.org/10.1136/bmjopen-2018-025445

de Cossart, L., Fish, D., 2005. Cultivating a thinking surgeon: New perspectives on clinical teaching, learning and assessment. tfm Publishing.

Elsey, C., Challinor, A., Monrouxe, L.V., 2016. Patients embodied and as-a-body within bedside teaching encounters: A video ethnographic study. Advances in Health Sciences Education, 1–24. https://doi.org/10.1007/s10459-016-9688-3

Gallagher, S., Payne, H., 2015. The role of embodiment and intersubjectivity in clinical reasoning. Body, Movement and Dance in Psychotherapy 10 (1), 68–78. https://doi.org/10.1080/17432979.2014.980320

Hager, P., Hodkinson, P., 2009. Moving beyond the metaphor of transfer of learning. British Educational Research Journal 35 (4), 619–638. https://doi.org/10.1080/01411920802642371

Hager, P., Lee, A., Reich, A., 2012. Problematising practice, reconceptualising learning and imagining change. In: Hager, P., Lee, A., Reich, A. (Eds.), Practice, learning and change: Practice-theory perspectives on professional learning. Springer, pp. 1–14.

Koufidis, C., Manninen, K., Nieminen, J., Wohlin, M., Silén, C., 2021. Unravelling the polyphony in clinical reasoning research in medical education. Journal of Evaluation in Clinical Practice 27 (2), 438–450. https://doi.org/10.1111/jep.13432

Koufidis, C., Manninen, K., Nieminen, J., Wohlin, M., Silen, C., 2022. Representation, interaction and interpretation: Making sense of the context in clinical reasoning. Medical Education 56, 98–109. https://doi.org/10.1111/medu.14545

Mamede, S., Schmidt, H.G., 2023. Deliberate reflection and clinical reasoning: Founding ideas and empirical findings. Medical Education 57 (1), 76–85. https://doi.org/10.1111/medu.14863

Nugus, P., Bridges, J., Braithwaite, J., 2009. Selling patients. BMJ 339 (2), b5201. https://doi.org/10.1136/bmj.b5201

Øberg, G.K., Normann, B., Gallagher, S., 2015. Embodied-enactive clinical reasoning in physical therapy. Physiotherapy Theory and Practice 31 (4), 244–252. https://doi.org/10.3109/09593985.2014.1002873

Paschal, K.A., Jensen, G.M., Mostrom, E., 2002. Building portfolios: A means for developing habits of reflective practice in physical therapy education. Journal of Physical Therapy Education 16 (3), 38–51.

Peters, A., Vanstone, M., Monteiro, S., Norman, G., Sherbino, J., Sibbald, M., 2017. Examining the influence of context and professional culture on clinical reasoning through rhetorical-narrative analysis. Qualitative Health Research 27 (6), 866–876. https://doi.org/10.1177/1049732316650418

Richards, J.B., Hayes, M.M., Schwartzstein, R.M., 2020. Teaching clinical reasoning and critical thinking: From cognitive theory to practical application. Chest 158 (4), 1617–1628. https://doi.org/10.1016/j.chest.2020.05.525

Rider, E.A., Keefer, C.H., 2006. Communication skills competencies: Definitions and a teaching toolbox. Medical Education 40 (7), 624–629. https://doi.org/10.1111/j.1365-2929.2006.02500.x

Tan, S.M., Ladyshewsky, R.K., Gardner, P., 2010. Using blogging to promote clinical reasoning and metacognition in undergraduate physiotherapy fieldwork programs. Australasian Journal of Educational Technology 26 (3), 355–368.

Verheijden, M., Giroldi, E., van den Eertwegh, V., Luijkx, M., van der Weijden, T., de Bruin, A., et al., 2023. Identifying characteristics of a skilled communicator in the clinical encounter. Medical Education 57 (5), 418–429.

Vermeir, P., Vandijck, D., Degroote, S., Peleman, R., Verhaeghe, R., Mortier, E., et al., 2015. Communication in healthcare: A narrative review of the literature and practical recommendations. International Journal of Clinical Practice 69 (11), 1257–1267. https://doi.org/10.1111/ijcp.12686

Windish, D.M., Price, E.G., Clever, S.L., Magaziner, J.L., Thomas, P.A., 2005. Teaching medical students the important connection between communication and clinical reasoning. Journal of General Internal Medicine 20 (12), 1108–1113.

Woodward-Kron, R., van Die, D., Webb, G., Pill, J., Elder, C., McNamara, T., et al., 2012. Perspectives from physiotherapy supervisors on student-patient communication. International Journal of Medical Education 3, 166–174. https://doi.org/10.5116/ijme.502f.6e18

42

LEARNING TO RESEARCH CLINICAL REASONING

KATHRYN N. HUGGETT ■ EMILY GREENBERGER ■
GAIL M. JENSEN ■ ANNA MAIO

CHAPTER OUTLINE

CHAPTER AIMS

The aims of this chapter are:

■ to discuss why educators should engage in research about clinical reasoning
■ to summarize common purposes and types of educational studies in the health sciences
■ to discuss considerations in selecting a conceptual framework to guide research
■ to describe early steps in determining the research design
■ to illustrate how an educator might propose to study a question from their teaching practice.

INTRODUCTION

Educational research may seem too far beyond the scope of customary activity for educators who develop and implement clinical reasoning curricula. Some educators feel unprepared to engage in educational research, citing lack of relevant social science research skills. There are at least three reasons, however, why educators should engage in research about clinical reasoning.

First, as educators and scholars, it is critical that we share descriptions of our work with others. Descriptive studies offer ideas and guidance to other educators who may be seeking a similar innovation or application of a new method. Second, justification studies permit us to compare educational interventions to answer the questions: 'Does it work?' and 'How well does it work?' (Cook et al., 2008). Finally, there is a rich history of scholarship describing theories of clinical reasoning, expertise and clinical decision-making methods. Clarification studies test predictions about these existing theories and models and answer questions such as: 'How does it work?' and 'Why does it work?' (Cook et al., 2008). Building on this work through justification studies allows us to better understand which theories apply to a particular context or setting, under what conditions and for whom.

Learning to research clinical reasoning can be the start of a new scholarly path. Traditionally, scientific inquiry pursued the creation of new knowledge. Ernest Boyer (1990, p. 24) challenged scholars to envision a wider understanding: 'What we urgently need today is a more inclusive view of what it means to be

465

a scholar—a recognition that knowledge is acquired through research, through synthesis, through practice and through teaching'. This is particularly true for expanding knowledge and understanding of clinical reasoning. For example, the clinical learning environment is often interdisciplinary and interprofessional, providing opportunities for the discovery of new relationships, techniques and approaches. The insights and questions that emerge in clinical practice also contribute to knowledge development through synthesis and these may advance knowledge in the form of policy papers and case reviews. Additionally, understanding how individuals and groups access information, draw upon prior experience and engage in clinical reasoning allows us to tailor our teaching and our system to be as inclusive and equitable as possible. New knowledge is also created through practical application, as questions emerge in practice and are explored when hypotheses are tested against clinical findings and pathophysiological principles. Likewise, the scholarship of practice can occur when technical skills are applied to develop quality indicators and innovations to improve healthcare systems and delivery. Finally, the scholarship of teaching and learning can enlarge knowledge of a clinical topic when educators create scholarly products to guide clinical practice such as textbooks, assessments and accreditation standards.

In this chapter, we offer ideas to help educators develop a research question supported by a conceptual framework. Next, we discuss early steps in determining the research design. Finally, we provide two case studies to illustrate how an educator might propose to study a question from their teaching practice. If you are new to educational research, do not be intimidated. If you have participated in basic science or clinical research, you already possess some of the skills and habits of mind required for educational research. Above all, use your skills of observation and stay open to new questions that emerge during your clinical teaching. These often set the foundation for studies that answer our own local questions and initiate a wider conversation in our field. See the examples in Case Studies 42.1 and 42.2.

DEVELOP A RESEARCH QUESTION

A question is the starting point and refining that question is critical to developing a project. A literature

CASE STUDY 42.1
Learning Clinical Reasoning

The director of an ambulatory clinic rotation has at least one teaching session devoted to the importance of antibiotic stewardship. The medical students have already learned that most upper respiratory infections, sinus infections and bronchitis are caused by viruses and rarely on presentation require antibiotics. Several of the clinic providers (including physicians, nurse practitioners, physician assistants) provide feedback that the students seem to understand the differential diagnosis but often still want to give antibiotics in these situations. The reasons seem unclear and some of the clinic providers speculate that these students may be responding to patients' requests for antibiotics. The course director initially surveys the students about their thought processes. The survey provides quantitative data indicating that most of the students acknowledge what they have learnt. Responses to other survey questions indicate that diagnostic uncertainty, office procedures, healthcare provider practices and patient requests may influence students' treatment plans. The survey responses alone do not provide sufficient insight into the reasons the students decide to treat with antibiotics. To understand better the clinical reasoning underlying the students' decision making, the director designs a study using a qualitative approach (grounded theory using interviews) to explore more deeply the various meanings underlying the factors identified in the survey. Examples of research questions that could be developed further include:

- What is the relationship between patients and students?
- How do patients pressurize students into prescribing antibiotics?
- How do students justify prescribing antibiotics in these settings?
- To what extent do students understand the notion of antibiotic stewardship?
- Do students encounter a hidden curriculum at their clinical placement sites, i.e. do providers demonstrate different prescribing practices?
- Do beliefs about prescribing antibiotics vary by profession?

CASE STUDY 42.2
Learning Clinical Reasoning

An academic hospitalist notices that medical students begin nearly all of their case presentations for patients of colour with a 'one-liner' that includes the race of the patient. For example, a student might begin: 'Ms Smith is a 34-year-old African American woman presenting with acute shortness of breath'. The hospitalist begins with a focus group of several students and asks them why they chose that information. The students report that they are modelling what they have seen in textbooks, clinical exam stems and what they have witnessed from medical residents. The hospitalist designs a translational study measuring how frequently medical students report patient race in clinical case presentations both before and after an educational session focussed on developing problem representations. In the educational session, the hospitalist instructs medical students to include information in the problem representation, otherwise known as the one-liner, which helps the listener form broad and accurate illness scripts and diagnostic schema without unnecessary language that may predispose to bias. Examples of research questions that could be developed further include:

- Have you experienced learners or colleagues who unintentionally incorporate bias in their case presentations? Why do you think this occurs?
- Where throughout the curriculum is the one-liner introduction to patient presentation formally taught and how can that approach be modified to be more inclusive and less biased? Start your analysis with the first-year physical diagnosis course and then proceed through the curriculum.
- How can you recruit other educators, staff and learners to model and reinforce a more inclusive and less biased problem representation?
- How could you evaluate the impact of your intervention over time? How could you evaluate it across different learning environments?
- Is there a way to empower everyone listening to a one-liner to speak up and suggest modifications to create a more inclusive and less biased environment?

- How can the intervention be structured so that the revised introduction also encourages learners to discuss what information should and should not be included to both broaden and narrow the differential diagnosis?
- Are there other research questions or designs you might approach for this case?

---

search is always an early step to refine a question, to see what has been studied and what still needs to be explored. Starting broad with a goal and thinking of it in terms of what you want to measure, replicate, discover or confirm begins the process. A working list of questions and ideas can be distilled by consulting and critiquing the literature. At a later date in the process, a method of inquiry is chosen. Keeping an open mind in this early phase is important.

A good question meets key criteria. Using a tool to assess questions is vital to development. One such tool is FINER (Hulley and Cummings, 1988). Using this acronym, F represents Feasible. Is the scope of the project possible and are there resources for the project (time and money)? I is Interesting. Why is it interesting to you and who else is interested who can help with resources and promotion? N identifies Novel. Has this been done before and how can this project be made unique? This is a signal to dive deeper into the literature. E is Ethical. Spend time thinking about your participants and any ethical issues that could arise. For example, a researcher may wish to conduct a think-aloud study to investigate how advanced nursing students solve complex cases and arrive at clinical decisions. The investigator is an educator who evaluates learners in a final capstone course and writes letters of recommendation. Thus, students may feel compelled to participate in the study. To address these ethical considerations, the study protocol must offer voluntary participation and ensure protections such as confidential data collection and de-identification of data before review by this researcher-teacher. The researcher-teacher must not be able to find out who provided data and who did not. R stands for Relevant. Your proposed project should be useful in some way and relate to the current state of health sciences education. Even if your project is historical, understanding how things were done in the past can help us understand why the present situation has come about in the way that it has.

IDENTIFY A CONCEPTUAL FRAMEWORK

Conceptual frameworks are an important resource in helping the researcher explain the significance of the research question. Although the terms 'conceptual framework' and 'theoretical framework' are often used interchangeably, Varpio et al. (2020) offer a useful distinction. They explain the conceptual framework as the researcher's 'argument justifying the need for the research study' (Varpio et al., 2020, p. 991). As such, the conceptual framework is a helpful structure to guide the selection of the study design and 'it is constructed to answer two questions: "Why is this research important?" and "What contributions might these findings make to what is already known?"' (Varpio et al., 2020, p. 990). In contrast, 'a theoretical framework is a logically developed and connected set of concepts and premises—developed from one or more theories—that a researcher creates to scaffold a study' (Varpio et al., 2020, p. 990). In health professions education research, theories are often drawn from multiple fields such as cognitive psychology, educational psychology, sociology and industrial and organizational psychology. Depending upon the purpose of the study (e.g. hypothesis testing or exploration of a phenomenon), the theories relevant to the research question will be identified and used in different ways and at different stages of the study. For example, if you are using qualitative research methods to explore a phenomenon that is not well described or understood, such as how health professions students describe their reasoning processes in their first semester of study, you would begin by interviewing and observing students. From this initial data collection, you could identify key concepts that might include how they describe their approach to reasoning and the processes they use to make decisions. To continue with this example, if you moved on to studying the development of clinical reasoning abilities of health professions students across all years of the educational programme, you might use concepts

from how learners organize knowledge (script theory) and dual-process theory (analytic and nonanalytic thinking), along with concepts you uncovered in your exploratory research from first-year students. For more information about theories informing educational research, we recommend consulting a textbook such as *Researching Medical Education* (Cleland and Durning, 2015).

REFLECTION POINT

Reflection Questions for Students

Here are some questions to guide your research planning:
1. What questions do I still have about clinical reasoning?
2. How could instruction for clinical reasoning be improved?
3. Where did the real learning occur?
4. What resources would have been useful to guide my learning?

Step 1: Get a Central Focus

In clinical reasoning research, an initial question for developing the framework is: What is the central question or problem? Are you interested in:

1. learner development of clinical reasoning abilities? (Schmidt and Mamede, 2015)
2. the teaching of clinical reasoning? (Schmidt and Mamede, 2015)
3. the assessment of clinical reasoning? (Thampy et al., 2019)
4. the clinical reasoning process used in the context of practice? (Thampy et al., 2019)
5. understanding types or approaches to clinical reasoning used? (Khatami et al., 2012)

When you have a central question or problem, consult one or two key references such as those listed. Then proceed to Step 2.

Step 2: Set Boundaries for the Framework

Once you have a central focus, which actors will be studied or relationship explored? In other words, what are the boundaries of the study (what is included and what is excluded and why)? You cannot study everything and setting boundaries for the framework or scaffold is a very important step in the process.

Step 3: Look to the Literature for Research and Theory

What do we already know about this problem in clinical reasoning from your profession and others? What are the recurring concepts, models and theories that you continue to see in the literature? Central to understanding the development of clinical reasoning abilities will be the learning sciences and educational theories. Which current learning science theories may be helpful in your research?

Learning theories that are currently used in clinical reasoning include cognitive theories. Currently popular is dual-process theory, which can be described simply as fast thinking (nonanalytic thinking; also called pattern recognition or type 1 thinking) or slow thinking (analytic thinking; also called type 2 thinking). Another example is cognitive load theory, which has to do with information processing and how much a learner can handle. Clinical reasoning research can also use noncognitive theories, such as those from social cognitive work, that are focussed on situativity theory, a framework that is based on knowledge, thinking and learning being situated in experience. Situativity theory contends that context is important; learning and thinking cannot be separated from the context and the interactions occurring in the learning environment and community of practice (Trowbridge et al., 2015).

Step 4: Make a Visual, One-Page Framework

Conceptual frameworks are sometimes best done as a graphic or visual. This helps you see the core concepts or constructs and the relationships among them. If you have more than one researcher, you may each want to develop an individual model and then come together to build a consensus model for the research.

REFLECTION POINT

Reflection Questions for Educators

Here are some questions to guide your research planning:
1. Did the instructional method and assessment support the learning objectives?

2. Did learners achieve the learning objectives as expected?
3. Are there key concepts or processes that consistently challenge learners?
4. What contributed to or detracted from the learning experience?

SELECT THE RESEARCH DESIGNS AND METHODS

Once you have identified an area of interest and developed your conceptual framework, you are ready to consider which type of research design and associated methods will lead to answering your type of research question. Ringsted et al. (2011) describe a 'research compass' model of design approaches that is very helpful for guiding initial decisions about which direction to take with research design, depending on the purpose of the study (Table 42.1).

Perhaps an even simpler place to start in selecting an appropriate research design is to consider which research paradigm is most suited to answer the research question. Research paradigms are commonly separated into qualitative, quantitative or mixed-method approaches to design. Qualitative approaches are well suited to answer open-ended exploratory research questions. Researchers working in the qualitative paradigm intentionally do not predetermine hypotheses related to what they expect or predict their possible outcomes to be. Rather, these designs have, as an outcome of the research, a description of 'what is there' in the phenomenon of interest or of what things mean to people. Quantitative approaches are well suited to answer closed-ended research questions; these are questions that test or measure 'what is there' as the outcome of research. The hypothesis being tested assumes that the entities being measured are there to begin with. Mixed-method approaches to design are often used when, to develop a deeper or more contextualized understanding of a situation, the researcher chooses to explore both closed-ended and open-ended questions that are closely related. It is helpful to consider that the quantitative aspects of a mixed-method design are intended to provide replicable evidence and therefore can contribute to the establishment of laws and principles, while the qualitative aspects,

TABLE 42.1
Research Design Directions With Associated Approaches

Category of Study	Purpose	Research Approaches	Types of Research Questions Answered
Explorative	Modelling: identification and explanation of elements and establishing relationships between those elements in phenomena; aims to understand the whole of a phenomenon rather than reduce data through statistical analysis	Descriptive e.g. action research, case studies Qualitative e.g. ethnography, grounded theory, phenomenology Psychometric e.g. focussed on measurement and/or development of a measurement instrument; establishment of validity (face, content, criterion, construct); establishment of reliability (repro-ducibility, internal consistency)	*What characterizes ...?* *How do theories of learning inform the observation of ...?* *What are students' perceptions of ...?* *What is the nature of ...?* *What is the validity and reliability of...?* *What are normative values for ...?*
Experimental	Justification: Highly controlled experiments involving homogeneous group comparisons; seek evidence of the effects of an intervention	Randomized controlled trials (RCTs)	*Does this intervention work?* *Is this new intervention better/more efficient than the way things have been traditionally done?*
Observational	Prediction: Examination of naturally occurring or static groups (heterogeneous), to predict an outcome or relationship; causal studies	Cohort: inquiry starts with the predictor variable (an exposure to a particular educational event or characteristic that is different between cohorts) Case-control: inquiry starts with criterion variable (outcome that is different between groups) Associational: cross-sectional studies that provide a snapshot of certain variables in a variety of people, to investigate how they are associated; no use of groups for comparison	*Does attending a programme that uses high-fidelity simulation activities predict future clinical competence?* *How do students who have educationally disadvantaged backgrounds perform in the first year of nursing school compared with students who do not have educationally disadvantaged backgrounds?* *What is the relationship between X (criterion variable) and Y (predictor variable)?*
Translational	Implementation: Knowledge and findings from research implemented in real-life complex settings with heterogeneous partici-pants; may involve evalua-tion of process and outcome	Knowledge creation (reviews): Investigations of prior research (e.g. systematic reviews, critical, narrative reviews) Knowledge implementation: Systematic efforts to change existing educational practices by distributing knowledge of and/or facilitating the implementation of new evidence-inspired educational practices Efficiency studies: address questions of what works, how and for whom in real-life settings	*What is the evidence base for this approach to curricular design?* *Does the provision of educational best-practice guidelines to the educators of a professional education program change teaching or assessment practices?* *Does this educational strategy work for first-year students in their early clinical rotations?*

Based on Ringsted, C., Hodges, B., Scherpbier, A., 2011. The research compass: An introduction to research in medical education: AMEE Guide No. 56. Med. Teach. 33, 695–709.

although not replicable, can provide essential context within which to understand the quantitative findings (Leppink, 2017).

DEVELOP THE RESEARCH DESIGN

After you have selected the appropriate research design, you can proceed to develop the plan for your study. Remember that the research design will help you answer your research questions and guide the investigation in a purposeful and systematic way. Although an in-depth examination of research design elements is beyond the scope of this chapter, here are some considerations to guide your planning. For quantitative studies, randomized controlled trials (RCTs) should be considered for relatively standard interventions. RCTs require the random assignment of participants to treatments and this randomization reduces bias. For this reason, RCTs are considered the gold standard in the clinical research paradigm. In educational settings, however, it is often difficult to randomize learners to different educational experiences. It is also challenging to standardize learning environments and experiences. Randomization will not control for sources of error such as variations in learner preparation and motivation, learning settings and intervention implementation. For these reasons, RCTs are recommended for situations in which the mechanism of learning is already understood, the outcome of the intervention is easily measured and accepted, the effect size of the intervention is small or the results from the trial may have a large effect. If any of these criteria are not met, it can be difficult to justify the cost of an RCT (Norman, 2010).

There are many alternatives to the RCT and it is not uncommon to use nonrandomized methods in education studies. In some educational settings, it is not appropriate to randomize learners. For example, if withholding the intervention or educational resource may disadvantage learners and jeopardize examination or course performance, it will be unfair to randomize learners. The complex design of health sciences education also makes it difficult to use the RCT model. Learners are often assigned to different sites, rotations and preceptors at different times. This makes it logistically difficult to randomize learners and minimize confounding influences. In these cases,

investigators must use other research design strategies to overcome potential sources of bias. Some examples include comparison groups, pretest/posttest, blinding of participants or teachers to the research hypothesis and increasing the sample size by waiting for several implementations of the intervention (Sullivan, 2011). Comparison groups offer an opportunity to investigate the outcome of an intervention when it is not feasible to create a control group. Comparison group designs may draw upon participants from other sites or historical groups (e.g. previous cohort). Another approach is to use a cross-over design in which control and experimental groups are created, but the groups switch halfway, thus ensuring each group receives the intervention. The pretest/posttest design is perhaps the most widely used research design for nonrandomized studies. This design provides comparison data because data are collected from the same group before and after the intervention. For a deeper explanation of these designs, their limitations and other approaches, consult an expert at your institution or resources such as the AMEE Guides published by the Association for Medical Education in Europe.

For quantitative and mixed-method studies, schedule early consultations with a statistician to ensure you plan for an appropriate sample size to ensure statistical power. The statistician can also provide guidance on your study design, data collection and management strategies and data analysis plan. For qualitative and mixed-method studies, be sure to consult an expert to help you select among many approaches, including case study, phenomenology, grounded theory, narrative and ethnography. Each approach has its own procedures and standards for participant selection, data collection, data analysis and quality control.

When you have finalized your research plan and have sufficient detail to describe the research design, instrumentation, data collection, sample and plan for data analysis, you are ready to submit a proposal for formal ethical approval. Nearly all educational research projects require formal ethical approval of some sort. The committees/organizations that provide ethical review can go by a variety of titles. For example, in North America they are generally called Institutional Review Boards.

While you await ethical approval for your project, continue to read the literature and prepare the infrastructure to support your project work. For example, consult with a librarian to expand your literature review and construct a bibliography, perhaps using an online bibliography and citation application. If you will be conducting interviews or observations, begin to identify time in your schedule and place a hold on these times. Similarly, consider reserving physical facilities such as clinical simulation centre space. This is also a good time to anticipate equipment needs (e.g. video cameras or software) and place orders, especially if the item may be limited or difficult to find. Finally, begin to create any necessary files, spreadsheets and databases to manage data collection.

The protocol for your project will guide you through implementation, but you may wish to consult with colleagues about strategies and tips to guide your work. Setting deadlines, scheduling periodic consultations with key study personnel and reserving time on your calendar for uninterrupted project work are simple but effective strategies. These strategies are also useful when you have completed data collection and analysis and proceed to the writing stage. Finally, be mindful of quality standards and journal guidelines when writing up your study findings. There are many helpful resources including the Association of American Medical Colleges' Review Criteria for Research Manuscripts (Durning and Carline, 2015) that include both a checklist and in-depth explanation of the criteria. For example, in the category 'Data Analysis and Statistics', there are six criteria, including 'Data analysis procedures are described in sufficient detail' and 'Power issues are considered in studies that make statistical inferences'. Although this checklist was designed for manuscript reviewers, it is equally valuable for authors. Using a checklist will make the process less daunting and ensure you do not omit an essential element in your manuscript.

Remember that most health sciences educators do not have training and expertise in education research and you are therefore not alone in seeking additional information and professional development. A growing number of institutions offer consultation, typically located in academies of educators, offices of research, departments of medical education or centres for teaching, learning and research. Many professional societies and organizations also offer professional development to foster educational research, including the American Educational Research Association (AERA), the Research Essential Skills in Medical Education (RESME) programme of the Association for Medical Education in Europe (AMEE), the International Association of Medical Science Educators (IAMSE) Medical Educator Fellowship programme and the Association of American Medical Colleges' (AAMC) Medical Education Research Certificate (MERC) programme.

CONCLUSION

The phenomenon of clinical reasoning is diverse enough, and rich enough, to be researched in many different ways. There are many disciplines and many theories that can be used, or combined, to provide a theoretical foundation for a research project. The nature of the research question will determine which theories will be most useful. The research question will also determine whether quantitative, qualitative or mixed methods will be appropriate. The case studies in this chapter provide two straightforward examples that can generate a number of research questions that can be researched in a variety of ways.

SUMMARY

In this chapter we have presented the following:

- Research about clinical reasoning is essential to understanding processes and conditions for optimal learning and assessment.
- A conceptual framework is a helpful structure for communicating the significance of your study and for thinking more deeply about the theories, constructs or variables and the relationships among them that you will be studying.
- The research design will help you answer your research questions and guide the investigation in a purposeful and systematic way.
- There are many alternatives to the RCT and it is not uncommon to use nonrandomized methods in education studies.

REFLECTION POINT

Research into clinical reasoning can bring many benefits. Research can generate new knowledge that helps us to gain a better understanding of clinical reasoning, a worthwhile goal in itself.
- How might you engage in research to improve your teaching and benefit students, teachers and ultimately patients?

REFERENCES

Boyer, E.L., 1990. Scholarship reconsidered: Priorities of the professoriate. Princeton University Press, Lawrenceville, NJ.

Cleland, J., Durning, S.J., 2015. Researching medical education. John Wiley & Sons.

Cook, D.A., Bordage, G., Schmidt, H.G., 2008. Description, justification and clarification: A framework for classifying the purposes of research in medical education. Medical Education 42, 128–133. https://doi.org/10.1111/j.1365-2923.2007.02974.x

Durning, S.J., Carline, J.D. (Eds.), 2015. Review criteria for research manuscripts, 2nd ed. Association of American Medical Colleges.

Hulley, S.B., Cummings, S.R. (Eds.), 1988. Designing clinical research: An epidemiologic approach. Lippincott Williams & Wilkins.

Khatami, S., MacEntee, M.I., Pratt, D.D., Collins, J.B., 2012. Clinical reasoning in dentistry: A conceptual framework for dental education. Journal of Dental Education 76, 1116–1128. https://doi.org/10.1002/j.0022-0337.2012.76.9.tb05366.x

Leppink, J., 2017. Revisiting the quantitative–qualitative-mixed methods labels: Research questions, developments, and the need for replication. Journal of Taibah University Medical Sciences 12, 97–101. https://doi.org/10.1016/j.jtumed.2016.11.008

Norman, G., 2010. Is experimental research passé? Advances in Health Science Education, Theory and Practice 15, 297–301. https://doi.org/10.1007/s10459-010-9243-6

Ringsted, C., Hodges, B., Scherpbier, A., 2011. 'The research compass': An introduction to research in medical education: AMEE Guide No. 56. Medical Teacher 33, 695–709. https://doi.org/10.3109/0142159X.2011.595436

Schmidt, H.G., Mamede, S., 2015. How to improve the teaching of clinical reasoning: A narrative review and a proposal. Medical Education 49 (10), 961–973. https://doi.org/10.1111/medu.12775

Sullivan, G.M., 2011. Getting off the 'gold standard': Randomized controlled trials and education research. Journal of Graduate Medical Education 3, 285–289. https://doi.org/10.4300/JGME-D-11-00147.1

Thampy, H., Willert, E., Ramani, S., 2019. Assessing clinical reasoning: Targeting the higher levels of the pyramid. Journal of General Internal Medicine 34 (8), 1631–1636. https://doi.org/10.1007/s11606-019-04953-4

Trowbridge, R., Rencic, J., Durning, S. (Eds.), 2015. Teaching clinical reasoning. American College of Physicians.

Varpio, L., Paradis, E., Uijtdehaage, S., Young, M., 2020. The distinctions between theory, theoretical framework, and conceptual framework. Academic Medicine 95 (7), 989–994. https://doi.org/10.1097/ACM.0000000000003075

43

CLINICAL DECISION MAKING, CULTURE AND HEALTH

MAREE SIMPSON ■ JENNIFER COX

CHAPTER OUTLINE

CHAPTER AIMS

The aims of this chapter are to:

- discuss the impact of culture and sub-cultures on the health of members of our communities
- consider those activities, beliefs, practices and roles that culture brings to a health interaction
- consider the impact of our own cultural background and our professional culture and those of people who come to our communities as migrants or as refugees who may have different understandings, needs and wants.

INTRODUCTION

So, What Is Culture in the 21st Century?

Like many words, 'culture' has been defined a number of different ways in different situations at different times. A current dictionary definition (Mirriam-Webster, n.d.) identifies culture as 'the customary beliefs, social forms, and material traits of a racial, religious, or social group, also the characteristic features of everyday existence (such as diversions or a way of life) shared by people in a place or time and the set of values, conventions, or social practices associated with a particular field, activity, or societal characteristic'. Further, other definitions include subgroups within a group of people, defined as 'the way of life, customs, and ideas of a particular group of people within a society that are different from the rest of that society' (Cambridge Dictionary, n.d.). This recognizes that not all people living in a certain area or nation adopt the mainstream culture and cultural practices with differences in spiritual, well-being, communication and health having perhaps most impact on health professionals' clinical decision making and practices.

From a health perspective, a World Health Organization Expert Group (Regional Office for Europe, 2015) agreed to embrace the United Nations Educational, Scientific and Cultural Organization's (UNESCO, 2001) definition of culture as described in the 2001 Universal Declaration on Cultural Diversity. This definition conceives of culture '… as a way of life rather than simply as religious, social or ethnic characteristics delimited by geopolitical boundaries, thus acknowledging the presence (and importance) of dynamic microcultures that exist everywhere, and that even the process of focusing on wellbeing is developing its own artefacts'.

Earlier this century, Kagawa-Singer (2011) identified the broad range of activities on which culture had an impact on health and disparity within Hammond's seven nested layers of culture (Hammond, 1978). These are Environment, Economy, Technology, Religion or world view, Language, Social structure, and Beliefs and values.

Most recently, Hernandez and Gibb (2020, p. 12) asserted that culture is '… a socially transmitted system of shared knowledge, beliefs and/or practices that varies across groups, and individuals within those groups, has been a critical mode of adaptation throughout the history of our species'. They further asserted that individual factors such as socioeconomic status, identified gender and moral and ethical views also have an impact, in addition to culture. The authors propose that identifying and understanding an individual's unique cultural experience plus their response to sociopolitical pressures can better prepare health professionals with those professional and communication skills and empathy that best results in culturally safe care.

Although these definitions of culture may vary across time and place, each, perhaps arguably, identifies that it has impacts on many aspects of life, especially a person's health. So, an individual's beliefs about health, illness and well-being, health and wellness practices, how help is sought and preferences for treatment vary by region, by nation and within nations, reflective of people who were raised in that area, people who migrated to that area and refugees who were accepted into that area. Potentially, additional challenges that migrants and/or refugees may face in addition to health and its institutional settings lie in legal systems and educational systems.

The Impacts of Culture on Health

Accepting that culture, individual factors and environments impact significantly on individuals, which types of impacts are recognized as having evidence-based support? There are many articles that identify the impacts of culture and individual factors on health and well-being, including practices such as circumcision, initiation rites, beliefs about activity such as formal exercise/swimming, dietary requirements and prohibitions such as the need for Halal foods and medicines, and varying perceptions on immunization. These are briefly outlined in the following text.

Hernandez and Gibb (2020) identified that in a diverse sample of pregnant women in New Zealand,

those women who disclosed experiencing ethnic-based discrimination were found to have higher levels of cortisol and, of concern, so were their infants. The 2018 Census conducted in New Zealand (Stats NZ, 2020) identified six major ethnic groups: those of European background (70.2%), Māori (16.5%), Pacific peoples (8.1%), Asian (15.1%), Middle Eastern/Latin American/African (1.5%) and 'other ethnicity' (1.2%).

Kahissay and colleagues (2017) explored perceptions of the causation of ill-health in rural north-eastern Ethiopia and established that illness was perceived to have many causes. They identified supernatural causes such as God or Allah, spirits in nature, environmental causes such as hygiene, sanitation and poverty, and societal causes such as breaking social taboos.

Further, Samatra (2019) explored the perceptions of Balinese healers about epilepsy. It was reported that the healers, who were Hindu males, understood epilepsy as both a medical and a spiritual illness. Samatra stated that none of the healers recognized epilepsy as a disease of the brain and that their management of this condition may have been influenced by this.

Liang and colleagues (2021) explored perceptions about Alzheimer's disease held by Asian Americans living in the United States. Using a sample of 2609 people representing diverse ethnic backgrounds (Chinese, Asian Indian, Korean, Vietnamese, Filipino and other Asians) and a broad age range (18–98 years), their research found that stigmatizing beliefs varied across ethnic backgrounds. For example, 63% of people from a Vietnamese background perceived Alzheimer's disease to be part of normal ageing and therefore may not seek medical help, whilst 10% of those from a Chinese background would feel embarrassed if their family member developed the condition.

Zolezzi and colleagues (2018) explored perceptions of mental health and stigma in Arab culture by undertaking a review of the literature and reporting stigmatizing beliefs, actions and attitudes towards people with mental illness. The majority of articles identified negative perceptions of mental illness and stigmatizing beliefs of causation such as God's punishment, being cursed or being influenced by magic. The researchers proposed that initiatives to enhance mental health literacy in the general public may benefit those living with mental health conditions who may be currently affected by stigma.

Some cultural practices, however, may be undertaken as a sport. For example, sumo, which is a national sport in Japan (Hagihara et al., 2018), involves participants known as *rikishi*, two of whom undertake matches in a ring-shaped venue, the *dohyo*. Current professional sumo wrestlers range from approximately 130 kilograms to over 180 kilograms in weight (Hagihara et al., 2018) though a very few are lighter (around 112 kg) and a very few are heavier (up to 212 kg). The wrestlers have a high kilojoule intake combined with a strenuous exercise programme (Nishizawa et al., 1976); however, Japanese sumo wrestlers have been identified as having high cardiovascular risk (Berglund et al., 2011; Kanda et al., 2009).

How Does Culture Affect Health Literacy, Self-Efficacy and Adherence to Disease Management?

Cultural, social and family influences shape attitudes and beliefs and therefore influence health literacy. Social determinants of health are well documented regarding the conditions over which the individual has little or no control but that affect their ability to participate fully in a health-literate society (Nielsen-Bohlman et al., 2004). These will be discussed briefly in the following sections.

HEALTH LITERACY

Health literacy refers to a person's ability to understand and act on health information (Institute of Medicine, Committee on Health Literacy, 2004). A growing body of evidence demonstrates that, compared with individuals with adequate health literacy skills, those with limited health literacy are more likely to misunderstand health information (Friedman et al., 2006), to have difficulty following medical instructions (Davis et al., 2006), to use healthcare services inappropriately or infrequently (Gazmararian et al., 1999; Sudore et al., 2006), to have worse physical and mental health (Wolf et al., 2005), to experience higher rates of hospitalization and to have a shorter life expectancy. Efforts to overcome limited health literacy have included developing plain language, patient-friendly education materials and navigation aids. Other strategies that can be used by healthcare professionals to improve patient health literacy levels (ACP Decisions, 2019, 2022), thereby aiding medical adherence and empowering patients to manage their own conditions better, include:

- remembering we had to LEARN medical terminology, disease state information, features of medicines and lots more,
- limiting the number of messages we give to patients (as a rule no more than between three and five pieces of information),
- clearly stating actions and behaviour(s),
- not assuming, e.g. what DOES three times a day mean? Check understanding and patient plans, help them remember (e.g. tie to meals) if suitable,
- supplementing instructions with written material (e.g. with pictures or flow charts),
- demonstrating devices,
- making directions easy to read for everyone, hence font size matters,
- asking open-ended questions and
- checking for understanding with open-ended questions.

Even those with adequate health literacy may still have difficulty adhering to advice from their healthcare professionals if that advice is perceived as culturally inappropriate (Case Study 43.1).

Self-Efficacy

Self-efficacy is generally defined as an individual's belief in their *own* ability to achieve a given outcome or level of attainment (Bandura, 1986) and is recognized as a key determinant in health behaviour. In this context, perceived self-efficacy influences exercise of control over the state of one's health (Zlatanović, 2016). Importantly, supportive associations with healthcare providers can help enhance the self-efficacy of patients to manage their treatment and/or condition, particularly those patients with lower education levels (Yeom and Lee, 2022), which impacts also health literacy.

Adherence to Medications and Condition Management

Chronic diseases are commonly managed by a multidisciplinary health team and use procedures, medications and lifestyle interventions. However, it is well recognized that patients may not accept these management activities or modalities for a variety of cultural and/or individual factors (Case Study 43.2). A recent study of medication adherence by Shahin and colleagues (2019) identified several personal and culturally based factors

CASE STUDY 43.1

Middle-Aged Female of Apparent Japanese Appearance

Mrs Keiko Watanabe is a 44-year-old married woman with diagnoses of dyslipidaemia and hypertension. She comes to your practice and seems unhappy and perhaps confused. Keiko has told you in the past that she was born and educated in Japan but moved to your region 18 months ago when her husband was promoted to regional manager in the Kawaii car company (a Japanese company with regional branches in the Asia-Pacific). You greet Keiko and ask what she seeks today. She tells you that another member of her health professional team has advised a Mediterranean diet for her to benefit her heart health. Keiko is concerned as she and her husband prefer Japanese traditional food.

Why might Keiko be concerned about a Mediterranean diet?

How much might it vary from the traditional diet Keiko prefers?

How could Keiko discuss her concerns with the other professional?

What could you suggest to assist?

REFLECTION POINT

Starting to Understand Our Patient With Type 2 Diabetes

- How well do you feel that Mr Hunter understands type 2 diabetes?
  - Does he understand that differences in his health status (being otherwise well or sick), activity level, diet and medicines both prescribed or bought by himself may all impact on his diabetes management and blood glucose levels?
  - Could Mr Hunter have other health conditions that might impact on his diabetes management?
  - Does he feel that following directions will or ought to lead to his desired outcome?
  - Which health practitioners may be best able to assist Mr Hunter?
  - What social support might Mr Hunter have and need?

CASE STUDY 43.2

Patient With Type 2 Diabetes

Mr Alexander Hunter, 62 years old, is a regular patient at your practice. Mr Hunter has told you that he prefers to be addressed as Alex, that he is a widower with two adult children who live with their families many hundreds of kilometres away.

He lives with type 2 diabetes that was diagnosed 7 months ago and tells you he is struggling to manage his condition: 'his blood sugars are all over the place'. He is frustrated because he is being an 'adherent' diabetic. He tells you he takes his medications, tests four times a day and records them as his doctor asked him to do. When you asked Mr Hunter why he has to record his blood glucose readings, he says that he doesn't understand WHY, but that he needed to record his BGL and that he just did.

What issues can you find in this case? How would you seek to assist Mr Hunter with these challenges?

Why would you make these recommendations?

This can be quite a challenging case, so it will be explored with a little support in the following section.

that were associated with adherence to medication regimes. Their systematic review was broadly based with 40% of articles ($n = 10$) examining perception of illness, 20% ($n = 5$) health literacy, 16% ($n = 4$) cultural beliefs, 12% ($n = 3$) self-efficacy, 16% ($n = 4$) spiritual and religious beliefs, as well as 20% ($n = 5$) illness knowledge. These researchers identified statistically significant associations between adherence to medications and personal and cultural factors 80% ($n = 20$) in the included studies (Shahin et al., 2019).

CULTURAL AWARENESS, SENSITIVITY, COMPETENCE, HUMILITY, SAFETY

Despite the growing interest in health literacy, little research has investigated health professionals' knowledge of health literacy or understanding the barriers to health literacy that patients face when navigating the healthcare system. Indigenous peoples in New Zealand (NZ), Canada and Australia experience numerous inequalities in health status and outcomes and international evidence reveals that Indigenous, minority and socio-economically disadvantaged populations have greater literacy needs. To address concerns in Indigenous health literacy, a two-pronged approach, inclusive of both education of health professionals and structural reform that reduces the demands placed on Indigenous patients by the system, are important steps towards reducing these inequalities.

Thus, healthcare practitioners, the health organizations and systems within which they practise all benefit from working systematically towards cultural safety for their patients and critical consciousness of their own beliefs, structures and practices and the impacts that result. Curtis and colleagues (2019) assert that this requires examining their own culture, cultural systems and power differentials rather than seeking to become aware or competent in the cultures of patients. They state that '…the objective of culturally safe activities needs to be linked to health equity and being socially accountable for providing culturally safe care as defined by their patients and their communities' (Curtis et al., 2019, p. 13).

Who Says What Is Culturally Safe and for Whom?

Although across the world there are many different ways of discussing cultural safety, there are commonalities which are well stated in the Australian Institute of Health and Welfare report (2022), addressing cultural safety for First Nations peoples within Australia in three modules: Module 1: Culturally respectful healthcare services; Module 2: Patient experiences of healthcare and Module 3: Access to healthcare services. A feature of these modules is that they each contain a number of domains and focus areas. For example, the domains or topics addressed in Module 2 are: communication, treated respectfully, unfair treatment and cultural barriers, empowerment, family inclusion, and leave events. Further, focus areas are specific issues relevant to and addressed within each domain.

The concept of cultural safety, however, has been around for some time and a commonly accepted definition arose from the Nursing Council of New Zealand (2020) which established '… effective nursing practice of a person or family from another culture is determined by that person or family… Unsafe cultural practice comprises any action which diminishes, demeans or disempowers the cultural identity and wellbeing of an individual.'

Further, the National Collaboration Centre for Indigenous Health in Canada proposed that culturally safe healthcare systems and environments are established through increasing movement from awareness to sensitivity to competence and finally to cultural safety. This requires, the Centre asserts, practitioners to be aware of their own values, beliefs and attitudes as these consciously or unconsciously shape their behaviours and can cause patients to feel rejected, judged or unsafe. The use of anti-racism tools and approaches has also been noted as critical to achieving culturally safe practice (Turpel-Lafond and Johnson, 2021).

WHY CULTURAL SAFETY IS IMPORTANT

Cultural safety emphasizes the culture of healthcare as a 'site for transformation' to address power imbalances, discrimination and the persistent impacts of historical injustices on health and healthcare. It has been examined in the literature as both a process and an outcome. As a process of considering culture in care, cultural safety implies critical reflection from healthcare providers and organizations to recognize and question their own biases and the balance of power in care relationships, as well as to implement consequent professional, organizational and system transformations to attend to power differentials. Importantly, cultural safety has been described as 'represent[ing] a key philosophical shift from providing care regardless of difference, to care that takes account of peoples' unique needs' (McGough et al., 2022, p. 36).

As an outcome determined by recipients or care, cultural safety refers to what people feel or experience when their cultural identity and worldview are acknowledged and respected through inclusive relationships, sincere commitment, dialogue, equitable partnership and shared decision making. Core to this is the anticipation that the person seeking cultural safety can guide/direct their needs and expectations or bring with them a translator, i.e. a person who can express what the patient wants/would prefer.

Expectations of Health Professionals

Globally, there are expectations that health professionals will provide a culturally safe environment for their patients whether they are First Nations peoples, migrants, refugees or people who identify as LGBTIQ+.

For example, within Australia, Principle 3 (Respectful and Culturally Safe Practice) of the Australian Health Practitioner Regulation Agency (AHPRA) Code of Conduct states:

Positive professional relationships are built on effective communication between a practitioner and the patient they are caring for. Good practice includes that you:

(a) communicate courteously, respectfully, compassionately and honestly with patients, their nominated partner, substitute decision maker, carers, family and friends;

(b) consider the age, maturity and intellectual capacity of young people and other groups that may have additional needs and provide information in a way that they can understand;

(c) are aware of health literacy issues and take health literacy into account when communicating with people;

(d) take all practical steps to meet the specific language, cultural, and communication needs of patients and their families, including by using translating and interpreting services where necessary, and being aware of how these needs affect understanding.

(AHPRA, 2022)

For Indigenous peoples, there is growing recognition that cultural needs are a vital component of healthcare provision. The challenge for health professionals and institutions is to ensure that these cultural needs are centralized and are not subsumed by clinical interventions (Hunter and Cook, 2020).

Interaction Versus Intervention

For health professionals, asking and answering questions is a fundamental component in the provision of appropriate management of patient issues. This enhances the appropriateness of differential diagnosis and of the treatment/intervention. A key activity is effective patient history taking. However, in that model patient–health professional interactions are traditionally led by the professional. Previous research in the field of psychotherapy has found that the relationship between the patient and therapist does have an influence on clinical outcomes (Hall et al., 2010). We would argue that patient-guided interactions are central to the provision of culturally safe healthcare. Such interactions can help gain a better understanding of health literacy levels, patient preferences and needs and, importantly, comfortable collaborative decision making (Fig. 43.1).

Viewing this relationship as a working alliance (Castonguay et al., 2006) is a useful approach for healthcare professionals and placing emphasis on 'interaction versus intervention' can offer a way

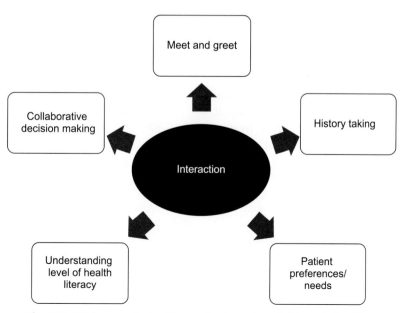

Fig. 43.1 ■ The central role of interaction in patient–clinician relationships.

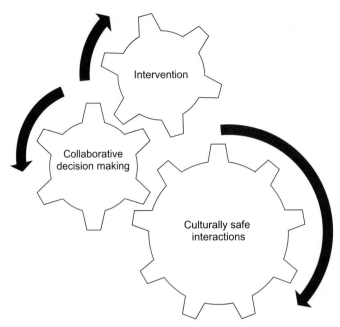

Fig. 43.2 ■ The interconnection between interaction and intervention in healthcare management.

forward that incorporates factors individual to each patient and their needs and wants. This is crucial as health registering bodies are increasingly explicitly expecting that health decision making and services occur within customized cultural safety requirements for each and every patient (Fig. 43.2).

SUMMARY

As health professionals, it is our responsibility to provide culturally safe healthcare. We benefit from exploring our own beliefs and practices and not generalizing or stereotyping our patients, even unconsciously. It is crucial that we interact rather than merely treat or intervene as all patients have individual backgrounds and cultures and we benefit from trying to understand all potential influences on their health. There are some wonderful examples in the following websites which challenge our assumptions and advocates for customizing.

Disclaimer: We are suggesting that you visit these sites to explore the impacts of making assumptions about a person's appearance, about potential unconscious bias and what they might actually like, want or need so that in practice we are less likely to stereotype or generalize. We do not in any way endorse any products that may be mentioned.

Please visit these links and explore your beliefs and practices:

Shazz: https://www.youtube.com/
watch?v=9al9dAyuC7w
Rebecca: https://www.youtube.com/
watch?v=f1jytX3FKJk
Jay: https://www.youtube.com/
watch?v=XWwN6KdtLEg
Arielle: https://www.youtube.com/
watch?v=o7QT6UIPIbE

REFERENCES

ACP Decisions, 2019. Four simple strategies for improving patient health literacy. https://www.acpdecisions.org/four-simple-strategies-for-improving-your-patients-health-literacy/.

ACP Decisions, 2022. Health literacy: A bridge to health equity. https://www.acpdecisions.org/health-literacy-a-bridge-to-health-equity/.

AHPRA, 2022. Australian Health Practitioner Regulation Agency (AHPRA) code of conduct. https://www.ahpra.gov.au/Resources/Code-of-conduct.aspx.

Australian Institute of Health and Welfare, 2022. Cultural safety in health care for Indigenous Australians: Monitoring framework [eReport (Web)](IHW 222). https://www.aihw.gov.au/reports/indigenous-australians/cultural-safety-health-care-framework/contents/monitoring-framework.

Bandura, A., 1986. Social foundations of thought and action: A social cognitive theory. Englewood Cliffs, NJ: Prentice-Hall.

Berglund, L., Sundgot-Borgen, J., Berglund, B., 2011. Adipositas athletica: A group of neglected conditions associated with medical risks. Scandinavian Journal of Medicine & Science in Sports 21 (5), 617–624.

Cambridge Dictionary, n.d. Culture. https://dictionary.cambridge.org/dictionary/english/culture

Castonguay, L.G., Constantino, M.J., Holtforth, M.G., 2006. The working alliance: Where are we and where should we go? *Psychotherapy: Theory, Research, Practice.* Training 43 (3), 271.

Curtis, E., Jones, R., Tipene-Leach, D., Walker, C., Loring, B., Paine, S.-J., et al., 2019. Why cultural safety rather than cultural competency is required to achieve health equity: A literature review and recommended definition. International Journal for Equity in Health 18 (1), 1–17.

Davis, T.C., Gazmararian, J., Kennen, E.M., 2006. Approaches to improving health literacy: Lessons from the field. Journal of Health Communication 11 (6), 551–554. https://doi.org/10.1080/10810730600835517

Friedman, D.B., Hoffman-Goetz, L., 2006. A systematic review of readability and comprehension instruments used for print and web-based cancer information. Health Education & Behavior, 33 (3), 352–272. https://doi.org/10.1177/1090198105277329

Gazmararian, J.A., Baker, S.D.W., Williams, M.V., Parker, R.M., Scott, T.L., Green, D.C., et al., 1999. Health literacy among Medicare enrollees in a managed care organization. JAMA 281 (6), 545–551. https://doi.org/10.1001/jama.281.6.545. PMID: 10022111

Hagihara, A., Onozuka, D., Hasegawa, M., Miyazaki, S., Nagata, T., 2018. Grand sumo tournaments and out-of-hospital cardiac arrests in Tokyo. Journal of the American Heart Association 7 (14), e009163.

Hall, A.M., Ferreira, P.H., Maher, C.G., Latimer, J., Ferreira, M.L., 2010. The influence of the therapist-patient relationship on treatment outcome in physical rehabilitation: A systematic review. Physical Therapy 90 (8), 1099–1110. https://doi.org/10.2522/ptj.20090245. Epub 2010 Jun 24. PMID: 20576715

Hammond, P.B, 1978. An introduction to cultural and social anthropology. New York: McMillan.

Hernandez, M., Gibb, J.K. 2020. Culture, behavior and health. Evolution, Medicine, and Public Health 2020 (1), 12–13.

Hunter, K., Cook, C., 2020. Indigenous nurses' practice realities of cultural safety and socioethical nursing. Nursing Ethics 27 (6), 1472–1483. https://doi.org/10.1177/0969733020940376

Institute of Medicine, Committee on Health Literacy, 2004. In: Kindig, D.A., Panzer, A.M., Nielsen-Bohlman, L.E. (Eds.), Health literacy: A prescription to end confusion. National Academies Press.

Kagawa-Singer, M., 2011. Impact of culture on health outcomes. Journal of Pediatric Hematology/Oncology 33, S90–S95.

Kahissay, M.H., Fenta, T.G., Boon, H., 2017. Beliefs and perception of ill-health causation: A socio-cultural qualitative study in rural North-Eastern Ethiopia. BMC Public Health 17 (1), 1–10.

Kanda, H., Hayakawa, T., Tsuboi, S., Mori, Y., Takahashi, T., Fukushima, T., 2009. Higher body mass index is a predictor of death among professional sumo wrestlers. Journal of Sports Science and Medicine 8 (4), 711–712.

Liang, J., Jang, Y., Aranda, M.P., 2021. Stigmatising beliefs about Alzheimer's disease: Findings from the Asian American Quality of Life Survey. Health & Social Care in the Community 29 (5), 1483–1490.

McGough, S., Wynaden, D., Gower, S., Duggan, R., Wilson, R., 2022. There is no health without Cultural Safety: why Cultural Safety matters. Contemporary Nurse 58 (1), 33–42. https://doi.org/10.1080/10376178.2022.2027254

Mirriam-Webster, n.d. Culture in Mirriam-Webster.com dictionary. Retrieved February 23 2023, from https://www.mirriam-webster.com/dictionary/culture

Nielsen-Bohlman, L., Panzer, A.M., Kindig, D.A.E., 2004. *Health literacy: A prescription to end confusion* (25009856). National Academies Press (US), Washington (DC). https://pubmed.ncbi.nlm.nih.gov/25009856/

Nishizawa, T., Akaoka, I., Nishida, Y., Kawaguchi, Y., Hayashi, E., Yoshimura, T., 1976. Some factors related to obesity in the Japanese sumo wrestler. The American Journal of Clinical Nutrition 29 (10), 1167–1174.

Nursing Council of New Zealand, 2020. Te Tiriti o Waitangi. https://www.nursingcouncil.org.nz/Public/Treaty_of_Waitangi/NCNZ/About-section/Te_Tiriti_o_Waitangi.aspx?hkey=36e3b0b6-da14-4186-bf0a-720446b56c52.

Samatra, D.P.G.P., 2019. Balinese traditional beliefs and epilepsy. Bali Medical Journal 8 (1), 255–258.

Shahin, W., Kennedy, G.A., Stupans, I., 2019. The impact of personal and cultural beliefs on medication adherence of patients with chronic illnesses: A systematic review. Patient Preference and Adherence 13, 1019.

Stats NZ, 2020. 2018 census ethnic group summaries. https://www.stats.govt.nz/news/ethnic-group-summaries-reveal-new-zealands-multicultural-make-up/.

Sudore, R.L., Mehta, K.M., Simonsick, E.M., Harris, T.B., Newman, A.B., Satterfield, S., et al., 2006. Limited literacy in older people and disparities in health and healthcare access. Journal of the American Geriatric Society 54 (5), 770–776. https://doi.org/10.1111/j.1532-5415.2006.00691.x. PMID: 16696742

Turpel-Lafond, M., Johnson, H., 2021. In plain sight: Addressing indigenous-specific racism and discrimination in B.C. Health Care. https://www.bcchr.ca/sites/default/files/group-opsei/in-plain-sight-full-report.pdf.

United Nations Educational, Scientific and Cultural Organization (UNESCO), 2001. Culture. https://www.unesco.org/en/culture.

Wolf, M.S., Gazmararian, J.A., Baker, D.W., 2005. Health literacy and functional health status among older adults. Archives of Internal Medicine 165 (17), 1946–1952. https://doi.org/10.1001/archinte.165.17.1946. PMID: 16186463

World Health Organization, Regional Office for Europe, 2015. Beyond bias: Exploring the cultural contexts of health and well-being measurement: First meeting of the expert group, Copenhagen, Denmark, 15–16 January 2015. https://apps.who.int/iris/handle/10665/182731.

Yeom, H.E., Lee, J., 2022. The association of education level with autonomy support, self-efficacy and health behaviour in patients with cardiovascular risk factors. Journal of Clinical Nursing 31 (11-12), 1547–1556.

Zlatanović, L., 2016. Self-efficacy and health behaviour: Some implications for medical anthropology. Glasnik Antropološkog društva Srbije 51, 17–25. https://doi.org/10.5937/gads51-12156

Zolezzi, M., Alamri, M., Shaar, S., Rainkie, D., 2018. Stigma associated with mental illness and its treatment in the Arab culture: A systematic review. International Journal of Social Psychiatry 64 (6), 597–609.

44

LEARNING ABOUT FACTORS INFLUENCING CLINICAL DECISION MAKING

MEGAN SMITH ■ JOY HIGGS

CHAPTER AIMS

The aims of this chapter are:

- to present a contemporary understanding of how clinical decision making can be influenced by contextual factors
- to reflect on the interaction between the decision makers' frame of reference and their decision making
- to assist novice health professionals to learn to account for these factors in their clinical decision making
- to assist educators to consider learning opportunities to develop clinical decision-making capability.

INTRODUCTION

Clinical decision making is both an outcome and a component of clinical reasoning. A contemporary understanding of decision making is that it is bound to the context in which it occurs (Durning et al., 2011). Quality healthcare occurs when practitioners are able to understand when factors influencing decision making contribute to errors, mistakes and potential adverse outcomes for healthcare participants and recipients, and when factors influencing decision making can be manipulated to enhance healthcare experiences or outcomes. Learning to make sound clinical decisions, therefore, requires the ability to learn to identify and understand how contextual factors influence decision making.

CLINICAL DECISION MAKING

Decision making refers to the process of making a choice between options as to categories (e.g. diagnoses, areas of responsibility), courses of action (e.g. clinical testing, communication, treatments) and judgements (e.g. evaluation of treatment outcomes). Clinical decision making by health professionals is a complex process, requiring more of individuals than making defined choices between limited options. Health professionals make decisions with multiple foci, in dynamic contexts, using a diverse knowledge base (including an increasing body of evidence-based literature), with multiple variables and individuals involved. In addition, clinical decisions are characterized by situations of uncertainty where not all the information needed to make them is, or can be, known. Clinical decision making may involve individual healthcare practitioners making decisions on behalf of patients or there may be a collaborative process, involving shared and parallel decision making with patients and teams of health professionals.

The collaborative nature of decision making means that we must consider factors that can influence individual practitioners and the teams they work in.

Learning to make clinical decisions involves an understanding of the nature of decision making in dynamic contexts (e.g. healthcare, industry and educational settings). These contexts include characteristics such as those described by Orasanu and Connolly (1993):

- problems that are ill-structured and made ambiguous by the presence of incomplete dynamic information and multiple interacting goals,
- decision-making environments that are uncertain and may change while decisions are being made,
- goals that may shift, compete or be ill-defined,
- decision making that occurs in the form of action–feedback loops, where actions result in effects and generate further information that decision makers have to react to and use in order to make further decisions,
- decision situations that contain elements of time pressure, personal stress and highly significant outcomes for the participants,
- multiple players who act together with different roles and
- organizational goals and norms that influence decision making.

REFLECTION POINT

Think about clinical decision making as a process of making choices. The decisions made may be small or large. The importance of considering carefully a range of factors that can influence such choices is generally much greater in the latter case.

Factors Influencing Decision Making

In this chapter we describe factors influencing decisions in terms of four key areas:

- the clinical task complexity,
- the internal context and capabilities of the decision maker,
- the decision-making environment and
- the level of shared decision making with clients.

These areas interact to shape the nature and outcomes of decision making (see Table 44.1). In this table, we have included reference to the shared nature of decision making, especially as it relates to decision making with clients.

A Model of Factors Influencing Clinical Decision Making

Smith (2006) explored clinical decision making by physiotherapists practising in acute care settings (hospitals). This research revealed decision making about individual patient care to be a complex and contextually dependent process. This illuminates the potential implications of the research for learning to make decisions more broadly.

This research generated a model of clinical decision making (see Fig. 44.1) in which:

- decision making is a process (where decisions are made about patients' healthcare problems, appropriate interventions, optimal modes of interaction and methods of evaluation) that is dependent upon attributes of the task such as difficulty, complexity and uncertainty,
- decision making involves a dynamic, reciprocal process of engaging with and managing environmental factors in the immediate context to identify and use these factors in making decisions and carrying out an optimal course of action,
- practitioner factors, such as their frames of reference, individual capabilities, and experience of decision making in the relevant work contexts, influence the decisions practitioners make,
- decision making is situated within a broader contextual ethos, with dimensions particular to the practice in the specific workplace and
- traversing all of these factors, to manage and make sense of them, requires four key capabilities: cognitive, emotional, social and reflexive.

Learning to Identify and Integrate Strategies for Dealing With Clinical Task Complexity Into Decision Making

The task of decision making is to make action-related choices (including, if necessary, deciding not to act). Decisions can be defined in terms of attributes such as stability, certainty, familiarity, urgency, congruence,

TABLE 44.1			
Interpretation of Factors Influencing Decision Making			

Practitioner's Personal and Professional Frame of Reference	Capabilities	Decision-Making Difficulty	
	Practitioner's level of decision-making expertise and knowledge	LOW ◄─────────────────────────► HIGH Task complexity Shared decision making Environmental challenges to decision making	
Range of individual practice models, personal frames of reference including values, beliefs and attitudes and personal dispositions particularly around interpersonal interactions	**Novice** Focus on: ■ process of reasoning ■ biomedical knowledge ■ hypothetico-deductive reasoning ■ practitioner-led reasoning ■ limited experience in reasoning and judgement	**Interaction With Context**	
		■ textbook approaches satisfy demands of low-difficulty and low-complexity tasks	■ insufficient knowledge, experience and reasoning capacity to deal with task and environment complexity ■ limited ability to deal with the human complexities of shared decision making
	Intermediate Focus on: ■ growing clinical knowledge and judgement ■ expanding clinical knowledge base ■ growing set of illness scripts based on clinical experience building on textbook learning ■ expanding interpersonal communication and collaboration skills	■ ability and experience-based confidence to explore more advanced reasoning approaches (e.g. pattern recognition, shared decision making) in simpler cases and contexts	■ limited ability to deal with highly complex cases and very challenging situations ■ reversion to hypothetico-deductive reasoning in unfamiliar and context situations
	Expert Focus on: ■ rich, extensive clinical knowledge base ■ many illness and instantiated scripts ■ well-developed clinical practice model ■ rich experience with involving patients in decision making	■ typically use advanced reasoning approaches built on clinical knowledge ■ much expertise and capacity to engage in shared decision making (if this is the chosen collaboration strategy)	■ considerable experience in working with a range of clients and situations makes experts highly capable of dealing with most complex cases and settings and working with a wide range of patients and patients' preferences for shared decision making

Based on: Boshuizen, H., Schmidt, H., 2008. The development of clinical reasoning expertise. In: Higgs, J., Jones, M., Loftus, S., Christensen, N. (Eds.), Clinical reasoning in the health professions (3rd ed.), Elsevier, pp. 113–121; Smith, M., Higgs, J., Ellis, E., 2008. Characteristics and processes of physiotherapy clinical decision making: A study of acute care cardiorespiratory physiotherapy. Physio. Res. Int., 13(4), 209–222.

risk, relevance and a number of additional variables (see Fig. 44.2). Smith's research found that these attributes shape clinical task complexity. These tasks can have poles of complexity (e.g. stable versus unstable, familiar versus unfamiliar), with further difficulty and complexity arising from the summation and interplay between attributes (Smith et al., 2008). The research found that attributes which made a decision relatively simple were familiarity, certainty, limited variables, stability, congruence and low risk. Decisions became more difficult if there was uncertainty, conflict, unfamiliarity, changing conditions, multiple relevant variables and high risk. Difficult decisions also had an ethical and emotional dimension that the participants found challenging.

Task complexity has an important relationship with the experiences of the decision maker which contributes to the perceived difficulty of decision making

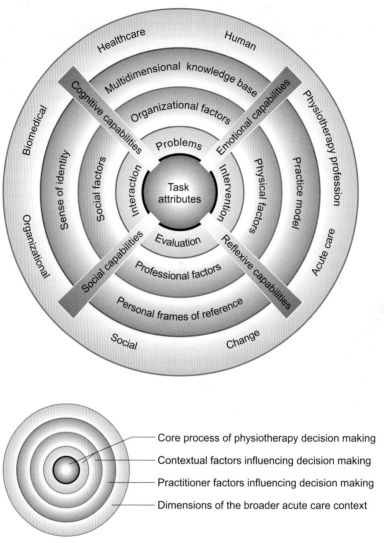

Core process of physiotherapy decision making

Contextual factors influencing decision making

Practitioner factors influencing decision making

Dimensions of the broader acute care context

Fig. 44.1 ■ Factors influencing physiotherapy decision making in acute care settings.

and learning to make decisions (McLellan et al., 2015; Parkes, 2017). Megan's research found that, when making decisions in acute care settings, participants responded to simple decisions by choosing a usual mode of practice, selecting an intervention that they found usually worked, and modifying their choice to fit the unique situation by adopting more creative and novel approaches to intervention. In contrast, when decisions were difficult, participants were more likely to experiment, draw upon the knowledge of other people, weigh up the competing aspects of the decision,

and follow protocols or rules and seek less opportunity for creativity (Smith et al., 2007). As we have illustrated in Table 44.1, the practitioner's level of expertise and their clinical experience are recognized to have an influence on these matters.

Novices learning to make decisions can be aided by learning to break down the clinical task to understand its complexity and context. Conceptualizing the complexity of decision tasks can provide opportunities for educators and facilitators to consider how to structure and scaffold learning for new practitioners. For

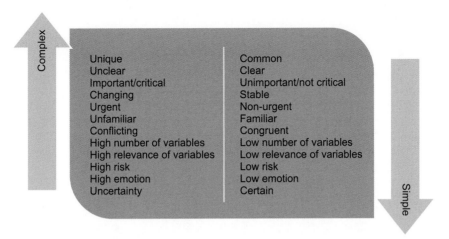

Fig. 44.2 ▪ Levels of clinical task complexity.

example, an educator working with new paramedicine students might choose an initial learning scenario with relatively low risk and that has stable variables with limited changes. With experience, as decision-making speed and accuracy improve the educator could vary the scenario to introduce additional, inconsistent and changing variables.

Learning About Your Capabilities and Experience as a Decision Maker

Smith's research (Smith et al., 2007) identified that practitioners' decision making was influenced by their capabilities, confidence, self-efficacy, emotions, frames of reference and degree of expertise. She found that therapists, in acute care settings, had a number of personal qualities and decision-making capabilities that enabled them to make effective decisions in relation to the nature of the task and the context of practice. The capabilities of the therapists in the study are illustrated in Fig. 44.3; these were categorized as cognitive, meta-cognitive/reflexive, social and emotional.

In her research, during clinical decision making by therapists, Smith revealed self-efficacy and confidence in decision making were important determinants of the decisions that were made. Their feelings and levels of self-efficacy resulted from: (1) evaluating their level of knowledge, particularly in comparison to the knowledge levels of other health professionals with whom they were working; (2) having experienced success and failure; and (3) knowing the likely responses

to interventions and the likelihood of adverse events occurring. When self-efficacy was higher, there was a greater willingness to take risks and greater confidence in decision making, as opposed to relying on others or deferring decision making. As an example of understanding emotional capability, she found decision makers' emotions and feelings of confidence and controllability influenced participants' decision making as they sought to control negative outcomes and emotions, particularly under conditions of risk and uncertainty.

An important attribute that influences decision making is the decision maker's level of expertise. Experts are considered to be superior decision makers, making decisions that are faster and more accurate and using their experience of similar situations to address more effectively, the perceived difficulty of decision-making tasks. A distinction is typically made between the extremes of novice and expert; however, individual practitioners are more appropriately viewed as being in varying degrees of transition between more and less experienced and expert. As such, they will demonstrate characteristics consistent with their own variable pathways towards expertise, dependent upon their unique experiences and the current clinical situation and task. In learning decision making, helping learners to understand how experience shapes decision making could be used to guide expectations of their decision making and the reflective learning activities that are used to learn from decision making.

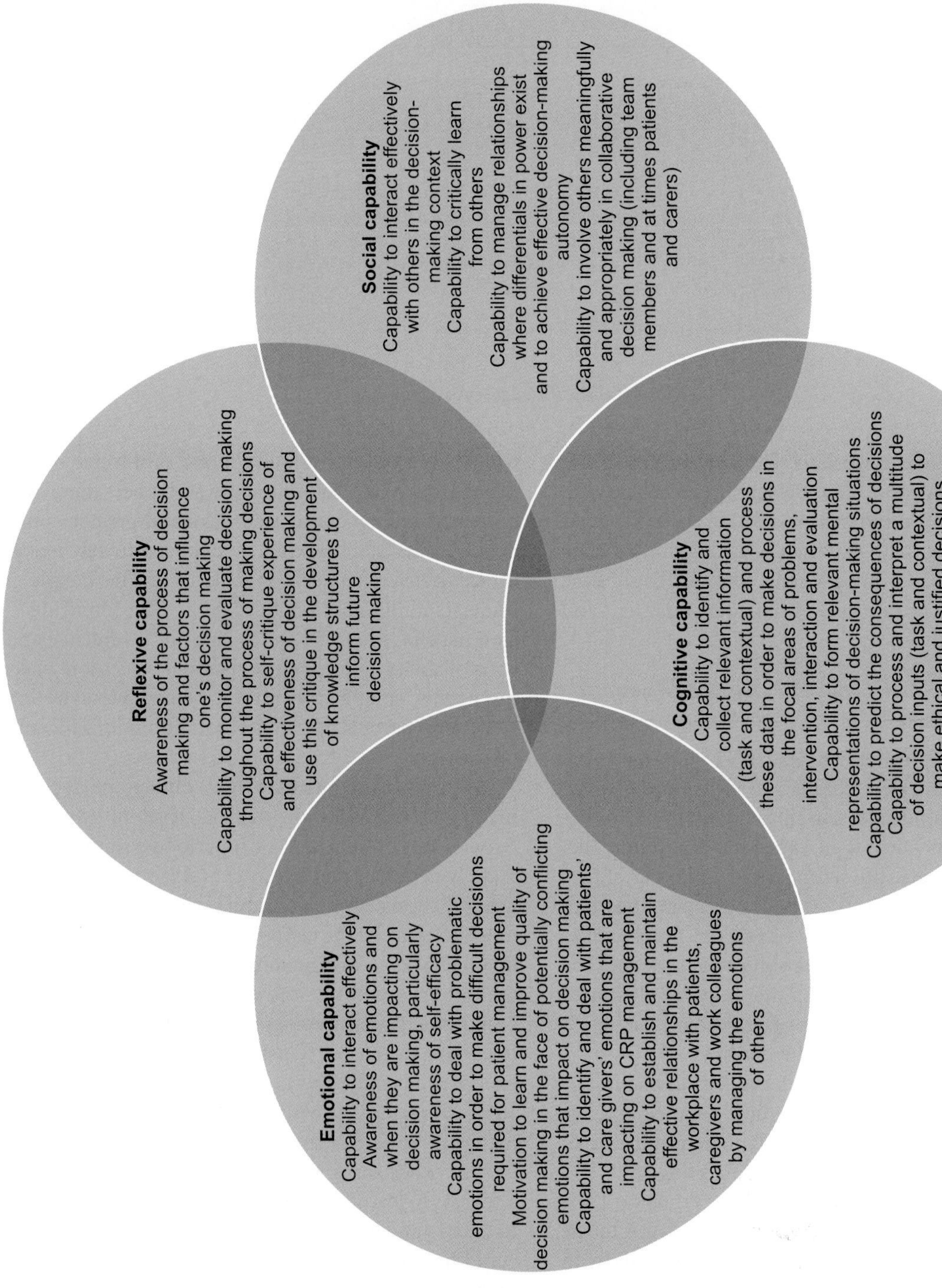

Social capability
Capability to interact effectively with others in the decision-making context
Capability to critically learn from others
Capability to manage relationships where differentials in power exist and to achieve effective decision-making autonomy
Capability to involve others meaningfully and appropriately in collaborative decision making (including team members and at times patients and carers)

Reflexive capability
Awareness of the process of decision making and factors that influence one's decision making
Capability to monitor and evaluate decision making throughout the process of making decisions
Capability to self-critique experience of and effectiveness of decision making and use this critique in the development of knowledge structures to inform future decision making

Cognitive capability
Capability to identify and collect relevant information (task and contextual) and process these data in order to make decisions in the focal areas of problems, intervention, interaction and evaluation
Capability to form relevant mental representations of decision-making situations
Capability to predict the consequences of decisions
Capability to process and interpret a multitude of decision inputs (task and contextual) to make ethical and justified decisions
Capability to make pragmatic decisions in the face of uncertainty and/or under-resourcing
Capability to adapt practice decisions to new and changing circumstances

Emotional capability
Capability to interact effectively
Awareness of emotions and when they are impacting on decision making, particularly awareness of self-efficacy
Capability to deal with problematic emotions in order to make difficult decisions required for patient management
Motivation to learn and improve quality of decision making in the face of potentially conflicting emotions that impact on decision making
Capability to identify and deal with patients' and care givers' emotions that are impacting on CRP management
Capability to establish and maintain effective relationships in the workplace with patients, caregivers and work colleagues by managing the emotions of others

Fig. 44.3 ■ Clinical reasoning capabilities to deal with the nature of the decision-making task and the decision context.

The more experienced therapists adopted an approach to decision making that was more specific, creative and refined towards the individual needs of patients and the unique contextual dimensions. Compared with less experienced therapists, they used more interpretation and critique in their decision making, being comparatively more confident and self-reliant. They handled uncertainty in decision making more effectively by adopting a higher level of practical certainty. This means they were better able to engage in wise risk-taking and possessed a greater knowledge base that decreased the relative uncertainty of decision making. Their knowledge base was broader and deeper than that of the novices and contained a greater level of experience-based knowledge. Their knowledge base was personalized and multidimensional; it included a better awareness of the limits of their knowledge and what could be known. More experienced therapists also had more advanced cognitive capabilities for decision making, being more flexible, adaptive and capable of predicting outcomes, as well as having higher levels of emotional capability. They were able to separate emotion from task and knew how to use their own personality in their decision making. They also had a higher awareness of patients' experiences of illness.

The frames of reference of more experienced practitioners are different from those of novices. Expert decision makers critically apply norms and criteria of decision making. Where novices choose simply to follow rules and value the safety of working within rules, experts understand the bases for the rules and thus apply them more variably and wisely. The more experienced therapists in this study had more developed personal theories of practice consisting of their own set of criteria for practice. These were more important than using rules and guidelines for practice derived from their university education or work-based protocols. The contrast was that less experienced practitioners framed decision making as needing to make the right decision, whereas more experienced practitioners sought optimal decisions given the circumstances.

More experienced practitioners were also more capable of managing the context, being more aware of the influences and better able to interact pragmatically with and manipulate contextual factors to achieve optimal decision outcomes. The knowledge base of experts has been found to extend beyond direct patient care,

to include knowledge of their work context in terms of the physical environment and organizational structures (Ebright et al., 2004).

REFLECTION POINT

- What are the key contextual factors you generally want to take into consideration for your patients?
- What impact do such factors make in relation to your clinical decision making, the patient's key concerns and treatment outcomes?

Learning About the External Context and Decision-Making Environments

A key focus in this research was to explore the influence of the external context of practice on decision making. The research showed that the therapists' decision making could not be separated from the context in which it occurred. They changed or modified decisions in response to contextual factors. They also learned the value of developing strategies to manage and control the context of their practice. In this way, the interaction between context and decision making was seen to be reciprocal, complex and dynamic. The influence of specific contextual factors upon decision making was dependent upon the unique features of the decision being undertaken at the time. Context was not a fixed entity but was found to be dynamic and variable. A key finding of this research was that contextual factors influencing practitioners' decision making could not be consistently ranked according to their prevalence or importance. Rather, different contextual factors assumed different importance according to the unique circumstances at a given time. We see through these findings that practitioners need to make decisions about their decision making (i.e. use metacognition) as well as making the decisions themselves (i.e. using cognition).

The broader context of clinical decision making can be seen to consist of different types of factors that become relevant to particular decisions; these include social, organizational and physical dimensions. In Table 44.2, these research findings have been applied to the implementation of a simulated learning activity that could be used to develop skills in clinical decision making. This includes a range of individual dispositional dimensions (such as emotion and motivation) (Durning et al., 2015)

TABLE 44.2

Using Simulated Learning Experiences to Assist Students to Learn Clinical Decision Making Under Different Environmental Conditions

Environmental Dimension	Example of Use During Simulation	Debrief: Positive Implications	Debrief: Negative Implications
Social	Learning decision making can be assisted by deliberately constructing social situations in scenarios involving varying perceived difficult decision making ■ allowing conferring with others to check their decision making ■ using others to generate novel perspectives ■ anchoring their decision making to decisions others made in the past	Debrief with learners about the positive role social interaction had on their decision making such as ■ using other individuals to check for errors, ■ using positive synergies arising from the combination of team members' knowledge and ■ recognizing that there is an increased likelihood of generating novel solutions and diverse perspectives when more people are consulted in decision making.	Debrief with learners about the negative role social interaction had on their decision making such as how they might ■ choose to do what others do to avoid social rejection, ■ take advantage of others' decision making rather than being responsible for their own decision making, perpetuate dominant workplace norms (people can be inhibited from offering or adopting different perspectives) and ■ not developing individual expertise.
Organizational systems	Introduce organizational variables into scenarios such as ■ variable workloads, ■ interruptions and ■ decision-making aids and guidelines.	Debrief on the effect of systems in place to guide decision making, such as clinical pathways, policies, protocols and system definitions and how these were relied upon in the decision making.	■ Where workload resulted in limited time availability, were any compromises made in the decisions that could be made? ■ What were the effects of systems on prioritization? ■ What were the effects of time pressures, such as less thinking time, less effective interventions, streamlining assessment, choosing less creative options for treatment, less time for offering patients choice in decision making and choosing interventions that would be adequate rather than optimal? ■ How did time pressures influence decision making by affecting the capacity of decision makers to develop rapport with patients? Did the learner feel he or she had the capacity to get to know patients and their condition? ■ How did interruptions add to the complexity of the decision-making process and affect the cognitive capacity to recall information and make decisions?
Physical	Adjusting scenarios to vary the physical environment ■ resources available such as the location and supply of equipment ■ room layout	What was the effect of familiarity on the efficiency of their decision making?	■ How effective was their response to limited resources?

and social and contextual dimensions of clinical reasoning (Ratcliffe and Durning, 2015).

REFLECTION POINT

■ What key messages about factors influencing decision making will be useful to aid your role as educator?

SUMMARY

Quality decision making is an essential component of good clinical practice. To understand, critique and improve clinical decision making, it is imperative that, in addition to understanding the elements of the immediate clinical problem, we make explicit the contextual factors that we need to take into account when making decisions. When seeking to improve decision making, a broad perspective needs to be adopted that considers factors such as the individual's decision-making attributes and the influence of the external context on decision making. As teachers, we need to explore our own, and our students', ability to use meta-cognition to appraise critically these factors in decision making in particular cases. We also need to consider how our decision-making practices need to evolve in response to patient, practitioner and environmental factors that impact on decisions and decision making.

Evidence-based practice is consistently advocated as a means for improving the quality of clinical practice. A broader perspective on factors influencing decision making illustrates how evidence-based practice needs to be integrated with the many other influences on practice. Consideration of personal, social and organizational dimensions of context is critical in optimizing the quality of clinical decision making. If we are to help learners develop effective decision making, we need to understand how we can best teach decision making that considers and manages the multiplicity of factors that influence it, rather than focussing only on the immediate clinical decision-making tasks of diagnosis and intervention.

REFERENCES

Boshuizen, H., Schmidt, H., 2008. The development of clinical reasoning expertise. In: Higgs, J., Jones, M., Loftus, S., Christensen, N. (Eds.), Clinical reasoning in the health professions, 3rd ed. Elsevier, pp. 113–121.

Durning, S., Artino, A.R., Pangaro, L., van der Vleuten, C.P., Schuwirth, L., 2011. Context and clinical reasoning: Understanding the perspective of the expert's voice. Medical Education 45 (9), 927–938. https://doi.org/10.1111/j.1365-2923.2011.04053.x

Durning, S., Rencic, J., Trowbridge, R., et al., 2015. Afterward teaching clinical reasoning – Where do we go from here? In: Trowbridge, R.I., Renic, J.J., Durning, S.J. (Eds.), Teaching clinical reasoning. Versa Press, pp. 235–238.

Ebright, P.R., Urden, L., Patterson, E.S., Chalko, B.A., 2004. Themes surrounding novice nurse near-miss and adverse-event situations. Journal of Nursing Administration 34 (11), 531–538. https://doi.org/10.1097/00005110-200411000-00010

McLellan, L., Yardley, S., Norris, B., de Bruin, A., Tully, M.P., Dornan, T., 2015. Preparing to prescribe: How do clerkship students learn in the midst of complexity? Advances in Health Sciences Education 20 (5), 1339–1354. https://doi.org/10.1007/s10459-015-9606-0

Orasanu, J., Connolly, T., 1993. The reinvention of decision making. In: Klein, G.A., Orasanu, J., Calderwood, R., Zsambok, C.E. (Eds.), Decision making in action: Models and methods. Ablex, pp. 3–20.

Parkes, A., 2017. The effect of individual and task characteristics on decision aid reliance. Behaviour and Information Technology 36 (2), 165–177. https://doi.org/10.1080/0144929X.2016.1209242

Ratcliffe, T., Durning, S., 2015. Theoretical concepts to consider in providing clinical reasoning instruction. In: Trowbridge, R.I., Renic, J.J., Durning, S.J. (Eds.), Teaching clinical reasoning. Versa Press, pp. 13–29.

Smith, M., 2006. Clinical decision making in acute care cardiopulmonary physiotherapy. [Doctoral thesis, The University of Sydney].

Smith, M., Higgs, J., Ellis, E., 2007. Physiotherapy decision making in acute cardiorespiratory care is influenced by factors related to the physiotherapist and the nature and context of the decision: A qualitative study. Australian Journal of Physiotherapy 53, 261–267. https://doi.org/10.1016/s0004-9514(07)70007-7

Smith, M., Higgs, J., Ellis, E., 2008. Characteristics and processes of physiotherapy clinical decision making: A study of acute care cardiorespiratory physiotherapy. Physiotherapy Research International 13 (4), 209–222.

45

PEER LEARNING TO DEVELOP CLINICAL REASONING ABILITIES

STEPHEN LOFTUS

CHAPTER AIMS

The aims of this chapter are:

- to introduce peer learning as an educational strategy to enhance professional education
- to discuss ways that peer learning can be used to facilitate the development of clinical reasoning
- to provide examples of peer learning activities that develop clinical reasoning in professional education.

INTRODUCTION

Many professional practitioners admit that they learned as much from their peers, their fellow students, as they ever did from their teachers. In recent decades, there has been a growing realization that learning from one's peers can be used as a powerful educational strategy (Boud and Cohen, 2014; Mazur, 1997). There are now several pedagogical strategies that make explicit use of peer learning. In this chapter, we will focus on the most popular in the education of health professionals: team-based learning (TBL), case-based learning (CBL) and problem-based learning (PBL). These techniques can be particularly useful ways to help students develop clinical reasoning skills at the same time as the students are learning the various forms of knowledge they need to practise their professions. The integration of factual knowledge with its use in clinical reasoning and making connections with clinical practice is the great strength of these strategies. However, a weakness of these approaches is that they must be designed, and implemented, with great care if they are to be successful. Teachers who want to make good use of these strategies need a thorough understanding of their theoretical foundations as well as managing the practicalities of designing and implementing them.

THEORETICAL FOUNDATIONS

There are several theoretical foundations that can be used to understand what is happening when these peer learning techniques are used. These foundations and their key points are summarized in Table 45.1.

Cognitive Psychology

The most common theory is probably cognitive psychology, which assumes that the human mind is similar to a computer in how it processes information. ten Cate (2018) provides a summary of how ideas on clinical

TABLE 45.1	
Theoretical Foundations and Key Points	
Theoretical Foundation	**Key Points**
Cognitive psychology	The brain is an information processor like a computer. Learning clinical reasoning is learning how to 'crunch the data'.
Narrative medicine	The patient's story accommodates multiple perspectives and complexity. Learning clinical reasoning is learning how to elicit and manage complex narratives.
Sociocultural psychology	We learn through interpersonal relationships. Learning clinical reasoning is learning how to internalize what is done in a social setting.

reasoning have developed over the years in cognitive psychology. However, the similarity of human cognition to computer information processing can be critiqued as superficial and unrealistic. The similarity may have been attractive in the 1960s when cognitive psychology was first developed and the first electronic computers offered an exciting new metaphor for reasoning of many kinds. In cognitive psychology, there is a strong emphasis on deductive reasoning, yet one can argue that much of human reasoning (including clinical reasoning is inductive). There are other theoretical frameworks that can be used and might be more useful.

Narrative Medicine

Clinical reasoning is often grounded in clinical cases and predominantly case-based and, therefore, narrative medicine offers a more realistic alternative to how we think about clinical reasoning and how it is learned (Ajjawi et al., 2009). In narrative reasoning, there is a complex mixture of deductive, inductive and abductive reasoning which is probably closer to how humans reason in the real world. This combination has strong parallels with what has been called analogical thinking (Hofstadter and Sander, 2013). There are other theoretical frameworks that can also be used.

Sociocultural Psychology

The sociocultural psychology of Vygotsky and Cole (1978) is based on the premise that we learn many

things in a social setting first and then gradually internalize them. We learn things interpsychologically first and then make these intra psychological. Vygotsky used the notion of the zone of proximal development (ZPD) to develop this idea. In the ZPD, a student can perform at the level of a competent practitioner if the proper scaffolding and support is given. With time and practice, as the student masters the performance and its underlying knowledge, the support can be gradually withdrawn until the students are fully competent on their own. This is precisely how some peer learning approaches, such as PBL, are designed to work (Loftus and Higgs, 2005). A group of students systematically work through a case to diagnose and plan the treatment of a patient. At first, they need a lot of support from the facilitator and each other. However, with time, as students work through many more cases and are exposed to clinical practice and build their theoretical and practical knowledge base, they can also develop their clinical reasoning skills. This means that the support can be gradually withdrawn until the students are competent on their own. A key aspect of these peer learning settings is that they promote active learning (e.g. the flipped classroom).

Active Learning

It is widely recognized today that passive pedagogies such as lectures can be very inefficient ways to help people learn. There is an acceptance that more active learning approaches need to be integrated into the curriculum, in addition to lectures. The flipped classroom is one way of thinking about active learning. Here, students must come to class prepared so that they can engage in processing and applying information rather than passively receiving it. Peer learning techniques can be effective ways of implementing a flipped classroom.

Peer learning techniques encourage students to engage with the knowledge to be learned and to apply that knowledge, especially in partnership with each other. Well-designed peer learning explicitly provides students the opportunity and the time to engage with the ideas and discuss them with each other and a facilitator. Students often comment that in these discussions they can discover that they have misunderstood an idea, especially when a new idea might be counterintuitive. Peer-learning techniques provide what can be described as a liminal space where students can try out new and challenging ideas (Derias et al., 2021). Misunderstandings can be brought to light. The idea of liminality comes from anthropology and describes the transitional state that persons enter when they change status in their communities, such as changing from child to adult. Applied to education, a liminal state is an opportunity for students to deal with the misunderstandings that can easily come from difficult new ideas. At the same time, students learn higher order ways of thinking with these ideas, such as the analyses, interpretations and syntheses required in clinical reasoning. The liminal state can be uncomfortable and challenging. Teachers/facilitators need to be present in order to help students with any misunderstandings and clinical reasoning that is going astray. The facilitator ensures that the small group setting is seen as a safe and supportive learning space where ignorance and misunderstandings can be articulated. Another strength of many peer learning techniques is that they foster self-directed learning and inquiry learning.

Self-Directed Learning

Self-directed learning is now seen as an important skill for many health professionals. In some countries, institutions need to demonstrate sufficient self-directed learning in the curriculum so that graduates have enough experience and expertise to make use of this ability throughout their careers in order to keep themselves up-to-date. Peer-learning techniques, such as PBL, require students to engage extensively in self-directed learning where they must not only gather relevant information but critique it and present it to their peers. Peer learning also promotes inquiry learning (see the immediate following Reflection Point).

REFLECTION POINT

Inquiry-based learning is usually described as having four levels (Banchi and Bell, 2008).
1. Students work to confirm information they have already been given.
2. Structured inquiry: the teacher provides the initial question and an outline of the procedure to answer the question. Students evaluate and analyse the information they find to formulate an explanation that will answer the question. TBL and CBL can be seen as mostly taking place at level 2.
3. Guided inquiry: the teacher provides only the question and the students must begin by first working out how to find the information they need. PBL can be seen as fitting into level 3.
4. Open (or true) inquiry: students formulate their own research questions and then work out how to answer them.
   - What forms of inquiry-based learning have you experienced?
   - If you are a teacher, what forms of inquiry-based learning does your institution provide? How well does it work?

Banchi and Bell (2008) claim that inquiry-based learning encourages students to be critically engaged in their own learning, where they actively seek out links between the different bodies of knowledge that they learn and how all this applies to the real world of professional practice. Students must not only obtain evidence that might answer the question but go on to explain how, and why, the evidence might answer the question. In the healthcare setting, inquiry-based learning is a robust way of encouraging clinical reasoning in a safe environment and where the connections between different kinds of knowledge can be fully explored and integrated. The different kinds of knowledge vary from biomedical science, such as the anatomy and pathophysiology of the heart, to social issues such as the management of a patient who, having been diagnosed with a heart problem, can no longer return to their own home and manage their own healthcare.

PEER-LEARNING STRATEGIES

Several peer-learning strategies are now used in higher education. They are normally used in small group teaching but some can be applied within a lecture with large numbers of people (Mazur, 1997). There are three peer-learning approaches that are popular in the education of health professionals: TBL, PBL and CBL. What they have in common is the emphasis on active learning and teamwork in small groups. PBL and CBL will be dealt with first as they have much in common. Of the three, the oldest and probably the best known technique is PBL (Klamen et al., 2022).

A PBL/CBL TRIGGER

A middle-aged woman brings her father, who is in his eighties, to see you, a new family practitioner. He is complaining of frequent headaches that started about a week ago. The woman answers nearly all the questions on behalf of her father who seems a little hesitant when trying to answer for himself.

Questions for a small group discussion include:
- What is the chief complaint?
- What are the possible causes, which are most likely, and which are most serious?
- Which questions in the medical history can help establish the differential diagnosis?
- What are the ethical implications of someone answering questions on behalf of another adult?

Problem-Based Learning

In PBL, the students are given a trigger, the basics of a clinical case (e.g. it can be as simple as an elderly man who presents with headache (see Case Study 45.1)).

The students brainstorm all the possible causes there could be of headache. They are then encouraged to follow the protocols of clinical reasoning for their profession to gather information that could help them reach a diagnosis and treatment plan. Each case will take two (or more) sessions to complete. Throughout the process the students are encouraged to identify areas of ignorance that might prevent them from fully understanding what is going on in the case. These areas of ignorance can be organized into learning issues. The students are given self-study time in the curriculum to find the knowledge they need to address the learning issues. This is shared among the group at the next meeting and they proceed with the case (see Case Study 45.2).

A key point is that, in PBL, there is an expectation that the students decide which learning issues they want to pursue. A controversial point is the extent of guidance the facilitator can provide to the students. The facilitator usually has knowledge of the learning goals of the case-writing team and what they want the students to gain from the case. There is a delicate balance to be maintained between giving the student

A PBL SESSION

Margot took her seat in the tutorial room. The facilitator soon arrived and began by asking the students to address the learning issues and the gaps in their knowledge that had emerged at the previous meeting. During their last session, the group had gathered information from the history and physical examination of the case and generated a list of hypotheses about potential alternative diagnoses. At today's session, each participant shared with the group what they had found out.

When Margot's turn came, she provided a copy of a review paper she had found on sarcoidosis, one of the group's hypotheses, and she summarized the key points of the paper. The others used these points to discuss whether or not sarcoidosis should still be an item on their differential diagnosis. The group continued moving through each member's information until they had come up with justifications for the reorganization of the differential diagnosis. They were then prompted to move on to the next phase of the patient assessment (the special tests) and gather more information about this particular case. The facilitator asked the group to justify the special tests they requested and to interpret the results when these were provided. Eventually, the group came up with a definitive diagnosis and discussed management options. Again, the facilitator prompted the group to justify their reasoning in selecting options.

At the end of their session, the facilitator asked participants to summarize what they had learned in terms of their medical knowledge, its application in their clinical reasoning and their teamwork.

group freedom to go their own way and providing enough guidance to ensure that they also learn what the teachers want them to learn from the case. This raises an important point about all these peer learning strategies. The job of facilitator needs some skill. There is some considerable overlap between PBL and CBL and the two are sometimes confused.

Case-Based Learning

A possible source of confusion between PBL and CBL is that many programmes that claim to be PBL have evolved over time to become more like CBL but have retained the name of PBL (Loftus, 2022). In CBL, the teachers lay out clear learning objectives and students are given pre-reading to do. When each session begins, the group is given a clinical trigger, similar to that in PBL. The group then systematically works through the case using their clinical reasoning protocols to come to a diagnosis and treatment plan. A big difference between PBL and CBL is that in CBL there is less emphasis on identifying areas of ignorance for further study, although this still occurs. There is more emphasis on applying and using the knowledge already given to explore the case and its ramifications. In CBL there tends to be more structure to each session and each case is usually completed within one session. A common variation is to explore a similar case within the session but with different features. For example, the first case might explore a particular pathology in an otherwise healthy young person with no co-morbidities. The variation might be to explore the same pathology in an older person who has significant co-morbidities that can complicate diagnosis and management. With both CBL and PBL careful design, planning and implementation are needed if they are to be successful.

Preparing for PBL/CBL

Teachers who are new to these techniques often try them as a stand-alone exercise to gain some experience and this is perfectly acceptable. However, these techniques are more often becoming a keystone pedagogy of an entire curriculum (Loftus, 2022). If this is going to be the case, careful planning needs to be done and the work involved is considerable. Full integration of these techniques can require complete reorganization of the curriculum. A long lead time will be needed. A year or more is not uncommon. There will need to be teams to design and write the cases and there will need to be teams of educators providing overall guidance. The cases have to fit within the curriculum and be integrated with other pedagogies, such as lectures and clinical experience. Design teams should be made up of experts who can provide appropriate input to each case. Such experts can include scientists, clinicians, ethicists, social workers and others. If the peer learning is interprofessional, other health professionals will need to provide input.

The Need for Detailed Planning

Clear goals for each case need to be laid out. The knowledge and reasoning needed to achieve the goals of each case should be articulated and documented. Each case should follow an accepted format so that there is consistency between cases and students and facilitators know what the procedure will be with each case. The planning should also include logistic details, such as clarifying where and when the sessions will occur. Each institution needs a sufficient number of rooms for small group learning so that a whole cohort of students can work through each case simultaneously. There will also be a need for professional development for all the teachers, both those who design and write the cases and those who will facilitate each small group.

Facilitator Roles

Facilitators need to be aware that they are not supposed to provide didactic teaching. As the old adage goes, they should be a 'guide on the side' and not a 'sage on the stage'. The facilitator's role is to ensure that the group stays on track and deals with the case in sufficient depth. There is an ongoing emphasis on clinical reasoning throughout each case. A good facilitator will do things such as ask the group to justify their decisions and consider how variations (such as different test results) might change the situation. Ideally, facilitators should be practitioners who can use their own clinical experience to contextualize cases for the group. However, many institutions must rely on others, such as biomedical scientists, or practitioners from other health professions to be facilitators. Some institutions use senior students as facilitators. This has the added advantage of giving students some experience of a teaching role. There is a growing recognition that we need to develop health professionals who can teach their juniors (ten Cate and Durning, 2007) and facilitating small group learning can be an excellent introduction.

Student Roles

The students too need to be taught what their role is and how to play the PBL/CBL 'game'. They need to realize that using the knowledge they are learning in realistic clinical reasoning is the main purpose of the exercise. The process of peer learning is more important than reaching the end goal of a diagnosis or treatment plan.

TABLE 45.2
Comparison of Features of PBL/CBL/TBL

Feature	PBL	CBL	TBL
Small group	Yes	Yes	Yes
Large group	No (but occasionally used for final debrief)	No	Yes
Preparatory learning	No	Yes	Yes
Sessions per case	Completed over 2 or more sessions	Completed in one session	Completed in one session
Self-directed learning	Between sessions	Before sessions	Before sessions
Structured sessions	Original design had strict structure (but now wide variations but follow clinical practice)	Flexible structure (but follow clinical practice)	Strict structure to sessions (little variation)

CBL, case-based learning; PBL, problem-based learning; TBL, team-based learning.

This is why students should be discouraged from seeking solutions to cases from more senior students and providing solutions to junior cohorts that follow them. If students are new to TBL, they will benefit from an introduction so that they can see how it works and what the benefits will be for them (Table 45.2).

Team-Based Learning

TBL has developed independently from PBL and CBL but has some similarities, especially in its use of the small group format, although this is usually in a large room where several groups can be present simultaneously (Parmelee, 2022). It is possible for one teacher to run a TBL session for several groups at the same time. TBL is an excellent example of the flipped class. Students are given preparatory material to read and know that they will be expected to apply that knowledge in the TBL class. It is also made clear that learning the information provided is the minimum preparation. Students are encouraged to identify their own learning objectives and to come to class as well-prepared as they can be. These classes tend to follow a common format.

First, each student completes an individual multiple choice test of their knowledge (*iRAT: independent Readiness Assurance Test*). This is followed by each small group answering the same multiple choice test but as a team (*tRAT: team Readiness Assurance Test*). The team is then provided with the answers. There can be discussion to clarify key concepts when misunderstandings become apparent.

The next phase is a *Group Application*. A set of questions are set for which there is no straightforward answer to be found in a textbook. Data can be provided that needs to be analysed, interpreted and/or synthesized with other information. The team must select an answer to each question that will be displayed (and probably justified) to the rest of the class. The questions frequently require each team to engage in some form of clinical reasoning. The point of the exercise is to generate the discussion in which concepts are applied and misunderstandings can emerge and be dealt with. These exercises are often done in a spirit of friendly competition against the other teams in the TBL.

Finally, there is an *Instructor Summary* where the teacher can reflect on what has been achieved and learned. Any remaining misunderstandings should be clarified at this point. Many teachers will also ask the students what else they might want to learn in order to become more expert. The very last stage of TBL will occur later in the course when learners are asked to provide constructive feedback to their peers about what each person contributed to the group process and how they might improve.

REFLECTION POINT

- For students: How much have you learned and do you learn from discussing ideas with other students?
- For teachers: What opportunities and support do we provide to encourage students to learn from each other?

CONSTRUCTIVE ALIGNMENT AND ASSESSMENT

All these peer learning techniques can be integrated into the curriculum and aligned with the goals and outcomes of an educational programme. The need for constructive alignment among all these elements is essential. One key point is that the type of learning involved in peer learning should also be prominently included in any assessments. It is widely accepted that students in the health professions are strategic in their learning and will only seriously study what is assessed. Students need to know that the assessments will require them to engage in the same intellectual activity (clinical reasoning) that is required in peer learning. Possible assessments include the Script Concordance Test (Charlin et al., 2000), Extended Matching Questions (Case and Swanson, 1993) and the Comprehensive Integrative Puzzle test (Ber, 2003). ten Cate (2018) uses these three in a combination which is a rigorous assessment of knowledge and clinical reasoning. Assessments can follow the development of a case. The students are given some information about a case and asked questions about the information given. For example, a question about the physical examination could be: 'What are the three most relevant physical examination procedures to be performed next?' A question about the results of the physical examination could be 'What physical findings would you expect if hypothesis 2 is true?' If students are aware that the assessment parallels, and is aligned with, their peer learning, they will have every incentive to engage with that peer learning.

SUMMARY

In this chapter, we have discussed:

- peer learning as an effective educational strategy to enhance the education of health professions students for discipline-specific knowledge and teaching and learning clinical reasoning skills,
- examples of peer learning activities in the health professions and
- the importance of careful design and constructive alignment of peer learning in the curriculum.

REFERENCES

Ajjawi, R., Loftus, S., Schmidt, H., Mamede, S., 2009. Clinical reasoning: The nuts and bolts of clinical education. In: Clinical education in the health professions, 7th ed. Elsevier, Churchill Livingstone, pp. 109–127.

Banchi, H., Bell, R., 2008. The many levels of inquiry. Science and Children 46 (2), 26.

Ber, R., 2003. The CIP (comprehensive integrative puzzle) assessment method. Med Teach 25 (2), 171–176. https://doi.org/10.1080/0142159031000092571

Boud, D., Cohen, R., 2014. Peer learning in higher education: Learning from and with each other. Routledge.

Case, S.M., Swanson, D.B., 1993. Extended-matching items: A practical alternative to free-response questions. Teaching and Learning in Medicine: An International Journal 5 (2), 107–115.

Charlin, B., Roy, L., Brailovsky, C., Goulet, F., van der Vleuten, C., 2000. The Script Concordance test: A tool to assess the reflective clinician. Teach Learn Med 12 (4), 189–195. https://doi.org/10.1207/S15328015TLM1204_5

Derias, N., Loftus, S., Kamel-ElSayed, S., 2021. Threshold concepts in preclinical medical education: Students' perceptions. Med Sci Educ 31 (2), 917–921. https://doi.org/10.1007/s40670-021-01258-2

Hofstadter, D.R., Sander, E., 2013. Surfaces and essences: Analogy as the fuel and fire of thinking. Basic Books.

Klamen, D., Suh, B., Tischkau, S., 2022. Problem-based learning. In: An introduction to medical teaching: The foundations of curriculum design, delivery, and assessment. Springer, pp. 115–131.

Loftus, S., 2022. Case-based learning. In: Huggett, K., Quesnelle, K., Jeffries, W. (Eds.), An introduction to medical teaching, 3rd ed. Springer, pp. 99–114. 10.1007/978-3-030-85524-6

Loftus, S., Higgs, J., 2005. Reconceptualising problem-based learning in a Vygotskian framework. Focus on Health Professional Education. A Multi-disciplinary Journal 7 (1), 1–14.

Mazur, E., 1997. Peer instruction: A user's manual. Prentice Hall, Upper Saddle River, NJ.

Parmelee, D., 2022. Team-Based Learning. In: Huggett, K.N., Quesnelle, K.M., Jeffries, W.B. (Eds.), An introduction to medical teaching. Innovation and Change in Professional Education, 3rd ed. Vol. 20. pp. 77–84 Springer, Cham. https://doi.org/10.1007/978-3-030-85524-6_6

ten Cate, O., 2018. Assessment of clinical reasoning using the CBCR test. In: Principles and practice of case-based clinical reasoning education: A method for preclinical students. Springer, pp. 85–94.

ten Cate, O., Durning, S., 2007. Dimensions and psychology of peer teaching in medical education. Med Teach 29 (6), 546–552. https://doi.org/10.1080/01421590701583816

Vygotsky, L.S., Cole, M., 1978. Mind in society: Development of higher psychological processes. Harvard University Press.

46

ASSESSING CLINICAL REASONING IN MEDICINE

GEOFFREY R. NORMAN ■ STEVEN J. DURNING

■ ■ ■ ■ ■ ■ ■ ■ ■ ■ ■ ■ ■ ■ ■ ■ ■ ■ ■

CHAPTER AIMS

The aims of this chapter are:

- to describe the developments in assessment of clinical reasoning
- to explain the possibilities and limitations in further developments.

INTRODUCTION

A central skill of a clinician is arriving at diagnoses and management by gathering data from history-taking, physical examination and laboratory tests. The process is described by a variety of terms in the literature, such as 'clinical reasoning' and 'decision making'. Many distinctions can be made, but perhaps the most important one is that reasoning focusses on the thought processes, with studies of clinicians and learners typically using psychological and observational methods. Decision making examines the optimal outcome of the process with studies using epidemiological data and methods such as decision analysis. More recent conceptualizations

of clinical reasoning often include the decision in the definition (e.g. decision making is a part of clinical reasoning); however, in this review we will restrict ourselves primarily on the process of diagnosis.

There has been increased interest in diagnostic error over the past decade, stimulated by two important documents from the Institute of Medicine in the United States: 'To Err Is Human', a review of management errors (Kohn et al., 2000), and 'Improving Diagnosis in Health Care' (Balogh et al., 2015). This increased interest has led to many studies and papers describing theories of clinical reasoning and subsequent educational strategies to reduce error (Croskerry, 2003; Norman, 2005).

Early Research on Clinical Reasoning

In the 1970s and 1980s, several studies showed that although expert clinicians systematically outperformed less experienced doctors on a variety of simulations of clinical diagnosis, there was little difference in the nature of problem-solving processes they used. This led to a new direction in fundamental research, guided by cognitive psychology (Eva, 2004; Norman, 2005; Regehr and Norman, 1996; Schmidt et al., 1990), which led to a further understanding that problem-solving ability is not a separate teachable skill and that it cannot be measured independently of relevant content knowledge. More important than the amount of knowledge are the ways in which it is structured, stored, accessed and retrieved (de Bruin et al., 2005). An essential facet in this storage and retrieval of knowledge is the understanding of the so-called deep structure – the fundamental ideas that shape our understanding of the problem (Chi et al., 1982). From this perspective, expertise is a function of how well the problem at hand is understood as a specific instance of the deep structure, which then allows us to understand differences and similarities between seemingly different problems. For example, there are similarities and differences between an aspirin overdose and hyperventilation; they may have different symptoms and aetiologies, but both cause a disturbance of the acid–base balance.

An alternative developmental theory of knowledge organization (Schmidt et al., 1990) proposes three different kinds of knowledge relevant to solving clinical problems. The most elementary is knowledge of disease processes and causal relationships, the basic science of medicine, followed by the acquisition of so-called 'illness scripts', which are quite literal, list-like structures relating signs and symptoms to disease prototypes. At the highest level of functioning, the expert uses a sophisticated form of pattern recognition, called 'nonanalytic' or 'exemplar-based' reasoning, characterized by speed and efficient use of information (Schmidt et al., 1990). It appears that pattern recognition is, in fact, recognition at a holistic level of the similarity between the present patient and previous patients (Hatala and Norman, 1999). More recent theories (Croskerry, 2003; Norman, 2005) collapse the distinction between process and knowledge and instead include a 'dual-process' model in which problems can be solved by both unconscious application of experiential knowledge (System 1) and conscious application of analytical knowledge (System 2).

The more experience a person has had with a given type of clinical problem, the more likely they are to use a faster and less effortful System 1 problem-solving process. However, if the solution is not recognized as a pattern, more effortful and analytical problem-solving

processes must be brought into play. Any individual will demonstrate a range of approaches, both within and across problems, depending on previous experience and exposure to similar problems. Problem-solving ability is, therefore, not a characteristic of the clinician but an interaction between the nature (including complexity) of the problem and the clinician's knowledge and problem-specific expertise. These insights help to explain the findings of idiosyncrasy and domain specificity of measures of 'problem solving' (Eva et al., 1998). A second apparently counterintuitive finding in the clinical reasoning literature is the finding that correct solutions are generally associated with, less, not more time on task (Sherbino et al., 2012). The explanation is simply that experts use more nonanalytical reasoning and pattern recognition and are, therefore, able to solve a problem more efficiently requiring less information than clinicians of more intermediate ability.

Research on Decision Making

Since the 1970s, research on decision making has taken a very different direction, driven by searches for optimal approaches to management decision making. A typical question might be whether a stent or bypass is a better approach, using epidemiological data, such as mortality, likelihood and severity of complications, etc. Rarely do human thinking processes enter into the assessment methodology. Rather, the goal is to use the health data to determine an optimal strategy, in terms of maximizing patient outcomes. There is one exception however; the 'heuristics and biases' literature originating in studies by Tversky and Kahneman in the 1970s and popularized more recently by Kahneman's bestseller, 'Thinking Fast and Slow' (Kahneman, 2011). This research typically takes the form of investigations of the extent to which human decision makers (doctors) are suboptimal in their decisions and the causes of these suboptimal decisions, typically framed as heuristics and biases used by the clinician (cf. Plous, 1993 for an overview); hence, there is some overlap with the clinical reasoning literature.

Implications for Assessment of Clinical Reasoning

Although the two domains of clinical reasoning and clinical decision making can appear to be different, in assessment the distinction blurs. In particular, assessment methods are somewhat agnostic regarding which is which and methods such as the 'Clinical Decision-Making—Key Features Approach' (Page and Bordage, 1995) routinely assess both dimensions within the same test.

Although we acknowledge that clinical reasoning can also be assessed with performance-based measures such as the OSCE (objective structured clinical examination) or in real-life clinical practice, it is first and foremost an activity of the mind.

REFLECTION POINT

No single assessment method will be able to capture the whole process of clinical reasoning and decision making. A combination of instruments will have to be used in an assessment program. In fact, a recent review of the literature in *Academic Medicine* concluded that there are many potential methods for assessing clinical reasoning and important factors to consider include what aspect of clinical reasoning is the focus of assessment and in what setting.

A HISTORICAL PERSPECTIVE ON ASSESSMENT

In the 1960s and 1970s, the focus was on the development of methods that assessed 'clinical problem-solving skills'. The main thrust was to mimic authentic clinical situations optimally in a paper-based format. One popular variant, the patient management problem (PMP), attempted to simulate the process by which a doctor obtained information from history and physical examination. A typical PMP began with an initial complaint and brief demographic details of the patient. The candidate was then requested to collect further data, sequentially in a branched fashion, e.g. with a 'rub out' pen that exposed the answer (or later on with computers). Then, the candidate could select investigations and/or make diagnostic and management decisions. A criterion panel of physicians would decide a priori on the weight assigned to each option, typically from +2 to −2. The candidate would then receive a variety of scores (proficiency, efficiency, competence, errors of

omission) based on various approaches to aggregating the weights over all components of the problem.

A number of psychometric problems with the PMP emerged (Swanson et al., 1987). First, different experts used different pathways to solve the same problem; therefore, it was difficult to get consensus on the scoring of each individual decision in the problem-solving process. Second, because the various scoring methods ultimately rewarded thoroughness and expert physicians relied more heavily on nonanalytic (System 1) reasoning, which proceeds rapidly by unconscious thinking rather than step-by-step, one piece of information at a time approach used by junior doctors, they often received higher scores than experts. A third problem was that studies that directly compared PMP performance with performance on the same problem with a live simulated (standardized) patient showed that people selected about twice as many data options in the PMP as they did with real patients, which was a fundamental threat to the validity of the method (Norman et al., 1982). Finally, the most striking and counterintuitive finding was that performance on one PMP was a poor predictor of performance on another PMP. Correlation across problems was typically around 0.1 to 0.3 (Norman et al., 1985), which seriously undermined the hypotheses that problem solving was a generic ability or skill, independently assessable of the underlying knowledge structure. The explanation of this phenomenon is referred to as content or case specificity (Elstein et al., 1978). Because candidates took too long to work through a single case of a PMP, typically 30 to 45 minutes, large numbers of cases and considerable testing time were needed to produce acceptably reliable results. This finding of case or domain specificity is not unique to PMPs but is also seen in other methods that assess clinical competence and performance.

A final consequence of these early studies was a renewed focus on knowledge as a prerequisite for clinical decision making and reasoning. Efficient measures of knowledge such as multiple-choice questions (MCQs) remain a mainstay of testing agencies because we now recognize, as we did not in the 1960s, that knowledge is central to expertise. Some studies, for example, have shown that written knowledge tests, oriented to the kind of clinical knowledge central to clinical practice, are better predictors of competence in medical practice 5 to 20 years later than more 'authentic' performance tests (Tamblyn et al., 2007; Wenghofer et al., 2009). The centrality of knowledge is not limited to medicine; research in the development of expertise in many domains comes to the same conclusions (Ericsson, 2007). Also, these studies suggest that highly authentic (and expensive) test situations do not automatically lead to useful assessment information. LaRochelle has shown that students can learn clinical reasoning using written cases just as effectively as they can with more realistic formats (LaRochelle et al., 2012). Norman et al. (2012) showed that low-fidelity simulations are as effective in learning transferrable skills as much more expensive high-fidelity simulations, a point we will refer to later.

FURTHER DEVELOPMENTS IN ASSESSMENT METHODS

The evidence thus far leads to a number of conclusions. First, assessment must be anchored in case-based material presented in a way that will induce and sample clinical reasoning activities (Schuwirth et al., 2001). Second, laboriously taking a student through the full data gathering and investigational phase of a real or simulated clinical case is an inefficient approach when the purpose is to evaluate clinical reasoning, because of content specificity. For example, up to 8 hours of testing time would be required to achieve reliable assessments with PMPs (Norcini et al., 1985), demonstrating that testing methods require more time-efficient sampling.

A useful distinction is between stimulus formats and response formats (Norman et al., 1996). The stimulus format refers to the task presented to the candidate. This may range from very simple short questions to complex and time-consuming tasks. The stimulus format typically ends with one or more questions asking the candidate to connect the information in the stimulus with the required response. Typical lead-ins are 'What is the most likely diagnosis?' or 'What are the most indicated next steps in the management?'

The response format refers to the way the response of the candidate is captured. It can consist of a short menu of options (MCQs), long extensive (computerized) menus, a short write-in format, a long write-in format (essay-type questions), an oral response or an observed behaviour either in a simulated environment (e.g. OSCE) or in a real-life context. Three developments, extended matching items (Case and Swanson, 1993), the key feature approach (Page et al., 1990) and the script concordance test (Charlin et al., 2000), exemplify the divergence of response approaches.

Multiple-Choice Questions and Extended-Matching Items

In their simplest format, clinical reasoning tasks can take the form of vignette-based MCQs. Short cases are presented that require a judgement or decision about data gathering, case management or any other phase of the clinical problem. These questions are, with some initial training, relatively easy to write, particularly because they come close to what clinicians do in actual clinical practice. The response format is a menu. The length of the menu does not need to be fixed but is usually as long as there are meaningful alternatives.

Another MCQ type, proposed by the US National Board of Medical Examiners (NBME), is the extended matching question (EMQ) (Case and Swanson, 1993). Students are presented with a series of brief case scenarios based on a single chief complaint (e.g. shortness of breath) and must select the most appropriate diagnosis or action from a menu of options. EMQs are relatively easy to construct. They represent clinical reasoning assessments in their simplest form, with an authentic stimulus in combination with a closed response. Reliability is similar to that of normal MCQs. Stimulus formats with richer (and longer) vignettes contain more 'measurement information' and contribute more to reliability than other vignettes. Longer menu response formats may appear to be better, but evidence suggests no advantage over simple four- or five-option MCQs. More complex response formats (e.g. using multiple best answers or allowing logical operators between different elements) and more complex scoring systems (such as penalties and partial credit) are not recommended. Simple single best answer formats and simple scoring systems are advised.

CASE STUDY 46.1

Virtual Patients in Student Assessment

Dr Dawson is a busy clinician with a huge interest in medical education and clinical reasoning. He is contacted by a friend, who has recently developed a new virtual reality engine and now suggests that Dr Dawson develop some authentic virtual patients. The friend suggests that they can use them to assess the clinical reasoning ability of medical students for their final examinations.

This thought is very appealing to Dr Dawson, given his interest in clinical reasoning, but he decides to ask for advice from medical education experts first. The medical education experts explain that the research into clinical reasoning and decision making has shown that fidelity/authenticity is not the same as validity and that the history of high-fidelity simulations for the assessment of clinical reasoning and decision making has been sobering. They explain that various concerns with this approach have been identified, with the most important being the so-called 'domain specificity'. So, regardless of how well designed the virtual reality engine and how authentic the simulation, it does not alter the fact that to get a reliable and valid assessment of a student's clinical decision making and reasoning ability, many cases need to be processed by the student. They further tell him that, up until now, the most promising developments have been with short cases and a limited number of questions per case and that low-fidelity simulations seem to be as valid as high-fidelity simulations for the assessment of clinical decision making and reasoning. Dr Dawson decides to read this literature himself and comes to the same conclusion. He is glad he has consulted the medical education experts and has thus avoided wasting considerable time and resources on an approach that has been demonstrated to be unsuccessful.

The lesson from this case is that much of the research outcome in the field of assessment of clinical decision making and clinical reasoning is counterintuitive and consulting people who have a good knowledge of this literature is helpful in preventing busy people from spending their precious time on unsuccessful approaches.

Excellent manuals for writing these MCQs are available through the NBME (2024).

Clinical Decision-Making (Key Feature Problem) Approach

Key features are the decisions pivotal to the successful outcome of the case, e.g. a particular diagnosis, a critical test or the next management steps. The basic idea behind key feature problems (KFPs) is to focus only on these essential aspects of clinical cases, allowing more cases to be asked per hour and providing more efficient sampling. Also, by asking essential decisions only, quick pattern recognition and expert efficiency are not 'penalized' as with PMPs. More detailed item construction tips are provided elsewhere (Farmer and Page, 2005; Page and Bordage, 1995; Schuwirth et al., 1999). Questions relating to the key features can use a variety of response formats (e.g. short-answer, MCQs or selection from longer menus of options), but they should be such that the candidate must read the whole case and synthesize the necessary information. The KFP allows 40 to 50 cases to be administered in the same time as needed for 12 to 15 PMPs. Studies so far have indicated substantially better reliability than with PMPs but, still, 2 to 5 hours of testing time may be required. Studies by the Medical Council of Canada showed a reliability of 0.80 with approximately 40 cases in 4 hours of testing time (Page and Bordage, 1995). One study showed that two to three items (questions) per case are optimal for maximum reliability (Norman et al., 2006); reading time will compromise reliability when fewer items are used and information redundancy will compromise reliability when more items are used.

Validity studies investigating correlations with other measures typically show moderate correlations. More compelling are studies using think-aloud strategies when comparing stimulus formats, showing that case-based stimulus formats elicit other cognitive processes than fact-oriented stimulus formats (Schuwirth et al., 2001). While the more factual questions elicited more or less simple black-and-white or 'yes/no' thinking steps, the case-based questions elicited probabilistic reasoning weighting different bits of information from the case against each other. Response formats that use menus instead of write-ins may cue the candidate to both correct and incorrect answers with slightly higher scores as a net effect, naturally depending on the number of alternatives in the menu (Schuwirth et al., 1996). Score correlations across these response formats, however, are invariably high.

A modern variation of the key feature format is the use of computers for test administration, allowing more flexible use of visual and audio information. Many variants of computer-based 'virtual patients' now exist. A recent systematic review (Cook et al., 2010) examined 50 studies of the use of virtual patients for learning reasoning and concluded that they have no systematic advantage over simpler formats.

Script Concordance Test

The assessment methods described earlier may have good psychometric properties, but many people feel that they do not fully capture the clinical reasoning process (e.g. Charlin et al., 2000). To fill this gap, Charlin et al. (2000) proposed a new type of assessment, the script concordance test (SCT), using cognitive expertise theory. The assumption is that most clinical problems are ill-defined, and experts are not always expected to collect exactly the same information. They challenged the MCQ formats because these always required agreed-upon solutions to well-defined problems (Charlin et al., 2000). SCT questions focus on essential decisions in a case like the KFP but allow for variability between experts. For this, Charlin suggested using ill-defined problems with a previously published aggregate scoring approach (Norman, 1985). A clinical scenario is presented that provides a challenge to the candidate because not all data are provided for solution of the problem. However, the question format is constrained to questions whose answers can be scaled on a +2 to −2 scale. An example is presented in Box 46.1.

The scoring reflects the variability experts demonstrate in the clinical reasoning process. Credits on each item are derived from the answers given by a reference panel, with each score being proportional to the number of reference panel members who have provided that answer. Studies into the validity of the SCT have been conducted and reliability studies show that a reliability of 0.80 can be reached with approximately 1 hour of testing using about 80 items.

REFLECTION POINT

For each case, there may not be a single best way of clinical reasoning. Assessment should focus on distinguishing between good or acceptable reasoning processes and bad or unacceptable reasoning processes.

CURRENT DEVELOPMENTS

Research Into Examiner Decision Making

Current theories acknowledge that analytical and nonanalytical processes work in conjunction and interact with each other continually (Norman, 2005) and any separation of these processes leads to oversimplification. Instead of trying to focus on single points in the process, modern assessment seeks to develop rigorous ways of assessing clinical reasoning heeding the complexity of the whole process. This means that they do not attempt to assess the single best reasoning process but acknowledge that there are multiple equally acceptable reasoning processes for any given case (Durning et al., 2013). There are also unacceptable solutions. Answer keys (descriptions of the correct answers) are not based on a single best solution but on defining boundaries between admissible and inadmissible solutions. Such boundaries are not clearly definable and much research is aimed at understanding the complexity associated with such reasoning (Checkland, 1985). Another consequence is a reappraisal of human judgement in assessment and the incorporation of qualitative approaches in assessment (Driessen et al., 2005). In this perspective, clinical reasoning expertise is now seen as the

---

BOX 46.1
X-RAY QUESTIONS

A 25-year-old male patient is admitted to the emergency department after a fall from a motorcycle with a direct impact to the pubis. Vital signs are normal. The X-ray reveals a fracture of the pelvis with a disjunction of the pubic symphysis. Followed by a series of questions like:

If you were thinking of:	And then you find:	This hypothesis becomes:
Urethral rupture	Urethral bleeding	−2 −1 0 +1 +2

ability to avoid overstepping boundaries of the 'problem space', the possession of a repertoire of strategies to manage the case (instead of a one-size-fits-all) and the agility to switch strategies or solutions.

This more nuanced view of assessment is clearly at odds with the traditional mechanistic approaches to scoring that characterize the methods we have reviewed. Human judgement must play a role in the assessment of clinical reasoning, including reappraisal in the literature of understanding the quality of human judgement and how it can be supported in valid assessment. Gingerich et al. (2011), for example, explored the different perceptions of different examiners, not from the viewpoint that differences equate to error but that different perspectives produce a more complete picture. Ginsburg et al. (2015) explored the 'narratives' that examiners use when providing judgement. In contrast to the biases and heuristics literature, these researchers celebrate the subtlety of human judgement, rather than disparage it (for an overview, see Plous, 1993). It remains somewhat unclear, however, how these findings can find their way into improved examiner judgement (Berendonk et al., 2013).

Focus on Diagnostic Outcome

There is an alternative perspective that arises from some of the findings we have reviewed.

1. The notion that the essential aspects of expertise in clinical reasoning lie in the processes of data gathering, data interpretation and diagnostic thinking has been at variance with the evidence for 50 years. Neufeld et al. (1981) showed that measures of the process of problem solving did not distinguish experts from novices. However, the nature of the diagnostic hypotheses, typically advanced in the first few minutes, was a strong predictor of diagnostic success. Similarly, Groves et al. (2003) showed that expert family physicians had more errors of data gathering than learners but were diagnostically superior.
2. As mentioned earlier, a recurrent finding in the literature is that success on one problem is a poor predictor of success on a second problem (Norcini, 2002). Again, an indication that the essence of diagnostic expertise lies more in relevant knowledge than general thinking skills.

3. LaRochelle et al. (2012) compared three learning formats (paper case, DVD, simulated patient) and showed that more realistic clinical simulations did not result in increased transfer performance on new clinical cases.
4. Schmidt and Mamede (2015) conducted a systematic review of strategies for learning clinical reasoning. One critical element was whether the case was presented as a single narrative or unfolded linearly to attempt to simulate the process of reasoning. The sequential strategy was largely ineffective; however, the whole case format resulted in effective learning.

The accumulation of these observations leads to the audacious conclusion that the preoccupation with measures of process (history-taking, relation between features and diagnoses and so on) is misplaced. Perhaps it is sufficient for an assessment method simply to count the number of times a candidate came up with the 'right' answer on a series of cases, in written form, presented as a whole. Such a strategy has one advantage over other, more complex methods – it can sample broadly and rapidly. Given the ubiquitous finding that clinical reasoning is not at all skill-like, but rather is massively case-specific, that may be sufficient (Monteiro et al., 2020).

GAPS AND REMEDIES
Dual Processing and Clinical Reasoning

The previous section has implications for the current state of the art. Although assessment methods to some degree mirror the various components of competence elucidated by fundamental research, this appears to occur haphazardly rather than by design. Basic research supports the dual-process model but by extension serves to underline that the two processes are very different, derive from different kinds of learning (formal rules and mechanisms for System 2, experience and exemplars for System 1) and warrant different assessment methods. As an example of the dilemma, the SCT, described earlier, purports to derive from research on clinical reasoning. However, its focus is entirely on the candidate's ability to 'correctly' (consistent with a panel of experts) enter the relation between features and diagnoses on a +2 to −2 scale.

Leaving aside the validity of reducing complex judgement processes to a simple arithmetic sum of weights, the focus is entirely on the interpretation of diagnostic cues. No attention is paid to data gathering, to the generation of hypotheses or to management decisions. As such, a test, whatever its psychometric properties, lacks face validity as a single measure of reasoning.

Theoretical Defects

A more glaring oversight arises from the dual processing model itself. Multiple studies (Neufeld et al., 1981) have shown that System 1 processing is central to the generation of hypotheses, which in turn are a major determinant of diagnostic success. But the very nature of System 1 processes precludes detailed examination of thinking based on analytic combination of elements such as arises in the SCT or the CRT; System 1 processes are not available to conscious introspection.

Such considerations lend support to the 'outcome only' approach advocated in the previous section. It is not really possible to identify strategies which are more or less optimal. So why try? If the candidate gets the right answer, do we care how they got there? It is perhaps more important to sample broadly to ensure that they have demonstrated success in a broad and representative sample of problems.

Management Decision Making

We earlier commented on the dearth of basic research around actual management decision making. To some degree, assessment may be in better shape. Measures like the key feature test, or even MCQs, are easily adapted to examine management decision making. Although they may not explore the thinking processes underlying these decisions, they remain a credible approach to assessing the appropriateness of management decisions.

IMPLICATIONS AND ADVICE

For the Reacher

The question remains as to what lessons can be drawn from these historical and ongoing developments. What should we educators do in day-to-day practice? Are there guidelines that could be developed from the findings allowing us to proceed with some forms of assessment of clinical reasoning? Unfortunately, there are no fixed answers and answers are quite different for

tests with different main purposes. However, there are several key points.

First, it is difficult to imagine a credible assessment of clinical competence that does not attempt to evaluate clinical reasoning. An assessment using less-than-perfect instruments is preferable to no assessment of this component at all. This validity issue must apply to the whole assessment procedure.

Second, perhaps one of the most ubiquitous findings from the literature is content and context specificity. General clinical reasoning skills or abilities simply do not exist. Nothing has emerged more recently that disproves this universal rule and so any credible assessment must be based on a substantial number of cases. A third compelling argument against discarding our imperfect instruments is the powerful relationship between assessment and student learning. Students will try to identify and study what they believe will be in their examinations (Cilliers et al., 2010), but they will also learn purely from taking the assessment (Larsen et al., 2008). This is inevitable, if not desirable, and requires a good match between the assessment and the expected outcomes of the course. This education effect may be as important as the psychometric properties.

Finally, because there are many ways to assess clinical reasoning and no single measure is the best measure, the choice is really yours. Which method appeals to you or your institution? How much effort do you wish to invest in writing simple or more complex stimulus formats? How many resources would you like to spend on the response format? What sort of reliability is required in your setting? What kind of effect do you strive for? What affinity or convention exists in your situation in relation to clinical reasoning assessment? Answers to these questions may vary across different education contexts. A deliberate and motivated choice among the many possibilities that the literature now has to offer is on your agenda. The simpler your selected approach, the more you can rely on existing technologies and procedures and the less you will need to invest in unique solutions.

SUMMARY

In this chapter, we have:

- described the developments in assessment of clinical reasoning and

- explained the possibilities and limitations in further developments.

REFLECTION POINT

Assessment of clinical reasoning is never an objective activity; it is a combination of information about a learner's clinical reasoning and an interpretation of this information. Interpretation is a process of expert human judgement.

REFERENCES

Balogh, E.P., Miller, B.T., Ball, J.R. (Eds.), 2015. Improving diagnosis in health care. National Academies Press.

Berendonk, C., Stalmeijer, R.E., Schuwirth, L.W.T., 2013. Expertise in performance assessment: Assessors' perspectives. Adv. Health Sci. Educ 18, 559–571. https://doi.org/10.1007/s10459-012-9392-x

Case, S.M., Swanson, D.B., 1993. Extended-matching items: A practical alternative to free response questions. Teach. Learn. Med. 5, 107–115.

Charlin, B., Roy, L., Brailovsky, C., et al., 2000. The script concordance test: A tool to assess the reflective clinician. Teach. Learn. Med. 12, 185–191. https://doi.org/10.1207/S15328015TLM1204_5

Checkland, P., 1985. From optimizing to learning: A development of systems thinking for the 1990s. J. Oper. Res. Soc. 36, 757–767.

Chi, M.T.H., Glaser, R., Rees, E., 1982. Expertise in problem solving. In: Sternberg, R.J. (Ed.), Advances in the psychology of human intelligence. Lawrence Erlbaum Associates, pp. 7–75.

Cilliers, F.J., et al., 2010. The mechanisms of impact of summative assessment on medical students' learning. Adv. Health Sci. Educ., 15, 695–715. https://doi.org/10.1007/s10459-010-9232-9

Cook, D.A., Erwin, P.J., Triola, M.M., 2010. Computerized virtual patients in health professions education: A systematic review and meta-analysis. Acad. Med. 85, 1589–1602. https://doi.org/10.1097/ACM.0b013e3181edfe13

Croskerry, P., 2003. The importance of cognitive errors in diagnosis and strategies to minimize them. Acad. Med. 78, 775–780. https://doi.org/10.1097/00001888-200308000-00003

de Bruin, A.B., Schmidt, H.G., Rikers, R.M., 2005. The role of basic science knowledge and clinical knowledge in diagnostic reasoning: A structural equation modelling approach. Acad. Med. 80, 765–773. https://doi.org/10.1097/00001888-200508000-00014

Driessen, E., van der Vleuten, C., Schuwirth, L., et al., 2005. The use of qualitative research criteria for portfolio assessment as an alternative to reliability evaluation: A case study. Med. Educ. 39, 214–220. https://doi.org/10.1111/j.1365-2929.2004.02059.x

Durning, S.J., Artino, A.R., Schuwirth, L., et al., 2013. Clarifying assumptions to enhance our understanding and assessment of clinical reasoning. Acad. Med. 88, 442–448. https://doi.org/10.1097/ACM.0b013e3182851b5b

Elstein, A.S., Schulmann, L.S., Sprafka, S.A., 1978. Medical problem-solving: An analysis of clinical reasoning. Harvard University Press.

Ericsson, K.A., 2007. An expert-performance perspective of research on medical expertise: The study of clinical performance. Med. Educ. 41, 1124–1130. https://doi.org/10.1111/j.1365-2923.2007.02946.x

Eva, K.W., et al., 1998. Exploring the etiology of content specificity: Factors influencing analogic transfer and problem solving. Acad. Med. 73 (10), s1–s5.

Eva, K.W., 2004. What every teacher needs to know about clinical reasoning. Med. Educ. 39, 98–106. https://doi.org/10.1111/j.1365-2929.2004.01972.x

Farmer, E.A., Page, G., 2005. A practical guide to assessing clinical decision-making skills using the key features approach. Med. Educ. 39, 1188–1194. https://doi.org/10.1111/j.1365-2929.2005.02339.x

Gingerich, A., Regehr, G., Eva, K., 2011. Rater-based assessments as social judgments: Rethinking the etiology of rater errors. Acad. Med. 86, S1–S7. https://doi.org/10.1097/ACM.0b013e31822a6cf8

Ginsburg, S., Regehr, G., Lingard, L., et al., 2015. Reading between the lines: Faculty interpretations of narrative evaluation comments. Med. Educ. 49, 296–306. https://doi.org/10.1111/medu.12637

Groves, M., O'Rourke, P., Alexander, H., 2003. Clinical reasoning: The relative contribution of identification, interpretation and hypothesis errors to misdiagnosis. Med Teach 25 (6), 621–625. https://doi.org/10.1080/01421590310001605688

Hatala, R., Norman, G.R., 1999. Influence of a single example upon subsequent electrocardiogram interpretation. Teach. Learn. Med. 11, 110–117.

Kahneman, D., 2011. Thinking, fast and slow. Macmillan.

Kohn, L.T., Corrigan, J.M., Donaldson, M.S., 2000. To err is human: Building a safer health system. National Academies Press.

Larsen, D., et al., 2008. Test-enhanced learning in medical education. Med. Ed. 42, 959–966. https://doi.org/10.1111/j.1365-2923.2008.03124.x

LaRochelle, J.S., Durning, S.J., Pangaro, L.N., et al., 2012. Impact of increased authenticity in instructional format on preclerkship students' performance: A two-year, prospective, randomized study. Acad. Med. 87, 1341–1347. https://doi.org/10.1097/ACM.0b013e31826735e2

Monteiro, S.D., Sherbino, J., Schmidt, H., Mamede, S., Ilgen, J., Norman, G., 2020. It's the destination: Diagnostic accuracy and reasoning. Adv Health Sci Educ Theory Pract 25, 19–29. https://doi.org/10.1007/s10459-019-09903-7

NBME (National Board of Medical Examiners), 2024. Assess and learn. NBME. https://www.nbme.org/educators/assess-learn

Neufeld, V.R., Norman, G.R., Feightner, J.W., Barrows, H.S., 1981. Clinical problem-solving by medical students: A cross-sectional and longitudinal analysis. Med Educ 15 (5), 315–322. https://doi.org/10.1111/j.1365-2923.1981.tb02495.x

Norcini, J.J., Swanson, D.B., Grosso, L.J., et al., 1985. Reliability, validity and efficiency of multiple choice question and patient management problem item formats in assessment of clinical competence. Med. Educ. 19, 238–247.

Norcini, J.J., 2002. The death of the long case? Br Med J 324 (7334), 408–409. https://doi.org/10.1136/bmj.324.7334.408

Norman, G.R., 1985. Objective measurement of clinical performance. Med Educ 19 (1), 43–47.

Norman, G.R., 2005. Research in clinical reasoning: Past history and current trends. Med. Educ. 39, 418–427. https://doi.org/10.1111/j.1365-2929.2005.02127.x

Norman, G., Bordage, G., Page, G., et al., 2006. How specific is case specificity? Med. Educ. 40, 618–623. https://doi.org/10.1111/j.1365-2929.2006.02511.x

Norman, G., Dore, K., Grierson, L., 2012. The minimal relationship between simulation fidelity and transfer of learning. Med. Educ. 46, 636–647. https://doi.org/10.1111/j.1365-2923.2012.04243.x

Norman, G., Swanson, D., Case, S., 1996. Conceptual and methodology issues in studies comparing assessment formats, issues in comparing item formats. Teach. Learn. Med. 8, 208–216.

Norman, G.R., Tugwell, P., Feightner, J.W., et al., 1985. Knowledge and clinical problem-solving. Med. Educ. 19, 344–356.

Norman, G.R., Tugwell, P., Feightner, J.W., 1982. A comparison of resident performance on real and simulated patients. Med. Educ. 57 (9), 708–715.

Page, G., Bordage, G., 1995. The Medical Council of Canada's key features project: A more valid written examination of clinical decision-making skills. Acad. Med. 70, 104–110.

Page, G., Bordage, G., Harasym, P., et al., 1990. A new approach to assessing clinical problem-solving skills by written examination: Conceptual basis and initial pilot test results. In: Bender, W., Hiemstra, R.J., Scherpbier, A., A. (Eds.), Teaching and assessing clinical competence: Proceedings of the Fourth Ottawa Conference. Boekwerk Publications.

Plous, S., 1993. The psychology of judgment and decision making. McGraw-Hill.

Regehr, G., Norman, G.R., 1996. Issues in cognitive psychology: Implications for professional education. Acad. Med. 71, 988–1001.

Schmidt, H.G., Norman, G.R., Boshuizen, H.P.A., 1990. A cognitive perspective on medical expertise: Theory and implications. Acad. Med. 65, 611–622.

Schmidt, H.G., Mamede, S., 2015. How to improve the teaching of clinical reasoning: A narrative review and a proposal. Med Educ 49 (10), 961–973. https://doi.org/10.1111/medu.12775

Schuwirth, L.W.T., Blackmore, D.E., Mom, E., et al., 1999. How to write short cases for assessing problem-solving skills. Med. Teach. 21, 144–150.

Schuwirth, L.W., van der Vleuten, C.P., Stoffers, H.E., et al., 1996. Computerized long-menu questions as an alternative to open-ended questions in computerized assessment. Med. Educ. 30, 50–55.

Schuwirth, L.W., Verheggen, M.M., van der Vleuten, C.P., et al., 2001. Do short cases elicit different thinking processes than factual knowledge questions do? Med. Educ. 35, 348–356. https://doi.org/10.1046/j.1365-2923.2001.00771.x

Sherbino, J., Dore, K.L., Wood, T.J., et al., 2012. The relationship between response time and diagnostic accuracy. Acad Med 87, 785–791. https://doi.org/10.1097/ACM.0b013e318253acbd

Swanson, D.B., Norcini, J.J., Grosso, L.J., 1987. Assessment of clinical competence: Written and computer-based simulations. Assess. Eval. Higher Educ. 12, 220–246.

Tamblyn, R., Abrahamowicz, M., Dauphinee, D., et al., 2007. Physician scores on a national clinical skills examination as predictors of complaints to medical regulatory authorities. JAMA 298, 993–1001. https://doi.org/10.1001/jama.298.9.993

Wenghofer, E., Klass, D., Abrahamowicz, M., et al., 2009. Doctor scores on national qualifying examinations predict quality of care in future practice. Med. Educ. 43, 1166–1173. https://doi.org/10.1111/j.1365-2923.2009.03534.x

47

CLINICAL REASONING EDUCATION
Looking to the Future

STEPHEN LOFTUS ■ GAIL M. JENSEN

■ ■

CHAPTER OUTLINE

CHAPTER AIMS

The aims of this chapter are:

- to identify key challenges in teaching and learning environments in clinical reasoning education
- to examine current trends in current education related to clinical reasoning
- to explore future directions that may be relevant for clinical reasoning education in the health professions

INTRODUCTION

'Practice sets the tasks and serves as the supreme judge of theory, as its truth criterion. It dictates how to construct the concepts and how to formulate the laws.' (Vygotsky, 1997, pp. 305–306).

Clinical reasoning is a central practice of most health professions. Indeed, it is sometimes referred to as the holy grail as it is regarded as *the* central practice (Gruppen, 2017). Yet as a defining characteristic of a profession, the complexity of clinical reasoning means that it is a demanding practice that requires a practitioner to be thinking on several different levels simultaneously. This requires a deeper examination of how we teach the practice of clinical reasoning. Because of this centrality and complexity, we believe that students would benefit from explicit teaching in clinical reasoning together with a deeper understanding of the learner and of how they learn clinical reasoning. Health professions education programmes need to include teaching and learning in clinical reasoning as a key factor in the curriculum. Students also need frequent and regular practice in clinical reasoning where they can get feedback on their performance and have the opportunity to develop some expertise by the time they graduate. In this concluding chapter on clinical reasoning education, we identify key challenges in our teaching and learning environments, explore current efforts in education and share new ideas for advancing student learning in clinical reasoning.

KEY CHALLENGES IN TEACHING AND LEARNING CLINICAL REASONING

Historically, most health professionals received little, if any, formal education in the practice of clinical reasoning. Clinical reasoning was effectively part of the so-called hidden curriculum. Students and novices certainly learned clinical reasoning and their teachers taught it, but almost as an aside. During the history of education in the health professions there seems to have been an assumption that the overwhelming need was for newcomers to a health profession to acquire knowledge, especially knowledge of the biomedical or foundation sciences. Another assumption seems to have been that once students had mastered detailed biomedical knowledge then applying this to clinical practice would be straightforward. The result has been that generations of students have struggled to learn clinical reasoning and many have learned it in a haphazard manner.

In the field of medicine, for example, the Flexner (1912) reforms in the early 20th century introduced a model of education where students were immersed in biomedical sciences for some years before being exposed to clinical practice and this model has been copied by many other health professions. Over the years, this model has become more problematic for several reasons. One of the problems is that there has been an explosion in the amount of biomedical knowledge that we have and decisions have had to be made about what must be included in the curriculum and what can be left out. The original disciplines of anatomy, biochemistry and physiology have been supplemented by others, all with a valid claim to a place in the curriculum of health professionals, such as neuroscience, genetics, molecular biology and health systems management. Other disciplines also claim to be important for the practice of health professionals, such as bioethics. Another problem is that basic science faculty often think in different ways to health professionals (Loftus, 2017). Scientists are seeking to understand biological mechanisms whereas health professionals want to help patients. For a health professional, understanding the mechanism is merely a means to an end. For a scientist, the goal is to understand the mechanism and no more. In addition, the emphasis on transmitting as much factual information as possible means there is less emphasis on the controversies and uncertainties within the sciences themselves.

Building on this, it is a common observation that students, who have devoted many months to acquiring biomedical scientific knowledge, struggle when they move out of the classroom and try to apply that knowledge in a clinical setting. Formal medical knowledge or foundational knowledge is often not well integrated with the acquisition of experiential knowledge over the continuum of health professions education (Cooke et al., 2010). Furthermore, the rapidly changing healthcare delivery environment means there is always a knowledge and skills gap and therefore clinicians need lifelong learning and problem solving as part of their daily clinical practice (Cutrer et al., 2017). Although there have been attempts to deal with these problems that have met with some success, we expect that these issues will continue into the future, together with other ideas that have yet to be seriously tested. We shall look at some of the current efforts to deal with these issues and then turn to some of the new ideas.

The strong emphasis on knowledge and certainty, visible in the way we assess our learners (knowledge-based examinations, finding the right answer), does little to help prepare students for the uncertainty and complexity of clinical practice. Clinicians need to be able to solve problems through uncovering the problem, understanding the context of the situation and navigating the other factors that are all part of their clinical reasoning abilities.

CURRENT EFFORTS: RENEWED EMPHASIS ON LEARNING

Some of the best known learning initiatives have transformed the curriculum in many institutions. These include initiatives such as problem-based learning (PBL), case-based learning (CBL) and team-based learning (TBL). There is a separate chapter on these approaches in this volume and readers are directed to this for more detail on their design and implementation. In Chapter 45, we emphasize that these initiatives have clinical reasoning as a central practice. Students, in groups, are encouraged to learn knowledge that they can apply immediately to clinical cases. The knowledge learned is immediately contextualized within healthcare practice. A PBL/CBL curriculum also introduces students to clinical contact from an early stage so that they can benefit from exposure to clinical experience. Students can see, at first hand, just how abstract and theoretical knowledge is applied and integrated in practice.

Without the clinical exposure there is a danger that classroom knowledge is seen as abstract theory that is unrelated to real-world practice (Loftus and Kinsella, 2021). Another important feature of these approaches is that they also emphasize the need for students to develop skills in finding relevant information, as and when they need it. In an age where vast amounts of information are now readily available, students need to develop high-level skills, not only in finding information, but in being able to critique it and judge how it might apply to the patient in front of them. All this is complicated by the realization that, in addition to new knowledge, there are regular reversals of existing knowledge. For example, some years ago, there was a widespread belief that children should be kept away from allergenic foods as long as possible. Now, there is a belief that children should be exposed to allergenic foods as early as possible. There are numerous other examples of such reversals. Health professionals need to develop the critical thinking skills to judge whether they should be early adopters of new knowledge in their practice or if they should be more cautious until the new knowledge is more firmly substantiated.

This ability to develop critical thinking skills and be able to make judgements in uncertain conditions requires the development of adaptive learners who develop clinical reasoning capability throughout their working lives. Adaptive learners are able to engage in active self-monitoring and critical reflection and to receive, as well as to seek, external feedback (Cutrer et al., 2017; Cutrer et al., 2020). They are motivated and skilled in learning from their experiences to change and grow. When needed, they can innovate, enabling themselves to continue to perform well when encountering complex, uncertain and novel situations. You can refer to Chapter 40 on developing clinical reasoning capability in this book for further examples of application.

We live at a time when artificial intelligence (AI) is starting to complicate the world of information technology. AI refers to the simulation of human intelligence processes by machines, particularly computer systems. The complications that AI introduces include efforts to deal with information overload. AI tools might inadvertently filter out relevant content. AI systems can also 'inherit' biases present in the data they are trained on. AI-driven decision-making processes might be difficult to understand and explain, especially when using complex algorithms such as deep neural networks. This complicates the evaluation and critique of the decisions made by these systems. The ability to critique information, how it is presented and how it might apply to patient care is more important than ever. This issue will engage educators for the foreseeable future as we navigate how AI will be incorporated into health professions education.

There is also an acceptance that it is only possible to teach a core of knowledge. Deciding what constitutes such a core is likely to be an ongoing issue that will engage educators on a regular basis because of the fluid and rapidly changing knowledge available. It is a common observation that knowledge is provisional. Educators struggle with making decisions about what learners need to know and what is nice for them to know. Content or declarative knowledge (facts and information) and procedural knowledge (application) need to be balanced with conceptual knowledge (enduring understanding) (Cutrer et al., 2020). Here is where the role of clinical cases and an explicit focus on clinical reasoning provide opportunities for learners to think on several different levels and integrate knowledge from different disciplines within the clinical setting in a manner that works for each patient (see Case Study 47.1).

NEW IDEAS IN HEALTH PROFESSIONS EDUCATION

There has been a steady evolution of thinking in education, some of which is controversial, and there are also new ideas that need to be tried and tested. A starting point is the contention that higher education should be thought of as developing students along three axes (Barnett and Coate, 2004). These axes are knowing, doing and being/becoming, also referred to as the three apprenticeships of professional education (habits of head, hand and heart) and they are shared by all health professions (Benner et al., 2010; Colby and Sullivan, 2008; Cooke et al., 2010; Jensen et al., 2019). One of the ongoing criticisms in health professions education is that professional formation or habits of heart (being) is the weakest compared with head and hand. The need for learners to demonstrate wise judgements under conditions of uncertainty is essential and requires knowing, doing and being (Sullivan, 2005). It is the integrative function of knowing, doing and being that results in wise judgement. We shall say more about wise judgement later. First, we shall take a look at an

CASE STUDY 47.1

The students thought that the paper-based case study was going to be straightforward when they heard it was about a man in his seventies presenting with chest pain. Although heart trouble was the first option they thought of, they realized that they had to distinguish it from several other possibilities that had to be considered. Even when they settled on heart disease as the most likely problem, they had to bring together and integrate knowledge from a range of disciplines. There were the basic sciences such as the anatomy, physiology and biochemistry of the heart. It turned out the patient had a family history of heart disease and the students were prompted to consider the interaction between genetics and environmental factors, such as lifestyle. There was also a possibility of rheumatic fever in the past and therefore microbiology also played a part in their thinking.

In the management of the case, other disciplines were needed such as pharmacology and therapeutics.

Social issues had to be brought into the management when students realized that the patient would not be safe continuing to live on his own. The students were also asked to think about the complexities of management when other co-morbidities were present such as emphysema and diabetes.

One of the students had recently seen a very similar case in the clinic. She shared her observations. It seemed that the patient had been very anxious and the doctor had devoted some extra time and effort to build up trust with the patient. The facilitator pointed out that the clinical reasoning involved must also include thinking about developing the relationship with a patient as a human being and how to manage each clinical encounter.

The students realized that to diagnose and manage this patient they needed to think on several levels simultaneously. Clinical reasoning is often complex.

---

important and evolving idea in health professions education and that is competency-based education (CBE).

The great strength of CBE is that it offers a straightforward theoretical basis for health professions education and clinical reasoning can be seen as a key competency. CBE emphasizes the mastery of specific skills, ensuring that students demonstrate mastery of basic concepts and tasks before moving on to more complex concepts and tasks. It also allows for personalized and flexible learning, so that teaching can be tailored to individual strengths, weaknesses and learning styles. CBE encourages regular assessment and providing plenty of feedback on performance for students. CBE also allows easy alignment with many of the demands of the workplace. Many technical procedures needed in the workplace can be articulated so that training can prepare students for those tasks and they can demonstrate their readiness for such tasks. However, there are several critiques of CBE.

One critique is that CBE claims to be personalized but implementing it on a large scale can lead to standardization that neglects individual student needs. Another critique is that designing valid and reliable assessments can be challenging and time-consuming.

There is also a risk that complex skills can be oversimplified so that measurable outcomes can be easily applied. This can lead to a lack of depth in teaching. Broader and deeper understanding of a subject might be sacrificed, particularly in areas that require critical thinking, creativity and synthesis of knowledge. Clinical reasoning is a good case in point. There are many practical tasks in clinical reasoning that lend themselves to a CBE approach, such as how well a student can follow the protocol for taking a pain history from a patient. However, clinical reasoning can often demand a great deal more from practitioners, especially when dealing with patients who may be unable, or unwilling, to cooperate and patients who have several co-morbidities. These demands are difficult to adapt to a conventional CBE approach.

Some of this critique of CBE has been articulated as a difference between education and training. Fish (2010) argues that adopting an educational approach rather than a training/technical approach is more appropriate for health professionals. She provides the example of performing a technical procedure, such as an endoscopy. The educational approach goes beyond competencies and encourages students to consider the wider context. Why is the procedure being done? If there are problems, what are the alternatives? How does this procedure fit within the overall well-being of the patient? As part of this educational approach, Fish encourages students to engage in deep reflective practice with their teachers to draw out the various lessons that can be learned from clinical experience beyond what went well and what did not (de Cossart et al., 2012). Their approach to reflective practice emphasizes articulating the nuances and subtleties that arise from coping with the complexities, the ambiguities and the uncertainties that come with real-world practice. This means that students will need individual mentoring as they learn their clinical reasoning and we shall say more about this later. Despite these criticisms, there is still a lot of support for CBE and the theory continues to develop and to be adapted.

There is renewed emphasis in CBE in the health professions as a core strategy to demonstrate public accountability and ensure the quality and safety of care received by patients (Holmboe, 2018; Thibault, 2020; Timmerberg et al., 2022). This renewed focus is grounded in outcomes assessment that is done in the workplace through performance-based assessment of entrustable professional activities (EPAs), that is, units of work that are observed from beginning to end and can be entrusted safely to a learner to do independently. This is not the implementation of task checklists. With adaptations such as EPAs, CBE is being seen as potentially a transformative strategy to facilitate the development of learners who become master adaptive learners and who are self-reflective, taking a meta-cognitive approach to learning based on self-regulation that will result in becoming an expert learner across a career (Cutrer et al., 2020; Holmboe, 2018; Jensen, 2022). Clinical reasoning is central to this development.

Clinical reasoning, whether we see it as a competency, or as a more complex, multidimensional capability, is foundational in all health professions for arriving at a diagnosis and implementing a management plan with patients. Yet, when it comes to curriculum development, we may discuss the importance of clinical reasoning as it is central and everywhere, but the reality is it often appears nowhere, since we often do not explicitly track or assess learners when it comes to clinical reasoning ability. If we agree that clinical reasoning is an essential ability for health professionals, then categorizing clinical reasoning as a core competency is important (Connor et al., 2020; Furze et al., 2022). Focussing on clinical reasoning as a competency in CBE will facilitate the development of curricula and hopefully move clinical reasoning education and research forward. The need for evidence-informed, structured and explicit teaching and assessment of clinical reasoning in health professions education will benefit not only from a focus on clinical reasoning as a core competency but also on an explicit curriculum. Chapter 34 on leading a faculty to do clinical reasoning in this book provides an example of how intentional leadership can facilitate organizational and curricular change.

When it comes to patient safety and quality care, technical skills are critical but not exclusive as it is the interdependence of all three apprenticeships (knowing, doing and being) that leads to competent performance (Cooke et al., 2010). For example, there are professional values, such as humility, moral agency, respect and integrity that cannot be assessed easily compared with technical skills. These professional values are qualities of habits of heart or being. They are not technical competencies nor are they simply behaviours that are observed and checked off. They are habits or dispositions that the learner consistently demonstrates (a way of being) (Benner and Purtilo, 2019). From this perspective, it can be argued that we need to move beyond CBE to a more holistic view of overall competence and capability. Other ideas that extend, or go beyond, CBE include the role of embodiment in learning clinical reasoning.

Embodiment

The concept of embodiment also offers openings for developing the education of health professionals (Loftus and Kinsella, 2021). The central idea of embodiment is that humans are not simply minds in possessions of bodies but that we are bodies and that much of what we know is embodied knowledge. The embodiment approach places great emphasis on the bodily experience of practice and what can be learned from it. The role that emotion can play in learning is seen as important. For example, it is now common practice for surgical teams to rehearse rare, but important, life-saving procedures in high-tech simulators. It is a common observation that intense emotion is generated in these settings even though the participants know that they are only treating mannequins. The (bodily) emotion is a key driver of learning in these settings. The participation in small group learning in TBL/CBL/PBL can also generate some emotional incentive as students usually want to show they are good team members with something to contribute. However, the lens of embodiment allows us to look a little deeper.

Dreyfus and Dorrance Kelly (2011) described situations where people had to react rapidly to deal with emergencies where there was little time for deliberation. Their claim was that our environment can 'call out' from us certain responses, but only if we are sensitive to the call and are already familiar with the affordances and meanings available in that context. The implication is that professional education must provide opportunities for students to practise in real and realistic settings. Professional practitioners, who develop the right (embodied) preparation, can then be in a position to discern rapidly what is going on in a professional setting. The training and education of professionals need to foster embodied knowledge. This can help students see work problems in the same way that experienced practitioners see them.

> *The skilled surgeon, for example, sees something more than a broken and bloody leg; he [sic] sees a particular kind of break, one that requires this precise surgical technique to fix it ... This vision of skill is essentially practical and embodied ... his ingenuity is practical, embodied, and in the moment.*
>
> *(Dreyfus and Dorrance Kelly, 2011, pp. 207-209)*

Such skills and embodied knowledge become part of an intuition that is anticipatory and allows the practitioner to be justifiably confident of what to do next. This is because, as Dreyfus and Dorrance Kelly note, 'The genuinely confident agent does not manufacture confidence, but receives it from the circumstances' (2011, p. 6). For this to happen, professional practitioners need education and experience that allow them to cultivate in themselves the skills and knowledge to discern the meanings of a situation that are already there in settings where these meanings are available to those trained to see them. Students need plenty of the experience provided in practice-based education (Higgs et al., 2010). The professional settings that provide such experience can then become an integral part of the budding practitioner's lifeworld. The importance of experience and learning for practice through practice cannot be emphasized enough here. However, it needs to be experience that is maximized for the purposes of education. Students (and junior practitioners) need mentors who can guide them through their experience, provide feedback and help them to learn whatever is available to be learned. Such an education can help students to move beyond the basics of clinical reasoning and can help them start developing clinical wisdom.

Clinical Wisdom

The idea of clinical wisdom can be interpreted in different ways. It is often seen, simplistically, as a more refined version of the routine propositional knowledge we can all learn from books. However, here is a quite different interpretation of what wisdom might be:

> *But when wisdom has shown up in my life, it's been less a body of knowledge and more a way of interacting, less the dropping of secret information, more a way of relating that helped me stumble to my own realizations. ... Wisdom has an embodied moral element.*
>
> *(Brooks, 2021; p. 23, emphasis added)*

From this perspective, wise people are those who can relate to others with deep (embodied) empathy. Brooks goes on to describe them as 'story editors'. This label applies to the best (wisest) health professionals. They help the rest of us to articulate our own life stories and reconsider them in new ways. They can do this because they have their own embodied experience that allows them to relate to the embodied experience of others. There is a sense of intercorporeality (sometimes called intercorporeity) that can be part of a deep attunement and meaningful interaction with the other (Merleau-Ponty, 1962). It is our belief that a (well-conducted) practice-based education can help students start to develop such wisdom in themselves. This is well summarized by Davey (2006):

What makes a practice a practice rather than a method is precisely the fact that it is based upon acquired and accumulated experience. The acquisition of discernment, judgment, and insight is based not so much upon what comes to us in a given experience but upon what comes to us by involvement and participation in a whole number of experiences … Experience of this order affords a wisdom.

(p. 245)

Two concepts related to clinical wisdom that have attracted attention in recent years are the neo-Aristotelian ideas of phronesis and praxis. Phronesis has been defined as 'something that develops through experience as a capacity to approach the unavoidable uncertainties of practice in a thoughtful and reflective way' (Kemmis, 2012, p. 147). Phronesis is the ability to make good judgements under conditions of complexity and uncertainty – judgements that are the best option for this particular patient in front of me now, at this particular time, in this particular place with the particular resources and expertise available. It is often said that phronesis cannot be taught, but we can provide students with the opportunity to learn it. For this to happen, students need lots of clinical experience and they need mentors who can help them reflect on their experiences and what can be learned from them. Mentors can also demonstrate their own expertise in action and share with students 'war stories' of the cases they have seen and the challenges they faced and discuss how they coped. The development of phronesis can lead to praxis. Carr (2009) defines this as 'morally committed action, guided by what is ethically right and proper, and in which, and through which, our values are given practical expression' (p. 60). Wise practitioners are comfortable working in a world of uncertainty and complexity and have the depth of character to do so. As Geva-May (2007) remarked:

Experts tend to be less certain of their judgments than nonexperts, as though expertise develops humility that allows for continuous critical assessment. This constant self-assessment leads to more perfected solutions.

(p. 138)

Developing practice wisdom requires this constant self-assessment together with the humility and willingness to learn from every case. By providing opportunities for this, encouraging it, and role modelling it, we can help our students develop the being/becoming aspect of their education that is so often ignored.

SUMMARY

We end this chapter where we began: where we see clinical reasoning as crucial to optimal patient care and essential for all health professions. The need for explicit structures and curricula for clinical reasoning cannot be overstated. While knowledge is essential, it is not a sufficient foundation for clinical reasoning. Making sense of the contextual factors through analytic and non-analytic approaches is necessary and requires a broadening of our theoretical lenses. Clinical reasoning education needs to help learners move beyond cognition and see it as contextually situated and socially mediated. This expanded view provides us with new opportunities for teaching and learning clinical reasoning.

REFERENCES

Barnett, R., Coate, K., 2004. Engaging the curriculum. McGraw-Hill Education.

Benner, P., Sutphen, M., Leonard, C., Day, L., 2010. Educating nurses: A call for radical transformation. Jossey-Bass.

Benner, P., Purtilo, R., 2019. Educating for professional responsibility: Integration across habits of head, hand, and heart. In: Jensen, G., Mostrom, E., Hack, L., Nordstrom, T., Gwyer, J. (Eds.), Educating physical therapists. Slack Inc.

Brooks, D., 2021. Wisdom isn't what you think it is. New York Times, 23.

Carr, W., 2009. Practice without theory? A postmodern perspective on professional practice. In: Green, B. (Ed.), Understanding and researching professional practice. Brill, pp. 55–64. 10.1163/9789087907327_005

Colby, A., Sullivan, W., 2008. Formation of professionalism and purpose: Perspectives from the preparation for the professions program. University of St Thomas Law Journal, 5404–426.

Connor, D., Durning, S., Rencic, J., 2020. Clinical reasoning as a core competency. Academic Medicine 95, 1166–1171. https://doi.org/10.1097/ACM.0000000000003027

Cooke, M., Irby, D., O'Brien, B., 2010. Educating physicians: Call for reform of medical school and residency. Jossey-Bass.

Cutrer, W., Miller, B., Pusic, M., Mejicano, G., Mangrulkar, R., Gruppen, L., et al., 2017. Fostering the development of master adaptive learners: A conceptual model to guide skill acquisition in medical education. Academic Medicine 92, 70–75.

Cutrer, W., Pusic, M., Gruppen, L., Hammoud, M., Santen, S., 2020. The master adaptive learner. Elsevier Health Sciences.

Davey, N., 2006. Unquiet understanding: Gadamer's philosophical hermeneutics. SUNY Press.

de Cossart, L., Fish, D., Hillman, K., 2012. Clinical reflection: A vital process for supporting the development of wisdom in doctors. Curr Opin Crit Care 18 (6), 712–717. https://doi.org/10.1097/MCC.0b013e328358e239

Dreyfus, H., Dorrance Kelly, S., 2011. All things shining: Reading the Western classics to find meaning in a secular age. Free Press.

Fish, D., 2010. Learning to practise interpretively: Exploring and developing practical rationality. In: Higgs, J., Fish, D., Goulter, I., Loftus, S., Reid, J.-A., Trede, F. (Eds.), Education for future practice. Sense, pp. 191–202.

Flexner, A., 1912. Medical education in Europe: A report to the Carnegie Foundation for the advancement of teaching. Carnegie Foundation for the Advancement of Teaching.

Furze, J., Black, L., McDevitt, A., Kobal, K., Durning, S., Jensen, G., 2022. Clinical reasoning: The missing core competency in physical therapy education and practice. Physical Therapy 102, 1–4. https://doi.org/10.1093/ptj/pzac093

Geva-May, I., 2007. "We seem to have always spoken in prose..." Policy analysis is a clinical profession: Implications for policy analysis practice and instruction. Policy Studies Journal 35 (2), 135–164.

Gruppen, L., 2017. Clinical reasoning: Defining it, teaching it, assessing it, studying it. Western Journal of Emergency Medicine 18, 5–7. https://doi.org/10.5811/westjem.2016.11.33191

Higgs, J., Fish, D., Goulter, I., Loftus, S., Reid, J., Trede, F. (Eds.) (2010) Education for future practice, Rotterdam, The Netherlands: Sense.

Holmboe, E., 2018. Competency-based medical education and the ghost of Kuhn: Reflections on the messy and meaningful work of transformation. Academic Medicine 93, 350–353. https://doi.org/10.1097/ACM.0000000000001866

Jensen, G., Mostrom, E., Hack, L., Nordstrom, T., Gwyer, J., 2019. Educating physical therapists. Slack Inc.

Jensen, G., 2022. Physical therapy education through the lens of the master adaptive learner. 24th Pauline Cerasoli Lecture. Journal of Physical Therapy Education 6, 348–358. https://doi.org/10.1097/JTE.0000000000000260

Kemmis, S., 2012. Phronesis, experience, and the primacy of praxis. In: Kinsella, E.A., Pitman, A. (Eds.), Phronesis as professional knowledge: Practical wisdom in the professions. Sense, pp. 147–161. 10.1007/978-94-6091-731-8_11

Loftus, S., 2017. Thinking like a scientist and thinking like a doctor. Medical Science Educator 28 (1), 251–254. https://doi.org/10.1007/s40670-017-0498-x

Loftus, S., Kinsella, E. A. (Eds.), 2021. Embodiment and professional education: Body, practice, pedagogy. Springer. https://doi.org/10.1007/978-981-16-4827-4

Merleau-Ponty, M., 1962. Phenomenology of perception (C. Smith, Trans.). Routledge.

Sullivan, W. M., (2005). Markets vs. professions: value added?. Daedalus 134 (3), 19–26.

Thibault, G., 2020. The future of health professions education: Emerging trends in the United States. FASEB Bioadvances 2, 685–694. https://doi.org/10.1096/fba.2020-00061

Timmerberg, J., Chesbro, S., Jensen, G., Dole, R., Jette, D., 2022. Competency-based education and practice in physical therapy: The time to act is now. Physical Therapy 102, 1–9. https://doi.org/10.1093/ptj/pzac018

Vygotsky, L.S., 1997. The historical meaning of the crisis in psychology: A methodological investigation. In: Rieber, R.W., Wollock, J. (Eds.), The collected works of LS Vygotsky, Vol. 3. Springer, pp. 233–343.

INDEX

Page numbers followed by '*f*' indicate figures, '*t*' indicate tables and '*b*' indicate boxes.